Essential Psychopharmacology
The Prescriber's Guide

Stephen M. Stahl, M.D., Ph.D.

Adjunct Professor of Psychiatry
University of California, San Diego

Chairman
Neuroscience Education Institute

Editorial assistant
Meghan M. Grady

With illustrations by
Nancy Muntner

Every effort has been made in preparing this book to provide accurate and up-to-date information that is in accord with accepted standards and practice at the time of publication. Nevertheless, the author, editors and publisher can make no warranties that the information contained herein is totally free from error, not least because clinical standards are constantly changing through research and regulation. The authors, editors and publisher therefore disclaim all liability for direct or consequential damages resulting from the use of material contained in this book. Readers are strongly advised to pay careful attention to information provided by the manufacturer of any drugs or equipment that they plan to use.

PUBLISHED BY THE PRESS SYNDICATE OF THE UNIVERSITY OF CAMBRIDGE
The Pitt Building, Trumpington Street, Cambridge, United Kingdom

CAMBRIDGE UNIVERSITY PRESS
The Edinburgh Building, Cambridge CB2 2RU, UK
40 West 20th Street, New York, NY 10011-4211, USA
477 Williamstown Road, Port Melbourne, VIC 3207, Australia
Ruiz de Alarcón 13, 28014 Madrid, Spain
Dock House, The Waterfront, Cape Town 8001, South Africa

http://www.cambridge.org

First published 2005

Printed in Canada

Typeset in Helvetica Condensed

Design and layout services: Page Designs International

*A catalog record for this book is available from
the British Library*

Library of Congress Cataloging-in-Publication Data
ISBN   0 521 01169 8   paperback

Essential Psychopharmacology
The Prescriber's Guide

The Prescriber's Guide is the latest addition to the *Essential Psychopharmacology* collection. In full color throughout, this volume presents to clinicians pragmatic guidance that complements the conceptual approach of *Essential Psychopharmacology.* With four or more pages for each of over 100 psychotropic drugs, Stephen Stahl gives all the information a prescriber needs to treat patients effectively. For each drug the information comes in five categories: *general therapeutics, dosing and use, side effects, special populations,* and *pearls. General Therapeutics* covers the class of drug, what the drug is prescribed for, how the drug works, how long it takes to work, what happens if it works, what happens if it doesn't, best augmentation/combination strategies, and any required tests. *Dosing and use* covers usual dosage, dosage forms, how to dose, dosing tips, overdose, long-term use, habit formation, how to stop, pharmacokinetics, drug interactions, warnings/precautions, and contraindications. *Side effects* covers how the drug causes side effects, notable side effects, life-threatening or dangerous side effects, weight gain, sedation, what to do about side effects, and best augmenting agents for side effects. *Special populations* covers renal impairment, hepatic impairment, cardiac impairment, the elderly, children and adolescents, and key phases of a woman's lifecycle. *Pearls* covers potential advantages, potential disadvantages, pearls, and suggested reading. Target icons appear next to key categories for each drug so that the prescriber can go easily and instantly to the information needed. Several indices are included, one consisting of a comprehensive list of both generic and proprietary names for all the drugs featured, one categorizing the generic drugs by use, and one listing the generic drugs by class.

Stephen M. Stahl is Adjunct Professor of Psychiatry at the University of California, San Diego, and Chairman, Neuroscience Education Institute, Carlsbad. He has conducted numerous research projects awarded by the National Institute of Mental Health, the Veteran's Administration, and the pharmaceutical industry. The author of more than 300 articles and chapters, Stephen Stahl is an internationally recognized clinician, researcher and teacher in psychiatry with subspecialty expertise in psychopharmacology.

From the reviews of *Essential Psychopharmacology*

"essential reading . . . I would thoroughly recommend this book to anyone who works with psychotropic drugs – or who has the task of teaching others about them!"
American Journal of Psychiatry

"Firmly grounded in contemporary neuroscience . . . an excellent and comprehensive account of the pharmacology of drugs currently used to treat psychiatric disorders. "
Psychological Medicine

"This masterful production will benefit a broad spectrum of readers, from students to knowledgeable and experienced psychopharmacologists."
Psychiatric Times

"Finally, an elega   basic scientist who is also a cli

To members of the Neuroscience Education Institute and prescribers of psychopharmacologic agents everywhere. Your relentless determination to find the best portfolio of treatments for each individual patient within your practice is my inspiration.

Table of contents

Introduction

This *Guide* is intended to complement *Essential Psychopharmacology*. *Essential Psychopharmacology* emphasizes mechanisms of action and how psychotropic drugs work upon receptors and enzymes in the brain. This *Guide* gives practical information on how to use these drugs in clinical practice.

It would be impossible to include all available information about any drug in a single work and no attempt is made here to be comprehensive. The purpose of this *Guide* is instead to integrate the art of clinical practice with the science of psychopharmacology. That means including only essential facts in order to keep things short. Unfortunately that also means excluding less critical facts as well as extraneous information, which may nevertheless be useful to the reader but would make the book too long and dilute the most important information. In deciding what to include and what to omit, the author has drawn upon common sense and 30 years of clinical experience with patients. He has also consulted with many experienced clinicians and analysed the evidence from controlled clinical trials and regulatory filings with government agencies.

In order to meet the needs of the clinician and to facilitate future updates of this *Guide,* the opinions of readers are sincerely solicited. Feedback can be emailed to feedback@neiglobal.com. Specifically, are the best and most essential psychotropic drugs included here? Do you find any factual errors? Are there agreements or disagreements with any of the opinions expressed here? Are there suggestions for any additional tips or pearls for future editions? Any and all suggestions and comments are welcomed.

All of the selected drugs are presented in the same design format in order to facilitate rapid access to information. Specifically, each drug is broken down into five sections, each designated by a unique color background: ■ therapeutics, ■ side effects, ■ dosing and use, ■ special populations, and ■ the art of psychopharmacology, followed by key references.

Therapeutics covers the brand names in major countries; the class of drug; what it is commonly prescribed and approved for by the United States Food and Drug Administration (FDA); how the drug works; how long it takes to work; what to do if it works or if it doesn't work; the best augmenting combinations for partial response or treatment resistance, and the tests (if any) that are required.

Side effects explains how the drug causes side effects; gives a list of notable, life threatening or dangerous side effects; gives a specific rating for weight gain or sedation, and advice about how to handle side effects, including best augmenting agents for side effects.

Dosing and use gives the usual dosing range; dosage forms; how to dose and dosing tips; symptoms of overdose; long-term use; if habit forming, how to stop; pharmacokinetics; drug interactions, when not to use and other warnings or precautions.

Special populations gives specific information about any possible renal, hepatic and cardiac impairments, and any precautions to be taken for treating the elderly, children, adolescents, and pregnant and breast-feeding women.

The art of psychopharmacology gives the author's opinions on issues such as the potential advantages and disadvantages of any one drug, the primary target symptoms, and clinical pearls to get the best out of a drug.

At the back of the *Guide* are several indices. The first is an index by drug name, giving both generic names (uncapitalized) and trade names (capitalized and followed by the generic name in parentheses). The second is an index of common uses for the generic drugs included in the *Guide* and is organized by disorder/symptom. Agents that are approved by the FDA for a particular use are shown in bold. The third index is organized by drug class, and lists all the agents that fall within each particular class. In addition to these indices there is a list of abbreviations and FDA definitions for the Pregnancy Categories A, B, C, D and X. A listing of the icons used in the *Guide* is included on pages xiii–xv.

Readers are encouraged to consult standard references[1] and comprehensive psychiatry and pharmacology textbooks for more in-depth information. They are also reminded that the art of psychopharmacology section is the author's opinion.

It is strongly advised that readers familiarize themselves with the standard use of these drugs before attempting any of the more exotic uses discussed, such as unusual drug combinations and doses. Reading about both drugs before augmenting one with the other is also strongly recommended. Today's psychopharmacologist should also regularly track blood pressure, weight and body mass index for most of their patients. The dutiful clinician will also check out the drug interactions of non-central-nervous-system (CNS) drugs with those that act in the CNS, including any prescribed by other clinicians.

Certain drugs may be for experts only and might include clozapine, thioridazine, pimozide, tacrine, pemoline, nefazodone, mesoridazine and MAO inhibitors, among others. Off-label uses not approved by the FDA and inadequately studied doses or combinations of drugs may also be for the expert only, who can weigh risks and benefits in the presence of sometimes vague and conflicting evidence. Pregnant or nursing women, or people with two or more psychiatric illnesses, substance abuse, and/or a concomitant medical illness may be suitable patients for the expert only. Controlled substances also require expertise. Use your best judgement as to your level of expertise and realize that we are all learning in this rapidly advancing field. The practice of medicine is often not so much a science as it is an art. It is important to stay within the standards of medical care for the field, and also within your personal comfort zone, while trying to help extremely ill and often difficult patients with medicines than can sometimes transform their lives and relieve their suffering.

Finally, this book is intended to be genuinely helpful for practitioners of psychopharmacology by providing them with the mixture of facts and opinions selected by the author. Ultimately, prescribing choices are the reader's responsibility. Every effort has been made in preparing this book to provide accurate and up-to-date information in accord with accepted standards and practice at the time of publication. Nevertheless, the psychopharmacology field is evolving rapidly and the author and publisher make no warranties that the information contained herein is totally free from error, not least because clinical standards are constantly changing through research and regulation. Furthermore, the author and publisher disclaim any responsibility for the continued currency of this information and disclaim all liability for any and all damages, including direct or consequential damages, resulting from the use of information contained in this book. Doctors recommending and patients using these drugs are strongly advised to pay careful attention to, and consult information provided by the manufacturer.

---

[1] For example, *Physician's Desk Reference* and *Martindale's*

List of icons

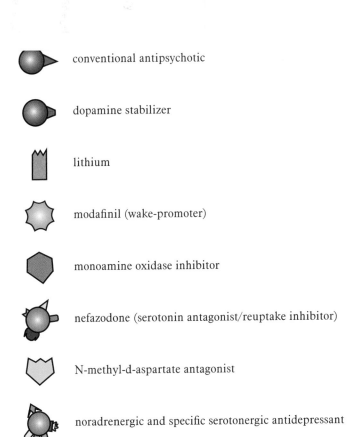

conventional antipsychotic

dopamine stabilizer

lithium

modafinil (wake-promoter)

monoamine oxidase inhibitor

nefazodone (serotonin antagonist/reuptake inhibitor)

N-methyl-d-aspartate antagonist

noradrenergic and specific serotonergic antidepressant

norepinephrine and dopamine reuptake inhibitor

 sedative hypnotic

 selective norepinephrine reuptake inhibitor

 selective serotonin reuptake inhibitor

 serotonin-dopamine antagonist

 serotonin and norepinephrine reuptake inhibitor

 serotonin 1A partial agonist

 stimulant

 trazodone (serotonin antagonist/reuptake inhibitor)

 tricyclic/tetracyclic antidepressant

 How the drug works, mechanism of action

 Best augmenting agents to add for partial response or treatment-resistance

 Life-threatening or dangerous side effects

Weight Gain: Degrees of weight gain associated with the drug, with unusual signifying that weight gain has been reported but is not expected; not unusual signifying that weight gain occurs in a significant minority; common signifying that many experience weight gain and/or it can be significant in amount; and problematic signifying that weight gain occurs frequently, can be significant in amount, and may be a health problem in some patients

Sedation: Degrees of sedation associated with the drug, with unusual signifying that sedation has been reported but is not expected; not unusual signifying that sedation occurs in a significant minority; common signifying that many experience sedation and/or it can be significant in amount; and problematic signifying that sedation occurs frequently, can be significant in amount, and may be a health problem in some patients

Tips for dosing based on the clinical expertise of the author

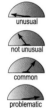

Drug interactions that may occur

Warnings and precautions regarding use of the drug

Dosing and other information specific to children and adolescents

Information regarding use of the drug during pregnancy

Clinical pearls of information based on the clinical expertise of the author

ALPRAZOLAM

Brands • Xanax, Xanax XR
see index for additional brand names

Generic? Yes (not for XR)

Class
• Benzodiazepine (anxiolytic)

Commonly Prescribed For
(bold for FDA approved)
• **Generalized anxiety disorder (IR)**
• **Panic disorder (IR and XR)**
• Other anxiety disorders
• Anxiety associated with depression
• Premenstrual dysphoric disorder
• Irritable bowel syndrome and other somatic symptoms associated with anxiety disorders
• Insomnia
• Acute mania (adjunctive)
• Acute psychosis (adjunctive)

 How The Drug Works
• Binds to benzodiazepine receptors at the GABA-A ligand-gated chloride channel complex
• Enhances the inhibitory effects of GABA
• Boosts chloride conductance through GABA-regulated channels
• Inhibits neuronal activity presumably in amygdala-centered fear circuits to provide therapeutic benefits in anxiety disorders

How Long Until It Works
• Some immediate relief with first dosing is common; can take several weeks with daily dosing for maximal therapeutic benefit

If It Works
• For short-term symptoms of anxiety – after a few weeks, discontinue use or use on an "as-needed" basis
• For chronic anxiety disorders, the goal of treatment is complete remission of symptoms as well as prevention of future relapses
• For chronic anxiety disorders, treatment most often reduces or even eliminates symptoms, but not a cure since symptoms can recur after medicine stopped

• For long-term symptoms of anxiety, consider switching to an SSRI or SNRI for long-term maintenance
• If long-term maintenance with a benzodiazepine is necessary, continue treatment for 6 months after symptoms resolve, and then taper dose slowly
• If symptoms reemerge, consider treatment with an SSRI or SNRI, or consider restarting the benzodiazepine; sometimes benzodiazepines have to be used in combination with SSRIs or SNRIs for best results

If It Doesn't Work
• Consider switching to another agent or adding an appropriate augmenting agent
• Consider psychotherapy, especially cognitive behavioral psychotherapy
• Consider presence of concomitant substance abuse
• Consider presence of alprazolam abuse
• Consider another diagnosis, such as a comorbid medical condition

 Best Augmenting Combos for Partial Response or Treatment-Resistance
• Benzodiazepines are frequently used as augmenting agents for antipsychotics and mood stabilizers in the treatment of psychotic and bipolar disorders
• Benzodiazepines are frequently used as augmenting agents for SSRIs and SNRIs in the treatment of anxiety disorders
• Not generally rational to combine with other benzodiazepines
• Caution if using as an anxiolytic concomitantly with other sedative hypnotics for sleep

Tests
• In patients with seizure disorders, concomitant medical illness, and/or those with multiple concomitant long-term medications, periodic liver tests and blood counts may be prudent

How Drug Causes Side Effects
• Same mechanism for side effects as for therapeutic effects – namely due to

excessive actions at benzodiazepine receptors
- Long-term adaptations in benzodiazepine receptors may explain the development of dependence, tolerance, and withdrawal
- Side effects are generally immediate, but immediate side effects often disappear in time

Notable Side Effects
✳ Sedation, fatigue, depression
✳ Dizziness, ataxia, slurred speech, weakness
✳ Forgetfulness, confusion
✳ Hyper-excitability, nervousness
- Rare hallucinations, mania
- Rare hypotension
- Hypersalivation, dry mouth

 Life Threatening or Dangerous Side Effects
- Respiratory depression, especially when taken with CNS depressants in overdose
- Rare hepatic dysfunction, renal dysfunction, blood dyscrasias

Weight Gain

unusual · not unusual · common · problematic
- Reported but not expected

Sedation

unusual · not unusual · common · problematic
- Occurs in significant minority
- Especially at initiation of treatment or when dose increases
- Tolerance often develops over time

What To Do About Side Effects
- Wait
- Wait
- Wait
- Lower the dose
- Switch to alprazolam XR
- Take largest dose at bedtime to avoid sedative effects during the day
- Switch to another agent
- Administer flumazenil if side effects are severe or life-threatening

Best Augmenting Agents for Side Effects
- Many side effects cannot be improved with an augmenting agent

DOSING AND USE

Usual Dosage Range
- Anxiety: alprazolam IR: 1–4 mg/day
- Panic: alprazolam IR: 5–6 mg/day
- Panic: alprazolam XR: 3–6 mg/day

Dosage Forms
- Alprazolam IR tablet 0.25 mg scored, 0.5 mg scored, 1 mg scored, 2 mg multi-scored
- Alprazolam IR solution, concentrate 1 mg/mL
- Alprazolam XR (extended-release) tablet 0.5 mg, 1 mg, 2 mg, 3 mg

How to Dose
- For anxiety, alprazolam IR should be started at 0.75–1.5 mg/day divided into 3 doses; increase dose every 3–4 days until desired efficacy is reached; maximum dose generally 4 mg/day
- For panic, alprazolam IR should be started at 1.5 mg/day divided into 3 doses; increase 1 mg or less every 3–4 days until desired efficacy is reached, increasing by smaller amounts for dosage over 4 mg/day; may require as much as 10 mg/day for desired efficacy in difficult cases
- For panic, alprazolam XR should be started at 0.5–1 mg/day once daily in the morning; dose may be increased by 1 mg/day every 3–4 days until desired efficacy is reached; maximum dose generally 10 mg/day

 Dosing Tips
- Use lowest possible effective dose for the shortest possible period of time (a benzodiazepine-sparing strategy)
- Assess need for continued treatment regularly
- Risk of dependence may increase with dose and duration of treatment
- For inter-dose symptoms of anxiety, can either increase dose or maintain same total daily dose but divide into more frequent

doses, or give as extended-release formulation
- Can also use an as-needed occasional "top up" dose for inter-dose anxiety
- Because panic disorder can require doses higher than 4 mg/day, the risk of dependence may be greater in these patients
- Some severely ill patients may require 8 mg/day or more
- Extended release formulation only needs to be taken once or twice daily
- Do not break or chew XR tablets as this will alter controlled release properties
- Frequency of dosing in practice is often greater than predicted from half-life, as duration of biological activity is often shorter than pharmacokinetic terminal half-life
- Alprazolam and alprazolam XR generally dosed about one tenth the dosage of diazepam
* Alprazolam and alprazolam XR generally dosed about twice the dosage of clonazepam

Overdose
- Fatalities have been reported both in monotherapy and in conjunction with alcohol; sedation, confusion, poor coordination, diminished reflexes, coma

Long-Term Use
- Risk of dependence, particularly for treatment periods longer than 12 weeks and especially in patients with past or current polysubstance abuse

Habit Forming
- Alprazolam is a Schedule IV drug
- Patients may develop dependence and/or tolerance with long-term use

How to Stop
- Seizures may rarely occur on withdrawal, especially if withdrawal is abrupt; greater risk for doses above 4 mg and in those with additional risks for seizures, including those with a history of seizures
- Taper by 0.5 mg every 3 days to reduce chances of withdrawal effects
- For difficult to taper cases, consider reducing dose much more slowly after reaching 3 mg/day, perhaps by as little as 0.25 mg per week or less

- For other patients with severe problems discontinuing a benzodiazepine, dosing may need to be tapered over many months (i.e., reduce dose by 1% every 3 days by crushing tablet and suspending or dissolving in 100 ml of fruit juice and then disposing of 1 ml while drinking the rest; 3–7 days later, dispose of 2 ml, and so on). This is both a form of very slow biological tapering and a form of behavioral desensitization
- Be sure to differentiate reemergence of symptoms requiring reinstitution of treatment from withdrawal symptoms
- Benzodiazepine-dependent anxiety patients and insulin-dependent diabetics are not addicted to their medications. When benzodiazepine-dependent patients stop their medication, disease symptoms can reemerge, disease symptoms can worsen (rebound), and/or withdrawal symptoms can emerge

Pharmacokinetics
- Metabolized by CYP450 3A4
- Inactive metabolites
- Elimination half-life 12–15 hours

 Drug Interactions
- Increased depressive effects when taken with other CNS depressants
- Inhibitors of CYP450 3A, such as nefazodone, fluvoxamine, fluoxetine, and even grapefruit juice, may decrease clearance of alprazolam and thereby raise alprazolam plasma levels and enhance sedative side effects; alprazolam dose may need to be lowered
- Thus, azole antifungal agents (such as ketoconazole and itraconazole), macrolide antibiotics, and protease inhibitors may also raise alprazolam plasma levels
- Inducers of CYP450 3A, such as carbamazepine, may increase clearance of alprazolam and lower alprazolam plasma levels and possibly reduce therapeutic effects

 Other Warnings/ Precautions
- Dosage changes should be made in collaboration with prescriber

- Use with caution in patients with pulmonary disease; rare reports of death after initiation of benzodiazepines in patients with severe pulmonary impairment
- History of drug or alcohol abuse often creates greater risk for dependency
- Hypomania and mania have occurred in depressed patients taking alprazolam
- Use only with extreme caution if patient has obstructive sleep apnea
- Some depressed patients may experience a worsening of suicidal ideation
- Some patients may exhibit abnormal thinking or behavioral changes similar to those caused by other CNS depressants (i.e., either depressant actions or disinhibiting actions)

Do Not Use

- If patient has narrow angle-closure glaucoma
- If patient is taking ketoconazole or itraconazole (azole antifungal agents)
- If there is a proven allergy to alprazolam or any benzodiazepine

SPECIAL POPULATIONS

Renal Impairment

- Drug should be used with caution

Hepatic Impairment

- Should begin with lower starting dose (0.5–0.75 mg/day in 2 or 3 divided doses)

Cardiac Impairment

- Benzodiazepines have been used to treat anxiety associated with acute myocardial infarction

Elderly

- Should begin with lower starting dose (0.5–0.75 mg/day in 2 or 3 divided doses) and be monitored closely

 Children and Adolescents

- Safety and efficacy not established but often used, especially short-term and at the lower end of the dosing scale
- Long-term effects of alprazolam in children/adolescents are unknown

- Should generally receive lower doses and be more closely monitored

 Pregnancy

- Risk Category D [positive evidence of risk to human fetus; potential benefits may still justify its use during pregnancy]
- Possible increased risk of birth defects when benzodiazepines taken during pregnancy
- Because of the potential risks, alprazolam is not generally recommended as treatment for anxiety during pregnancy, especially during the first trimester
- Drug should be tapered if discontinued
- Infants whose mothers received a benzodiazepine late in pregnancy may experience withdrawal effects
- Neonatal flaccidity has been reported in infants whose mothers took a benzodiazepine during pregnancy
- Seizures, even mild seizures, may cause harm to the embryo/fetus

Breast Feeding

- Some drug is found in mother's breast milk
- ✱ Recommended either to discontinue drug or bottle feed
- Effects on infant have been observed and include feeding difficulties, sedation, and weight loss

THE ART OF PSYCHOPHARMACOLOGY

Potential Advantages

- Rapid onset of action
- Less sedation than some other benzodiazepines
- Availability of an XR formulation with longer duration of action

Potential Disadvantages

- Euphoria may lead to abuse
- Abuse especially risky in past or present substance abusers

Primary Target Symptoms

- Panic attacks
- Anxiety

Pearls

✳ One of the most popular benzodiazepines for anxiety, especially among primary care physicians and psychiatrists
• Is a very useful adjunct to SSRIs and SNRIs in the treatment of numerous anxiety disorders
• Not effective for treating psychosis as a monotherapy, but can be used as an adjunct to antipsychotics
• Not effective for treating bipolar disorder as a monotherapy, but can be used as an adjunct to mood stabilizers and antipsychotics
• May both cause depression and treat depression in different patients
• Risk of seizure is greatest during the first 3 days after discontinuation of alprazolam, especially in those with prior seizures, head injuries, or withdrawal from drugs of abuse
• Clinical duration of action may be shorter than plasma half-life, leading to dosing more frequently than 2–3 times daily in some patients, especially for immediate release alprazolam
• Adding fluvoxamine, fluoxetine, or nefazodone can increase alprazolam levels and make the patient very sleepy unless the alprazolam dose is lowered by half or more

• When using to treat insomnia, remember that insomnia may be a symptom of some other primary disorder itself, and thus warrant evaluation for comorbid psychiatric and/or medical conditions
✳ Alprazolam XR may be less sedating than immediate release alprazolam
✳ Alprazolam XR may be dosed less frequently than immediate release alprazolam, and lead to less inter-dose breakthrough symptoms and less "clock-watching" in anxious patients
• Slower rises in plasma drug levels for alprazolam XR have the potential to reduce euphoria/abuse liability, but this has not been proven
• Slower falls in plasma drug levels for alprazolam XR have the potential to facilitate drug discontinuation by reducing withdrawal symptoms, but this has not been proven
✳ Alprozolam XR generally has longer biological duration of action than clonazepam
✳ If clonazepam can be considered a "long-acting alprazolam-like anxiolytic", then alprazolam XR can be considered "an even longer-acting clonazepam-like anxiolytic" with the potential of improved tolerability features in terms of less euphoria, abuse, dependence, and withdrawal problems, but this has not been proven

Suggested Reading

DeVane CL, Ware MR, Lydiard RB. Pharmacokinetics, pharmacodynamics, and treatment issues of benzodiazepines: alprazolam, adinazolam, and clonazepam. Psychopharmacol Bull 1991;27:463–73.

Greenblatt DJ, Wright CE. Clinical pharmacokinetics of alprazolam. Therapeutic implications. Clin Pharmacokinet 1993; 24:453–71.

Jonas JM, Cohon MS. A comparison of the safety and efficacy of alprazolam versus other agents in the treatment of anxiety, panic, and depression: a review of the literature. J Clin Psychiatry 1993;54 (Suppl):25–45.

Klein E. The role of extended-release benzodiazepines in the treatment of anxiety: a risk-benefit evaluation with a focus on extended-release alprazolam. J Clin Psychiatry 2002;63 (Suppl 14):27–33.

Speigel DA. Efficacy studies of alprazolam in panic disorder. Psychopharmacol Bull 1998; 34:191–5.

AMISULPRIDE

THERAPEUTICS

Brands • Solian
see index for additional brand names

Generic? No

Class
• Atypical antipsychotic (benzamide; possibly a dopamine stabilizer and dopamine partial agonist)

Commonly Prescribed For
(bold for FDA approved)
• Schizophrenia, acute and chronic (outside of U.S., especially Europe)
• Dysthymia

How The Drug Works
• Theoretically blocks presynaptic dopamine 2 receptors at low doses
• Theoretically blocks postsynaptic dopamine 2 receptors at higher doses
✳ May be a partial agonist at dopamine 2 receptors, which would theoretically reduce dopamine output when dopamine concentrations are high and increase dopamine output when dopamine concentrations are low
• Blocks dopamine 3 receptors, which may contribute to its clinical actions
✳ Unlike other atypical antipsychotics, amisulpride does not have potent actions at serotonin receptors

How Long Until It Works
• Psychotic symptoms can improve within 1 week, but it may take several weeks for full effect on behavior as well as on cognition and affective stabilization
• Classically recommended to wait at least 4–6 weeks to determine efficacy of drug, but in practice some patients require up to 16–20 weeks to show a good response, especially on cognitive symptoms

If It Works
• Most often reduces positive symptoms in schizophrenia but does not eliminate them
• Can improve negative symptoms, as well as aggressive, cognitive, and affective symptoms in schizophrenia

• Most schizophrenic patients do not have a total remission of symptoms but rather a reduction of symptoms by about a third
• Perhaps 5–15% of schizophrenic patients can experience an overall improvement of greater than 50–60%, especially when receiving stable treatment for more than a year
• Such patients are considered super-responders or "awakeners" since they may be well enough to be employed, live independently, and sustain long-term relationships
• Continue treatment until reaching a plateau of improvement
• After reaching a satisfactory plateau, continue treatment for at least a year after first episode of psychosis
• For second and subsequent episodes of psychosis, treatment may need to be indefinite
• Even for first episodes of psychosis, it may be preferable to continue treatment indefinitely to avoid subsequent episodes

If It Doesn't Work
• Try one of the other first-line atypical antipsychotics (risperidone, olanzapine, quetiapine, ziprasidone, aripiprazole)
• If two or more antipsychotic monotherapies do not work, consider clozapine
• If no atypical antipsychotic is effective, consider higher doses or augmentation with valproate or lamotrigine
• Some patients may require treatment with a conventional antipsychotic
• Consider noncompliance and switch to another antipsychotic with fewer side effects or to an antipsychotic that can be given by depot injection
• Consider initiating rehabilitation and psychotherapy
• Consider presence of concomitant drug abuse

 Best Augmenting Combos for Partial Response or Treatment-Resistance
• Valproic acid (valproate, divalproex, divalproex ER)
• Augmentation of amisulpride has not been systematically studied

- Other mood stabilizing anticonvulsants (carbamazepine, oxcarbazepine, lamotrigine)
- Lithium
- Benzodiazepines

Tests

✳ Although risk of diabetes and dyslipidemia with amisulpride has not been systematically studied, monitoring as for all other atypical antipsychotics is suggested

Before starting an atypical antipsychotic

✳ Weigh all patients and track BMI during treatment
- Get baseline personal and family history of obesity, dyslipidemia, hypertension, and cardiovascular disease
- Get waistline circumference (at umbilicus), blood pressure, fasting plasma glucose, and fasting lipid profile
- Determine if patient is
  - overweight (BMI 25.0–29.9)
  - obese (BMI ≥30)
  - has pre-diabetes (fasting plasma glucose 100–125 mg/dl)
  - has diabetes (fasting plasma glucose >126 mg/dl)
  - has hypertension (BP >140/90 mm Hg)
  - has dyslipidemia (increased total cholesterol, LDL cholesterol, and triglycerides; decreased HDL cholesterol)
- Treat or refer such patients for treatment, including nutrition and weight management, physical activity counseling, smoking cessation, and medical management

Monitoring after starting an atypical antipsychotic

✳ BMI monthly for 3 months, then quarterly
- Blood pressure, fasting plasma glucose, fasting lipids within 3 months and then annually, but earlier and more frequently for patients with diabetes or who have gained >5% initial weight
- Treat or refer for treatment and consider switching to another atypical antipsychotic for patients who become overweight, obese, pre-diabetic, diabetic, hypertensive, or dyslipidemic while receiving an atypical antipsychotic

✳ Even in patients without known diabetes, be vigilant for the rare but life threatening onset of diabetic ketoacidosis, which always requires immediate treatment by monitoring for the rapid onset of polyuria, polydipsia, weight loss, nausea, vomiting, dehydration, rapid respiration, weakness and clouding of sensorium, even coma

- EKGs may be useful for selected patients (e.g., those with personal or family history of QTc prolongation; cardiac arrhythmia; recent myocardial infarction; uncompensated heart failure; or taking agents that prolong QTc interval such as pimozide, thioridazine, selected antiarrhythmics, moxifloxacin, sparfloxacin, etc.)
- Patients at risk for electrolyte disturbances (e.g., patients on diuretic therapy) should have baseline and periodic serum potassium and magnesium measurements

SIDE EFFECTS

How Drug Causes Side Effects

- By blocking dopamine 2 receptors in the striatum, it can cause motor side effects, especially at high doses
- By blocking dopamine 2 receptors in the pituitary, it can cause elevations in prolactin
- Mechanism of weight gain and possible increased incidence of diabetes and dyslipidemia with atypical antipsychotics is unknown

Notable Side Effects

✳ Extrapyramidal symptoms
✳ Galactorrhea, amenorrhea
✳ Atypical antipsychotics may increase the risk for diabetes and dyslipidemia, although the specific risks associated with amisulpride are unknown
- Insomnia, sedation, agitation, anxiety
- Constipation, weight gain
- Rare tardive dyskinesia

 Life Threatening or Dangerous Side Effects

- Rare neuroleptic malignant syndrome
- Rare seizures
- Dose-dependent QTc prolongation

Weight Gain

unusual not unusual common problematic

• Occurs in significant minority

Sedation

unusual not unusual common problematic

• Many experience and/or can be significant in amount, especially at high doses

What To Do About Side Effects
• Wait
• Wait
• Wait
• Lower the dose
• For motor symptoms, add an anticholinergic agent
• Take more of the dose at bedtime to help reduce daytime sedation
• Weight loss, exercise programs, and medical management for high BMIs, diabetes, dyslipidemia
• Switch to another atypical antipsychotic

Best Augmenting Agents for Side Effects
• Benztropine or trihexyphenidyl for motor side effects
• Many side effects cannot be improved with an augmenting agent

DOSING AND USE

Usual Dosage Range
• Schizophrenia: 400–800 mg/day in 2 doses
• Negative symptoms only: 50–300 mg/day
• Dysthymia: 50 mg/day

Dosage Forms
• Different formulations may be available in different markets
• Tablet 50 mg, 100 mg, 200 mg, 400 mg
• Oral solution 100 mg/mL

How to Dose
• Initial 400–800 mg/day in 2 doses; daily doses above 400 mg should be divided in 2; maximum generally 1200 mg/day

 Dosing Tips
✱ Efficacy for negative symptoms in schizophrenia may be achieved at lower doses, while efficacy for positive symptoms may require higher doses
• Patients receiving low doses may only need to take the drug once daily
✱ For dysthymia and depression, use only low doses
✱ Dose-dependent QTc prolongation, so use with caution, especially at higher doses (>800 mg/day)
✱ Amisulpride may accumulate in patients with renal insufficiency, requiring lower dosing or switching to another antipsychotic to avoid QTc prolongation in these patients

Overdose
• Sedation, coma, hypotension, extrapyramidal symptoms

Long-Term Use
• Amisulpride is used for both acute and chronic schizophrenia treatment

Habit Forming
• No

How to Stop
• Slow down-titration (over 6 to 8 weeks), especially when simultaneously beginning a new antipsychotic while switching (i.e., cross-titration)
• Rapid discontinuation may lead to rebound psychosis and worsening of symptoms

Pharmacokinetics
• Elimination half-life approximately 12 hours
• Excreted largely unchanged

 Drug Interactions
• Can decrease the effects of levodopa, dopamine agonists
• Can increase the effects of antihypertensive drugs
• CNS effects may be increased if used with a CNS depressant
• May enhance QTc prolongation of other drugs capable of prolonging QTc interval

- Since amisulpride is only weakly metabolized, few drug interactions that could raise amisulpride plasma levels are expected

 Other Warnings/ Precautions

- Use cautiously in patients with alcohol withdrawal or convulsive disorders because of possible lowering of seizure threshold
- If signs of neuroleptic malignant syndrome develop, treatment should be immediately discontinued
- Because amisulpride may dose-dependently prolong QTc interval, use with caution in patients who have bradycardia or who are taking drugs that can induce bradycardia (e.g., beta blockers, calcium channel blockers, clonidine, digitalis)
- Because amisulpride may dose-dependently prolong QTc interval, use with caution in patients who have hypokalemia and/or hypomagnesemia or who are taking drugs that can induce hypokalemia and/or magnesemia (e.g., diuretics, stimulant laxatives, intravenous amphotericin B, glucocorticoids, tetracosactide)
- Use only with caution if at all in Parkinson's disease or Lewy Body dementia, especially at high doses

Do Not Use

- If patient has pheochromocytoma
- If patient has prolactin-dependent tumor
- If patient is pregnant or nursing
- If patient is taking agents capable of significantly prolonging QTc interval (e.g., pimozide; thioridazine; selected antiarrhythmics such as quinidine, disopyramide, amiodarone, and sotalol; selected antibiotics such as moxifloxacin and sparfloxacin)
- If there is a history of QTc prolongation or cardiac arrhythmia, recent acute myocardial infarction, uncompensated heart failure
- If patient is taking cisapride, intravenous erythromycin, or pentamidine
- In children
- If there is a proven allergy to amisulpride

Renal Impairment

- Use with caution; drug may accumulate
- Amisulpride is eliminated by the renal route; in cases of severe renal insufficiency, the dose should be decreased and intermittent treatment or switching to another antipsychotic should be considered

Hepatic Impairment

- Use with caution, but dose adjustment not generally necessary

Cardiac Impairment

- Amisulpride produces a dose-dependent prolongation of QTc interval, which may be enhanced by the existence of bradycardia, hypokalemia, congenital or acquired long QTc interval, which should be evaluated prior to administering amisulpride
- Use with caution if treating concomitantly with a medication likely to produce prolonged bradycardia, hypokalemia, slowing of intracardiac conduction, or prolongation of the QTc interval
- Avoid amisulpride in patients with a known history of QTc prolongation, recent acute myocardial infarction, and uncompensated heart failure

Elderly

- Some patients may be more susceptible to sedative and hypotensive effects

 Children and Adolescents

- Efficacy and safety not established under age 18

 Pregnancy

- Although animal studies have not shown teratogenic effect, amisulpride is not recommended for use during pregnancy
- Psychotic symptoms may worsen during pregnancy and some form of treatment may be necessary
- Amisulpride may be preferable to anticonvulsant mood stabilizers if treatment is required during pregnancy

Breast Feeding

- Unknown if amisulpride is secreted in human breast milk, but all psychotropics assumed to be secreted in breast milk
- ✴ Recommended either to discontinue drug or bottle feed

Potential Advantages

- Not as clearly associated with weight gain as some other atypical antipsychotics
- For patients who are responsive to low dose activation effects that reduce negative symptoms and depression

Potential Disadvantages

- Patients who have difficulty being compliant with twice daily dosing
- Patients for whom elevated prolactin may not be desired (e.g., possibly pregnant patients; pubescent girls with amenorrhea; postmenopausal women with low estrogen who do not take estrogen replacement therapy)
- Patients with severe renal impairment

Primary Target Symptoms

- Positive symptoms of psychosis
- Negative symptoms of psychosis
- Depressive symptoms

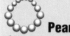

Pearls

- ✴ Efficacy has been particularly well demonstrated in patients with predominantly negative symptoms
- ✴ The increase in prolactin caused by amisulpride may cause menstruation to stop
- Some treatment-resistant patients with inadequate responses to clozapine may benefit from amisulpride augmentation of clozapine
- Risks of diabetes and dyslipidemia not well studied, but does not seem to cause as much weight gain as some other atypical antipsychotics
- Has atypical antipsychotic properties (i.e., antipsychotic action without a high incidence of extrapyramidal symptoms), especially at low doses, but not a serotonin dopamine antagonist

- Mediates its atypical antipsychotic properties via novel actions on dopamine receptors, perhaps dopamine stabilizing partial agonist actions on dopamine 2 receptors
- May be more of a dopamine 2 antagonist than aripiprazole, but less of a dopamine 2 antagonist than other atypical or conventional antipsychotics
- Low dose activating actions may be beneficial for negative symptoms in schizophrenia
- Very low doses may be useful in dysthymia
- Compared to sulpiride, amisulpride has better oral bioavailability and more potency, thus allowing lower dosing, less weight gain, and fewer extrapyramidal symptoms
- Compared to other atypical antipsychotics with potent serotonin 2A antagonism, amisulpride may have more extrapyramidal symptoms and prolactin elevation, but may still be classified as an atypical antipsychotic, particularly at low doses
- Patients have very similar antipsychotic responses to any conventional antipsychotic, which is different from atypical antipsychotics where antipsychotic responses of individual patients can occasionally vary greatly from one atypical antipsychotic to another
- Patients with inadequate responses to atypical antipsychotics may benefit from a trial of augmentation with a conventional antipsychotic or switching to a conventional antipsychotic
- However, long-term polypharmacy with a combination of a conventional antipsychotic with an atypical antipsychotic may combine their side effects without clearly augmenting the efficacy of either
- Although a frequent practice by some prescribers, adding two conventional antipsychotics together has little rationale and may reduce tolerability without clearly enhancing efficacy

AMISULPRIDE

Suggested Reading

Burns T, Bale R. Clinical advantages of amisulpride in the treatment of acute schizophrenia. J Int Med Res 2001; 29 (6): 451–66.

Curran MP, Perry CM. Spotlight on amisulpride in schizophrenia. CNS Drugs 2002; 16 (3): 207–11.

Leucht S, Pitschel-Walz G, Engel RR, Kissling W. Amisulpride, an unusual "atypical" antipsychotic: a meta-analysis of randomized controlled trials. Am J Psychiatry 2002; 159 (2): 180–90.

Brands • Elavil
see index for additional brand names

Generic? Yes

Class

- Tricyclic antidepressant (TCA)
- Serotonin and norepinephrine/
  noradrenaline reuptake inhibitor

Commonly Prescribed For

(bold for FDA approved)
- **Depression**
- **Endogenous depression**
- ✳ Neuropathic pain/chronic pain
- ✳ Fibromyalgia
- ✳ Headache
- ✳ Low back pain/neck pain
- Anxiety
- Insomnia
- Treatment-resistant depression

How The Drug Works

- Boosts neurotransmitters serotonin and norepinephrine/noradrenaline
- Blocks serotonin reuptake pump (serotonin transporter), presumably increasing serotonergic neurotransmission
- Blocks norepinephrine reuptake pump (norepinephrine transporter), presumably increasing noradrenergic neurotransmission
- Presumably desensitizes both serotonin 1A receptors and beta adrenergic receptors
- Since dopamine is inactivated by norepinephrine reuptake in frontal cortex, which largely lacks dopamine transporters, amitriptyline can increase dopamine neurotransmission in this part of the brain

How Long Until It Works

- May have immediate effects in treating insomnia or anxiety
- Onset of therapeutic actions usually not immediate, but often delayed 2 to 4 weeks
- If it is not working within 6 to 8 weeks for depression, it may require a dosage increase or it may not work at all
- May continue to work for many years to prevent relapse of symptoms

If It Works

- The goal of treatment of depression is complete remission of current symptoms as well as prevention of future relapses
- The goal of treatment of chronic pain conditions such as neuropathic pain, fibromyalgia, headaches, low back pain, and neck pain is to reduce symptoms as much as possible, especially in combination with other treatments
- Treatment of depression most often reduces or even eliminates symptoms, but not a cure since symptoms can recur after medicine stopped
- Treatment of chronic pain conditions such as neuropathic pain, fibromyalgia, headache, low back pain, and neck pain may reduce symptoms, but rarely eliminates them completely, and is not a cure since symptoms can recur after medicine is stopped
- Continue treatment of depression until all symptoms are gone (remission)
- Once symptoms of depression are gone, continue treating for 1 year for the first episode of depression
- For second and subsequent episodes of depression, treatment may need to be indefinite
- Use in anxiety disorders and chronic pain conditions such as neuropathic pain, fibromyalgia, headache, low back pain, and neck pain may also need to be indefinite, but long-term treatment is not well studied in these conditions

If It Doesn't Work

- Many depressed patients only have a partial response where some symptoms are improved but others persist (especially insomnia, fatigue, and problems concentrating)
- Other depressed patients may be nonresponders, sometimes called treatment-resistant or treatment-refractory
- Consider increasing dose, switching to another agent or adding an appropriate augmenting agent
- Consider psychotherapy
- Consider evaluation for another diagnosis or for a comorbid condition (e.g., medical illness, substance abuse, etc.)
- Some patients may experience apparent lack of consistent efficacy due to activation of latent or underlying bipolar disorder, and

require antidepressant discontinuation and a switch to a mood stabilizer

Best Augmenting Combos for Partial Response or Treatment-Resistance

- Lithium, buspirone, thyroid hormone (for depression)
- Gabapentin, tiagabine, other anticonvulsants, even opiates if done by experts while monitoring carefully in difficult cases (for chronic pain)

Tests

- None for healthy individuals
- ✳ Since tricyclic and tetracyclic antidepressants are frequently associated with weight gain, before starting treatment, weigh all patients and determine if the patient is already overweight (BMI 25.0–29.9) or obese (BMI ≥30)
- Before giving a drug that can cause weight gain to an overweight or obese patient, consider determining whether the patient already has pre-diabetes (fasting plasma glucose 100–125 mg/dl), diabetes (fasting plasma glucose >126 mg/dl), or dyslipidemia (increased total cholesterol, LDL cholesterol and triglycerides; decreased HDL cholesterol), and treat or refer such patients for treatment, including nutrition and weight management, physical activity counseling, smoking cessation, and medical management
- ✳ Monitor weight and BMI during treatment
- ✳ While giving a drug to a patient who has gained >5% of initial weight, consider evaluating for the presence of pre-diabetes, diabetes, or dyslipidemia, or consider switching to a different antidepressant
- EKGs may be useful for selected patients (e.g., those with personal or family history of QTc prolongation; cardiac arrhythmia; recent myocardial infarction; uncompensated heart failure; or taking agents that prolong QTc interval such as pimozide, thioridazine, selected antiarrhythmics, moxifloxacin, sparfloxacin, etc.)
- Patients at risk for electrolyte disturbances (e.g., patients on diuretic therapy) should have baseline and periodic serum potassium and magnesium measurements

SIDE EFFECTS

How Drug Causes Side Effects

- Anticholinergic activity may explain sedative effects, dry mouth, constipation, and blurred vision
- Sedative effects and weight gain may be due to antihistamine properties
- Blockade of alpha adrenergic 1 receptors may explain dizziness, sedation, and hypotension
- Cardiac arrhythmias and seizures, especially in overdose, may be caused by blockade of ion channels

Notable Side Effects

- Blurred vision, constipation, urinary retention, increased appetite, dry mouth, nausea, diarrhea, heartburn, unusual taste in mouth, weight gain
- Fatigue, weakness, dizziness, sedation, headache, anxiety, nervousness, restlessness
- Sexual dysfunction (impotence, change in libido)
- Sweating, rash, itching

Life Threatening or Dangerous Side Effects

- Paralytic ileus, hyperthermia (TCAs + anticholinergic agents)
- Lowered seizure threshold and rare seizures
- Orthostatic hypotension, sudden death, arrhythmias, tachycardia
- QTc prolongation
- Hepatic failure, extrapyramidal symptoms
- Increased intraocular pressure
- Rare induction of mania and activation of suicidal ideation

Weight Gain

unusual   not unusual   common   problematic

- Many experience and/or can be significant in amount
- Can increase appetite and carbohydrate craving

Sedation

unusual   not unusual   common   problematic

- Many experience and/or can be significant in amount

- Tolerance to sedative effects may develop with long-term use

What To Do About Side Effects
- Wait
- Wait
- Wait
- Lower the dose
- Switch to an SSRI or newer antidepressant

Best Augmenting Agents for Side Effects
- Many side effects cannot be improved with an augmenting agent

DOSING AND USE

Usual Dosage Range
- 50–150 mg/day

Dosage Forms
- Capsule 25 mg, 50 mg, 100 mg

How to Dose
- Initial 25 mg/day at bedtime; increase by 25 mg every 3–7 days
- 75 mg/day in divided doses; increase to 150 mg/day; maximum 300 mg/day

 Dosing Tips
- If given in a single dose, should generally be administered at bedtime because of its sedative properties
- If given in split doses, largest dose should generally be given at bedtime because of its sedative properties
- If patients experience nightmares, split dose and do not give large dose at bedtime
- Patients treated for chronic pain may only require lower doses
- If intolerable anxiety, insomnia, agitation, akathisia, or activation occur either upon dosing initiation or discontinuation, consider the possibility of activated bipolar disorder, and switch to a mood stabilizer or an atypical antipsychotic

Overdose
- Death may occur; CNS depression, convulsions, cardiac dysrhythmias, severe hypotension, ECG changes, coma

Long-Term Use
- Safe

Habit Forming
- No

How to Stop
- Taper to avoid withdrawal effects
- Even with gradual dose reduction, some withdrawal symptoms may appear within the first 2 weeks
- Many patients tolerate 50% dose reduction for 3 days, then another 50% reduction for 3 days, then discontinuation
- If withdrawal symptoms emerge during discontinuation, raise dose to stop symptoms and then restart withdrawal much more slowly

Pharmacokinetics
- Substrate for CYP450 2D6 and 1A2
- Plasma half-life 10–28 hours
- Metabolized to an active metabolite, nortriptyline, which is predominantly a norepinephrine reuptake inhibitor, by demethylation via CYP450 1A2

 Drug Interactions
- Tramadol increases the risk of seizures in patients taking TCAs
- Use of TCAs with anticholinergic drugs may result in paralytic ileus or hyperthermia
- Fluoxetine, paroxetine, bupropion, duloxetine, and other CYP450 2D6 inhibitors may increase TCA concentrations
- Fluvoxamine, a CYP450 1A2 inhibitor, can decrease the conversion of amitriptyline to nortriptyline and increase amitriptyline plasma concentrations
- Cimetidine may increase plasma concentrations of TCAs and cause anticholinergic symptoms
- Phenothiazines or haloperidol may raise TCA blood concentrations
- May alter effects of antihypertensive drugs; may inhibit hypotensive effects of clonidine
- Use of TCAs with sympathomimetic agents may increase sympathetic activity
- Methylphenidate may inhibit metabolism of TCAs
- Activation and agitation, especially following switching or adding

antidepressants, may represent the induction of a bipolar state, especially a mixed dysphoric bipolar II condition sometimes associated with suicidal ideation, and require the addition of lithium, a mood stabilizer or an atypical antipsychotic, and/or discontinuation of amitriptyline

 Other Warnings/ Precautions

- Add or initiate other antidepressants with caution for up to 2 weeks after discontinuing amitriptyline
- Generally, do not use with MAO inhibitors, including 14 days after MAOIs are stopped; do not start an MAOI until 2 weeks after discontinuing amitriptyline, but see Pearls
- Use with caution in patients with history of seizures, urinary retention, narrow angle-closure glaucoma, hyperthyroidism
- TCAs can increase QTc interval, especially at toxic doses, which can be attained not only by overdose but also by combining with drugs that inhibit TCA metabolism via CYP450 2D6, potentially causing torsade de pointes-type arrhythmia or sudden death
- Because TCAs can prolong QTc interval, use with caution in patients who have bradycardia or who are taking drugs that can induce bradycardia (e.g., beta blockers, calcium channel blockers, clonidine, digitalis)
- Because TCAs can prolong QTc interval, use with caution in patients who have hypokalemia and/or hypomagnesemia, or who are taking drugs that can induce hypokalemia and/or magnesemia (e.g., diuretics, stimulant laxatives, intravenous amphotericin B, glucocorticoids, tetracosactide)

Do Not Use

- If patient is recovering from myocardial infarction
- If patient is taking agents capable of significantly prolonging QTc interval (e.g., pimozide, thioridazine, selected antiarrhythmics, moxifloxacin, sparfloxacin)
- If there is a history of QTc prolongation or cardiac arrhythmia, recent acute myocardial infarction, uncompensated heart failure
- If patient is taking drugs that inhibit TCA metabolism, including CYP450 2D6 inhibitors, except by an expert
- If there is reduced CYP450 2D6 function, such as patients who are poor 2D6 metabolizers, except by an expert and at low doses
- If there is a proven allergy to amitriptyline or nortriptyline

SPECIAL POPULATIONS

Renal Impairment

- Use with caution; may need to lower dose

Hepatic Impairment

- Use with caution; may need to lower dose

Cardiac Impairment

- TCAs have been reported to cause arrhythmias, prolongation of conduction time, orthostatic hypotension, sinus tachycardia, and heart failure, especially in the diseased heart
- Myocardial infarction and stroke have been reported with TCAs
- TCAs produce QTc prolongation, which may be enhanced by the existence of bradycardia, hypokalemia, congenital or acquired long QTc interval, which should be evaluated prior to administering amitriptyline
- Use with caution if treating concomitantly with a medication likely to produce prolonged bradycardia, hypokalemia, slowing of intracardiac conduction, or prolongation of the QTc interval
- Avoid TCAs in patients with a known history of QTc prolongation, recent acute myocardial infarction, and uncompensated heart failure
- TCAs may cause a sustained increase in heart rate in patients with ischemic heart disease and may worsen (decrease) heart rate variability, an independent risk of mortality in cardiac populations
- Since SSRIs may improve (increase) heart rate variability in patients following a myocardial infarct and may improve survival as well as mood in patients with acute angina or following a myocardial infarction, these are more appropriate

agents for cardiac population than tricyclic/tetracyclic antidepressants

✳ Risk/benefit ratio may not justify use of TCAs in cardiac impairment

Elderly

- May be more sensitive to anticholinergic, cardiovascular, hypotensive, and sedative effects
- Initial dose 50 mg/day; increase gradually up to 100 mg/day

Children and Adolescents

- Use with caution, observing for activation of known or unknown bipolar disorder and/or suicidal ideation, and strongly consider informing parents or guardian of this risk so they can help observe child or adolescent patients
- Not generally recommended for use under age 12
- Several studies show lack of efficacy of TCAs for depression
- May be used to treat enuresis or hyperactive/impulsive behaviors
- Some cases of sudden death have occurred in children taking TCAs
- Adolescents: initial dose 50 mg/day; increase gradually up to 100 mg/day

Pregnancy

- Risk Category C [some animal studies show adverse effects, no controlled studies in humans]
- Crosses the placenta
- Adverse effects have been reported in infants whose mothers took a TCA (lethargy, withdrawal symptoms, fetal malformations)
- Must weigh the risk of treatment (first trimester fetal development, third trimester newborn delivery) to the child against the risk of no treatment (recurrence of depression, maternal health, infant bonding) to the mother and child
- For many patients this may mean continuing treatment during pregnancy

Breast Feeding

- Some drug is found in mother's breast milk
- ✳ Recommended either to discontinue drug or bottle feed

- Immediate postpartum period is a high-risk time for depression, especially in women who have had prior depressive episodes, so drug may need to be reinstituted late in the third trimester or shortly after childbirth to prevent a recurrence during the postpartum period
- Must weigh benefits of breast feeding with risks and benefits of antidepressant treatment versus non-treatment to both the infant and the mother
- For many patients this may mean continuing treatment during breast feeding

THE ART OF PSYCHOPHARMACOLOGY

Potential Advantages

- Patients with insomnia
- Severe or treatment-resistant depression
- Patients with a wide variety of chronic pain syndromes

Potential Disadvantages

- Pediatric and geriatric patients
- Patients concerned with weight gain
- Cardiac patients

Primary Target Symptoms

- Depressed mood
- Symptoms of anxiety
- Somatic symptoms
- Chronic pain
- Insomnia

Pearls

- Was once one of the most widely prescribed agents for depression
- Remains one of the most favored TCAs for treating headache and a wide variety of chronic pain syndromes, including neuropathic pain, fibromyalgia, migraine, neck pain, and low back pain
- ✳ Preference of some prescribers for amitriptyline over other tricyclic/tetracyclic antidepressants for the treatment of chronic pain syndromes is based more upon art and anecdote rather than controlled clinical trials, since many TCAs/tetracylics may be effective for chronic pain syndromes
- Tricyclic antidepressants are no longer generally considered a first-line treatment

option for depression because of their side effect profile

✳ Amitriptyline has been shown to be effective in primary insomnia

- TCAs may aggravate psychotic symptoms
- Alcohol should be avoided because of additive CNS effects
- Underweight patients may be more susceptible to adverse cardiovascular effects
- Children, patients with inadequate hydration, and patients with cardiac disease may be more susceptible to TCA-induced cardiotoxicity than healthy adults
- For the expert only: although generally prohibited, a heroic but potentially dangerous treatment for severely treatment-resistant patients is to give a tricyclic/tetracyclic antidepressant other than clomipramine simultaneously with an MAO inhibitor for patients who fail to respond to numerous other antidepressants
- If this option is elected, start the MAOI with the tricyclic/tetracyclic antidepressant simultaneously at low doses after appropriate drug washout, then alternately increase doses of these agents every few days to a week as tolerated
- Although very strict dietary and concomitant drug restrictions must be observed to prevent hypertensive crises and serotonin syndrome, the most common side effects of MAOI/tricyclic or tetracyclic combinations may be weight gain and orthostatic hypotension
- Patients on TCAs should be aware that they may experience symptoms such as photosensitivity or blue-green urine
- SSRIs may be more effective than TCAs in women, and TCAs may be more effective than SSRIs in men
- Since tricyclic/tetracyclic antidepressants are substrates for CYP450 2D6, and 7% of the population (especially Caucasians) may have a genetic variant leading to reduced activity of 2D6, such patients may not safely tolerate normal doses of tricyclic/tetracyclic antidepressants and may require dose reduction
- Phenotypic testing may be necessary to detect this genetic variant prior to dosing with a tricyclic/tetracyclic antidepressant, especially in vulnerable populations such as children, elderly, cardiac populations, and those on concomitant medications
- Patients who seem to have extraordinarily severe side effects at normal or low doses may have this phenotypic CYP450 2D6 variant and require low doses or switching to another antidepressant not metabolized by 2D6

Suggested Reading

Anderson IM. Meta-analytical studies on new antidepressants. Br Med Bull 2001; 57:161–178.

Anderson IM. Selective serotonin reuptake inhibitors versus tricyclic antidepressants: a meta-analysis of efficacy and tolerability. J Aff Disorders 2000;58:19–36.

Barbui C, Hotopf M. Amitriptyline v. the rest: still the leading antidepressant after 40 years of randomised controlled trials. Br J Psychiatry 2001;178:129–144.

Bryson HM, Wilde MI. Amitriptyline. A review of its pharmacological properties and therapeutic use in chronic pain states. Drugs Aging 1996;8:459–76.

AMOXAPINE

THERAPEUTICS

Brands • Asendin
see index for additional brand names

Generic? Yes

Class

- Tricyclic antidepressant (TCA), sometimes classified as a tetracyclic antidepressant
- Norepinephrine/noradrenaline reuptake inhibitor
- Serotonin 2A antagonist
- Parent drug and especially an active metabolite are dopamine 2 antagonists

Commonly Prescribed For
(bold for FDA approved)
- **Neurotic or reactive depressive disorder**
- **Endogenous and psychotic depressions**
- **Depression accompanied by anxiety or agitation**
- Depressive phase of bipolar disorder
- Anxiety
- Insomnia
- Neuropathic pain/chronic pain
- Treatment-resistant depression

How The Drug Works
- Boosts neurotransmitter norepinephrine/noradrenaline
- Blocks norepinephrine reuptake pump (norepinephrine transporter), presumably increasing noradrenergic neurotransmission
- Since dopamine is inactivated by norepinephrine reuptake in frontal cortex, which largely lacks dopamine transporters, amoxapine can thus increase dopamine neurotransmission in this part of the brain
- A more potent inhibitor of norepinephrine reuptake pump than serotonin reuptake pump (serotonin transporter)
- At high doses may also boost neurotransmitter serotonin and presumably increase serotonergic neurotransmission
- Blocks dopamine 2 receptors, reducing positive symptoms of psychosis

How Long Until It Works
- Onset of therapeutic actions usually not immediate, but often delayed 2 to 4 weeks

- If it is not working within 6 to 8 weeks for depression, it may require a dosage increase or it may not work at all
- May continue to work for many years to prevent relapse of symptoms

If It Works
- The goal of treatment is complete remission of current symptoms as well as prevention of future relapses
- Treatment most often reduces or even eliminates symptoms, but not a cure since symptoms can recur after medicine stopped
- Continue treatment until all symptoms are gone (remission)
- Once symptoms gone, continue treating for 1 year for the first episode of depression
- For second and subsequent episodes of depression, treatment may need to be indefinite
- Use in anxiety disorders may also need to be indefinite

If It Doesn't Work
- Many patients only have a partial response where some symptoms are improved but others persist (especially insomnia, fatigue, and problems concentrating)
- Other patients may be nonresponders, sometimes called treatment-resistant or treatment-refractory
- Consider increasing dose, switching to another agent or adding an appropriate augmenting agent
- Consider psychotherapy
- Consider evaluation for another diagnosis or for a comorbid condition (e.g., medical illness, substance abuse, etc.)
- Some patients may experience apparent lack of consistent efficacy due to activation of latent or underlying bipolar disorder, and require antidepressant discontinuation and a switch to a mood stabilizer

Best Augmenting Combos for Partial Response or Treatment-Resistance
- Lithium, buspirone, thyroid hormone

Tests
- None for healthy individuals
- ✱ Since tricyclic and tetracyclic antidepressants are frequently associated with weight gain, before starting treatment,

weigh all patients and determine if the patient is already overweight (BMI 25.0–29.9) or obese (BMI ≥30)

- Before giving a drug that can cause weight gain to an overweight or obese patient, consider determining whether the patient already has pre-diabetes (fasting plasma glucose 100–125 mg/dl), diabetes (fasting plasma glucose >126 mg/dl), or dyslipidemia (increased total cholesterol, LDL cholesterol and triglycerides; decreased HDL cholesterol), and treat or refer such patients for treatment, including nutrition and weight management, physical activity counseling, smoking cessation, and medical management

✳ Monitor weight and BMI during treatment

✳ While giving a drug to a patient who has gained >5% of initial weight, consider evaluating for the presence of pre-diabetes, diabetes, or dyslipidemia, or consider switching to a different antidepressant

- EKGs may be useful for selected patients (e.g., those with personal or family history of QTc prolongation; cardiac arrhythmia; recent myocardial infarction; uncompensated heart failure; or taking agents that prolong QTc interval such as pimozide, thioridazine, selected antiarrhythmics, moxifloxacin, sparfloxacin, etc.)

- Patients at risk for electrolyte disturbances (e.g., patients on diuretic therapy) should have baseline and periodic serum potassium and magnesium measurements

SIDE EFFECTS

How Drug Causes Side Effects

- Anticholinergic activity may explain sedative effects, dry mouth, constipation, and blurred vision
- Sedative effects and weight gain may be due to antihistamine properties
- Blockade of alpha adrenergic 1 receptors may explain dizziness, sedation, and hypotension
- Cardiac arrhythmias and seizures, especially in overdose, may be caused by blockade of ion channels

Notable Side Effects

- Blurred vision, constipation, urinary retention, increased appetite, dry mouth, nausea, diarrhea, heartburn, unusual taste in mouth, weight gain
- Fatigue, weakness, dizziness, sedation, headache, anxiety, nervousness, restlessness
- Sexual dysfunction, sweating

✳ Can cause extrapyramidal symptoms, akathisia, and theoretically, tardive dyskinesia

 Life Threatening or Dangerous Side Effects

- Paralytic ileus, hyperthermia (TCAs/tetracyclics + anticholinergic agents)
- Lowered seizure threshold and rare seizures
- Orthostatic hypotension, sudden death, arrhythmias, tachycardia
- QTc prolongation
- Hepatic failure, extrapyramidal symptoms
- Increased intraocular pressure
- Rare induction of mania and activation of suicidal ideation

Weight Gain

unusual   not unusual   common   problematic

- Many experience and/or can be significant in amount
- Can increase appetite and carbohydrate craving

Sedation

unusual   not unusual   common   problematic

- Many experience and/or can be significant in amount
- Tolerance to sedative effect may develop with long-term use

What To Do About Side Effects

- Wait
- Wait
- Wait
- Lower the dose
- Switch to an SSRI or newer antidepressant

Best Augmenting Agents for Side Effects

- Many side effects cannot be improved with an augmenting agent
- May use anticholinergics for extrapyramidal symptoms, or switch to another antidepressant

DOSING AND USE

Usual Dosage Range
- 200–300 mg/day

Dosage Forms
- Tablets 25 mg, 50 mg, 100 mg, 150 mg

How to Dose
- Initial 25 mg 2–3 times/day; increase gradually to 100 mg 2–3 times/day or a single dose at bedtime; maximum 400 mg/day (may dose up to 600 mg/day in inpatients)

 Dosing Tips

- If given in a single dose, should generally be administered at bedtime because of its sedative properties
- If given in split doses, largest dose should generally be given at bedtime because of its sedative properties
- If patients experience nightmares, split dose and do not give large dose at bedtime
- If intolerable anxiety, insomnia, agitation, akathisia, or activation occur either upon dosing initiation or discontinuation, consider the possibility of activated bipolar disorder, and switch to a mood stabilizer or an atypical antipsychotic

Overdose
- Death may occur; convulsions, cardiac dysrhythmias, severe hypotension, CNS depression, coma, changes in ECG

Long-Term Use
- Generally safe
- Some patients may develop withdrawal dyskinesias when discontinuing amoxapine after long-term use

Habit Forming
- Some patients may develop tolerance

How to Stop
- Taper to avoid withdrawal effects
- Even with gradual dose reduction some withdrawal symptoms may appear within the first 2 weeks
- Many patients tolerate 50% dose reduction for 3 days, then another 50% reduction for 3 days, then discontinuation
- If withdrawal symptoms emerge during discontinuation, raise dose to stop symptoms and then restart withdrawal much more slowly

Pharmacokinetics
- Substrate for CYP450 2D6
- Half-life of parent drug approximately 8 hours
- ✳ 7- and 8-hydroxymetabolites are active and possess serotonin 2A and dopamine 2 antagonist properties, similar to atypical antipsychotics
- ✳ Amoxapine is the N-desmethyl metabolite of the conventional antipsychotic loxapine
- Half-life of the active metabolites approximately 24 hours

 Drug Interactions

- Tramadol increases the risk of seizures in patients taking TCAs
- Use of TCAs/tetracyclics with anticholinergic drugs may result in paralytic ileus or hyperthermia
- Fluoxetine, paroxetine, bupropion, duloxetine, and other CYP450 2D6 inhibitors may increase TCA/tetracyclic concentrations
- Cimetidine may increase plasma concentrations of TCAs/tetracyclics and cause anticholinergic symptoms
- Phenothiazines or haloperidol may raise TCA/tetracyclic blood concentrations
- May alter effects of antihypertensive drugs; may inhibit hypotensive effects of clonidine
- Use of TCAs/tetracyclics with sympathomimetic agents may increase sympathetic activity
- Methylphenidate may inhibit metabolism of TCAs/tetracyclics
- Activation and agitation, especially following switching or adding antidepressants, may represent the induction of a bipolar state, especially a mixed dysphoric bipolar II condition

sometimes associated with suicidal ideation, and require the addition of lithium, a mood stabilizer or an atypical antipsychotic, and/or discontinuation of amoxapine

Other Warnings/ Precautions

- Add or initiate other antidepressants with caution for up to 2 weeks after discontinuing amoxapine
- Generally, do not use with MAO inhibitors, including 14 days after MAOIs are stopped; do not start an MAOI until 2 weeks after discontinuing amoxapine, but see Pearls
- Use with caution in patients with history of seizure, urinary retention, narrow angle-closure glaucoma, hyperthyroidism
- TCAs/tetracyclics can increase QTc interval, especially at toxic doses, which can be attained not only by overdose but also by combining with drugs that inhibit its metabolism via CYP450 2D6, potentially causing torsade de pointes-type arrhythmia or sudden death
- Because TCAs/tetracyclics can prolong QTc interval, use with caution in patients who have bradycardia or who are taking drugs that can induce bradycardia (e.g., beta blockers, calcium channel blockers, clonidine, digitalis)
- Because TCAs/tetracyclics can prolong QTc interval, use with caution in patients who have hypokalemia and/or hypomagnesemia, or who are taking drugs that can induce hypokalemia and/or magnesemia (e.g., diuretics, stimulant laxatives, intravenous amphotericin B, glucocorticoids, tetracosactide)

Do Not Use

- If patient is recovering from myocardial infarction
- If patient is taking agents capable of significantly prolonging QTc interval (e.g., pimozide, thioridazine, selected antiarrhythmics, moxifloxacin, sparfloxacin)
- If there is a history of QTc prolongation or cardiac arrhythmia, recent acute myocardial infarction, uncompensated heart failure

- If patient is taking drugs that inhibit TCA/tetracyclic metabolism, including CYP450 2D6 inhibitors, except by an expert
- If there is reduced CYP450 2D6 function, such as patients who are poor 2D6 metabolizers, except by an expert and at low doses
- If there is a proven allergy to amoxapine or loxapine

SPECIAL POPULATIONS

Renal Impairment

- Use with caution – may require lower than usual adult dose

Hepatic Impairment

- Use with caution – may require lower than usual adult dose

Cardiac Impairment

- TCAs/tetracyclics have been reported to cause arrhythmias, prolongation of conduction time, orthostatic hypotension, sinus tachycardia, and heart failure, especially in the diseased heart
- Myocardial infarction and stroke have been reported with TCAs/tetracyclics
- TCAs/tetracyclics produce QTc prolongation, which may be enhanced by the existence of bradycardia, hypokalemia, congenital or acquired long QTc interval, which should be evaluated prior to administering amoxapine
- Use with caution if treating concomitantly with a medication likely to produce prolonged bradycardia, hypokalemia, slowing of intracardiac conduction, or prolongation of the QTc interval
- Avoid TCAs/tetracyclics in patients with a known history of QTc prolongation, recent acute myocardial infarction, and uncompensated heart failure
- TCAs/tetracyclics may cause a sustained increase in heart rate in patients with ischemic heart disease and may worsen (decrease) heart rate variability, an independent risk of mortality in cardiac populations
- Since SSRIs may improve (increase) heart rate variability in patients following a myocardial infarct and may improve survival as well as mood in patients with acute angina or following a myocardial

infarction, these are more appropriate agents for cardiac population than tricyclic/tetracyclic antidepressants
✳ Risk/benefit ratio may not justify use of TCAs/tetracyclics in cardiac impairment

Elderly
• May be more sensitive to anticholinergic, cardiovascular, hypotensive, and sedative effects
• Initial dose 25 mg/day at bedtime; increase by 25 mg/day each week; maximum dose 300 mg/day

 Children and Adolescents
• Use with caution, observing for activation of known or unknown bipolar disorder and/or suicidal ideation, and strongly consider informing parents or guardian of this risk so they can help observe child or adolescent patients
• Not generally recommended for use under age 16
• Several studies show lack of efficacy of TCAs/tetracyclics for depression
• May be used to treat enuresis or hyperactive/impulsive behaviors
• Some cases of sudden death have occurred in children taking TCAs/tetracyclics
• Adolescents: initial 25–50 mg/day; increase gradually to 100 mg/day in divided doses or single dose at bedtime

Pregnancy
• Risk Category C [some animal studies show adverse effects, no controlled studies in humans]
• Amoxapine crosses the placenta
• Adverse effects have been reported in infants whose mothers took a TCA (lethargy, withdrawal symptoms, fetal malformations)
• Evaluate for treatment with an antidepressant with a better risk/benefit ratio

Breast Feeding
• Some drug is found in mother's breast milk
✳ Recommended either to discontinue drug or bottle feed

• Immediate postpartum period is a high-risk time for depression, especially in women who have had prior depressive episodes, so drug may need to be reinstituted late in the third trimester or shortly after childbirth to prevent a recurrence during the postpartum period
• Evaluate for treatment with an antidepressant with a better risk/benefit ratio

THE ART OF PSYCHOPHARMACOLOGY

Potential Advantages
• Severe or treatment-resistant depression
• Treatment-resistant psychotic depression

Potential Disadvantages
• Pediatric and geriatric patients
• Patients concerned with weight gain
• Cardiac patients
• Patients with Parkinson's disease or tardive dyskinesia

Primary Target Symptoms
• Depressed mood

 Pearls
• Tricyclic/tetracyclic antidepressants are no longer generally considered a first-line treatment option for depression because of their side effect profile
• Tricyclic/tetracyclic antidepressants continue to be useful for severe or treatment-resistant depression
✳ Because of potential extrapyramidal symptoms, akathisia, and theoretical risk of tardive dyskinesia, first consider other TCAs/tetracyclics for long-term use in general and for treatment of chronic patients
• TCAs may aggravate psychotic symptoms
• Alcohol should be avoided because of additive CNS effects
• Underweight patients may be more susceptible to adverse cardiovascular effects
• Children, patients with inadequate hydration, and patients with cardiac disease may be more susceptible to TCA-induced cardiotoxicity than healthy adults

- For the expert only: although generally prohibited, a heroic but potentially dangerous treatment for severely treatment-resistant patients is to give a tricyclic/tetracyclic antidepressant other than clomipramine simultaneously with an MAO inhibitor for patients who fail to respond to numerous other antidepressants
- Use of MAOIs with clomipramine is always prohibited because of the risk of serotonin syndrome and death
- Amoxapine may be the preferred trycyclic/tetracyclic antidepressant to combine with an MAOI in heroic cases due to its theoretically protective 5HT2A antagonist properties
- If this option is elected, start the MAOI with the tricyclic/tetracyclic antidepressant simultaneously at low doses after appropriate drug washout, then alternately increase doses of these agents every few days to a week as tolerated
- Although very strict dietary and concomitant drug restrictions must be observed to prevent hypertensive crises and serotonin syndrome, the most common side effects of MAOI/tricyclic or tetracyclic combinations may be weight gain and orthostatic hypotention
- Patients on TCAs/tetracyclics should be aware that they may experience symptoms such as photosensitivity or blue-green urine
- SSRIs may be more effective than TCAs/tetracyclics in women, and TCAs/tetracyclics may be more effective than SSRIs in men
* May cause some motor effects, possibly due to effects on dopamine receptors
* Amoxapine may have a faster onset of action than some other antidepressants
* May be pharmacologically similar to an atypical antipsychotic in some patients
* At high doses, patients who form high concentrations of active metabolites may have akathisia, extrapyramidal symptoms, and possibly develop tardive dyskinesia
* Structurally and pharmacologically related to the antipsychotic loxapine
- Since tricyclic/tetracyclic antidepressants are substrates for CYP450 2D6, and 7% of the population (especially Caucasians) may have a genetic variant leading to reduced activity of 2D6, such patients may not safely tolerate normal doses of tricyclic/tetracyclic antidepressants and may require dose reduction
- Phenotypic testing may be necessary to detect this genetic variant prior to dosing with a tricyclic/tetracyclic antidepressant, especially in vulnerable populations such as children, elderly, cardiac populations, and those on concomitant medications
- Patients who seem to have extraordinarily severe side effects at normal or low doses may have this phenotypic CYP450 2D6 variant and require low doses or switching to another antidepressant not metabolized by 2D6

Suggested Reading

Anderson IM. Meta-analytical studies on new antidepressants. Br Med Bull 2001; 57:161–178.

Anderson IM. Selective serotonin reuptake inhibitors versus tricyclic antidepressants: a meta-analysis of efficacy and tolerability. J Aff Disorders 2000;58:19–36.

Hayes PE, Kristoff CA. Adverse reactions to five new antidepressants. Clin Pharm 1986; 5:471–80.

Jue SG, Dawson GW, Brogden RN. Amoxapine: a review of its pharmacology and efficacy in depressed states. Drugs 1982; 24:1–23.

ARIPIPRAZOLE

THERAPEUTICS

Brands • Abilify
see index for additional brand names

Generic? Not in U.S., Europe, or Japan

Class
- Dopamine partial agonist (dopamine stabilizer, atypical antipsychotic, third generation antipsychotic; sometimes included as a second generation antipsychotic; also a mood stabilizer)

Commonly Prescribed For
(bold for FDA approved)
- **Schizophrenia**
- **Maintaining stability in schizophrenia**
- Other psychotic disorders
- Acute mania
- Bipolar maintenance
- Bipolar depression
- Behavioral disturbances in dementias
- Behavioral disturbances in children and adolescents
- Disorders associated with problems with impulse control

How The Drug Works
✳ Partial agonism at dopamine 2 receptors
- Theoretically reduces dopamine output when dopamine concentrations are high, thus improving positive symptoms and mediating antipsychotic actions
- Theoretically increases dopamine output when dopamine concentrations are low, thus improving cognitive, negative, and mood symptoms
- Actions at dopamine 3 receptors could theoretically contribute to aripiprazole's efficacy
- Partial agonism at 5HT1A receptors may be relevant at clinical doses
- Blockade of serotonin type 2A receptors may contribute at clinical doses to cause enhancement of dopamine release in certain brain regions, thus reducing motor side effects and possibly improving cognitive and affective symptoms

How Long Until It Works
- Psychotic symptoms can improve within 1 week, but it may take several weeks for full effect on behavior as well as on cognition and affective stabilization
- Classically recommended to wait at least 4–6 weeks to determine efficacy of drug, but in practice some patients require up to 16–20 weeks to show a good response, especially on cognitive symptoms

If It Works
- Most often reduces positive symptoms in schizophrenia but does not eliminate them
- Can improve negative symptoms, as well as aggressive, cognitive, and affective symptoms in schizophrenia
- Most schizophrenic patients do not have a total remission of symptoms but rather a reduction of symptoms by about a third
- Perhaps 5–15% of schizophrenic patients can experience an overall improvement of greater than 50–60%, especially when receiving stable treatment for more than a year
- Such patients are considered super-responders or "awakeners" since they may be well enough to be employed, live independently, and sustain long-term relationships
- Many bipolar patients may experience a reduction of symptoms by half or more
- Continue treatment until reaching a plateau of improvement
- After reaching a satisfactory plateau, continue treatment for at least a year after first episode of psychosis
- For second and subsequent episodes of psychosis, treatment may need to be indefinite
- Even for first episodes of psychosis, it may be preferable to continue treatment indefinitely to avoid subsequent episodes
- Treatment may not only reduce mania but also prevent recurrences of mania in bipolar disorder

If It Doesn't Work
- Try one of the other atypical antipsychotics (risperidone, olanzapine, quetiapine, ziprasidone, amisulpride)
- If two or more antipsychotic monotherapies do not work, consider clozapine
- If no first-line atypical antipsychotic is effective, consider higher doses or augmentation with valproate or lamotrigine

- Some patients may require treatment with a conventional antipsychotic
- Consider noncompliance and switch to another antipsychotic with fewer side effects or to an antipsychotic that can be given by depot injection
- Consider initiating rehabilitation and psychotherapy
- Consider presence of concomitant drug abuse

 Best Augmenting Combos for Partial Response or Treatment-Resistance

- Valproic acid (valproate, divalproex, divalproex ER)
- Other mood stabilizing anticonvulsants (carbamazepine, oxcarbazepine, lamotrigine)
- Lithium
- Benzodiazepines

Tests

Before starting an atypical antipsychotic

✳ Weigh all patients and track BMI during treatment
- Get baseline personal and family history of obesity, dyslipidemia, hypertension, and cardiovascular disease
✳ Get waist circumference (at umbilicus), blood pressure, fasting plasma glucose, and fasting lipid profile
- Determine if the patient is
  - overweight (BMI 25.0–29.9)
  - obese (BMI ≥30)
  - has pre-diabetes (fasting plasma glucose 100–125 mg/dl)
  - has diabetes (fasting plasma glucose >126 mg/dl)
  - has hypertension (BP >140/90 mm Hg)
  - has dyslipidemia (increased total cholesterol, LDL cholesterol, and triglycerides; decreased HDL cholesterol)
- Treat or refer such patients for treatment, including nutrition and weight management, physical activity counseling, smoking cessation, and medical management

Monitoring after starting an atypical antipsychotic

✳ BMI monthly for 3 months, then quarterly
✳ Blood pressure, fasting plasma glucose, fasting lipids within 3 months and then annually, but earlier and more frequently

for patients with diabetes or who have gained >5% of initial weight
- Treat or refer for treatment and consider switching to another atypical antipsychotic for patients who become overweight, obese, pre-diabetic, diabetic, hypertensive, or dyslipidemic while receiving an atypical antipsychotic
✳ Even in patients without known diabetes, be vigilant for the rare but life threatening onset of diabetic ketoacidosis, which always requires immediate treatment, by monitoring for the rapid onset of polyuria, polydipsia, weight loss, nausea, vomiting, dehydration, rapid respiration, weakness and clouding of sensorium, even coma

SIDE EFFECTS

How Drug Causes Side Effects

- By blocking alpha 1 adrenergic receptors, it can cause dizziness, sedation, and hypotension
- Partial agonist actions at dopamine 2 receptors in the striatum can cause motor side effects, such as akathisia (occasionally)
- Partial agonist actions at dopamine 2 receptors can also cause nausea, occasional vomiting, and activating side effects
✳ Mechanism of any possible weight gain is unknown; weight gain is not common with aripiprazole and may thus have a different mechanism from atypical antipsychotics for which weight gain is common or problematic
✳ Mechanism of any possible increased incidence of diabetes or dyslipidemia is unknown; early experience suggests these complications are not clearly associated with aripiprazole and if present may therefore have a different mechanism from that of atypical antipsychotics associated with an increased incidence of diabetes and dyslipidemia

Notable Side Effects

✳ Dizziness, insomnia, akathisia, activation
✳ Nausea, vomiting
- Orthostatic hypotension, occasionally during initial dosing
- Constipation

- Headache, asthenia, sedation
- Theoretical risk of tardive dyskinesia

 Life Threatening or Dangerous Side Effects
- Rare neuroleptic malignant syndrome (much reduced risk compared to conventional antipsychotics)
- Rare seizures

Weight Gain

unusual   not unusual   common   problematic

- Reported in a few patients, especially those with low BMIs, but not expected
- Less frequent and less severe than for most other antipsychotics

Sedation

unusual   not unusual   common   problematic

- Reported in a few patients but not expected
- May be less than for some other antipsychotics, but never say never
- Can be activating at moderate to high doses

What To Do About Side Effects
- Wait
- Wait
- Wait
- Reduce the dose
- Anticholinergics may reduce akathisia when present
- Weight loss, exercise programs, and medical management for high BMIs, diabetes, dyslipidemia
- Switch to another atypical antipsychotic

Best Augmenting Agents for Side Effects
- Benztropine or trihexyphenidyl for motor side effects and akathisia
- Many side effects cannot be improved with an augmenting agent

DOSING AND USE

Usual Dosage Range
- 15–30 mg/day

Dosage Forms
- Tablet 5 mg, 10 mg, 15 mg, 20 mg, 30 mg

How to Dose
- Initial approved recommendation is 15 mg/day; maximum approved dose 30 mg/day

 Dosing Tips
- ✳ **For some, less may be more:** frequently, patients not acutely psychotic may need to be dosed lower (e.g., 5–10 mg/day) in order to avoid akathisia and activation and for maximum tolerability
- **For others, more may be more:** rarely, patients may need to be dosed higher than 30 mg/day for optimum efficacy
- Consider cutting 5 mg tablet in half (tablets not scored) for children and adolescents, as well as for adults very sensitive to side effects
- ✳ Although studies suggest patients switching to aripiprazole from another antipsychotic can do well with rapid switch or with cross-titration, clinical experience suggests many patients may do best by adding a full dose of aripiprazole to the maintenance dose of the first antipsychotic for several days prior to slow down-titration of the first antipsychotic
- Rather than raise the dose above these levels in acutely agitated patients requiring acute antipsychotic actions, consider augmentation with a benzodiazepine or conventional antipsychotic, either orally or intramuscularly
- Rather than raise the dose above these levels in partial responders, consider augmentation with a mood stabilizing anticonvulsant, such as valproate or lamotrigine
- Children and elderly should generally be dosed at the lower end of the dosage spectrum
- Less expensive than some antipsychotics, more expensive than others depending on dose administered
- Due to its very long half-life, aripiprazole will take longer to reach steady state when

initiating dosing, and longer to wash out when stopping dosing, than other atypical antipsychotics

Overdose
- No fatalities have been reported; sedation, vomiting

Long-Term Use
- Approved to delay relapse in long-term treatment of schizophrenia
- Often used for long-term maintenance in bipolar disorder and various behavioral disorders

Habit Forming
- No

How to Stop
- Slow down-titration (over 6 to 8 weeks), especially when simultaneously beginning a new antipsychotic while switching (i.e., cross-titration)
- Rapid discontinuation could theoretically lead to rebound psychosis and worsening of symptoms

Pharmacokinetics
- Metabolized primarily by CYP450 2D6 and CYP450 3A4
- Mean elimination half-life 75 hours (aripiprazole) and 94 hours (major metabolite dehydro-aripiprazole)

 Drug Interactions
- Ketaconazole and possibly other CYP450 3A4 inhibitors such as nefazodone, fluvoxamine, and fluoxetine may increase plasma levels of aripiprazole
- Carbamazepine and possibly other inducers of CYP450 3A4 may decrease plasma levels of aripiprazole
- Quinidine and possibly other inhibitors of CYP450 2D6 such as paroxetine, fluoxetine, and duloxetine may increase plasma levels of aripiprazole
- Aripiprazole may enhance the effects of antihypertensive drugs
- Aripiprazole may antagonize levodopa, dopamine agonists

 Other Warnings/ Precautions
- Use with caution in patients with conditions that predispose to hypotension (dehydration, overheating)
- Dysphagia has been associated with antipsychotic use, and aripiprazole should be used cautiously in patients at risk for aspiration pneumonia

Do Not Use
- If there is a proven allergy to aripiprazole

Renal Impairment
- Dose adjustment not necessary

Hepatic Impairment
- Dose adjustment not necessary

Cardiac Impairment
- Use in patients with cardiac impairment has not been studied, so use with caution because of risk of orthostatic hypotension

Elderly
- Dose adjustment generally not necessary, but some elderly patients may tolerate lower doses better

 Children and Adolescents
- Not officially recommended for patients under age 18
- Clinical experience and early data suggest aripiprazole may be safe and effective for behavioral disturbances in children and adolescents, especially at lower doses
- Children and adolescents using aripiprazole may need to be monitored more often than adults and may tolerate lower doses better

 Pregnancy
- Risk Category C [some animal studies show adverse effects, no controlled studies in humans]
- Psychotic symptoms may worsen during pregnancy and some form of treatment may be necessary

- Aripiprazole may be preferable to anticonvulsant mood stabilizers if treatment is required during pregnancy

Breast Feeding
- Unknown if aripiprazole is secreted in human breast milk, but all psychotropics assumed to be secreted in breast milk
- ✳ Recommended either to discontinue drug or bottle feed
- Infants of women who choose to breast feed while on aripiprazole should be monitored for possible adverse effects

THE ART OF PSYCHOPHARMACOLOGY

Potential Advantages
- Some cases of psychosis and bipolar disorder refractory to treatment with other antipsychotics
- ✳ Patients concerned about gaining weight
- ✳ Patients with diabetes
- Patients requiring rapid onset of antipsychotic action without dosage titration

Potential Disadvantages
- Patients in whom sedation is desired
- May be more difficult to dose for children, elderly, or "off label" uses

Primary Target Symptoms
- Positive symptoms of psychosis
- Negative symptoms of psychosis
- Cognitive symptoms
- Unstable mood
- Aggressive symptoms

 Pearls

- ✳ Well accepted in clinical practice when wanting to avoid weight gain because less weight gain than most other antipsychotics
- ✳ Well accepted in clinical practice when wanting to avoid sedation because less sedation than most other antipsychotics at all doses
- ✳ Can even be activating, which can be reduced by lowering the dose or starting at a lower dose
- A moderately priced atypical antipsychotic within the therapeutic dosing range
- ✳ May not have diabetes or dyslipidemia risk, but monitoring is still indicated
- Anecdotal reports of utility in treatment-resistant cases
- Has a very favorable tolerability profile in clinical practice
- Favorable tolerability profile leading to "off-label" uses for many indications other than schizophrenia (e.g., acute bipolar mania; bipolar II disorder, including hypomanic, mixed, rapid cycling, and depressed phases; treatment-resistant depression; anxiety disorders)

 Suggested Reading

Marder SR, McQuade RD, Stock E, Kaplita S, Marcus R, Safferman AZ, Saha A, Ali M, Iwamoto T. Aripiprazole in the treatment of schizophrenia: safety and tolerability in short-term, placebo-controlled trials. Schizophr Res 2003;61(2–3):123–36.

Sajatovic M. Treatment for mood and anxiety disorders: quetiapine and aripiprazole. Curr Psychiatry Rep 2003;5:320–6.

Shapiro DA, Renock S, Arrington E, Chiodo LA, Liu LX, Sibley DR, Roth BL, Mailman R. Aripiprazole, a novel atypical antipsychotic drug with a unique and robust pharmacology. Neuropsychopharmacology 2003;28:1400–11.

Stahl SM. Dopamine system stabilizers, aripiprazole, and the next generation of antipsychotics, part 1: "Goldilocks" actions at dopamine receptors. J Clin Psychiatry 2001;62:841–2.

Stahl SM. Dopamine system stabilizers, aripiprazole, and the next generation of antipsychotics, part 2: illustrating their mechanism of action. J Clin Psychiatry 2001;62 (12):923–4.

ATOMOXETINE

THERAPEUTICS

Brands • Strattera
see index for additional brand names

Generic? No

 Class
• Selective norepinephrine reuptake inhibitor (NRI)

Commonly Prescribed For
(bold for FDA approved)
• **Attention deficit hyperactivity disorder (ADHD) in adults and children over 6**
• Treatment-resistant depression

 How The Drug Works
• Boosts neurotransmitters norepinephrine/noradrenaline and dopamine
• Blocks norepinephrine reuptake pumps, also known as norepinephrine transporters
• Presumably this increases noradrenergic neurotransmission
• Since dopamine is inactivated by norepinephrine reuptake in frontal cortex, which largely lacks dopamine transporters, atomoxetine can also increase dopamine neurotransmission in this part of the brain

How Long Until It Works
✳ Onset of therapeutic actions in ADHD can be seen as early as the first day of dosing
• Therapeutic actions may continue to improve for 4 to 8 weeks
• If it is not working within 6 to 8 weeks, it may not work at all

If It Works
• The goal of treatment of ADHD is reduction of symptoms of inattentiveness, motor hyperactivity, and/or impulsiveness that disrupt social, school, and/or occupational functioning
• Continue treatment until all symptoms are under control or improvement is stable and then continue treatment indefinitely as long as improvement persists
• Reevaluate the need for treatment periodically
• Treatment for ADHD begun in childhood may need to be continued into adolescence

and adulthood if continued benefit is documented

If It Doesn't Work
• Consider adjusting dose or switching to another agent
• Consider behavioral therapy
• Consider the presence of noncompliance and counsel patient and parents
• Consider evaluation for another diagnosis or for a comorbid condition (e.g., bipolar disorder, substance abuse, medical illness, etc.)
• Some patients may experience apparent lack of consistent efficacy due to activation of latent or underlying bipolar disorder, and require atomoxetine discontinuation and a switch to a mood stabilizer

 Best Augmenting Combos for Partial Response or Treatment-Resistance
✳ Best to attempt other monotherapies prior to augmenting
• SSRIs, SNRIs, or mirtazapine for treatment-resistant depression (use combinations of antidepressants with atomoxetine with caution as this may theoretically activate bipolar disorder and suicidal ideation)
• Mood stabilizers or atypical antipsychotics for comorbid bipolar disorder
• For the expert, can combine with modafinil, methylphenidate, or amphetamine for ADHD

Tests
• None recommended for healthy patients
• May be prudent to monitor blood pressure and pulse when initiating treatment and until dosage increments have stabilized

SIDE EFFECTS

How Drug Causes Side Effects
• Norepinephrine increases in parts of the brain and body and at receptors other than those that cause therapeutic actions (e.g., unwanted actions of norepinephrine on acetylcholine release causing decreased appetite, increased heart rate and blood pressure, dry mouth, urinary retention, etc.)

- Most side effects are immediate but often go away with time
- Lack of enhancing dopamine activity in limbic areas theoretically explains atomoxetine's lack of abuse potential

Notable Side Effects

✳ Sedation, fatigue
✳ Decreased appetite
- Increased heart rate (6–9 beats/min)
- Increased blood pressure (2–4 mm Hg)
- Insomnia, dizziness, anxiety, agitation, aggression, irritability
- Dry mouth, constipation, nausea, vomiting, abdominal pain, dyspepsia
- Urinary hesitancy, urinary retention (older men)
- Dysmenorrhea, sweating
- Sexual dysfunction (men: decreased libido, erectile disturbance, impotence, ejaculatory dysfunction, abnormal orgasm; women: decreased libido, abnormal orgasm)

 Life Threatening or Dangerous Side Effects

- Increased heart rate and hypertension
- Orthostatic hypotension
- Hypomania and, theoretically, rare induction of mania and activation of suicidal ideation

Weight Gain

unusual   not unusual   common   problematic

- Reported but not expected
- Patients may experience weight loss

Sedation

unusual   not unusual   common   problematic

- Occurs in significant minority

What To Do About Side Effects

- Wait
- Wait
- Wait
- Lower the dose
- If giving once daily, can change to split dose twice daily
- In a few weeks, switch or add other drugs

Best Augmenting Agents for Side Effects

- For urinary hesitancy, give an alpha 1 blocker such as tamsulosin
- Often best to try another monotherapy prior to resorting to augmentation strategies to treat side effects
- Many side effects are dose-dependent (i.e., they increase as dose increases, or they reemerge until tolerance re-develops)
- Many side effects are time-dependent (i.e., they start immediately upon dosing and upon each dose increase, but go away with time)
- Activation and agitation may represent the induction of a bipolar state, especially a mixed dysphoric bipolar II condition sometimes associated with suicidal ideation, and require the addition of lithium, a mood stabilizer or an atypical antipsychotic, and/or discontinuation of atomoxetine

---

DOSING AND USE

Usual Dosage Range

- 90 mg/day, 1.2 mg/kg/day

Dosage Forms

- Capsule 10 mg, 18 mg, 25 mg, 40 mg, 60 mg

How to Dose

- For children 70 kg or less: initial dose 0.5 mg/kg/day; after 3 days can increase to 1.2 mg/kg/day either once in the morning or divided; maximum dose 1.4 mg/kg/day or 100 mg/day, whichever is less
- For adults and children over 70 kg: initial dose 40 mg/day; after 3 days can increase to 80 mg/day once in the morning or divided; after 2–4 weeks can increase to 100 mg/day if necessary; maximum daily dose 100 mg

 Dosing Tips

- Can be given once a day in the morning
✳ Efficacy with once-daily dosing despite a half-life of 5 hours suggests therapeutic effects persist beyond direct pharmacologic effects, unlike stimulants

whose effects are generally closely correlated with plasma drug levels
- Once-daily dosing may increase gastrointestinal side effects
- Starting dose is half of therapeutic dose
- Lower starting dose allows detection of those patients who may be especially sensitive to side effects such as tachycardia and increased blood pressure
- Patients especially sensitive to the side effects of atomoxetine may include those individuals deficient in the enzyme that metabolizes atomoxetine, CYP450 2D6 (i.e., 7% of the population, especially Caucasians)
- In such individuals, use half the usual dose of atomoxetine if tolerated
- Other individuals may require up to 1.8 mg/kg total daily dose

Overdose
- No fatalities have been reported; sedation, agitation, hyperactivity, abnormal behavior, gastrointestinal symptoms

Long-Term Use
- Safe

Habit Forming
- No

How to Stop
- Taper not necessary

Pharmacokinetics
- Metabolized by CYP450 2D6
- Half-life approximately 5 hours

 Drug Interactions
- Tramadol increases the risk of seizures in patients taking an antidepressant
- Plasma concentrations of atomoxetine may be increased by drugs that inhibit CYP450 2D6 (e.g., paroxetine, fluoxetine), so atomoxetine dose may need to be reduced if co-administered
- Co-administration of atomoxetine and albuterol may lead to increases in heart rate and blood pressure
- Co-administration with methylphenidate does not increase cardiovascular side effects beyond those seen with methylphenidate alone

- Do not use with MAO inhibitors, including 14 days after MAOIs are stopped

 Other Warnings/ Precautions
- Growth (height and weight) should be monitored during treatment with atomoxetine; for patients who are not growing or gaining weight satisfactorily, interruption of treatment should be considered
- Use with caution in patients with hypertension, tachycardia, cardiovascular disease, or cerebrovascular disease
- Use with caution in patients with bipolar disorder
- Use with caution in patients with urinary retention, benign prostatic hypertrophy
- Use with caution with antihypertensive drugs

Do Not Use
- If patient is taking an MAO inhibitor
- If patient has narrow angle-closure glaucoma
- If there is a proven allergy to atomoxetine

SPECIAL POPULATIONS

Renal Impairment
- Dose adjustment not generally necessary

Hepatic Impairment
- For patients with moderate liver impairment, dose should be reduced to 50% of normal dose
- For patients with severe liver impairment, dose should be reduced to 25% of normal dose

Cardiac Impairment
- Use with caution because atomoxetine can increase heart rate and blood pressure

Elderly
- Some patients may tolerate lower doses better

 Children and Adolescents
- Approved to treat ADHD in children over age 6
- Recommended dose is 1.2 mg/kg/day

Pregnancy

- Risk Category C [some animal studies show adverse effects, no controlled studies in humans]
- Use in women of childbearing potential requires weighing potential benefits to the mother against potential risks to the fetus
- ✱ For ADHD patients, atomoxetine should generally be discontinued before anticipated pregnancies

Breast Feeding

- Unknown if atomoxetine is secreted in human breast milk, but all psychotropics assumed to be secreted in breast milk
- ✱ Recommend either to discontinue drug or bottle feed

THE ART OF PSYCHOPHARMACOLOGY

Potential Advantages

- No known abuse potential

Potential Disadvantages

- May not act as rapidly as stimulants when initiating treatment in some patients

Primary Target Symptoms

- Concentration, attention span
- Motor hyperactivity
- Depressed mood

Pearls

- ✱ Unlike other agents approved for ADHD, atomoxetine does not have abuse potential and is not a scheduled substance
- ✱ Despite its name as a selective norepinephrine reuptake inhibitor, atomoxetine enhances both dopamine and norepinephrine in frontal cortex, presumably accounting for its therapeutic actions on attention and concentration
- Since dopamine is inactivated by norepinephrine reuptake in frontal cortex, which largely lacks dopamine transporters, atomoxetine can increase dopamine as well as norepinephrine in this part of the brain, presumably causing therapeutic actions in ADHD
- Since dopamine is inactivated by dopamine reuptake in nucleus accumbens, which largely lacks norepinephrine transporters, atomoxetine does not increase dopamine in this part of the brain, presumably explaining why atomoxetine lacks abuse potential
- Preliminary studies and atomoxetine's known mechanism of action as a selective norepinephrine reuptake inhibitor suggest its efficacy as an antidepressant
- Pro-noradrenergic actions may be theoretically useful for the treatment of chronic pain
- Atomoxetine's mechanism of action and its potential antidepressant actions suggest it has the potential to de-stabilize latent or undiagnosed bipolar disorder, similar to the known actions of proven antidepressants
- Thus, administer with caution to ADHD patients who may also have bipolar disorder
- Unlike stimulants, atomoxetine may not exacerbate tics in Tourette's Syndrome patients with comorbid ADHD
- Urinary retention in men over 50 with borderline urine flow has been observed with other agents with potent norepinephrine reuptake blocking properties (e.g., reboxetine, milnacipran), so administer atomoxetine with caution to these patients
- Atomoxetine was originally called tomoxetine but the name was changed to avoid potential confusion with tamoxifen, which might lead to errors in drug dispensing

Suggested Reading

Kratochvil CJ, Vaughan BS, Harrington MJ, Burke WJ. Atomoxetine: a selective noradrenaline reuptake inhibitor for the treatment of attention-deficit/hyperactivity disorder. Expert Opin Pharmacother 2003;4(7):1165–74.

Michelson D, Adler L, Spencer T, Reimherr FW, West SA, Allen AJ, Kelsey D, Wernicke J, Dietrich A, Milton D. Atomoxetine in adults with ADHD: two randomized, placebo-controlled studies. Biol Psychiatry 2003;53(2):112–20.

Simpson D, Perry CM. Atomoxetine. Paediatr Drugs 2003;5(6):407–15.

Wernicke JF, Kratochvil CJ. Safety profile of atomoxetine in the treatment of children and adolescents with ADHD. J Clin Psychiatry 2002;63 Suppl 12:50–5.

BUPROPION

THERAPEUTICS

Brands • Wellbutrin, Wellbutrin SR, Wellbutrin XL
• Zyban
see index for additional brand names

Generic? Yes (bupropion and bupropion SR)

Class
• NDRI (norepinephrine dopamine reuptake inhibitor); antidepressant; smoking cessation treatment

Commonly Prescribed For
(bold for FDA approved)
• **Major depressive disorder (bupropion, bupropion SR, and bupropion XL)**
• **Nicotine addiction (bupropion SR)**
• Bipolar depression
• Attention deficit / hyperactivity disorder
• Sexual dysfunction

How The Drug Works
• Boosts neurotransmitters norepinephrine/noradrenaline and dopamine
• Blocks norepinephrine reuptake pump (norepinephrine transporter), presumably increasing norepinephrine neurotransmission
• Since dopamine is inactivated by norepinephrine reuptake in frontal cortex, which largely lacks dopamine transporters, bupropion can increase dopamine neurotransmission in this part of the brain
• Blocks dopamine reuptake pump (dopamine transporter), presumably increasing dopaminergic neurotransmission

How Long Until It Works
• Onset of therapeutic actions usually not immediate, but often delayed 2 to 4 weeks
• If it is not working within 6 to 8 weeks for depression, it may require a dosage increase or it may not work at all
• May continue to work for many years to prevent relapse of symptoms

If It Works
• The goal of treatment of depression is complete remission of current symptoms as well as prevention of future relapses
• Treatment of depression most often reduces or even eliminates symptoms, but is not a cure since symptoms can recur after medicine stopped
• Continue treatment of depression until all symptoms are gone (remission)
• Once symptoms of depression are gone, continue treating for 1 year for the first episode of depression
• For second and subsequent episodes of depression, treatment may need to be indefinite
• Treatment for nicotine addiction should consist of a single treatment for 6 weeks

If It Doesn't Work
• Many patients only have a partial response where some symptoms are improved but others persist (especially insomnia, fatigue, and problems concentrating)
• Other patients may be nonresponders, sometimes called treatment-resistant or treatment-refractory
• Some patients who have an initial response may relapse even though they continue treatment, sometimes called "poop-out"
• Consider increasing dose, switching to another agent or adding an appropriate augmenting agent
• Consider psychotherapy
• Consider evaluation for another diagnosis or for a comorbid condition (e.g., medical illness, substance abuse, etc.)
• Some patients may experience apparent lack of consistent efficacy due to activation of latent or underlying bipolar disorder, and require antidepressant discontinuation and a switch to a mood stabilizer, although this may be a less frequent problem with bupropion than with other antidepressants

Best Augmenting Combos for Partial Response or Treatment-Resistance
• Trazodone for residual insomnia
• Benzodiazepines for residual anxiety
✳ Can be added to SSRIs to reverse SSRI-induced sexual dysfunction, SSRI-induced apathy (use combinations of antidepressants with caution as this may

activate bipolar disorder and suicidal ideation)

✳ Can be added to SSRIs to treat partial responders

✳ Often used as an augmenting agent to mood stabilizers and/or atypical antipsychotics in bipolar depression

• Mood stabilizers or atypical antipsychotics can also be added to bupropion for psychotic depression or treatment-resistant depression

• Hypnotics for insomnia

• Mirtazapine, modafinil, atomoxetine (add with caution and at lower doses since bupropion could theoretically raise atomoxetine levels) both for residual symptoms of depression and attention deficit disorder

Tests
• None for healthy individuals

SIDE EFFECTS

How Drug Causes Side Effects
• Side effects are probably caused in part by actions of norepinephrine and dopamine in brain areas with undesired effects (e.g., insomnia, tremor, agitation, headache, dizziness)

• Side effects are probably also caused in part by actions of norepinephrine in the periphery with undesired effects (e.g., sympathetic and parasympathetic effects such as dry mouth, constipation, nausea, anorexia, sweating)

• Most side effects are immediate but often go away with time

Notable Side Effects
• Dry mouth, constipation, nausea, weight loss, anorexia

• Insomnia, dizziness, headache, agitation, tremor, abdominal pain, tinnitus

• Sweating

• Hypertension (rare)

Life Threatening or Dangerous Side Effects
• Rare seizures (higher incidence for immediate release than for sustained release; risk increases with doses above the recommended maximums; risk

increases for patients with predisposing factors)

• Hypomania (more likely in bipolar patients but perhaps less common than with some other antidepressants)

• Rare induction of mania and activation of suicidal ideation

Weight Gain

unusual   not unusual   common   problematic
• Reported but not expected

Sedation

unusual   not unusual   common   problematic
• Reported but not expected

What To Do About Side Effects
• Wait
• Wait
• Wait
• Keep dose as low as possible
• Take no later than mid-afternoon to avoid insomnia
• Switch to another drug

Best Augmenting Agents for Side Effects
• Often best to try another antidepressant monotherapy prior to resorting to augmentation strategies to treat side effects

• Trazodone or a hypnotic for drug-induced insomnia

• Mirtazapine for insomnia, agitation, and gastrointestinal side effects

• Benzodiazepines or buspirone for drug-induced anxiety, agitation

• Many side effects are dose-dependent (i.e., they increase as dose increases, or they reemerge until tolerance re-develops)

• Many side effects are time-dependent (i.e., they start immediately upon dosing and upon each dose increase, but go away with time)

• Activation and agitation may represent the induction of a bipolar state, especially a mixed dysphoric bipolar II condition sometimes associated with suicidal ideation, and require the addition of lithium, a mood stabilizer or an atypical antipsychotic, and/or discontinuation of bupropion

DOSING AND USE

Usual Dosage Range
- Bupropion: 225–450 mg in 3 divided doses (maximum single dose 150 mg)
- Bupropion SR: 200–450 mg in 2 divided doses (maximum single dose 200 mg)
- Bupropion XL: 150–450 mg once daily

Dosage Forms
- Bupropion: tablet 75 mg, 100 mg
- Bupropion SR (sustained release): tablet 100 mg, 150 mg, 200 mg
- Bupropion XL (extended release): tablet 150 mg, 300 mg

How to Dose
- Depression: for bupropion immediate release, dosing should be in divided doses, starting at 75 mg twice daily, increasing to 100 mg twice daily, then to 100 mg 3 times daily; maximum dose 450 mg per day
- Depression: for bupropion SR, initial dose 100 mg twice a day, increase to 150 mg twice a day after at least 3 days; wait 4 weeks or longer to ensure drug effects before increasing dose; maximum dose 400 mg total per day
- Depression: for bupropion XL, initial dose 150 mg once daily in the morning; can increase to 300 mg QD after 4 days; maximum dose 450 mg once daily
- Nicotine addiction [for bupropion SR]: Initial dose 150 mg/day once a day, increase to 150 mg twice a day after at least 3 days; maximum dose 300 mg/day; bupropion treatment should begin 1–2 weeks before smoking is discontinued

 Dosing Tips
- XL formulation has replaced immediate release and SR formulations as the preferred option
- XL is best dosed once a day, whereas SR is best dosed twice daily, and immediate release is best dosed 3 times daily
- Dosing higher than 450 mg/day (400 mg/day SR) increases seizure risk
- Patients who do not respond to 450 mg/day should discontinue use or get blood levels of bupropion and its major active metabolite 6-hydroxy-bupropion
- If levels of parent drug and active metabolite are low despite dosing at 450 mg/day, experts can prudently increase dosing beyond the therapeutic range while monitoring closely, informing the patient of the potential risk of seizures and weighing risk benefit ratios in difficult-to-treat patients
- When used for bipolar depression, it is usually as an augmenting agent to mood stabilizers, lithium, and/or atypical antipsychotics
- For smoking cessation, may be used in conjunction with nicotine replacement therapy
- Do not break or chew SR or XL tablets as this will alter controlled release properties
- The more anxious and agitated the patient, the lower the starting dose, the slower the titration, and the more likely the need for a concomitant agent such as trazodone or a benzodiazepine
- If intolerable anxiety, insomnia, agitation, akathisia, or activation occur either upon dosing initiation or discontinuation, consider the possibility of activated bipolar disorder and switch to a mood stabilizer or an atypical antipsychotic

Overdose
- Rarely lethal; seizures, cardiac disturbances, hallucinations, loss of consciousness

Long-Term Use
- For smoking cessation, treatment for up to 6 months has been found effective

Habit Forming
- No

How to Stop
- Tapering is prudent to avoid withdrawal effects, but no well-documented tolerance, dependence, or withdrawal reactions

Pharmacokinetics
- Inhibits CYP450 2D6
- Parent half-life 10–14 hours
- Metabolite half-life 20–27 hours

 Drug Interactions
- Tramadol increases the risk of seizures in patients taking an antidepressant
- Can increase tricyclic antidepressant levels; use with caution with tricyclic

antidepressants or when switching from a TCA to bupropion

- Can be fatal when combined with MAO inhibitors, so do not use with MAO inhibitors or for at least 14 days after MAOIs are stopped
- Do not start an MAO inhibitor for at least two weeks after discontinuing bupropion
- Via CYP450 2D6 inhibition, bupropion could theoretically interfere with the analgesic actions of codeine, and increase the plasma levels of some beta blockers and of atomoxetine
- Via CYP450 2D6 inhibition, bupropion could theoretically increase concentrations of thioridazine and cause dangerous cardiac arrhythmias

 Other Warnings/ Precautions

- Use cautiously with other drugs that increase seizure risk (TCAs, lithium, phenothiazines, thioxanthenes, some antipsychotics)
- Bupropion should be used with caution in patients taking levodopa or amantadine, as these agents can potentially enhance dopamine neurotransmission and be activating
- Do not use if patient has severe insomnia
- Use with caution in patients with bipolar disorder unless treated with concomitant mood stabilizing agent
- Monitor patients for activation of suicidal ideation, especially children and adolescents

Do Not Use

- Zyban in combination with any formulation of Wellbutrin
- If patient has history of seizures
- If patient is anorexic or bulimic, either currently or in the past, but see Pearls
- If patient is abruptly discontinuing alcohol or sedative use
- If patient has had recent head injury
- If patient has a nervous system tumor
- If patient is taking an MAO inhibitor
- If patient is taking thioridazine
- If there is a proven allergy to bupropion

Renal Impairment

- Lower initial dose, perhaps give less frequently
- Drug concentration may be increased
- Patient should be monitored closely

Hepatic Impairment

- Lower initial dose, perhaps give less frequently
- Patient should be monitored closely
- In severe hepatic cirrhosis, bupropion XL should be administered at no more than 150 mg every other day

Cardiac Impairment

- Limited available data
- Evidence of rise in supine blood pressure
- Use with caution

Elderly

- Some patients may tolerate lower doses better

 Children and Adolescents

- Use with caution, observing for activation of known or unknown bipolar disorder and/or suicidal ideation, and strongly consider informing parents or guardian of this risk so they can help observe child or adolescent patients
- Safety and efficacy have not been established
- May be used for ADHD in children or adolescents
- May be used for smoking cessation in adolescents
- Preliminary research suggests efficacy in comorbid depression and ADHD
- Dosage may follow adult pattern for adolescents
- Children may require lower doses initially, with a maximum dose of 300 mg/day

 Pregnancy

- Risk Category B [animal studies do not show adverse effects; no controlled studies in humans]
- Pregnant women wishing to stop smoking may consider behavioral therapy before pharmacotherapy

- Not generally recommended for use during pregnancy, especially during first trimester
- Must weigh the risk of treatment (first trimester fetal development, third trimester newborn delivery) to the child against the risk of no treatment (recurrence of depression, maternal health, infant bonding) to the mother and child
- For many patients this may mean continuing treatment during pregnancy

Breast Feeding

- Some drug is found in mother's breast milk
- If child becomes irritable or sedated, breast feeding or drug may need to be discontinued
- Immediate postpartum period is a high-risk time for depression, especially in women who have had prior depressive episodes, so drug may need to be reinstituted late in the third trimester or shortly after childbirth to prevent a recurrence during the postpartum period
- Must weigh benefits of breast feeding with risks and benefits of antidepressant treatment versus non-treatment to both the infant and the mother
- For many patients, this may mean continuing treatment during breast feeding

THE ART OF PSYCHOPHARMACOLOGY

Potential Advantages

- Retarded depression
- Atypical depression
- Bipolar depression
- Patients concerned about sexual dysfunction
- Patients concerned about weight gain

Potential Disadvantages

- Patients experiencing weight loss associated with their depression
- Patients who are excessively activated

Primary Target Symptoms

- Depressed mood
- Sleep disturbance, especially hypersomnia
- Cravings associated with nicotine withdrawal
- Cognitive functioning

 Pearls

- ✳ May be effective if SSRIs have failed or for SSRI "poop-out"
- Less likely to produce hypomania than some other antidepressants
- ✳ May improve cognitive slowing/pseudodementia
- ✳ Reduces hypersomnia and fatigue
- Approved to help reduce craving during smoking cessation
- Anecdotal use in attention deficit disorder
- May cause sexual dysfunction only infrequently
- May exacerbate tics
- Bupropion may not be as effective in anxiety disorders as many other antidepressants
- Prohibition for use in eating disorders is related to past observations when bupropion immediate release was dosed at especially high levels to low body weight patients with active anorexia nervosa
- Current practice suggests that patients of normal BMI without additional risk factors for seizures can benefit from bupropion, especially if given prudent doses of the XL formulation; such treatment should be administered by experts, and patients should be monitored closely and informed of the potential risks
- The active enantiomer of the principle active metabolite (+6-hydroxy-bupropion) is in clinical development as a novel antidepressant

Suggested Reading

Ferry L, Johnston JA. Efficacy and safety of bupropion SR for smoking cessation: data from clinical trials and five years of postmarketing experience. Int J Clin Pract 2003;57(3):224–30.

Hirschfeld RM. Efficacy of SSRIs and newer antidepressants in severe depression: comparison with TCAs. Journal of Clinical Psychiatry 1999;60:326–335.

Horst WD, Preskorn SH. Mechanisms of action and clinical characteristics of three atypical antidepressants: venlafaxine, nefazodone, bupropion. Journal of Affective Disorders 1998;51:237–254.

Masand PS, Gupta S. Long-term side effects of newer-generation antidepressants: SSRIs, venlafaxine, nefazodone, bupropion, and mirtazapine. Ann Clin Psychiatry 2002;14(3):175–82.

Nieuwstraten CE, Dolovich LR. Bupropion versus selective serotonin-reuptake inhibitors for treatment of depression. Ann Pharmacother 2001;35(12):1608–13.

BUSPIRONE

THERAPEUTICS

Brands • BuSpar
see index for additional brand names

Generic? Yes

 Class
• Anxiolytic (azapirone; serotonin 1A partial agonist; serotonin stabilizer)

Commonly Prescribed For
(bold for FDA approved)
• **Management of anxiety disorders**
• **Short-term treatment of symptoms of anxiety**
• Mixed anxiety and depression
• Treatment-resistant depression (adjunctive)

 How The Drug Works
• Binds to serotonin type 1A receptors
• Partial agonist actions post-synaptically may theoretically diminish serotonergic activity and contribute to anxiolytic actions
• Partial agonist actions at presynaptic somatodendritic serotonin autoreceptors may theoretically enhance serotonergic activity and contribute to antidepressant actions

How Long Until It Works
• Generally takes within 2–4 weeks to achieve efficacy
• If it is not working within 6 to 8 weeks, it may require a dosage increase or it may not work at all

If It Works
• The goal of treatment is complete remission of symptoms as well as prevention of future relapses
• Treatment most often reduces or even eliminates symptoms, but not a cure since symptoms can recur after medicine stopped
• Chronic anxiety disorders may require long-term maintenance with buspirone to control symptoms

If It Doesn't Work
• Consider switching to another agent (a benzodiazepine or antidepressant)

 Best Augmenting Combos for Partial Response or Treatment-Resistance
• Sedative hypnotic for insomnia
• Buspirone is often given as an augmenting agent to SSRIs or SNRIs

Tests
• None for healthy individuals

SIDE EFFECTS

How Drug Causes Side Effects
• Serotonin partial agonist actions in parts of the brain and body and at receptors other than those that cause therapeutic actions

Notable Side Effects
✳ Dizziness, headache, nervousness, sedation, excitement
• Nausea
• Restlessness

 Life Threatening or Dangerous Side Effects
• Rare cardiac symptoms

Weight Gain

| unusual | not unusual | common | problematic |

• Reported but not expected

Sedation

| unusual | not unusual | common | problematic |

• Occurs in significant minority

What To Do About Side Effects
• Wait
• Wait
• Wait
• Lower the dose
• Give total daily dose divided into 3, 4, or more doses
• Switch to another agent

Best Augmenting Agents for Side Effects
• Many side effects cannot be improved with an augmenting agent

DOSING AND USE

Usual Dosage Range
• 20–30 mg/day

Dosage Forms
• Tablet 5 mg scored, 10 mg scored, 15 mg multi-scored, 30 mg multi-scored

How to Dose
• Initial 15 mg twice a day; increase in 5 mg/day increments every 2–3 days until desired efficacy is reached; maximum dose generally 60 mg/day

 Dosing Tips
• Requires dosing 2–3 times a day for full effect

Overdose
• No deaths reported in monotherapy; sedation, dizziness, small pupils, nausea, vomiting

Long-Term Use
• Limited data suggest that it is safe

Habit Forming
• No

How to Stop
• Taper generally not necessary

Pharmacokinetics
• Metabolized primarily by CYP450 3A4
• Elimination half-life approximately 2–3 hours

 Drug Interactions
• Do not use with MAO inhibitors, including 14 days after MAOIs are stopped
• CYP450 3A4 inhibitors (e.g., fluxotine, fluvoxamine, nefazodone) may reduce clearance of buspirone and raise its plasma levels, so the dose of buspirone may need to be lowered when given concomitantly with these agents
• CYP450 3A4 inducers (e.g., carbamazepine) may increase clearance of buspirone, so the dose of buspirone may need to be raised
• Buspirone may increase plasma concentrations of haloperidol

• Buspirone may raise levels of nordiazepam, the active metabolite of diazepam, which may result in increased symptoms of dizziness, headache, or nausea

 Other Warnings/ Precautions
• None

Do Not Use
• If patient is taking an MAO inhibitor
• If there is a proven allergy to buspirone

SPECIAL POPULATIONS

Renal Impairment
• Use with caution
• Not recommended for patients with severe renal impairment

Hepatic Impairment
• Use with caution
• Not recommended for patients with severe hepatic impairment

Cardiac Impairment
• Buspirone has been used to treat hostility in patients with cardiac impairment

Elderly
• Some patients may tolerate lower doses better

 Children and Adolescents
• Studies in children 6–17 do not show significant reduction in anxiety symptoms in GAD
• Safety profile in children encourages use

 Pregnancy
• Risk Category B [animal studies do not show adverse effects, no controlled studies in humans]
• Not generally recommended in pregnancy, but may be safer than some other options

Breast Feeding
• Some drug is found in mother's breast milk
• Trace amounts may be present in nursing children whose mothers are on buspirone

- If child becomes irritable or sedated, breast feeding or drug may need to be discontinued

THE ART OF PSYCHOPHARMACOLOGY

Potential Advantages
- Safety profile
- Lack of dependence, withdrawal
- Lack of sexual dysfunction or weight gain

Potential Disadvantages
- Takes 4 weeks for results, whereas benzodiazepines have immediate effects

Primary Target Symptoms
- Anxiety

Pearls
❋ Buspirone does not appear to cause dependence and shows virtually no withdrawal symptoms

- May have less severe side effects than benzodiazepines
❋ Buspirone generally lacks sexual dysfunction
- Buspirone may reduce sexual dysfunction associated with generalized anxiety disorder and with serotonergic antidepressants
- Sedative effects may be more likely at doses above 20 mg/day
- May have less anxiolytic efficacy than benzodiazepines for some patients
- Buspirone is generally reserved as an augmenting agent to treat anxiety
- A new controlled-release azapirone related to buspirone is in late clinical testing as an antidepressant (gepirone ER)

Suggested Reading

Apter JT, Allen LA. Buspirone: future directions. J Clin Psychopharmacol 1999; 19:86–93.

Mahmood I, Sahaiwalla C. Clinical pharmacokinetics and pharmacodynamics of buspirone, an anxiolytic drug. Clin Pharmacokinet 1999;36:277–87.

Pecknold JC. A risk-benefit assessment of buspirone in the treatment of anxiety disorders. Drug Saf 1997;16:118–32.

Sramek JJ, Hong WW, Hamid S, Nape B, Cutler NR. Meta-analysis of the safety and tolerability of two dose regimens of buspirone in patients with persistent anxiety. Depress Anxiety 1999;9:131–4.

CARBAMAZEPINE

Brands • Tegretol
• Carbatrol
see index for additional brand names

Generic? Yes (not for extended release
formulation)

 Class

• Anticonvulsant, antineuralgic for chronic
pain, voltage-sensitive sodium channel
antagonist

Commonly Prescribed For
(bold for FDA approved)
• **Partial seizures with complex
symptomatology**
• **Generalized tonic-clonic seizures (grand
mal)**
• **Mixed seizure patterns**
• **Pain associated with true trigeminal
neuralgia**
• Glossopharyngeal neuralgia
• Bipolar disorder
• Psychosis, schizophrenia (adjunctive)

 How The Drug Works

* Acts as a use-dependent blocker of
voltage-sensitive sodium channels
* Interacts with the open channel
conformation of voltage-sensitive sodium
channels
* Interacts at a specific site of the alpha
pore-forming subunit of voltage-sensitive
sodium channels
• Inhibits release of glutamate

How Long Until It Works
• For acute mania, effects should occur
within a few weeks
• May take several weeks to months to
optimize an effect on mood stabilization
• Should reduce seizures by 2 weeks

If It Works
• The goal of treatment is complete
remission of symptoms (e.g., seizures,
mania, pain)
• Continue treatment until all symptoms are
gone or until improvement is stable and
then continue treating indefinitely as long
as improvement persists

• Continue treatment indefinitely to avoid
recurrence of mania and seizures
• Treatment of chronic neuropathic pain
most often reduces but does not eliminate
pain and is not a cure since symptoms
usually recur after medicine stopped

If It Doesn't Work (for bipolar disorder)
* Many patients only have a partial
response where some symptoms are
improved but others persist or continue to
wax and wane without stabilization of
mood
• Other patients may be nonresponders,
sometimes called treatment-resistant or
treatment-refractory
• Consider increasing dose, switching to
another agent or adding an appropriate
augmenting agent
• Consider adding psychotherapy
• Consider biofeedback or hypnosis for pain
• For bipolar disorder, consider the presence
of noncompliance and counsel patient
• Switch to another mood stabilizer with
fewer side effects or to extended release
carbamazepine
• Consider evaluation for another diagnosis
or for a comorbid condition (e.g., medical
illness, substance abuse, etc.)

 **Best Augmenting Combos
for Partial Response or
Treatment-Resistance**

• Carbamazepine is itself a second-line
augmenting agent for numerous other
anticonvulsants, lithium, and atypical
antipsychotics in treating bipolar disorder
• Carbamazepine is itself a second or third-
line augmenting agent for atypical
antipsychotics in treating schizophrenia

Tests
* Before starting: blood count, liver, kidney,
and thyroid function tests
• During treatment: blood count every
2 weeks for 2 months, then every
3 months throughout treatment
• During treatment: liver, kidney, and thyroid
function tests every 6–12 months
• Consider monitoring sodium levels
because of possibility of hyponatremia

SIDE EFFECTS

How Drug Causes Side Effects
- CNS side effects theoretically due to excessive actions at voltage-sensitive sodium channels
- Major metabolite (carbamazepine-10, 11 epoxide) may be the cause of many side effects
- Mild anticholinergic effects may contribute to sedation, blurred vision

Notable Side Effects
- ❊ Sedation, dizziness, confusion, unsteadiness, headache
- ❊ Nausea, vomiting, diarrhea
- Blurred vision
- ❊ Benign leukopenia (transient; in up to 10%)
- ❊ Rash

 ### Life Threatening or Dangerous Side Effects
- ❊ Rare aplastic anemia, agranulocytosis (unusual bleeding or bruising, mouth sores, infections, fever, sore throat)
- ❊ Rare severe dermatologic reactions (Stevens Johnson syndrome)
- Rare cardiac problems
- Rare induction of psychosis or mania
- ❊ SIADH (syndrome of inappropriate antidiuretic hormone secretion) with hyponatremia
- Increased frequency of generalized convulsions (in patients with atypical absence seizures)

Weight Gain

unusual | not unusual | common | problematic

- Occurs in significant minority

Sedation

unusual | not unusual | common | problematic

- Frequent and can be significant in amount
- Some patients may not tolerate it
- Dose-related
- Can wear off with time, but commonly does not wear off at high doses

What To Do About Side Effects
- Wait
- Wait
- Wait

- Take with food or split dose to avoid gastrointestinal effects
- Extended release carbamazepine can be sprinkled on soft food
- Take at night to reduce daytime sedation
- Switch to another agent or to extended release carbamazepine

Best Augmenting Agents for Side Effects
- Many side effects cannot be improved with an augmenting agent

DOSING AND USE

Usual Dosage Range
- 400–1200 mg/day
- Under age 6: 10–20 mg/kg/day

Dosage Forms
- Tablet 100 mg chewable, 200 mg
- Extended release tablet 100 mg, 200 mg, 400 mg
- Extended release capsule 200 mg, 300 mg
- Oral suspension 100 mg/5mL (450 mL)

How to Dose
- For bipolar disorder and seizures (ages 13 and older): initial 200 mg twice daily (tablet) or 1 teaspoon (100 mg) 4 times a day (suspension); each week increase by up to 200 mg/day in divided doses (2 doses for extended release formulation, 3–4 doses for other tablets); maximum dose generally 1200 mg/day for adults and 1000 mg/day for children under age 15; maintenance dose generally 800–1200 mg/day for adults; some patients may require up to 1600 mg/day
- Seizures (under age 13): see Children and Adolescents
- Trigeminal neuralgia: initial 100 mg twice daily (tablet) or 0.5 teaspoon (50 mg) 4 times a day; each week increase by up to 200 mg/day in divided doses (100 mg every 12 hours for tablet formulations, 50 mg 4 times a day for suspension formulation); maximum dose generally 1200 mg/day
- Lower initial dose and slower titration should be used for carbamazepine suspension

Dosing Tips

- Higher peak levels occur with the suspension formulation than with the same dose of the tablet formulation, so suspension should generally be started at a lower dose and titrated slowly
- Take carbamazepine with food to avoid gastrointestinal effects
- ✷ Slow dose titration may delay onset of therapeutic action but enhance tolerability to sedating side effects
- Should titrate slowly in the presence of other sedating agents, such as other anticonvulsants, in order to best tolerate additive sedative side effects
- ✷ Can sometimes minimize the impact of carbamazepine upon the bone marrow by dosing slowly and monitoring closely when initiating treatment; initial trend to leukopenia/neutropenia may reverse with continued conservative dosing over time and allow subsequent dosage increases with careful monitoring
- ✷ Carbamazepine often requires a dosage adjustment upward with time, as the drug induces its own metabolism, thus lowering its own plasma levels over the first several weeks to months of treatment
- Do not break or chew carbamazepine extended release tablets as this will alter controlled release properties

Overdose

- Can be fatal (lowest known fatal dose in adults is 3.2 g, in adolescents is 4 g, and in children is 1.6 g); nausea, vomiting, involuntary movements, irregular heartbeat, urinary retention, trouble breathing, sedation, coma

Long-Term Use

- May lower sex drive
- Monitoring of liver, kidney, thyroid functions, blood counts and sodium may be required

Habit Forming

- No

How to Stop

- Taper; may need to adjust dosage of concurrent medications as carbamazepine is being discontinued

- ✷ Rapid discontinuation may increase the risk of relapse in bipolar disorder
- Epilepsy patients may seize upon withdrawal, especially if withdrawal is abrupt
- Discontinuation symptoms uncommon

Pharmacokinetics

- Metabolized in the liver, primarily by CYP450 3A4
- Renally excreted
- Active metabolite (carbamazepine-10,11 epoxide)
- Initial half-life 26–65 hours (35–40 hours for extended release formulation); half-life 12–17 hours with repeated doses
- Half-life of active metabolite is approximately 34 hours
- ✷ Is not only a substrate for CYP450 3A4, but also an inducer of CYP450 3A4
- ✷ Thus, carbamazepine induces its own metabolism, often requiring an upward dosage adjustment

Drug Interactions

- Enzyme-inducing antiepileptic drugs (carbamazepine itself as well as phenobarbital, phenytoin, and primidone) may increase the clearance of carbamazepine and lower its plasma levels
- CYP450 3A4 inducers, such as carbamazepine itself, can lower the plasma levels of carbamazepine
- CYP450 3A4 inhibitors, such as nefazodone, fluvoxamine, and fluoxetine, can increase plasma levels of carbamazepine
- Carbamazepine can increase plasma levels of clomipramine, phenytoin, primidone
- Carbamazepine can decrease plasma levels of acetaminophen, clozapine, benzodiazepines, dicumarol, doxycycline, theophylline, warfarin, and haloperidol as well as other anticonvulsants such as phensuximide, methsuximide, ethosuximide, phenytoin, tiagabine, topiramate, lamotrigine, and valproate
- Carbamazepine can decrease plasma levels of hormonal contraceptives and adversely affect their efficacy
- Combined use of carbamazepine with other anticonvulsants may lead to altered thyroid function

• Combined use of carbamazepine and lithium may increase risk of neurotoxic effects

• Depressive effects are increased by other CNS depressants (alcohol, MAOIs, other anticonvulsants, etc.)

• Combined use of carbamazepine suspension with liquid formulations of chlorpromazine has been shown to result in excretion of an orange rubbery precipitate; because of this, combined use of carbamazepine suspension with any liquid medicine is not recommended

 Other Warnings/ Precautions

✳ Patients should be monitored carefully for signs of unusual bleeding or bruising, mouth sores, infections, fever, or sore throat, as the risk of aplastic anemia and agranulocytosis with carbamazepine use is 5–8 times greater than in the general population (risk in the untreated general population is 6 patients per one million per year for agranulocytosis and 2 patients per one million per year for aplastic anemia)

• Because carbamazepine has a tricyclic chemical structure, it is not recommended to be taken with MAOIs, including 14 days after MAOIs are stopped; do not start an MAOI until 2 weeks after discontinuing carbamazepine

• May exacerbate narrow angle-closure glaucoma

• Because carbamazepine can lower plasma levels of hormonal contraceptives, it may also reduce their effectiveness

• May need to restrict fluid intake because of risk of developing syndrome of inappropriate antidiuretic hormone secretion, hyponatremia and its complications

• Use with caution in patients with mixed seizure disorders that include atypical absence seizures because carbamazepine has been associated with increased frequency of generalized convulsions in such patients

Do Not Use

• If patient is taking an MAOI

• If patient has history of bone marrow suppression

• If there is a proven allergy to any tricyclic compound

• If there is a proven allergy to carbamazepine

SPECIAL POPULATIONS

Renal Impairment

• Carbamazepine is renally secreted, so the dose may need to be lowered

Hepatic Impairment

• Drug should be used with caution

• Rare cases of hepatic failure have occurred

Cardiac Impairment

• Drug should be used with caution

Elderly

• Some patients may tolerate lower doses better

• Elderly patients may be more susceptible to adverse effects

 Children and Adolescents

• Approved use for epilepsy; therapeutic range of total carbamazepine in plasma is considered the same for children and adults

• Ages 6–12: initial dose 100 mg twice daily (tablets) or 0.5 teaspoon (50 mg) 4 times a day (suspension); each week increase by up to 100 mg/day in divided doses (2 doses for extended release formulation, 3–4 doses for all other formulations); maximum dose generally 1000 mg/day; maintenance dose generally 400–800 mg/day

• Ages 5 and younger: initial 10–20 mg/kg/day in divided doses (2–3 doses for tablet formulations, 4 doses for suspension); increase weekly as needed; maximum dose generally 35 mg/kg/day

 Pregnancy

• Risk category D [positive evidence of risk to human fetus; potential benefits may still justify its use during pregnancy]

✳ Use during first trimester may raise risk of neural tube defects (e.g., spina bifida) or other congenital anomalies

- Use in women of childbearing potential requires weighing potential benefits to the mother against the risks to the fetus
❋ If drug is continued, perform tests to detect birth defects
❋ If drug is continued, start on folate 1 mg/day early in pregnancy to reduce risk of neural tube defects
- Use of anticonvulsants in combination may cause a higher prevalence of teratogenic effects than anticonvulsant monotherapy
- Taper drug if discontinuing
- Seizures, even mild seizures, may cause harm to the embryo/fetus
❋ For bipolar patients, carbamazepine should generally be discontinued before anticipated pregnancies
- Recurrent bipolar illness during pregnancy can be quite disruptive
- For bipolar patients, given the risk of relapse in the postpartum period, some form of mood stabilizer treatment may need to be restarted immediately after delivery if patient is unmedicated during pregnancy
❋ Atypical antipsychotics may be preferable to lithium or anticonvulsants such as carbamazepine if treatment of bipolar disorder is required during pregnancy
- Bipolar symptoms may recur or worsen during pregnancy and some form of treatment may be necessary

Breast Feeding
- Some drug is found in mother's breast milk
❋ Recommended either to discontinue drug or bottle feed
- If drug is continued while breast feeding, infant should be monitored for possible adverse effects, including hematological effects
- If infant shows signs of irritability or sedation, drug may need to be discontinued
- Some cases of neonatal seizures, respiratory depression, vomiting, and diarrhea have been reported in infants whose mothers received carbamazepine during pregnancy
❋ Bipolar disorder may recur during the postpartum period, particularly if there is a history of prior postpartum episodes of either depression or psychosis

- Relapse rates may be lower in women who receive prophylactic treatment for postpartum episodes of bipolar disorder
- Atypical antipsychotics and anticonvulsants such as valproate may be safer than carbamazepine during the postpartum period when breast feeding

---

THE ART OF PSYCHOPHARMACOLOGY

Potential Advantages
- Treatment-resistant bipolar and psychotic disorders

Potential Disadvantages
- Patients who do not wish to or cannot comply with blood testing and close monitoring
- Patients who cannot tolerate sedation
- Pregnant patients

Primary Target Symptoms
- Incidence of seizures
- Unstable mood, especially mania
- Pain

 Pearls
- Carbamazepine is the first anticonvulsant widely used for the treatment of bipolar disorder
❋ Due to the emergence of anticonvulsants with better documentation of efficacy and better tolerability, use in bipolar disorder is declining
❋ An extended release formulation has better evidence of efficacy and improved tolerability in bipolar disorder than does immediate release carbamazepine
- Dosage frequency as well as sedation, diplopia, confusion, and ataxia may be reduced with extended release carbamazepine
- Risk of serious side effects is greatest in the first few months of treatment
- Common side effects such as sedation often abate after a few months
❋ May be effective in patients who fail to respond to lithium or other mood stabilizers
❋ Especially preferred as a second or third-line treatment for mania

- Not clearly effective for the depressed phase of bipolar disorder
- Can be complicated to dose
- Can be complicated to use with concomitant medications

- Although less well investigated in bipolar disorder, oxcarbazepine, a structural analog of carbamazepine, may be better tolerated and thus an appropriate alternative to carbamazepine

 Suggested Reading

Brambilla P, Barale F, Soares JC. Perspectives on the use of anticonvulsants in the treatment of bipolar disorder. Int J Neuropsychopharmacol. 2001; 4: 421–46.

Leucht S, McGrath J, White P, Kissling W. Carbamazepine for schizophrenia and schizoaffective psychoses. Cochrane Database Syst Rev. 2002;(3):CD001258.

Marson AG, Williamson PR, Hutton JL, Clough HE, Chadwick DW. Carbamazepine versus valproate monotherapy for epilepsy. Cochrane Database Syst Rev. 2000; (3): CD001030.

Weisler RH, Kalali AH, Ketter TA. A multicenter, randomized, double-blind, placebo-controlled trial of extended-release carbamazepine capsules as monotherapy for bipolar disorder patients with manic or mixed episodes. J Clin Psychiatry 2004; 65: 478–84.

CHLORDIAZEPOXIDE

THERAPEUTICS

Brands
- Limbitrol
- Librium
- Librax

see index for additional brand names

Generic? Yes

 Class
- Benzodiazepine (anxiolytic)

Commonly Prescribed For
(bold for FDA approved)
- **Anxiety disorders**
- **Symptoms of anxiety**
- **Preoperative apprehension and anxiety**
- **Withdrawal symptoms of acute alcoholism**

 How The Drug Works
- Binds to benzodiazepine receptors at the GABA-A ligand-gated chloride channel complex
- Enhances the inhibitory effects of GABA
- Boosts chloride conductance through GABA-regulated channels
- Inhibits neuronal activity presumably in amygdala-centered fear circuits to provide therapeutic benefits in anxiety disorders

How Long Until It Works
- Some immediate relief with first dosing is common; can take several weeks with daily dosing for maximal therapeutic benefit

If It Works
- For short-term symptoms of anxiety – after a few weeks, discontinue use or use on an "as-needed" basis
- For chronic anxiety disorders, the goal of treatment is complete remission of symptoms as well as prevention of future relapses
- For chronic anxiety disorders, treatment most often reduces or even eliminates symptoms, but not a cure since symptoms can recur after medicine stopped
- For long-term symptoms of anxiety, consider switching to an SSRI or SNRI for long-term maintenance
- If long-term maintenance with a benzodiazepine is necessary, continue treatment for 6 months after symptoms resolve, and then taper dose slowly
- If symptoms reemerge, consider treatment with an SSRI or SNRI, or consider restarting the benzodiazepine; sometimes benzodiazepines have to be used in combination with SSRIs or SNRIs for best results

If It Doesn't Work
- Consider switching to another agent or adding an appropriate augmenting agent
- Consider psychotherapy, especially cognitive behavioral psychotherapy
- Consider presence of concomitant substance abuse
- Consider presence of chlordiazepoxide abuse
- Consider another diagnosis, such as a comorbid medical condition

 Best Augmenting Combos for Partial Response or Treatment-Resistance
- Benzodiazepines are frequently used as augmenting agents for antipsychotics and mood stabilizers in the treatment of psychotic and bipolar disorders
- Benzodiazepines are frequently used as augmenting agents for SSRIs and SNRIs in the treatment of anxiety disorders
- Not generally rational to combine with other benzodiazepines
- Caution if using as an anxiolytic concomitantly with other sedative hypnotics for sleep

Tests
- In patients with seizure disorders, concomitant medical illness, and/or those with multiple concomitant long-term medications, periodic liver tests and blood counts may be prudent

SIDE EFFECTS

How Drug Causes Side Effects
- Same mechanism for side effects as for therapeutic effects – namely due to excessive actions at benzodiazepine receptors
- Long-term adaptations in benzodiazepine receptors may explain the development of dependence, tolerance, and withdrawal

- Side effects are generally immediate, but immediate side effects often disappear in time

Notable Side Effects

✳ Sedation, fatigue, depression
✳ Dizziness, ataxia, slurred speech, weakness
✳ Forgetfulness, confusion
✳ Hyper-excitability, nervousness
✳ Pain at injection site
- Rare hallucinations, mania
- Rare hypotension
- Hypersalivation, dry mouth

 ### Life Threatening or Dangerous Side Effects

- Respiratory depression, especially when taken with CNS depressants in overdose
- Rare hepatic dysfunction, renal dysfunction, blood dyscrasias

Weight Gain

unusual   not unusual   common   problematic

- Reported but not expected

Sedation

unusual   not unusual   common   problematic

- Many experience and/or can be significant in amount
- Especially at initiation of treatment or when dose increases
- Tolerance often develops over time

What To Do About Side Effects

- Wait
- Wait
- Wait
- Lower the dose
- Take largest dose at bedtime to avoid sedative effects during the day
- Switch to another agent
- Administer flumazenil if side effects are severe or life-threatening

Best Augmenting Agents for Side Effects

- Many side effects cannot be improved with an augmenting agent

Usual Dosage Range

- Oral: mild to moderate anxiety: 15–40 mg/day in 3–4 doses
- Oral: severe anxiety: 60–100 mg/day in 3–4 doses

Dosage Forms

- Capsule 5 mg, 10 mg, 25 mg
- Injectable 100 mg/5 mL

How to Dose

- Injectable: acute/severe anxiety: initial 50–100 mg; 25–50 mg 3–4 times/day if necessary
- Injectable: alcohol withdrawal: initial 50–100 mg; repeat after 2 hours if necessary
- Injectable: preoperative: 50–100 mg 1 hour before surgery
- Patients who receive injectable chlordiazepoxide should be observed for up to 3 hours

 ### Dosing Tips

✳ One of the few benzodiazepines available in an injectable formulation
- Chlordiazepoxide injection is intended for acute use; patients who require longer treatment should be switched to the oral formulation
- Use lowest possible effective dose for the shortest possible period of time (a benzodiazepine-sparing strategy)
- Assess need for continued treatment regularly
- Risk of dependence may increase with dose and duration of treatment
- For inter-dose symptoms of anxiety, can either increase dose or maintain same total daily dose but divide into more frequent doses
- Can also use an as-needed occasional "top up" dose for inter-dose anxiety
- Because anxiety disorders can require higher doses, the risk of dependence may be greater in these patients
- Some severely ill patients may require doses higher than the generally recommended maximum dose
- Frequency of dosing in practice is often greater than predicted from half-life, as duration of biological activity is often shorter than pharmacokinetic terminal half-life

Overdose
- Fatalities can occur; hypotension, tiredness, ataxia, confusion, coma

Long-Term Use
- Evidence of efficacy for up to 16 weeks
- Risk of dependence, particularly for treatment periods longer than 12 weeks, and especially in patients with past or current polysubstance abuse

Habit Forming
- Chlordiazepoxide is a Schedule IV drug
- Patients may develop dependence and/or tolerance with long-term use

How to Stop
- Patients with history of seizure may seize upon withdrawal, especially if withdrawal is abrupt
- Taper by 10 mg every 3 days to reduce chances of withdrawal effects
- For difficult to taper patients, consider reducing dose much more slowly after reaching 20 mg/day, perhaps by as little as 5 mg per week or less
- For other patients with severe problems discontinuing a benzodiazepine, dosing may need to be tapered over many months (i.e., reduce dose by 1% every 3 days by crushing tablet and suspending or dissolving in 100 ml of fruit juice and then disposing of 1 ml while drinking the rest; 3–7 days later, dispose of 2 ml, and so on). This is both a form of very slow biological tapering and a form of behavioral desensitization
- Be sure to differentiate reemergence of symptoms requiring reinstitution of treatment from withdrawal symptoms
- Benzodiazepine-dependent anxiety patients and insulin-dependent diabetics are not addicted to their medications. When benzodiazepine-dependent patients stop their medication, disease symptoms can reemerge, disease symptoms can worsen (rebound), and/or withdrawal symptoms can emerge

Pharmacokinetics
- Elimination half-life 24–48 hours

 Drug Interactions
- Increased depressive effects when taken with other CNS depressants

 Other Warnings/ Precautions
- Dosage changes should be made in collaboration with prescriber
- Use with caution in patients with pulmonary disease; rare reports of death after initiation of benzodiazepines in patients with severe pulmonary impairment
- History of drug or alcohol abuse often creates greater risk for dependency
- Some depressed patients may experience a worsening of suicidal ideation
- Some patients may exhibit abnormal thinking or behavioral changes similar to those caused by other CNS depressants (i.e., either depressant actions or disinhibiting actions)

Do Not Use
- If patient has narrow angle-closure glaucoma
- If there is a proven allergy to chlordiazepoxide or any benzodiazepine

SPECIAL POPULATIONS

Renal Impairment
- Oral: Initial 10–20 mg/day in 2–4 doses; increase as needed
- Injectable: 25–50 mg

Hepatic Impairment
- Oral: Initial 10–20 mg/day in 2–4 doses; increase as needed
- Injectable: 25–50 mg

Cardiac Impairment
- Benzodiazepines have been used to treat anxiety associated with acute myocardial infarction

Elderly
- Oral: Initial 10–20 mg/day in 2–4 doses; increase as needed
- Injectable: 25–50 mg
- Elderly patients may be more sensitive to sedative effects

 Children and Adolescents
- Oral: Not recommended under age 6

- Oral: Initial 10–20 mg/day in 2–4 doses; may increase to 20–30 mg/day in 2–3 doses if ineffective
- Injectable: Not recommended under age 12
- Injectable: 25–50 mg
- Hyperactive children should be monitored for paradoxical effects
- Long-term effects of chlordiazepoxide in children/adolescents are unknown
- Should generally receive lower doses and be more closely monitored

Pregnancy

- Risk Category D [positive evidence of risk to human fetus; potential benefits may still justify its use during pregnancy]
- Possible increased risk of birth defects when benzodiazepines taken during pregnancy
- Because of the potential risks, chlordiazepoxide is not generally recommended as treatment for anxiety during pregnancy, especially during the first trimester
- Drug should be tapered if discontinued
- Infants whose mothers received a benzodiazepine late in pregnancy may experience withdrawal effects
- Neonatal flaccidity has been reported in infants whose mothers took a benzodiazepine during pregnancy
- Seizures, even mild seizures, may cause harm to the embryo/fetus

Breast Feeding

- Unknown if chlordiazepoxide is secreted in human breast milk, but all psychotropics assumed to be secreted in breast milk
- ✳ Recommended either to discontinue drug or bottle feed

- Effects of benzodiazepines on nursing infants have been reported and include feeding difficulties, sedation, and weight loss

THE ART OF PSYCHOPHARMACOLOGY

Potential Advantages
- Rapid onset of action

Potential Disadvantages
- Euphoria may lead to abuse
- Abuse especially risky in past or present substance abusers

Primary Target Symptoms
- Panic attacks
- Anxiety

Pearls

- Can be a useful adjunct to SSRIs and SNRIs in the treatment of numerous anxiety disorders, but not used as frequently as some other benzodiazepines
- Not effective for treating psychosis as a monotherapy, but can be used as an adjunct to antipsychotics
- Not effective for treating bipolar disorder as a monotherapy, but can be used as an adjunct to mood stabilizers and antipsychotics
- Can both cause depression and treat depression in different patients
- When using to treat insomnia, remember that insomnia may be a symptom of some other primary disorder itself, and thus warrant evaluation for comorbid psychiatric and/or medical conditions
- ✳ Remains a viable treatment option for alcohol withdrawal

Suggested Reading

Baskin SI, Esdale A. Is chlordiazepoxide the rational choice among benzodiazepines? Pharmacotherapy 1982;2:110–9.

Erstad BL, Cotugno CL. Management of alcohol withdrawal. Am J Health Syst Pharm 1995;52:697–709.

Fraser AD. Use and abuse of the benzodiazepines. Ther Drug Monit 1998; 20:481–9.

Murray JB. Effects of valium and librium on human psychomotor and cognitive functions. Genet Psychol Monogr 1984;109(2D Half):167–97.

CHLORPROMAZINE

THERAPEUTICS

Brands • Thorazine
see index for additional brand names

Generic? Yes

 Class
- Conventional antipsychotic (neuroleptic, phenothiazine, dopamine 2 antagonist, antiemetic)

Commonly Prescribed For
(bold for FDA approved)
- **Schizophrenia**
- **Nausea, vomiting**
- **Restlessness and apprehension before surgery**
- **Acute intermittent porphyria**
- **Manifestations of manic type of manic-depressive illness**
- **Tetanus (adjunct)**
- **Intractable hiccups**
- **Combativeness and/or explosive hyperexcitable behavior (in children)**
- **Hyperactive children who show excessive motor activity with accompanying conduct disorders consisting of some or all of the following symptoms: impulsivity, difficulty sustaining attention, aggressivity, mood lability, and poor frustration tolerance**
- **Psychosis**
- Bipolar disorder

 How The Drug Works
- Blocks dopamine 2 receptors, reducing positive symptoms of psychosis and improving other behaviors
- Combination of dopamine D2, histamine H1, and cholinergic M1 blockade in the vomiting center may reduce nausea and vomiting

How Long Until It Works
- Psychotic symptoms can improve within 1 week, but it may take several weeks for full effect on behavior
- Actions on nausea and vomiting are immediate

If It Works
- Most often reduces positive symptoms in schizophrenia but does not eliminate them
- Most schizophrenic patients do not have a total remission of symptoms but rather a reduction of symptoms by about a third
- Continue treatment in schizophrenia until reaching a plateau of improvement
- After reaching a satisfactory plateau, continue treatment for at least a year after first episode of psychosis in schizophrenia
- For second and subsequent episodes of psychosis in schizophrenia, treatment may need to be indefinite
- Reduces symptoms of acute psychotic mania but not proven as a mood stabilizer or as an effective maintenance treatment in bipolar disorder
- After reducing acute psychotic symptoms in mania, switch to a mood stabilizer and/or an atypical antipsychotic for mood stabilization and maintenance

If It Doesn't Work
- Consider trying one of the first-line atypical antipsychotics (risperidone, olanzapine, quetiapine, ziprasidone, aripiprazole, amisulpride)
- Consider trying another conventional antipsychotic
- If 2 or more antipsychotic monotherapies do not work, consider clozapine

 Best Augmenting Combos for Partial Response or Treatment-Resistance
- Augmentation of conventional antipsychotics has not been systematically studied
- Addition of a mood stabilizing anticonvulsant such as valproate, carbamazepine, or lamotrigine may be helpful in both schizophrenia and bipolar mania
- Augmentation with lithium in bipolar mania may be helpful
- Addition of a benzodiazepine, especially short-term for agitation

Tests
✳ Since conventional antipsychotics are frequently associated with weight gain, before starting treatment, weigh all patients and determine if the patient is already

overweight (BMI 25.0–29.9) or obese (BMI ≥30)
- Before giving a drug that can cause weight gain to an overweight or obese patient, consider determining whether the patient already has pre-diabetes (fasting plasma glucose 100–125 mg/dl), diabetes (fasting plasma glucose >126 mg/dl), or dyslipidemia (increased total cholesterol, LDL cholesterol and triglycerides; decreased HDL cholesterol), and treat or refer such patients for treatment, including nutrition and weight management, physical activity counseling, smoking cessation, and medical management
* Monitor weight and BMI during treatment
* While giving a drug to a patient who has gained >5% of initial weight, consider evaluating for the presence of pre-diabetes, diabetes, or dyslipidemia, or consider switching to a different antipsychotic
- Should check blood pressure in the elderly before starting and for the first few weeks of treatment
- Monitoring elevated prolactin levels of dubious clinical benefit
- Phenothiazines may cause false positive phenylketonuria results

SIDE EFFECTS

How Drug Causes Side Effects
- By blocking dopamine 2 receptors in the striatum, it can cause motor side effects
- By blocking dopamine 2 receptors in the pituitary, it can cause elevations in prolactin
- By blocking dopamine 2 receptors excessively in the mesocortical and mesolimbic dopamine pathways, especially at high doses, it can cause worsening of negative and cognitive symptoms (neuroleptic-induced deficit syndrome)
- Anticholinergic actions may cause sedation, blurred vision, constipation, dry mouth
- Antihistaminic actions may cause sedation, weight gain
- By blocking alpha 1 adrenergic receptors, it can cause dizziness, sedation, and hypotension
- Mechanism of weight gain and any possible increased incidence of diabetes or dyslipidemia with conventional antipsychotics is unknown

Notable Side Effects
* Neuroleptic-induced deficit syndrome
* Akathisia
* Priapism
* Extrapyramidal symptoms, Parkinsonism, tardive dyskinesia
* Galactorrhea, amenorrhea
- Dizziness, sedation, impaired memory
- Dry mouth, constipation, urinary retention, blurred vision
- Decreased sweating
- Sexual dysfunction
- Hypotension, tachycardia, syncope
- Weight gain

Life Threatening or Dangerous Side Effects
- Rare neuroleptic malignant syndrome
- Rare jaundice, agranulocytosis
- Rare seizures

Weight Gain

unusual   not unusual   **common**   problematic
- Many experience and/or can be significant in amount

Sedation

unusual   not unusual   common   **problematic**
- Tolerance to sedation can develop over time

What To Do About Side Effects
- Wait
- Wait
- Wait
- For motor symptoms, add an anticholinergic agent
- Reduce the dose
- For sedation, give at night
- Switch to an atypical antipsychotic
- Weight loss, exercise programs, and medical management for high BMIs, diabetes dyslipidemia

Best Augmenting Agents for Side Effects
- Benztropine or trihexyphenidyl for motor side effects

- Sometimes amantadine can be helpful for motor side effects
- Benzodiazepines may be helpful for akathisia
- Many side effects cannot be improved with an augmenting agent

DOSING AND USE

Usual Dosage Range
- 200–800 mg/day

Dosage Forms
- Tablet 10 mg, 25 mg, 50 mg, 100 mg, 200 mg
- Capsule 30 mg, 75 mg, 150 mg
- Ampul 25 mg/mL; 1 mL, 2 mL
- Vial 25 mg/mL; 10 mL
- Liquid 10 mg/5 mL
- Suppository 25 mg, 100 mg

How to Dose
- Psychosis: increase dose until symptoms are controlled; after 2 weeks reduce to lowest effective dose
- Psychosis (intramuscular): varies by severity of symptoms and inpatient/outpatient status

 Dosing Tips
- Low doses may have more sedative actions than antipsychotic actions
- Low doses have been used to provide short-term relief of daytime agitation and anxiety and to enhance sedative hypnotic actions in non-psychotic patients, but other treatment options such as atypical antipsychotics are now preferred
- Higher doses may induce or worsen negative symptoms of schizophrenia
- Ampuls and vials contain sulfites that may cause allergic reactions, particularly in patients with asthma
- One of the few antipsychotics available as a suppository

Overdose
- Extrapyramidal symptoms, sedation, hypotension, coma, respiratory depression

Long-Term Use
- Some side effects may be irreversible (e.g., tardive dyskinesia)

Habit Forming
- No

How to Stop
- Slow down-titration of oral formulation (over 6 to 8 weeks), especially when simultaneously beginning a new antipsychotic while switching (i.e., cross-titration)
- Rapid oral discontinuation may lead to rebound psychosis and worsening of symptoms
- If antiparkinson agents are being used, they should be continued for a few weeks after chlorpromazine is discontinued

Pharmacokinetics
- Half-life approximately 8–33 hours

 Drug Interactions
- May decrease the effects of levodopa, dopamine agonists
- May increase the effects of antihypertensive drugs except for guanethidine, whose antihypertensive actions chlorpromazine may antagonize
- Additive effects may occur if used with CNS depressants
- Some pressor agents (e.g., epinephrine) may interact with chlorpromazine to lower blood pressure
- Alcohol and diuretics may increase the risk of hypotension
- Reduces effects of anticoagulants
- May reduce phenytoin metabolism and increase phenytoin levels
- Plasma levels of chlorpromazine and propranolol may increase if used concomitantly
- Some patients taking a neuroleptic and lithium have developed an encephalopathic syndrome similar to neuroleptic malignant syndrome

 Other Warnings/ Precautions
- If signs of neuroleptic malignant syndrome develop, treatment should be immediately discontinued

- Use cautiously in patients with alcohol withdrawal or convulsive disorders because of possible lowering of seizure threshold
- Use with caution in patients with respiratory disorders, glaucoma, or urinary retention
- Avoid extreme heat exposure
- Avoid undue exposure to sunlight
- Antiemetic effect of chlorpromazine may mask signs of other disorders or overdose; suppression of cough reflex may cause asphyxia
- Use only with caution if at all in Parkinson's disease or Lewy Body dementia

Do Not Use

- If patient is in a comatose state
- If patient is taking metrizamide or large doses of CNS depressants
- If there is a proven allergy to chlorpromazine
- If there is a known sensitivity to any phenothiazine

SPECIAL POPULATIONS

Renal Impairment
- Use with caution

Hepatic Impairment
- Use with caution

Cardiac Impairment
- Cardiovascular toxicity can occur, especially orthostatic hypotension

Elderly
- Lower doses should be used and patient should be monitored closely
- Often do not tolerate sedating actions of chlorpromazine

 Children and Adolescents
- Can be used cautiously in children or adolescents over 1 with severe behavioral problems
- Oral – 0.25 mg/lb every 4–6 hours as needed; rectal – 0.5 mg/lb every 6–8 hours as needed; IM – 0.25 mg/lb every

6–8 hours as needed; maximum 40 mg/day (under 5), 75 mg/day (5–12)
- Do not use if patient shows signs of Reye's syndrome
- Generally consider second-line after atypical antipsychotics

 Pregnancy
- Risk Category C [some animal studies show adverse effects, no controlled studies in humans]
- Reports of extrapyramidal symptoms, jaundice, hyperreflexia, hyporeflexia in infants whose mothers took a phenothiazine during pregnancy
- Chlorpromazine should generally not be used during the first trimester
- Chlorpromazine should only be used during pregnancy if clearly needed
- Psychotic symptoms may worsen during pregnancy and some form of treatment may be necessary
- Atypical antipsychotics may be preferable to conventional antipsychotics or anticonvulsant mood stabilizers if treatment is required during pregnancy

Breast Feeding
- Some drug is found in mother's breast milk
- Effects on infant have been observed (dystonia, tardive dyskinesia, sedation)
- ✳ Recommended either to discontinue drug or bottle feed

THE ART OF PSYCHOPHARMACOLOGY

Potential Advantages
- Intramuscular formulation for emergency use
- Patients who require sedation for behavioral control

Potential Disadvantages
- Patients with tardive dyskinesia
- Children
- Elderly
- Patients who wish to avoid sedation

Primary Target Symptoms
- Positive symptoms of psychosis
- Motor and autonomic hyperactivity
- Violent or aggressive behavior

Pearls

- Chlorpromazine is one of the earliest classical conventional antipsychotics
- Chlorpromazine has a broad spectrum of efficacy, but risk of tardive dyskinesia and the availability of alternative treatments make its utilization outside of psychosis a short-term and second-line treatment option
- Chlorpromazine is a low potency phenothiazine
- Sedative actions of low potency phenothiazines are an important aspect of their therapeutic actions in some patients and side effect profile in others
- Conventional antipsychotics are much less expensive than atypical antipsychotics
- Low potency phenothiazines like chlorpromazine have a greater risk of cardiovascular side effects

- Patients have very similar antipsychotic responses to any conventional antipsychotic, which is different from atypical antipsychotics where antipsychotic responses of individual patients can occasionally vary greatly from one atypical antipsychotic to another
- Patients with inadequate responses to atypical antipsychotics may benefit from a trial of augmentation with a conventional antipsychotic such as chlorpromazine or from switching to a conventional antipsychotic such as chlorpromazine
- However, long-term polypharmacy with a combination of a conventional antipsychotic such as chlorpromazine with an atypical antipsychotic may combine their side effects without clearly augmenting the efficacy of either

 Suggested Reading

Davis JM, Chen N, Glick ID. A meta-analysis of the efficacy of second-generation antipsychotics. Arch Gen Psychiatry 2003;60:553–64.

Frankenburg FR. Choices in antipsychotic therapy in schizophrenia. Harv Rev Psychiatry 1999;6:241–9.

Gocke E. Review of the genotoxic properties of chlorpromazine and related phenothiazines. Mutat Res 1996;366:9–21.

Leucht S, Wahlbeck K, Hamann J, Kissling W. New generation antipsychotics versus low-potency conventional antipsychotics: a systematic review and meta-analysis. The Lancet 2003;361:1581–9.

Thomley B, Adams CE, Awad G. Chlorpromazine versus placebo for schizophrenia. Cochrane Database Syst Rev 2000;(2):CD000284.

Tohen M, Jacobs TG, Feldman PD. Onset of action of antipsychotics in the treatment of mania. Bipolar Disord 2000;2(3 Pt 2):261–8.

CITALOPRAM

THERAPEUTICS

Brands • Celexa
see index for additional brand names

Generic? In Australia and some European countries, but not in U.S.

Class

- SSRI (selective serotonin reuptake inhibitor); often classified as an antidepressant, but it is not just an antidepressant

Commonly Prescribed For
(bold for FDA approved)

- **Depression**
- Premenstrual dysphoric disorder (PMDD)
- Obsessive-compulsive disorder (OCD)
- Panic disorder
- Generalized anxiety disorder
- Posttraumatic stress disorder (PTSD)
- Social anxiety disorder (social phobia)

How The Drug Works

- Boosts neurotransmitter serotonin
- Blocks serotonin reuptake pump (serotonin transporter)
- Desensitizes serotonin receptors, especially serotonin 1A autoreceptors
- Presumably increases serotonergic neurotransmission
- ✻ Citalopram also has mild antagonist actions at H1 histamine receptors
- ✻ Citalopram's inactive R enantiomer may interfere with the therapeutic actions of the active S enantiomer at serotonin reuptake pumps

How Long Until It Works

- Onset of therapeutic actions usually not immediate, but often delayed 2 to 4 weeks
- If it is not working within 6 to 8 weeks, it may require a dosage increase or it may not work at all
- May continue to work for many years to prevent relapse of symptoms

If It Works

- The goal of treatment is complete remission of current symptoms as well as prevention of future relapses

- Treatment most often reduces or even eliminates symptoms, but not a cure since symptoms can recur after medicine stopped
- Continue treatment until all symptoms are gone (remission) or significantly reduced (e.g., OCD, PTSD)
- Once symptoms are gone, continue treating for 1 year for the first episode of depression
- For second and subsequent episodes of depression, treatment may need to be indefinite
- Use in anxiety disorders may also need to be indefinite

If It Doesn't Work

- Many patients only have a partial response where some symptoms are improved but others persist (especially insomnia, fatigue, and problems concentrating in depression)
- Other patients may be nonresponders, sometimes called treatment-resistant or treatment-refractory
- Some patients who have an initial response may relapse even though they continue treatment, sometimes called "poop-out"
- Consider increasing dose, switching to another agent or adding an appropriate augmenting agent
- Consider psychotherapy
- Consider evaluation for another diagnosis or for a comorbid condition (e.g., medical illness, substance abuse, etc.)
- Some patients may experience apparent lack of consistent efficacy due to activation of latent or underlying bipolar disorder, and require antidepressant discontinuation and a switch to a mood stabilizer

Best Augmenting Combos for Partial Response or Treatment-Resistance

- Trazodone, especially for insomnia
- Bupropion, mirtazapine, reboxetine, or atomoxetine (add with caution and at lower doses since citalopram could theoretically raise atomoxetine levels); use combinations of antidepressants with caution as this may activate bipolar disorder and suicidal ideation
- Modafinil, especially for fatigue, sleepiness, and lack of concentration
- Mood stabilizers or atypical antipsychotics for bipolar depression, psychotic

depression, treatment-resistant depression, or treatment-resistant anxiety disorders
- Benzodiazepines
- If all else fails for anxiety disorders, consider gabapentin or tiagabine
- Hypnotics for insomnia
- Classically, lithium, buspirone, or thyroid hormone

Tests
- None for healthy individuals

SIDE EFFECTS

How Drug Causes Side Effects
- Theoretically due to increases in serotonin concentrations at serotonin receptors in parts of the brain and body other than those that cause therapeutic actions (e.g., unwanted actions of serotonin in sleep centers causing insomnia, unwanted actions of serotonin in the gut causing diarrhea, etc.)
- Increasing serotonin can cause diminished dopamine release and might contribute to emotional flattening, cognitive slowing, and apathy in some patients
- Most side effects are immediate but often go away with time, in contrast to most therapeutic effects which are delayed and are enhanced over time
- ✳ Citalopram's unique mild antihistamine properties may contribute to sedation and fatigue in some patients

Notable Side Effects
- Sexual dysfunction (men: delayed ejaculation, erectile dysfunction; men and women: decreased sexual desire, anorgasmia)
- Gastrointestinal (decreased appetite, nausea, diarrhea, constipation, dry mouth)
- Mostly central nervous system (insomnia but also sedation, agitation, tremors, headache, dizziness)
- Note: patients with diagnosed or undiagnosed bipolar or psychotic disorders may be more vulnerable to CNS-activating actions of SSRIs
- Autonomic (sweating)
- Bruising and rare bleeding
- Rare hyponatremia (mostly in elderly patients and generally reversible on discontinuation of citalopram)

- SIADH (syndrome of inappropriate antidiuretic hormone secretion)

 Life Threatening or Dangerous Side Effects
- Rare seizures
- Rare induction of mania and activation of suicidal ideation

Weight Gain

unusual   not unusual   common   problematic

- Reported but not expected
- Citalopram has been associated with both weight gain and weight loss in various studies, but is relatively weight neutral overall

Sedation

unusual   not unusual   common   problematic

- Occurs in significant minority

What To Do About Side Effects
- Wait
- Wait
- Wait
- Take in the morning if nighttime insomnia
- Take at night if daytime sedation
- In a few weeks, switch to another agent or add other drugs

Best Augmenting Agents for Side Effects
- Often best to try another SSRI or another antidepressant monotherapy prior to resorting to augmentation strategies to treat side effects
- Trazodone or a hypnotic for insomnia
- Bupropion, sildenafil, vardenafil, or tadalafil for sexual dysfunction
- Bupropion for emotional flattening, cognitive slowing, or apathy
- Mirtazapine for insomnia, agitation, and gastrointestinal side effects
- Benzodiazepines for jitteriness and anxiety, especially at initiation of treatment and especially for anxious patients
- Many side effects are dose-dependent (i.e., they increase as dose increases, or they reemerge until tolerance re-develops)
- Many side effects are time-dependent (i.e., they start immediately upon dosing and

upon each dose increase, but go away with time)
• Activation and agitation may represent the induction of a bipolar state, especially a mixed dysphoric bipolar II condition sometimes associated with suicidal ideation, and require the addition of lithium, a mood stabilizer or an atypical antipsychotic, and/or discontinuation of citalopram

DOSING AND USE

Usual Dosage Range
• 20–60 mg/day

Dosage Forms
• Tablets 10 mg, 20 mg scored, 40 mg scored

How to Dose
• Initial 20 mg/day; increase by 20 mg/day after 1 or more weeks until desired efficacy is reached; maximum usually 60 mg/day; single dose administration, morning or evening

 Dosing Tips
• Tablets are scored, so to save costs, give 10 mg as half of 20 mg tablet or 20 mg as half of 40 mg tablet, since the tablets cost about the same in many markets
• Many patients respond better to 40 mg than to 20 mg
• Given once daily, any time of day when best tolerated by the individual
• If intolerable anxiety, insomnia, agitation, akathisia, or activation occur either upon dosing initiation or discontinuation, consider the possibility of activated bipolar disorder and switch to a mood stabilizer or an atypical antipsychotic

Overdose
• Rare fatalities have been reported with citalopram overdose, both alone and in combination with other drugs
• Vomiting, sedation, heart rhythm disturbances, dizziness, sweating, nausea, tremor
• Rarely amnesia, confusion, coma, convulsions

Long-Term Use
• Safe

Habit Forming
• No

How to Stop
• Taper not usually necessary
• However, tapering to avoid potential withdrawal reactions generally prudent
• Many patients tolerate 50% dose reduction for 3 days, then another 50% reduction for 3 days, then discontinuation
• If withdrawal symptoms emerge during discontinuation, raise dose to stop symptoms and then restart withdrawal much more slowly

Pharmacokinetics
• Parent drug has 23–45 hour half-life
• Weak inhibitor of CYP450 2D6

 Drug Interactions
• Tramadol increases the risk of seizures in patients taking an antidepressant
• Can increase tricyclic antidepressant levels; use with caution with tricyclic antidepressants
• Can cause a fatal "serotonin syndrome" when combined with MAO inhibitors, so do not use with MAO inhibitors or at least for 14 days after MAOIs are stopped
• Do not start an MAO inhibitor for at least 2 weeks after discontinuing citalopram
• May displace highly protein bound drugs (e.g., warfarin)
• Can rarely cause weakness, hyperreflexia, and incoordination when combined with sumatriptan or possibly other triptans, requiring careful monitoring of patient
• Via CYP450 2D6 inhibition, citalopram could theoretically interfere with the analgesic actions of codeine, and increase the plasma levels of some beta blockers and of atomoxetine
• Via CYP450 2D6 inhibition, citalopram could theoretically increase concentrations of thioridazine and cause dangerous cardiac arrhythmias

Other Warnings/ Precautions

- Use with caution in patients with history of seizures
- Use with caution in patients with bipolar disorder unless treated with concomitant mood stabilizing agent
- Monitor patients for activation of suicidal ideation, especially children and adolescents

Do Not Use

- If patient is taking an MAO inhibitor
- If patient is taking thioridazine
- If there is a proven allergy to citalopram or escitalopram

SPECIAL POPULATIONS

Renal Impairment

- No dose adjustment for mild to moderate impairment
- Use cautiously in patients with severe impairment

Hepatic Impairment

- Recommended dose 20 mg/day; can be raised to 40 mg/day for nonresponders
- May need to dose cautiously at the lower end of the dose range in some patients for maximal tolerability

Cardiac Impairment

- Clinical experience suggests that citalopram is safe in these patients
- Treating depression with SSRIs in patients with acute angina or following myocardial infarction may reduce cardiac events and improve survival as well as mood

Elderly

- 20 mg/day; 40 mg/day for nonresponders
- May need to dose at the lower end of the dose range in some patients for maximal tolerability
- Citalopram may be an especially well-tolerated SSRI in the elderly

 Children and Adolescents

- Use with caution, observing for activation of known or unknown bipolar disorder and/or suicidal ideation, and strongly consider informing parents or guardian of this risk so they can help observe child or adolescent patients
- Not specifically approved, but preliminary data suggest citalopram is safe and effective in children and adolescents with OCD and with depression

 Pregnancy

- Risk Category C [some animal studies show adverse effects, no controlled studies in humans]
- Not generally recommended for use during pregnancy, especially during first trimester
- Nonetheless, continuous treatment during pregnancy may be necessary and has not been proven to be harmful to the fetus
- At delivery there may be more bleeding in the mother and transient irritability or sedation in the newborn
- Must weigh the risk of treatment (first trimester fetal development, third trimester newborn delivery) to the child against the risk of no treatment (recurrence of depression, maternal health, infant bonding) to the mother and child
- For many patients, this may mean continuing treatment during pregnancy
- Neonates exposed to SSRIs or SNRIs late in the third trimester have developed complications requiring prolonged hospitalization, respiratory support, and tube feeding; reported symptoms are consistent with either a direct toxic effect of SSRIs and SNRIs or, possibly, a drug discontinuation syndrome, and include respiratory distress, cyanosis, apnea, seizures, temperature instability, feeding difficulty, vomiting, hypoglycemia, hypotonia, hypertonia, hyperreflexia, tremor, jitteriness, irritability, and constant crying

Breast Feeding

- Some drug is found in mother's breast milk
- Trace amounts may be present in nursing children whose mothers are on citalopram
- If child becomes irritable or sedated, breast feeding or drug may need to be discontinued
- Immediate postpartum period is a high-risk time for depression, especially in women who have had prior depressive episodes,

so drug may need to be reinstituted late in the third trimester or shortly after childbirth to prevent a recurrence during the postpartum period
• Must weigh benefits of breast feeding with risks and benefits of antidepressant treatment versus non-treatment to both the infant and the mother
• For many patients, this may mean continuing treatment during breast feeding

THE ART OF PSYCHOPHARMACOLOGY

Potential Advantages
• Elderly patients
• Patients excessively activated or sedated by other SSRIs

Potential Disadvantages
• May require dosage titration to attain optimal efficacy
• Can be sedating in some patients

Primary Target Symptoms
• Depressed mood
• Anxiety
• Panic attacks, avoidant behavior, re-experiencing, hyperarousal
• Sleep disturbance, both insomnia and hypersomnia

 Pearls

✻ May be more tolerable than some other antidepressants
• May have less sexual dysfunction than some other SSRIs
• May be especially well tolerated in the elderly
✻ May be less well tolerated than escitalopram
• Documentation of efficacy in anxiety disorders is less comprehensive than for escitalopram and other SSRIs
• Can cause cognitive and affective "flattening"
• Some evidence suggests that citalopram treatment during only the luteal phase may be more effective than continuous treatment for patients with PMDD
• SSRIs may be less effective in women over 50, especially if they are not taking estrogen
• SSRIs may be useful for hot flushes in perimenopausal women
• Nonresponse to citalopram in elderly may require consideration of mild cognitive impairment or Alzheimer disease

 Suggested Reading

Bezchlibnyk-Butler K, Aleksic I, Kennedy SH. Citalopram – a review of pharmacological and clinical effects. Journal of Psychiatry and Neuroscience 2000;25:241–254.

Edwards JG, Anderson I. Systematic review and guide to selection of selective serotonin reuptake inhibitors. Drugs 1999;57:507–533.

Keller MB. Citalopram therapy for depression: a review of 10 years of European experience and data from U.S. clinical trials. Journal of Clinical Psychiatry 2000;61:896–908.

Pollock BG. Citalopram: a comprehensive review. Expert Opin Pharmacother 2001;2:681–98.

Stahl SM. Placebo-controlled comparison of the selective serotonin reuptake inhibitors citalopram and sertraline. Biol Psychiatry 2000;48:894–901.

CLOMIPRAMINE

Brands • Anafranil
see index for additional brand names

Generic? Yes

Class

- Tricyclic antidepressant (TCA)
- Parent drug is a potent serotonin reuptake inhibitor
- Active metabolite is a potent norepinephrine/noradrenaline reuptake inhibitor

Commonly Prescribed For

(bold for FDA approved)
* **Obsessive-compulsive disorder**
- Depression
* Severe and treatment-resistant depression
* Cataplexy syndrome
- Anxiety
- Insomnia
- Neuropathic pain/chronic pain

How The Drug Works

- Boosts neurotransmitters serotonin and norepinephrine/noradrenaline
- Blocks serotonin reuptake pump (serotonin transporter), presumably increasing serotonergic neurotransmission
- Blocks norepinephrine reuptake pump (norepinephrine transporter), presumably increasing noradrenergic neurotransmission
- Presumably desensitizes both serotonin 1A receptors and beta adrenergic receptors
- Since dopamine is inactivated by norepinephrine reuptake in frontal cortex, which largely lacks dopamine transporters, clomipramine can increase dopamine neurotransmission in this part of the brain

How Long Until It Works

- May have immediate effects in treating insomnia or anxiety
- Onset of therapeutic actions in depression usually not immediate, but often delayed 2 to 4 weeks
- Onset of therapeutic action in OCD can be delayed 6 to 12 weeks

- If it is not working within 6 to 8 weeks for depression, it may require a dosage increase or it may not work at all
- If it is not working within 12 weeks for OCD, it may not work at all
- May continue to work for many years to prevent relapse of symptoms

If It Works

- The goal of treatment of depression is complete remission of current symptoms as well as prevention of future relapses
- Treatment most often reduces or even eliminates symptoms, but not a cure since symptoms can recur after medicine stopped
- Although the goal of treatment of OCD is also complete remission of symptoms, this may be less likely than in depression
- The goal of treatment of chronic neuropathic pain is to reduce symptoms as much as possible, especially in combination with other treatments
- Continue treatment of depression until all symptoms are gone (remission)
- Once symptoms of depression are gone, continue treating for 1 year for the first episode of depression
- For second and subsequent episodes of depression, treatment may need to be indefinite
- Use in OCD may also need to be indefinite, starting from the time of initial treatment
- Use in other anxiety disorders and chronic pain may also need to be indefinite, but long-term treatment is not well studied in these conditions

If It Doesn't Work

- Many patients only have a partial response where some symptoms are improved but others persist (especially insomnia, fatigue, and problems concentrating)
- Other patients may be nonresponders, sometimes called treatment-resistant or treatment-refractory
- Consider increasing dose, switching to another agent or adding an appropriate augmenting agent
- Consider psychotherapy, especially behavioral therapy in OCD
- Consider evaluation for another diagnosis or for a comorbid condition (e.g., medical illness, substance abuse, etc.)
- Some patients may experience apparent lack of consistent efficacy due to activation

of latent or underlying bipolar disorder, and require antidepressant discontinuation and a switch to a mood stabilizer

 Best Augmenting Combos for Partial Response or Treatment-Resistance

- Lithium, buspirone, hormone (for depression and OCD)
- For the expert: consider cautious addition of fluvoxamine for treatment-resistant OCD
- Thyroid hormone (for depression)
- Atypical antipsychotics (for OCD)

Tests

* None for healthy individuals, although monitoring of plasma drug levels is potentially available at specialty laboratories for the expert
* Since tricyclic and tetracyclic antidepressants are frequently associated with weight gain, before starting treatment, weigh all patients and determine if the patient is already overweight (BMI 25.0–29.9) or obese (BMI ≥30)
- Before giving a drug that can cause weight gain to an overweight or obese patient, consider determining whether the patient already has pre-diabetes (fasting plasma glucose 100–125 mg/dl), diabetes (fasting plasma glucose >126 mg/dl), or dyslipidemia (increased total cholesterol, LDL cholesterol and triglycerides; decreased HDL cholesterol), and treat or refer such patients for treatment, including nutrition and weight management, physical activity counseling, smoking cessation, and medical management
* Monitor weight and BMI during treatment
* While giving a drug to a patient who has gained >5% of initial weight, consider evaluating for the presence of pre-diabetes, diabetes, or dyslipidemia, or consider switching to a different antidepressant
- EKGs may be useful for selected patients (e.g., those with personal or family history of QTc prolongation; cardiac arrhythmia; recent myocardial infarction; uncompensated heart failure; or taking agents that prolong QTc interval such as pimozide, thioridazine, selected antiarrhythmics, moxifloxacin, sparfloxacin, etc.)
- Patients at risk for electrolyte disturbances (e.g., patients on diuretic therapy) should have baseline and periodic serum potassium and magnesium measurements

How Drug Causes Side Effects

- Anticholinergic activity may explain sedative effects, dry mouth, constipation, and blurred vision
- Sedative effects and weight gain may be due to antihistamine properties
- Blockade of alpha adrenergic 1 receptors may explain dizziness, sedation, and hypotension
- Cardiac arrhythmias and seizures, especially in overdose, may be caused by blockade of ion channels

Notable Side Effects

- Blurred vision, constipation, urinary retention, increased appetite, dry mouth, nausea, diarrhea, heartburn, unusual taste in mouth, weight gain
- Fatigue, weakness, dizziness, sedation, headache, anxiety, nervousness, restlessness
- Sexual dysfunction, sweating

 Life Threatening or Dangerous Side Effects

- Paralytic ileus, hyperthermia (TCAs + anticholinergic agents)
- Lowered seizure threshold and rare seizures
- Orthostatic hypotension, sudden death, arrhythmias, tachycardia
- QTc prolongation
- Hepatic failure, extrapyramidal symptoms
- Increased intraocular pressure
- Rare induction of mania and activation of suicidal ideation

Weight Gain

unusual   not unusual   **common**   problematic

- Many experience and/or can be significant in amount
- Can increase appetite and carbohydrate craving

Sedation

unusual   not unusual   **common**   problematic

- Many experience and/or can be significant in amount
- Tolerance to sedative effect may develop with long-term use

What To Do About Side Effects
- Wait
- Wait
- Wait
- Lower the dose
- Switch to an SSRI or newer antidepressant

Best Augmenting Agents for Side Effects
- Many side effects cannot be improved with an augmenting agent

DOSING AND USE

Usual Dosage Range
- 100 mg/day – 200 mg/day

Dosage Forms
- Capsule 25 mg, 50 mg, 75 mg

How to Dose
- Initial 25 mg/day; increase over 2 weeks to 100 mg/day; maximum dose generally 250 mg/day

 Dosing Tips
- If given in a single dose, should generally be administered at bedtime because of its sedative properties
- If given in split doses, largest dose should generally be given at bedtime because of its sedative properties
- If patients experience nightmares, split dose and do not give large dose at bedtime
- Patients treated for chronic pain may only require lower doses
- ✱ Patients treated for OCD may often require doses at the high end of the range (e.g., 200–250 mg/day)
- Risk of seizure increases with dose, especially with clomipramine at doses above 250 mg/day
- ✱ Dose of 300 mg may be associated with up to 7/1000 incidence of seizures, a generally unacceptable risk
- If intolerable anxiety, insomnia, agitation, akathisia, or activation occur either upon dosing initiation or discontinuation, consider the possibility of activated bipolar disorder, and switch to a mood stabilizer or an atypical antipsychotic

Overdose
- Death may occur; convulsions, cardiac dysrhythmias, severe hypotension, CNS depression, coma, changes in ECG

Long-Term Use
- Limited data but appears to be efficacious and safe long-term

Habit Forming
- No

How to Stop
- Taper to avoid withdrawal effects
- Even with gradual dose reduction some withdrawal symptoms may appear within the first 2 weeks
- Many patients tolerate 50% dose reduction for 3 days, then another 50% reduction for 3 days, then discontinuation
- If withdrawal symptoms emerge during discontinuation, raise dose to stop symptoms and then restart withdrawal much more slowly

Pharmacokinetics
- Substrate for CYP450 2D6 and 1A2
- Metabolized to an active metabolite, desmethyl-clomipramine, a predominantly norepinephrine reuptake inhibitor, by demethylation via CYP450 1A2
- Half-life approximately 17–28 hours

 Drug Interactions
- Tramadol increases the risk of seizures in patients taking TCAs
- Use of TCAs with anticholinergic drugs may result in paralytic ileus or hyperthermia
- Fluoxetine, paroxetine, bupropion, duloxetine, and other CYP450 2D6 inhibitors may increase TCA concentrations
- Fluvoxamine, a CYP450 1A2 inhibitor, can decrease the conversion of clomipramine to desmethyl-clomipramine, and increase clomipramine plasma concentrations
- Cimetidine may increase plasma concentrations of TCAs and cause anticholinergic symptoms
- Phenothiazines or haloperidol may raise TCA blood concentrations
- May alter effects of antihypertensive drugs
- Use of TCAs with sympathomimetic agents may increase sympathetic activity

- TCAs may inhibit hypotensive effects of clonidine
- Methylphenidate may inhibit metabolism of TCAs
- Activation and agitation, especially following switching or adding antidepressants, may represent the induction of a bipolar state, especially a mixed dysphoric bipolar II condition sometimes associated with suicidal ideation, and require the addition of lithium, a mood stabilizer or an atypical antipsychotic, and/or discontinuation of clomipramine

 Other Warnings/ Precautions

- Add or initiate other antidepressants with caution for up to 2 weeks after discontinuing clomipramine
- Generally, do not use with MAO inhibitors, including 14 days after MAOIs are stopped; do not start an MAOI until 2 weeks after discontinuing clomipramine, but see Pearls
- Use with caution in patients with history of seizures, urinary retention, narrow angle-closure glaucoma, hyperthyroidism
- TCAs can increase QTc interval, especially at toxic doses, which can be attained not only by overdose but also by combining with drugs that inhibit TCA metabolism via CYP450 2D6, potentially causing torsade de pointes-type arrhythmia or sudden death
- Because TCAs can prolong QTc interval, use with caution in patients who have bradycardia or who are taking drugs that can induce bradycardia (e.g., beta blockers, calcium channel blockers, clonidine, digitalis)
- Because TCAs can prolong QTc interval, use with caution in patients who have hypokalemia and/or hypomagnesemia or who are taking drugs that can induce hypokalemia and/or magnesemia (e.g., diuretics, stimulant laxatives, intravenous amphotericin B, glucocorticoids, tetracosactide)

Do Not Use

- If patient is recovering from myocardial infarction
- If patient is taking agents capable of significantly prolonging QTc interval (e.g., pimozide, thioridazine, selected antiarrhythmics, moxifloxacin, sparfloxacin)
- If there is a history of QTc prolongation or cardiac arrhythmia, recent acute myocardial infarction, uncompensated heart failure
- If patient is taking drugs that inhibit TCA metabolism, including CYP450 2D6 inhibitors, except by an expert
- If there is reduced CYP450 2D6 function, such as patients who are poor 2D6 metabolizers, except by an expert and at low doses
- If there is a proven allergy to clomipramine

Renal Impairment
- Use with caution

Hepatic Impairment
- Use with caution

Cardiac Impairment
- TCAs have been reported to cause arrhythmias, prolongation of conduction time, orthostatic hypotension, sinus tachycardia, and heart failure, especially in the diseased heart
- Myocardial infarction and stroke have been reported with TCAs
- TCAs produce QTc prolongation, which may be enhanced by the existence of bradycardia, hypokalemia, congenital or acquired long QTc interval, which should be evaluated prior to administering clomipramine
- Use with caution if treating concomitantly with a medication likely to produce prolonged bradycardia, hypokalemia, slowing of intracardiac conduction, or prolongation of the QTc interval
- Avoid TCAs in patients with a known history of QTc prolongation, recent acute myocardial infarction, and uncompensated heart failure
- TCAs may cause a sustained increase in heart rate in patients with ischemic heart disease and may worsen (decrease) heart rate variability, an independent risk of mortality in cardiac populations
- Since SSRIs may improve (increase) heart rate variability in patients following a

myocardial infarct and may improve survival as well as mood in patients with acute angina or following a myocardial infarction, these are more appropriate agents for cardiac population than tricyclic/tetracyclic antidepressants

✱ Risk/benefit ratio may not justify use of TCAs in cardiac impairment

Elderly
• May be more sensitive to anticholinergic, cardiovascular, hypotensive, and sedative effects
• Dose may need to be lower than usual adult dose, at least initially

Children and Adolescents
• Use with caution, observing for activation of known or unknown bipolar disorder and/or suicidal ideation, and strongly consider informing parents or guardian of this risk so they can help observe child or adolescent patients
• Not recommended for use under age 10
• Several studies show lack of efficacy of TCAs for depression
• May be used to treat enuresis or hyperactive/impulsive behaviors
• Effective for OCD in children
• Some cases of sudden death have occurred in children taking TCAs
• Dose in children/adolescents should be titrated to a maximum of 100 mg/day or 3 mg/kg/day after 2 weeks, after which dose can then be titrated up to a maximum of 200 mg/day or 3 mg/kg/day

Pregnancy
• Risk Category C [some animal studies show adverse effects, no controlled studies in humans]
• Clomipramine crosses the placenta
• Adverse effects have been reported in infants whose mothers took a TCA (lethargy, withdrawal symptoms, fetal malformations)
• Must weigh the risk of treatment (first trimester fetal development, third trimester newborn delivery) to the child against the risk of no treatment (recurrence of depression, worsening of OCD, maternal

health, infant bonding) to the mother and child
• For many patients this may mean continuing treatment during pregnancy

Breast Feeding
• Some drug is found in mother's breast milk
✱ Recommended either to discontinue drug or bottle feed
• Immediate postpartum period is a high-risk time for depression and worsening of OCD, especially in women who have had prior depressive episodes or OCD symptoms, so drug may need to be reinstituted late in the third trimester or shortly after childbirth to prevent a recurrence or exacerbation during the postpartum period
• Must weigh benefits of breast feeding with risks and benefits of antidepressant treatment versus non-treatment to both the infant and the mother
• For many patients this may mean continuing treatment during breast feeding

THE ART OF PSYCHOPHARMACOLOGY

Potential Advantages
• Patients with insomnia
• Severe or treatment-resistant depression
• Patients with comorbid OCD and depression
• Patients with cataplexy

Potential Disadvantages
• Pediatric and geriatric patients
• Patients concerned with weight gain
• Cardiac patients
• Patients with seizure disorders

Primary Target Symptoms
• Depressed mood
• Obsessive thoughts
• Compulsive behaviors

Pearls
✱ The only TCA with proven efficacy in OCD
• Normally, clomipramine (CMI), a potent serotonin reuptake blocker, at steady state is metabolized extensively to its active metabolite desmethyl-clomipramine (de-CMI), a potent nonadrenaline reuptake blocker, by the enzyme CYP450 1A2

- Thus, at steady state, plasma drug activity is generally more noradrenergic (with higher de-CMI levels) than serotonergic (with lower parent CMI levels)
- Addition of the SSRI and CYP450 1A2 inhibitor fluvoxamine blocks this conversion and results in higher CMI levels than de-CMI levels
- For the expert only: addition of the SSRI fluvoxamine to CMI in treatment-resistant OCD can powerfully enhance serotonergic activity, not only due to the inherent additive pharmacodynamic serotonergic activity of fluvoxamine added to CMI, but also due to a favorable pharmacokinetic interaction inhibiting CYP450 1A2 and thus converting CMI's metabolism to a more powerful serotonergic portfolio of parent drug
* One of the most favored TCAs for treating severe depression
- Tricyclic antidepressants are no longer generally considered a first-line treatment option for depression because of their side effect profile
- Tricyclic antidepressants continue to be useful for severe or treatment-resistant depression
- Tricyclic antidepressants are often a first-line treatment option for chronic pain
* Unique among TCAs, clomipramine has a potentially fatal interaction with MAOIs in addition to the danger of hypertension characteristic of all MAOI-TCA combinations
* A potentially fatal serotonin syndrome with high fever, seizures, and coma, analogous to that caused by SSRIs and MAOIs, can occur with clomipramine and SSRIs, presumably due to clomipramine's potent serotonin reuptake blocking properties
- TCAs may aggravate psychotic symptoms
- Alcohol should be avoided because of additive CNS effects
- Underweight patients may be more susceptible to adverse cardiovascular effects
- Children, patients with inadequate hydration, and patients with cardiac disease may be more susceptible to TCA-induced cardiotoxicity than healthy adults
- Patients on TCAs should be aware that they may experience symptoms such as photosensitivity or blue-green urine
- SSRIs may be more effective than TCAs in women, and TCAs may be more effective than SSRIs in men
- Since tricyclic/tetracyclic antidepressants are substrates for CYP450 2D6, and 7% of the population (especially Caucasians) may have a genetic variant leading to reduced activity of 2D6, such patients may not safely tolerate normal doses of tricyclic/tetracyclic antidepressants and may require dose reduction
- Phenotypic testing may be necessary to detect this genetic variant prior to dosing with a tricyclic/tetracyclic antidepressant, especially in vulnerable populations such as children, elderly, cardiac populations, and those on concomitant medications
- Patients who seem to have extraordinarily severe side effects at normal or low doses may have this phenotypic CYP450 2D6 variant and require low doses or switching to another antidepressant not metabolized by 2D6

 Suggested Reading

Anderson IM. Meta-analytical studies on new antidepressants. Br Med Bull 2001; 57:161–178.

Anderson IM. Selective serotonin reuptake inhibitors versus tricyclic antidepressants: a meta-analysis of efficacy and tolerability. J Aff Disorders 2000;58:19–36.

Cox BJ, Swinson RP, Morrison B, Lee PS. Clomipramine, fluoxetine, and behavior therapy in the treatment of obsessive-compulsive disorder: a meta-analysis. J Behav Ther Exp Psychiatry 1993;24:149–53.

Feinberg M. Clomipramine for obsessive-compulsive disorder. Am Fam Physician 1991; 43:1735–8.

CLONAZEPAM

THERAPEUTICS

Brands • Klonopin
see index for additional brand names

Generic? Yes (not for disintegrating wafer)

 Class
• Benzodiazepine (anxiolytic, anticonvulsant)

Commonly Prescribed For
(bold for FDA approved)
• **Panic disorder, with or without agoraphobia**
• **Lennox-Gastaut syndrome (petit mal variant)**
• **Akinetic seizure**
• **Myoclonic seizure**
• **Absence seizure (petit mal)**
• Atonic seizures
• Other seizure disorders
• Other anxiety disorders
• Acute mania (adjunctive)
• Acute psychosis (adjunctive)
• Insomnia

 How The Drug Works
• Binds to benzodiazepine receptors at the GABA-A ligand-gated chloride channel complex
• Enhances the inhibitory effects of GABA
• Boosts chloride conductance through GABA-regulated channels
• Inhibits neuronal activity presumably in amygdala-centered fear circuits to provide therapeutic benefits in anxiety disorders
• Inhibitory actions in cerebral cortex may provide therapeutic benefits in seizure disorders

How Long Until It Works
• Some immediate relief with first dosing is common; can take several weeks with daily dosing for maximal therapeutic benefit

If It Works
• For short-term symptoms of anxiety – after a few weeks, discontinue use or use on an "as-needed" basis
• For chronic anxiety disorders, the goal of treatment is complete remission of symptoms as well as prevention of future relapses

• For chronic anxiety disorders, treatment most often reduces or even eliminates symptoms, but not a cure since symptoms can recur after medicine stopped
• For long-term symptoms of anxiety, consider switching to an SSRI or SNRI for long-term maintenance
• If long-term maintenance with a benzodiazepine is necessary, continue treatment for 6 months after symptoms resolve, and then taper dose slowly
• If symptoms reemerge, consider treatment with an SSRI or SNRI, or consider restarting the benzodiazepine; sometimes benzodiazepines have to be used in combination with SSRIs or SNRIs for best results
• For long-term treatment of seizure disorders, development of tolerance dose escalation and loss of efficacy necessitating adding or switching to other anticonvulsants is not uncommon

If It Doesn't Work
• Consider switching to another agent or adding an appropriate augmenting agent
• Consider psychotherapy, especially cognitive behavioral psychotherapy
• Consider presence of concomitant substance abuse
• Consider presence of clonazepam abuse
• Consider another diagnosis such as a comorbid medical condition

 Best Augmenting Combos for Partial Response or Treatment-Resistance
• Benzodiazepines are frequently used as augmenting agents for antipsychotics and mood stabilizers in the treatment of psychotic and bipolar disorders
• Benzodiazepines are frequently used as augmenting agents for SSRIs and SNRIs in the treatment of anxiety disorders
• Not generally rational to combine with other benzodiazepines
• Caution if using as an anxiolytic concomitantly with other sedative hypnotics for sleep
• Clonazepam is commonly combined with other anticonvulsants for the treatment of seizure disorders

Tests
- In patients with seizure disorders, concomitant medical illness, and/or those with multiple concomitant long-term medications, periodic liver tests and blood counts may be prudent

SIDE EFFECTS

How Drug Causes Side Effects
- Same mechanism for side effects as for therapeutic effects – namely due to excessive actions at benzodiazepine receptors
- Long-term adaptations in benzodiazepine receptors may explain the development of dependence, tolerance, and withdrawal
- Side effects are generally immediate, but immediate side effects often disappear in time

Notable Side Effects
- ❋ Sedation, fatigue, depression
- ❋ Dizziness, ataxia, slurred speech, weakness
- ❋ Forgetfulness, confusion
- ❋ Hyper-excitability, nervousness
- Rare hallucinations, mania
- Rare hypotension
- Hypersalivation, dry mouth

Life Threatening or Dangerous Side Effects
- Respiratory depression, especially when taken with CNS depressants in overdose
- Rare hepatic dysfunction, renal dysfunction, blood dyscrasias
- Grand mal seizures

Weight Gain

unusual   not unusual   common   problematic

- Reported but not expected

Sedation

unusual   not unusual   common   problematic

- Occurs in significant minority
- Especially at initiation of treatment or when dose increases
- Tolerance often develops over time

What To Do About Side Effects
- Wait
- Wait
- Wait
- Lower the dose
- Take largest dose at bedtime to avoid sedative effects during the day
- Switch to another agent
- Administer flumazenil if side effects are severe or life-threatening

Best Augmenting Agents for Side Effects
- Many side effects cannot be improved with an augmenting agent

DOSING AND USE

Usual Dosage Range
- Seizures: dependent on individual response of patient, up to 20 mg/day
- Panic: 0.5–2 mg/day either as divided doses or once at bedtime

Dosage Forms
- Tablet 0.5 mg scored, 1 mg, 2 mg
- Disintegrating (wafer): 0.125 mg, 0.25 mg, 0.5 mg, 1 mg, 2 mg

How to Dose
- Seizures – 1.5 mg divided into 3 doses, raise by 0.5 mg every 3 days until desired effect is reached; divide into 3 even doses or else give largest dose at bedtime; maximum dose generally 20 mg/day
- Panic – 1 mg/day; start at 0.25 mg divided into 2 doses, raise to 1 mg after 3 days; dose either twice daily or once at bedtime; maximum dose generally 4 mg/day

Dosing Tips
- For anxiety disorders, use lowest possible effective dose for the shortest possible period of time (a benzodiazepine sparing strategy)
- Assess need for continuous treatment regularly
- Risk of dependence may increase with dose and duration of treatment
- For inter-dose symptoms of anxiety, can either increase dose or maintain same daily dose but divide into more frequent doses

- Can also use an as-needed occasional "top-up" dose for inter-dose anxiety
- Because seizure disorder can require doses much higher than 2 mg/day, the risk of dependence may be greater in these patients
- Because panic disorder can require doses somewhat higher than 2 mg/day, the risk of dependence may be greater in these patients than in anxiety patients maintained at lower doses
- Some severely ill seizure patients may require more than 20 mg/day
- Some severely ill panic patients may require 4 mg/day or more
- Frequency of dosing in practice is often greater than predicted from half-life, as duration of biological activity is often shorter than pharmacokinetic terminal half-life
* Clonazepam is generally dosed half the dosage of alprazolam
- Escalation of dose may be necessary if tolerance develops in seizure disorders
- Escalation of dose usually not necessary in anxiety disorders, as tolerance to clonazepam does not generally develop in the treatment of anxiety disorders
* Available as an oral disintegrating wafer

Overdose
- Rarely fatal in monotherapy; sedation, confusion, coma, diminished reflexes

Long-Term Use
- May lose efficacy for seizures; dose increase may restore efficacy
- Risk of dependence, particularly for treatment periods longer than 12 weeks and especially in patients with past or current polysubstance abuse

Habit Forming
- Clonazepam is a Schedule IV drug
- Patients may develop dependence and/or tolerance with long-term use

How to Stop
- Patients with history of seizures may seize upon withdrawal, especially if withdrawal is abrupt
- Taper by 0.25 mg every 3 days to reduce chances of withdrawal effects
- For difficult to taper cases, consider reducing dose much more slowly after

reaching 1.5 mg/day, perhaps by as little as 0.125 mg per week or less
- For other patients with severe problems discontinuing a benzodiazepine, dosing may need to be tapered over many months (i.e., reduce dose by 1% every 3 days by crushing tablet and suspending or dissolving in 100 ml of fruit juice and then disposing of 1 ml while drinking the rest; 3–7 days later, dispose of 2 ml, and so on). This is both a form of very slow biological tapering and a form of behavioral desensitization
- Be sure to differentiate reemergence of symptoms requiring reinstitution of treatment from withdrawal symptoms
- Benzodiazepine-dependent anxiety patients and insulin-dependent diabetics are not addicted to their medications. When benzodiazepine-dependent patients stop their medication, disease symptoms can reemerge, disease symptoms can worsen (rebound), and/or withdrawal symptoms can emerge

Pharmacokinetics
- Long half-life compared to other benzodiazepine anxiolytics (elimination half-life approximately 30–40 hours)

 Drug Interactions
- Increased depressive effects when taken with other CNS depressants
- Inhibitors of CYP450 3A4 may affect the clearance of clonazepam, but dosage adjustment usually not necessary
- Flumazenil (used to reverse the effects of benzodiazepines) may precipitate seizures and should not be used in patients treated for seizure disorders with clonazepam
- Use of clonazepam with valproate may cause absence status

 Other Warnings/ Precautions
- Dosage changes should be made in collaboration with prescriber
- Use with caution in patients with pulmonary disease; rare reports of death after initiation of benzodiazepines in patients with severe pulmonary impairment
- History of drug or alcohol abuse often creates greater risk for dependency

- Clonazepam may induce grand mal seizures in patients with multiple seizure disorders
- Use only with extreme caution if patient has obstructive sleep apnea
- Some depressed patients may experience a worsening of suicidal ideation
- Some patients may exhibit abnormal thinking or behavioral changes similar to those caused by other CNS depressants (i.e., either depressant actions or disinhibiting actions)

Do Not Use
- If patient has narrow angle-closure glaucoma
- If patient has severe liver disease
- If there is a proven allergy to clonazepam or any benzodiazepine

SPECIAL POPULATIONS

Renal Impairment
- Dose should be reduced

Hepatic Impairment
- Dose should be reduced

Cardiac Impairment
- Benzodiazepines have been used to treat anxiety associated with acute myocardial infarction

Elderly
- Should receive lower doses and be monitored

Children and Adolescents
- Seizures – up to 10 years or 30 kg – 0.01–0.03 mg/kg/day divided into 2–3 doses; maximum dose 0.05 mg/kg/day
- Safety and efficacy not established in panic disorder
- For anxiety, children and adolescents should generally receive lower doses and be more closely monitored
- Long-term effects of clonazepam in children/adolescents are unknown

Pregnancy
- Risk Category D [positive evidence of risk to human fetus; potential benefits may still justify its use during pregnancy, especially for seizure disorders]
- Possible increased risk of birth defects when benzodiazepines taken during pregnancy
- Because of the potential risks, clonazepam is not generally recommended as treatment for anxiety during pregnancy, especially during the first trimester
- Drug should be tapered if discontinued
- Infants whose mothers received a benzodiazepine late in pregnancy may experience withdrawal effects
- Neonatal flaccidity has been reported in infants whose mothers took a benzodiazepine during pregnancy
- Seizures, even mild seizures, may cause harm to the embryo/fetus

Breast Feeding
- Some drug is found in mother's breast milk
- ✳ Recommended either to discontinue drug or bottle feed
- Effects on infant have been observed and include feeding difficulties, sedation, and weight loss

THE ART OF PSYCHOPHARMACOLOGY

Potential Advantages
- Rapid onset of action
- Less sedation than some other benzodiazepines
- Longer duration of action than some other benzodiazepines
- Availability of oral disintegrating wafer

Potential Disadvantages
- Development of tolerance may require dose increases, especially in seizure disorders
- Abuse especially risky in past or present substance abusers

Primary Target Symptoms
- Frequency and duration of seizures
- Spike and wave discharges in absence seizures (petit mal)
- Panic attacks
- Anxiety

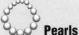 **Pearls**

❋ One of the most popular benzodiazepines for anxiety, especially among psychiatrists
• Is a very useful adjunct to SSRIs and SNRIs in the treatment of numerous anxiety disorders
• Not effective for treating psychosis as a monotherapy, but can be used as an adjunct to antipsychotics
• Not effective for treating bipolar disorder as a monotherapy, but can be used as an adjunct to mood stabilizers and antipsychotics
• Generally used as second-line treatment for petit mal seizures if succinimides are ineffective
• Can be used as an adjunct or as monotherapy for seizure disorders
• Clonazepam is the only benzodiazepine that is used as a solo maintenance treatment for seizure disorders

❋ Easier to taper than some other benzodiazepines because of long half-life
❋ May have less abuse potential than some other benzodiazepines
❋ May cause less depression, euphoria, or dependence than some other benzodiazepines
❋ Clonazepan is often considered a "longer-acting alprazolam-like anxiolytic" with improved tolerability features in terms of less euphoria, abuse, dependence, and withdrawal problems, but this has not been proven
• When using to treat insomnia, remember that insomnia may be a symptom of some other primary disorder itself, and thus warrant evaluation for comorbid psychiatric and/or medical conditions

 Suggested Reading

Davidson JR, Moroz G. Pivotal studies of clonazepam in panic disorder. Psychopharmacol Bull 1998;34:169–74.

DeVane CL, Ware MR, Lydiard RB. Pharmacokinetics, pharmacodynamics, and treatment issues of benzodiazepines: alprazolam, adinazolam, and clonazepam. Psychopharmacol Bull 1991;27:463–73.

Iqbal MM, Sobhan T, Ryals T. Effects of commonly used benzodiazepines on the fetus, the neonate, and the nursing infant. Psychiatr Serv 2002;53:39–49.

Panayiotopoulos CP. Treatment of typical absence seizures and related epileptic syndromes. Paediatr Drugs 2001;3:379–403.

CLONIDINE

THERAPEUTICS

Brands
- Duraclon (injection)
- Catapres
- Catapres-TTS (Clonidine Transdermal Therapeutic System)
- Clorpres

see index for additional brand names

Generic? Yes (not for transdermal)

Class
- Antihypertensive; centrally acting alpha 2 agonist hypotensive agent

Commonly Prescribed For
(bold for FDA approved)
- **Hypertension**
- Attention deficit hyperactivity disorder
- Tourette's syndrome
- Substance withdrawal, including opiates and alcohol
- Anxiety disorders, including PTSD and social anxiety disorder
- Clozapine-induced hypersalivation
- Menopausal flushing
- Severe pain in cancer patients that is not adequately relieved by opioid analgesics alone (combination with opiates)

How The Drug Works
- For hypertension, stimulates alpha 2 adrenergic receptors in the brain stem, reducing sympathetic outflow from the CNS and decreasing peripheral resistance, renal vascular resistance, heart rate, and blood pressure
- An imidazoline, so also interacts at imidazoline receptors
* For CNS uses, presumably has central actions on either pre- or postsynaptic alpha 2 receptors, and/or actions at imidazoline receptors may cause behavioral changes in numerous conditions (unknown and speculative)

How Long Until It Works
- Blood pressure may be lowered 30–60 minutes after first dose; greatest reduction seen after 2–4 hours
- May take several weeks to control blood pressure adequately
- For CNS uses, can take a few weeks to see therapeutic benefits

If It Works
- For hypertension, continue treatment indefinitely and check blood pressure regularly
- For CNS uses, continue to monitor continuing benefits as well as blood pressure

If It Doesn't Work (for CNS indications)
* Since clonidine is a second-line and experimental treatment for CNS disorders, many patients may not respond
- Consider adjusting dose or switching to another agent with better evidence for CNS efficacy

Best Augmenting Combos for Partial Response or Treatment-Resistance
- Best to attempt another monotherapy prior to augmenting for CNS uses
- Chlorthalidone, thiazide-type diuretics, and furosemide for hypertension
- Possibly combination with stimulants (with caution as benefits of combination poorly documented and there are some reports of serious adverse events)
- Combinations for CNS uses should be for the expert, while monitoring the patient closely, and when other treatment options have failed

Tests
- Blood pressure should be checked regularly during treatment

SIDE EFFECTS

How Drug Causes Side Effects
- Excessive actions on alpha 2 receptors and/or on imidazoline receptors

Notable Side Effects
* Dry mouth
* Dizziness, constipation, sedation
- Weakness, fatigue, impotence, loss of libido, insomnia, headache
- Major depression
- Dermatologic reactions (especially with transdermal clonidine)

- Hypotension, occasional syncope
- Tachycardia
- Nervousness, agitation
- Nausea, vomiting

 Life Threatening or Dangerous Side Effects

- Sinus bradycardia, atrioventricular block
- During withdrawal, hypertensive encephalopathy, cerebrovascular accidents, and death (rare)

Weight Gain

unusual   not unusual   common   problematic

- Reported but not expected

Sedation

unusual   not unusual   common   problematic

- Many experience and/or can be significant in amount
- Some patients may not tolerate it
- Can abate with time

What To Do About Side Effects

- Wait
- Take larger dose at bedtime to avoid daytime sedation
- Switch to another medication with better evidence of efficacy
- ✻ For withdrawal and discontinuation reactions, may need to reinstate clonidine and taper very slowly when stabilized

Best Augmenting Agents for Side Effects

- Dose reduction or switching to another agent may be more effective since most side effects cannot be improved with an augmenting agent

DOSING AND USE

Usual Dosage Range

- 0.2–0.6 mg/day in divided doses

Dosage Forms

- Tablet 0.1 mg scored, 0.2 mg scored, 0.3 mg scored
- Topical (7 day administration) 0.1 mg/24 hours, 0.2 mg/24 hours, 0.3 mg/24 hours

- Injection 100 mg/mL, 500 mg/mL

How to Dose

- Oral: initial 0.1 mg in 2 divided doses, morning and night; can increase by 0.1 mg/day each week; maximum dose generally 2.4 mg/day
- Topical: apply once every 7 days in hairless area; change location with each application
- Injection: initial 30 mcg/hr; maximum 40 mcg/hr; 500 mg/mL must be diluted

 Dosing Tips

- Adverse effects are dose-related and usually transient
- The last dose of the day should occur at bedtime so that blood pressure is controlled overnight
- If clonidine is terminated abruptly, rebound hypertension may occur within 2–4 days
- Using clonidine in combination with another antihypertensive agent may attenuate the development of tolerance to clonidine's antihypertensive effects
- The likelihood of severe discontinuation reactions with CNS and cardiovascular symptoms may be greater after administration of high doses of clonidine
- ✻ In patients who have developed localized contact sensitization to transdermal clonidine, continuing transdermal dosing on other skin areas or substituting with oral clonidine may be associated with the development of a generalized skin rash, urticaria, or angioedema
- ✻ If administered with a beta blocker, stop the beta blocker first for several days before the gradual discontinuation of clonidine in cases of planned discontinuation

Overdose

- Hypotension, hypertension, miosis, respiratory depression, seizures, bradycardia, hypothermia, coma, sedation, decreased reflexes, weakness, irritability, dysrhythmia

Long-Term Use

- Patients may develop tolerance to the antihypertensive effects
- ✻ Studies have not established the utility of clonidine for long-term CNS uses

✳ Be aware that forgetting to take clonidine or running out of medication can lead to abrupt discontinuation and associated withdrawal reactions and complications

Habit Forming
• Reports of some abuse by opiate addicts
• Reports of some abuse by non-opioid dependent patients

How to Stop
✳ Discontinuation reactions are common and sometimes severe
• Sudden discontinuation can result in nervousness, agitation, headache, and tremor, with rapid rise in blood pressure
• Rare instances of hypertensive encephalopathy, cerebrovascular accident, and death have been reported after clonidine withdrawal
• Taper over 2–4 days or longer to avoid rebound effects (nervousness, increased blood pressure)
• If administered with a beta blocker, stop the beta blocker first for several days before the gradual discontinuation of clonidine

Pharmacokinetics
• Half-life 12–16 hours
• Metabolized by the liver
• Excreted renally

 Drug Interactions
• The likelihood of severe discontinuation reactions with CNS and cardiovascular symptoms may be greater when clonidine is combined with beta blocker treatment
• Increased depressive and sedative effects when taken with other CNS depressants
• Tricyclic antidepressants may reduce the hypotensive effects of clonidine
• Corneal lesions in rats increased by use of clonidine with amitriptyline
• Use of clonidine with agents that affect sinus node function or AV nodal function (e.g., digitalis, calcium channel blockers, beta blockers) may result in bradycardia or AV block

 Other Warnings/ Precautions
• There have been cases of hypertensive encephalopathy, cerebrovascular accidents, and death after abrupt discontinuation
• If used with a beta blocker, the beta blocker should be stopped several days before tapering clonidine
• In patients who have developed localized contact sensitization to transdermal clonidine, continuing transdermal dosing on other skin areas or substituting with oral clonidine may be associated with the development of a generalized skin rash, urticaria, or angioedema
• Injection is not recommended for use in managing obstetrical, postpartum or peri-operative pain

Do Not Use
• If there is a proven allergy to clonidine

SPECIAL POPULATIONS

Renal Impairment
• Use with caution and possibly reduce dose

Hepatic Impairment
• Use with caution

Cardiac Impairment
• Use with caution in patients with recent myocardial infarction, severe coronary insufficiency, cerebrovascular disease

Elderly
• Elderly patients may tolerate a lower initial dose better
• Elderly patients may be more sensitive to sedative effects

 Children and Adolescents
• Safety and efficacy not established under age 12
• Children may be more sensitive to hypertensive effects of withdrawing treatment
✳ Because children commonly have gastrointestinal illnesses that lead to vomiting, they may be more likely to abruptly discontinue clonidine and therefore be more susceptible to

hypertensive episodes resulting from abrupt inability to take medication
- Children may be more likely to experience CNS depression with overdose and may even exhibit signs of toxicity with 0.1 mg of clonidine
- ADHD: initial 0.05 mg at bedtime; titrate over 2–4 weeks; usual dose 0.05–4 mg/day
- Injection may be used in pediatric cancer patients with severe pain unresponsive to other medications

Pregnancy
- Risk Category C [some animal studies show adverse effects, no controlled studies in humans]
- Use in women of childbearing potential requires weighing potential benefits to the mother against potential risks to the fetus
* For ADHD patients, clonidine should generally be discontinued before anticipated pregnancies

Breast Feeding
- Some drug is found in mother's breast milk
- No adverse effects have been reported in nursing infants
- If irritability or sedation develop in nursing infant, may need to discontinue drug or bottle feed

THE ART OF PSYCHOPHARMACOLOGY

Potential Advantages
- For numerous CNS indications when conventional treatments have failed (investigational)

Potential Disadvantages
- Poor documentation of efficacy for most off-label uses
- Withdrawal reactions
- Noncompliant patients
- Patients on concomitant CNS medications

Primary Target Symptoms
- High blood pressure
- Miscellaneous CNS, behavioral, and psychiatric symptoms

Pearls
* Although not approved for ADHD, clonidine has been shown to be effective treatment for this disorder in several published studies
* As monotherapy for ADHD, may be inferior to other options, including stimulants and desipramine
- As monotherapy or in combination with methylphenidate for ADHD with conduct disorder or oppositional defiant disorder, may improve aggression, oppositional, and conduct disorder symptoms
- Clonidine is sometimes used in combination with stimulants to reduce side effects and enhance therapeutic effects on motor hyperactivity
- Doses of 0.1 mg in 3 divided doses have been reported to reduce stimulant-induced insomnia as well as impulsivity
- Considered a third-line treatment option now for ADHD
* Clonidine may also be effective for treatment of tic disorders, including Tourette's syndrome
- May suppress tics especially in severe Tourette's syndrome, and may be even better at reducing explosive violent behaviors in Tourette's syndrome
- Sedation is often unacceptable in various patients despite improvement in CNS symptoms and leads to discontinuation of treatment, especially for ADHD and Tourette's syndrome
- Considered an investigational treatment for most other CNS applications
- May block the autonomic symptoms in anxiety and panic disorders (e.g., palpitations, sweating) and improve subjective anxiety as well
- May be useful in decreasing the autonomic arousal of PTSD
- May be useful as an as needed medication for stage fright or other predictable socially phobic situations
- May also be useful when added to SSRIs for reducing arousal and dissociative symptoms in PTSD
- May block autonomic symptoms of opioid withdrawal (e.g., palpitations, sweating) especially in inpatients, but muscle aches, irritability, and insomnia may not be well suppressed by clonidine

- May be useful in decreasing the hypertension, tachycardia, and tremulousness associated with alcohol withdrawal, but not the seizures or delirium tremens in complicated alcohol withdrawal
- Clonidine may improve social relationships, affectual responses, and sensory responses in autistic disorder
- Clonidine may reduce the incidence of menopausal flushing
- Growth hormone response to clonidine may be reduced during menses
- Clonidine stimulates growth hormone secretion (no chronic effects have been observed)

- Alcohol may reduce the effects of clonidine on growth hormone
- ✺ Guanfacine is a related centrally active alpha 2 agonist hypotensive agent that has been used for similar CNS applications but has not been as widely investigated or used as clonidine
- ✺ Guanfacine may be tolerated better than clonidine in some patients (e.g., sedation) or it may work better in some patients for CNS applications than clonidine, but no head-to-head trials

Suggested Reading

Burris JF. The USA experience with the clonidine transdermal therapeutic system. Clin Auton Res. 1993; 3: 391–6.

Gavras I, Manolis AJ, Gayras H. The alpha2-adrenergic receptors in hypertension and heart failure: experimental and clinical studies. J Hypertens. 2001; 19: 2115–24.

Guay DR. Adjunctive agents in the management of chronic pain. Pharmacotherapy. 2001; 21: 1070–81.

Silver LB. Alternative (nonstimulant) medications in the treatment of attention-deficit/hyperactivity disorder in children. Pediatr Clin North Am. 1999; 46: 965–75.

CLORAZEPATE

THERAPEUTICS

Brands • Azene
• Tranxene
see index for additional brand names

Generic? Yes

Class
• Benzodiazepine (anxiolytic)

Commonly Prescribed For
(bold for FDA approved)
• **Anxiety disorder**
• **Symptoms of anxiety**
• **Acute alcohol withdrawal**
• Partial seizures (adjunct)

 How The Drug Works
• Binds to benzodiazepine receptors at the GABA-A ligand-gated chloride channel complex
• Enhances the inhibitory effects of GABA
• Boosts chloride conductance through GABA-regulated channels
• Inhibits neuronal activity presumably in amygdala-centered fear circuits to provide therapeutic benefits in anxiety disorders

How Long Until It Works
• Some immediate relief with first dosing is common; can take several weeks with daily dosing for maximal therapeutic benefit

If It Works
• For short-term symptoms of anxiety – after a few weeks, discontinue use or use on an "as-needed" basis
• For chronic anxiety disorders, the goal of treatment is complete remission of symptoms as well as prevention of future relapses
• For chronic anxiety disorders, treatment most often reduces or even eliminates symptoms, but not a cure since symptoms can recur after medicine stopped
• For long-term symptoms of anxiety, consider switching to an SSRI or SNRI for long-term maintenance
• If long-term maintenance with a benzodiazepine is necessary, continue treatment for 6 months after symptoms resolve, and then taper dose slowly

• If symptoms reemerge, consider treatment with an SSRI or SNRI, or consider restarting the benzodiazepine; sometimes benzodiazepines have to be used in combination with SSRIs or SNRIs for best results

If It Doesn't Work
• Consider switching to another agent or adding an appropriate augmenting agent
• Consider psychotherapy, especially cognitive behavioral psychotherapy
• Consider presence of concomitant substance abuse
• Consider presence of clorazepate abuse
• Consider another diagnosis, such as a comorbid medical condition

 Best Augmenting Combos for Partial Response or Treatment-Resistance
• Benzodiazepines are frequently used as augmenting agents for antipsychotics and mood stabilizers in the treatment of psychotic and bipolar disorders
• Benzodiazepines are frequently used as augmenting agents for SSRIs and SNRIs in the treatment of anxiety disorders
• Not generally rational to combine with other benzodiazepines
• Caution if using as an anxiolytic concomitantly with other sedative hypnotics for sleep

Tests
• In patients with seizure disorders, concomitant medical illness, and/or those with multiple concomitant long-term medications, periodic liver tests and blood counts may be prudent

SIDE EFFECTS

How Drug Causes Side Effects
• Same mechanism for side effects as for therapeutic effects – namely due to excessive actions at benzodiazepine receptors
• Long-term adaptations in benzodiazepine receptors may explain the development of dependence, tolerance, and withdrawal
• Side effects are generally immediate, but immediate side effects often disappear in time

Notable Side Effects

* ✳ Sedation, fatigue, depression
* ✳ Dizziness, ataxia, slurred speech, weakness
* ✳ Forgetfulness, confusion
* ✳ Hyper-excitability, nervousness
* Rare hallucinations, mania
* Rare hypotension
* Hypersalivation, dry mouth

 ### Life Threatening or Dangerous Side Effects

* Respiratory depression, especially when taken with CNS depressants in overdose
* Rare hepatic dysfunction, renal dysfunction, blood dyscrasias

Weight Gain

unusual / not unusual / common / problematic

* Reported but not expected

Sedation

unusual / not unusual / common / problematic

* Many experience and/or can be significant in amount
* Especially at initiation of treatment or when dose increases
* Tolerance often develops over time

What To Do About Side Effects

* Wait
* Wait
* Wait
* Lower the dose
* Take largest dose at bedtime to avoid sedative effects during the day
* Switch to another agent
* Administer flumazenil if side effects are severe or life-threatening

Best Augmenting Agents for Side Effects

* Many side effects cannot be improved with an augmenting agent

DOSING AND USE

Usual Dosage Range

* Anxiety: 15–60 mg/day in divided doses
* Alcohol withdrawal: 30–60 mg/day in divided doses

Dosage Forms

* Tablet 3.75 mg scored, 7.5 mg scored, 15 mg scored, 22.5 mg single dose, 11.25 mg single dose half strength

How to Dose

* Anxiety: Initial 15 mg/day in divided doses; adjust dose as needed on subsequent days; single dose tablet may be given once daily at bedtime after patient is stable; maximum generally 90 mg/day
* Alcohol withdrawal: Initial 30 mg, then 30–60 mg in divided doses; second day 45–90 mg in divided doses; third day 22.5–45 mg in divided doses; fourth day 15–30 mg in divided doses; after fourth day decrease dose gradually and discontinue when patient is stable; maximum generally 90 mg/day
* Epilepsy: Initial 7.5 mg 3 times/day; increase by 7.5 mg weekly; maximum generally 90 mg/day

 ### Dosing Tips

* Use lowest possible effective dose for the shortest possible period of time (a benzodiazepine-sparing strategy)
* Assess need for continued treatment regularly
* Risk of dependence may increase with dose and duration of treatment
* For inter-dose symptoms of anxiety, can either increase dose or maintain same total daily dose but divide into more frequent doses
* Can also use an as-needed occasional "top up" dose for inter-dose anxiety
* Because anxiety disorders can require higher doses, the risk of dependence may be greater in these patients
* Frequency of dosing in practice is often greater than predicted from half-life, as duration of biological activity is often shorter than pharmacokinetic terminal half-life

Overdose

* Fatalities can occur; hypotension, tiredness, ataxia, confusion, coma

Long-Term Use
- Evidence of efficacy for up to 16 weeks
- Risk of dependence, particularly for periods longer than 12 weeks and especially in patients with past or current polysubstance abuse

Habit Forming
- Clorazepate is a Schedule IV drug
- Patients may develop dependence and/or tolerance with long-term use

How to Stop
- Patients with history of seizure may seize upon withdrawal, especially if withdrawal is abrupt
- Taper by 7.5 mg every 3 days to reduce chances of withdrawal effects
- For difficult to taper cases, consider reducing dose much more slowly after reaching 30 mg/day, perhaps by as little as 3.75 mg per week or less
- For other patients with severe problems discontinuing a benzodiazepine, dosing may need to be tapered over many months (i.e., reduce dose by 1% every 3 days by crushing tablet and suspending or dissolving in 100 ml of fruit juice and then disposing of 1 ml while drinking the rest; 3–7 days later, dispose of 2 ml, and so on). This is both a form of very slow biological tapering and a form of behavioral desensitization
- Be sure to differentiate reemergence of symptoms requiring reinstitution of treatment from withdrawal symptoms
- Benzodiazepine-dependent anxiety patients and insulin-dependent diabetics are not addicted to their medications. When benzodiazepine-dependent patients stop their medication, disease symptoms can reemerge, disease symptoms can worsen (rebound), and/or withdrawal symptoms can emerge

Pharmacokinetics
- Elimination half-life 40–50 hours

 Drug Interactions
- Increased depressive effects when taken with other CNS depressants

 Other Warnings/ Precautions
- Dosage changes should be made in collaboration with prescriber
- Use with caution in patients with pulmonary disease; rare reports of death after initiation of benzodiazepines in patients with severe pulmonary impairment
- History of drug or alcohol abuse often creates greater risk for dependency
- Some depressed patients may experience a worsening of suicidal ideation
- Some patients may exhibit abnormal thinking or behavioral changes similar to those caused by other CNS depressants (i.e., either depressant actions or disinhibiting actions)

Do Not Use
- If patient has narrow angle-closure glaucoma
- If there is a proven allergy to clorazepate or any benzodiazepine

SPECIAL POPULATIONS

Renal Impairment
- Initial 7.5–15 mg/day in divided doses or in 1 dose at bedtime

Hepatic Impairment
- Initial 7.5–15 mg/day in divided doses or in 1 dose at bedtime

Cardiac Impairment
- Benzodiazepines have been used to treat anxiety associated with acute myocardial infarction

Elderly
- Initial 7.5–15 mg/day in divided doses or in 1 dose at bedtime

 Children and Adolescents
- Not recommended for use under age 9
- Recommended initial dose: 7.5 mg twice a day

Pregnancy

- Risk Category D [positive evidence of risk to human fetus; potential benefits may still justify its use during pregnancy]
- Possible increased risk of birth defects when benzodiazepines taken during pregnancy
- Because of the potential risks, clorazepate is not generally recommended as treatment for anxiety during pregnancy, especially during the first trimester
- Drug should be tapered if discontinued
- Infants whose mothers received a benzodiazepine late in pregnancy may experience withdrawal effects
- Neonatal flaccidity has been reported in infants whose mothers took a benzodiazepine during pregnancy
- Seizures, even mild seizures, may cause harm to the embryo/fetus

Breast Feeding

- Some drug is found in mother's breast milk
- ✱ Recommended either to discontinue drug or bottle feed
- Effects of benzodiazepines on nursing infants have been reported and include feeding difficulties, sedation, and weight loss

---

THE ART OF PSYCHOPHARMACOLOGY

Potential Advantages

- Rapid onset of action

Potential Disadvantages

- Euphoria may lead to abuse
- Abuse especially risky in past or present substance abusers

Primary Target Symptoms

- Panic attacks
- Anxiety
- Incidence of seizures (adjunct)

Pearls

- Can be very useful as an adjunct to SSRIs and SNRIs in the treatment of numerous anxiety disorders
- Not effective for treating psychosis as a monotherapy, but can be used as an adjunct to antipsychotics
- Not effective for treating bipolar disorder as a monotherapy, but can be used as an adjunct to mood stabilizers and antipsychotics
- ✱ More commonly used than some other benzodiazepines for treating alcohol withdrawal
- May both cause depression and treat depression in different patients
- When using to treat insomnia, remember that insomnia may be a symptom of some other primary disorder itself, and thus warrant evaluation for comorbid psychiatric and/or medical conditions

---

Suggested Reading

Griffith JL, Murray GB. Clorazepate in the treatment of complex partial seizures with psychic symptomatology. J Nerv Ment Dis 1985;173:185–6.

Kiejna A, Kantorska-Janiec M, Malyszczak K. [The use of chlorazepate dipotassium (Tranxene) in the states of restlessness and agitation]. Psychiatr Pol 1997;31:753–60.

Mielke L, Breinbauer B, Schubert M, Kling M, Entolzner E, Hargasser S, Hipp R. [Comparison of the effectiveness of orally administered clorazepate dipotassium and nordiazepam on preoperative anxiety]. Anaesthesiol Reanim 1995;20:144–8.

Rickels K, Schweizer E, Csanalosi I, Case WG, Chung H. Long-term treatment of anxiety and risk of withdrawal. Prospective comparison of clorazepate and buspirone. Arch Gen Psychiatry 1988;45:444–50.

CLOZAPINE

THERAPEUTICS

Brands • Clozaril
• Leponex
see index for additional brand names

Generic? Yes

Class

• Atypical antipsychotic (serotonin-dopamine antagonist; second generation antipsychotic; also a mood stabilizer)

Commonly Prescribed For
(bold for FDA approved)
• **Treatment-resistant schizophrenia**
• **Reduction in risk of recurrent suicidal behavior in patients with schizophrenia or schizoaffective disorder**
• Treatment-resistant bipolar disorder
• Violent aggressive patients with psychosis and other brain disorders not responsive to other treatments

How The Drug Works

• Blocks dopamine 2 receptors, reducing positive symptoms of psychosis and stabilizing affective symptoms
• Blocks serotonin 2A receptors, causing enhancement of dopamine release in certain brain regions and thus reducing motor side effects and possibly improving cognitive and affective symptoms
• Interactions at a myriad of other neurotransmitter receptors may contribute to clozapine's efficacy
✳ Specifically, interactions at 5HT2C and 5HT1A receptors may contribute to efficacy for cognitive and affective symptoms in some patients
• Mechanism of efficacy for psychotic patients who do not respond to conventional antipsychotics is unknown

How Long Until It Works

• Psychotic symptoms can improve within 1 week, especially with first-line use, but often takes several weeks for full effect on behavior as well as on cognition and affective stabilization, especially in treatment-resistant cases
• Classically recommended to wait at least 4–6 weeks to determine efficacy of drug, but in practice patients often require up to 16–20 weeks to show a good response, especially in treatment-resistant cases

If It Works

• As for other antipsychotics, most often reduces positive symptoms in schizophrenia but does not eliminate them
✳ However, clozapine may reduce positive symptoms in patients who do not respond to other antipsychotics, especially other conventional antipsychotics
• Can improve negative symptoms, as well as aggressive, cognitive, and affective symptoms in schizophrenia
• Most schizophrenic patients do not have a total remission of symptoms but rather a reduction of symptoms by about a third
• Many patients with bipolar disorder and other disorders with psychotic, aggressive, violent, impulsive, and other types of behavioral disturbances may respond to clozapine when other agents have failed
• Perhaps 5–15% of schizophrenic patients can experience an overall improvement of greater than 50–60%, especially when receiving stable treatment for more than a year
✳ Such patients are considered super-responders or "awakeners" since they may be well enough to be employed, live independently, and sustain long-term relationships; super-responders are anecdotally reported more often with clozapine than with some other antipsychotics
• Continue treatment until reaching a plateau of improvement
• After reaching a satisfactory plateau, continue treatment for at least a year after first episode of psychosis
• For second and subsequent episodes of psychosis, treatment may need to be indefinite
• Even for first episodes of psychosis, it may be preferable to continue treatment indefinitely to avoid subsequent episodes
• Treatment may not only reduce mania but also prevent recurrences of mania in bipolar disorder

If It Doesn't Work

• Some patients may respond better if switched to a conventional antipsychotic

✳ Some patients may require augmentation with a conventional antipsychotic or with an atypical antipsychotic (especially risperidone or amisulpride), but these are the most refractory of all psychotic patients and such treatment is very expensive

✳ Consider augmentation with valproate or lamotrigine

• Consider noncompliance and switch to another antipsychotic with fewer side effects or to an antipsychotic that can be given by depot injection

• Consider initiating rehabilitation and psychotherapy

• Consider presence of concomitant drug abuse

 ### Best Augmenting Combos for Partial Response or Treatment-Resistance

• Valproic acid (valproate, divalproex, divalproex ER)
• Lamotrigine
• Other mood stabilizing anticonvulsants (carbamazepine, oxcarbazepine)
• Conventional antipsychotics
• Benzodiazepines
• Lithium

Tests

✳ Complete blood count before treatment, weekly for 6 months of treatment, and biweekly thereafter

Before starting an atypical antipsychotic

✳ Weigh all patients and track BMI during treatment

• Get baseline personal and family history of obesity, dyslipidemia, hypertension, and cardiovascular disease

✳ Get waist circumference (at umbilicus), blood pressure, fasting plasma glucose, and fasting lipid profile

• Determine if the patient is
  • overweight (BMI 25.0–29.9)
  • obese (BMI ≥30)
  • has pre-diabetes (fasting plasma glucose 100–125 mg/dl)
  • has diabetes (fasting plasma glucose >126 mg/dl)
  • has hypertension (BP >140/90 mm Hg)
  • has dyslipidemia (increased total cholesterol, LDL cholesterol, and triglycerides; decreased HDL cholesterol)

• Treat or refer such patients for treatment, including nutrition and weight management, physical activity counseling, smoking cessation, and medical management

Monitoring after starting an atypical antipsychotic

✳ BMI monthly for 3 months, then quarterly

✳ Blood pressure, fasting plasma glucose, fasting lipids within 3 months and then annually, but earlier and more frequently for patients with diabetes or who have gained >5% of initial weight

• Treat or refer for treatment and consider switching to another atypical antipsychotic for patients who become overweight, obese, pre-diabetic, diabetic, hypertensive, or dyslipidemic while receiving an atypical antipsychotic

✳ Even in patients without known diabetes, be vigilant for the rare but life threatening onset of diabetic ketoacidosis, which always requires immediate treatment, by monitoring for the rapid onset of polyuria, polydipsia, weight loss, nausea, vomiting, dehydration, rapid respiration, weakness and clouding of sensorium, even coma

• Liver function testing, electrocardiogram, general physical exam, and assessment of baseline cardiac status before starting treatment

• Liver tests may be necessary during treatment in patients who develop nausea, vomiting, or anorexia

✳ Electrocardiograms and cardiac evaluation to rule out myocarditis may be necessary during treatment in patients who develop shortness of breath or chest pain

SIDE EFFECTS

How Drug Causes Side Effects

• By blocking histamine 1 receptors in the brain, it can cause sedation and possibly weight gain

• By blocking alpha 1 adrenergic receptors, it can cause dizziness, sedation, and hypotension

• By blocking muscarinic 1 receptors, it can cause dry mouth, constipation, and sedation

- By blocking dopamine 2 receptors in the striatum, it can cause motor side effects (very rare)
- Mechanism of weight gain and increased incidence of diabetes and dyslipidemia with atypical antipsychotics is unknown

Notable Side Effects

＊ Probably increases risk for diabetes and dyslipidemia
＊ Increased salivation (can be severe)
＊ Sweating
- Dizziness, sedation, headache, tachycardia, hypotension
- Nausea, constipation, dry mouth, weight gain
- Rare tardive dyskinesia (no reports have directly implicated clozapine in the development of tardive dyskinesia)

 Life Threatening or Dangerous Side Effects

- Hyperglycemia, in some cases extreme and associated with ketoacidosis or hyperosmolar coma or death, has been reported in patients taking atypical antipsychotics
- Agranulocytosis (includes flu-like symptoms or signs of infection)
- Seizures (risk increases with dose)
- Neuroleptic malignant syndrome (more likely when clozapine is used with another agent)
- Pulmonary embolism (may include deep vein thrombosis or respiratory symptoms)
- Myocarditis

Weight Gain

unusual   not unusual   common   problematic

- Frequent and can be significant in amount
- Can become a health problem in some
- More than for some other antipsychotics, but never say always as not a problem in everyone

Sedation

unusual   not unusual   common   problematic

- Frequent and can be significant in amount
- Some patients may not tolerate it

- More than for some other antipsychotics, but never say always as not a problem in everyone
- Can wear off over time
- Can reemerge as dose increases and then wear off again over time

What To Do About Side Effects

- Patients must inform prescriber immediately of any flu-like symptoms, muscle rigidity, altered mental status, irregular pulse or blood pressure
- Take at bedtime to help reduce daytime sedation
- Sedation may wear off with time
- Start dosing low and increase slowly as side effects wear off at each dosing increment
- Weight loss, exercise programs, and medical management for high BMIs, diabetes, dyslipidemia
- Switch to another agent

Best Augmenting Agents for Side Effects

- Many side effects cannot be improved with an augmenting agent

DOSING AND USE

Usual Dosage Range

- 300–450 mg/day

Dosage Forms

- Tablet 25 mg scored, 100 mg scored

How to Dose

- Initial 25 mg in 2 divided doses; increase by 25–50 mg/day each day until desired efficacy is reached; maintenance dose 300–450 mg/day; doses above 300 mg/day should be divided; increases in doses above 450 mg/day should be made weekly; maximum dose generally 900 mg/day

 Dosing Tips

- Prescriptions are generally given 1 week at a time for the first 6 months of treatment because of the risk of agranulocytosis; after 6 months prescriptions can generally be given 2 weeks at a time

✳ Treatment should be suspended if absolute neutrophil count falls below 1,000/mm³
• Treatment should be suspended if white blood cell count falls below 2,000/mm³
• Treatment should be suspended if eosinophil count rises above 4,000/mm³, and continued once it falls below 3,000/mm³
• If treatment is discontinued for more than 2 days, it may need to be reinitiated at a lower dose and slowly increased in order to maximize tolerability
• Plasma half-life suggests twice daily administration, but in practice it may be given once a day at night
• Doses over 550 mg/day may require concomitant anticonvulsant administration to reduce the chances of a seizure
✳ Rebound psychosis may occur unless dose is very slowly tapered, by 100 mg/week or less

Overdose
• Sometimes lethal; changes in heart rhythm, excess salivation, respiratory depression, altered state of consciousness

Long-Term Use
• Treatment to reduce risk of suicidal behavior should be continued for at least 2 years
• Often used for long-term maintenance in treatment-resistant schizophrenia

Habit Forming
• No

How to Stop
• Slow down-titration (over 6 to 8 weeks), especially when simultaneously beginning a new antipsychotic while switching (i.e., cross-titration)
✳ Rapid discontinuation may lead to rebound psychosis and worsening of symptoms

Pharmacokinetics
• Half-life 5–16 hours
• Metabolized by multiple CYP450 enzymes, including 1A2, 2D6, and 3A4

Drug Interactions
• Dose may need to be reduced if given in conjunction with CYP450 1A2 inhibitors (e.g., fluvoxamine)
• Dose may need to be raised if given in conjunction with CYP450 1A2 inducers (e.g., cigarette smoke)
• CYP450 2D6 inhibitors (e.g., paroxetine, fluoxetine, duloxetine) can raise clozapine levels, but dosage adjustment usually not necessary
• CYP450 3A4 inhibitors (e.g., nefazodone, fluvoxamine, fluoxetine) can raise clozapine levels, but dosage adjustment usually not necessary
• Clozapine may enhance effects of antihypertensive drugs

Other Warnings/ Precautions
• Possible association between myocarditis and cardiomyopathy and clozapine use, even in physically healthy individuals
• Should not be used in conjunction with agents that are known to cause agranulocytosis
• Use with caution in patients with glaucoma
• Use with caution in patients with enlarged prostate

Do Not Use
• In patients with myeloproliferative disorder
• In patients with uncontrolled epilepsy
• In patients with granulocytopenia
• In patients with CNS depression
• If there is a proven allergy to clozapine

SPECIAL POPULATIONS

Renal Impairment
• Should be used with caution

Hepatic Impairment
• Should be used with caution

Cardiac Impairment
• Should be used with caution, particularly if patient is taking concomitant medication

Elderly
• Some patients may tolerate lower doses better

 Children and Adolescents
• Safety and efficacy have not been established
• Preliminary research has suggested efficacy in early-onset treatment-resistant schizophrenia
• Children and adolescents taking clozapine should be monitored more often than adults

 Pregnancy
• Risk Category B [animal studies do not show adverse effects, no controlled studies in humans]
• Psychotic symptoms may worsen during pregnancy and some form of treatment may be necessary
• Clozapine should be used only when the potential benefits outweigh potential risks to the fetus

Breast Feeding
• Unknown if clozapine is secreted in human breast milk, but all psychotropics assumed to be secreted in breast milk
✳ Recommended either to discontinue drug or bottle feed
• Infants of women who choose to breast feed while on clozapine should be monitored for possible adverse effects

THE ART OF PSYCHOPHARMACOLOGY

Potential Advantages
✳ Treatment-resistant schizophrenia
✳ Violent, aggressive patients
✳ Patients with tardive dyskinesia
✳ Patients with suicidal behavior

Potential Disadvantages
✳ Patients with diabetes, obesity
• Patients with cardiac impairment

Primary Target Symptoms
• Positive symptoms of psychosis
• Negative symptoms of psychosis
• Cognitive symptoms

• Affective symptoms
• Suicidal behavior
• Violence and aggression

 Pearls
✳ Not a first-line treatment choice in most countries
✳ Most efficacious but most dangerous
✳ Documented efficacy in treatment-refractory schizophrenia
• May reduce violence and aggression in difficult cases, including forensic cases
✳ Reduces suicide in schizophrenia
• May reduce substance abuse
• May improve tardive dyskinesia
• Little or no prolactin elevation, motor side effects, or tardive dyskinesia
• Clinical improvements often continue slowly over several years
• Cigarette smoke can decrease clozapine levels and patients may be at risk for relapse if they begin or increase smoking

Suggested Reading

Iqbal MM, Rahman A, Husain Z, Mahmud SZ, Ryan WG, Feldman JM. Clozapine: a clinical review of adverse effects and management. Ann Clin Psychiatry 2003;15:33–48.

Lieberman JA. Maximizing clozapine therapy: managing side effects. J Clin Psychiatry 1998;59 (suppl 3):38–43.

Schulte P. What is an adequate trial with clozapine?: therapeutic drug monitoring and time to response in treatment-refractory schizophrenia. Clin Pharmacokinet 2003;42:607–18.

Wagstaff A, Perry C. Clozapine: in prevention of suicide in patients with schizophrenia or schizoaffective disorder. CNS Drugs 2003;17:273–80

Wahlbeck K, Cheine M, Essali A, Adams C. Evidence of clozapine's effectiveness in schizophrenia: a systematic review and meta-analysis of randomized trials. Am J Psychiatry 1999;156:990–999.

D-AMPHETAMINE

THERAPEUTICS

Brands • Dexedrine
• Dexedrine Spansules
• Dextro Stat
see index for additional brand names

Generic? Yes

 Class
• Stimulant

Commonly Prescribed For
(bold for FDA approved)
• **Attention deficit hyperactivity disorder (ages 3–16)**
• **Narcolepsy**
• Treatment-resistant depression

 How The Drug Works
* Increases norepinephrine and especially dopamine actions by blocking their reuptake and facilitating their release
• Enhancement of dopamine and norepinephrine actions in certain brain regions may improve attention, concentration, executive function and wakefulness (e.g. dorsolateral prefrontal cortex)
• Enhancement of dopamine actions in other brain regions (e.g., basal ganglia) may improve hyperactivity
• Enhancement of dopamine and norepinephrine in yet other brain regions (e.g., medial prefrontal cortex, hypothalamus) may improve depression, fatigue, and sleepiness

How Long Until It Works
• Some immediate effects can be seen with first dosing
• Can take several weeks to attain maximum therapeutic benefit

If It Works (for ADHD)
• The goal of treatment of ADHD is reduction of symptoms of inattentiveness, motor hyperactivity, and/or impulsiveness that disrupt social, school, and/or occupational functioning
• Continue treatment until all symptoms are under control or improvement is stable and then continue treatment indefinitely as long as improvement persists

• Reevaluate the need for treatment periodically
• Treatment for ADHD begun in childhood may need to be continued into adolescence and adulthood if continued benefit is documented

If It Doesn't Work (for ADHD)
• Consider adjusting dose or switching to another formulation of d-amphetamine or to another agent
• Consider behavioral therapy
• Consider the presence of noncompliance and counsel patient and parents
• Consider evaluation for another diagnosis or for a comorbid condition (e.g., bipolar disorder, substance abuse, medical illness, etc.)
* Some ADHD patients and some depressed patients may experience lack of consistent efficacy due to activation of latent or underlying bipolar disorder, and require either augmenting with a mood stabilizer or switching to a mood stabilizer

 Best Augmenting Combos for Partial Response or Treatment-Resistance
* Best to attempt other monotherapies prior to augmenting
• For the expert, can combine immediate release formulation with a sustained release formulation of d-amphetamine for ADHD
• For the expert, can combine with modafinil or atomoxetine for ADHD
• For the expert, can occasionally combine with atypical antipsychotics in highly treatment-resistant cases of bipolar disorder or ADHD
• For the expert, can combine with antidepressants to boost antidepressant efficacy in highly treatment-resistant cases of depression while carefully monitoring patient

Tests
• Blood pressure should be monitored regularly
• In children, monitor weight and height

SIDE EFFECTS

How Drug Causes Side Effects
- Increases in norepinephrine peripherally can cause autonomic side effects, including tremor, tachycardia, hypertension, and cardiac arrhythmias
- Increases in norepinephrine and dopamine centrally can cause CNS side effects such as insomnia, agitation, psychosis and substance abuse

Notable Side Effects
- ✻ Insomnia, headache, exacerbation of tics, nervousness, irritability, overstimulation, tremor, dizziness
- Anorexia, nausea, dry mouth, constipation, diarrhea, weight loss
- Can temporarily slow normal growth in children (controversial)
- Sexual dysfunction long-term (impotence, libido changes) but can also improve sexual dysfunction short-term

 Life Threatening or Dangerous Side Effects
- Psychotic episodes, especially with parenteral abuse
- Seizures
- Palpitations, tachycardia, hypertension
- Rare activation of hypomania, mania, or suicidal ideation (controversial)

Weight Gain

unusual / not unusual / common / problematic
- Reported but not expected
- Some patients may experience weight loss

Sedation

unusual / not unusual / common / problematic
- Reported but not expected
- Activation much more common than sedation

What To Do About Side Effects
- Wait
- Adjust dose
- Switch to a long-acting stimulant
- Switch to another agent
- For insomnia, avoid dosing in afternoon/evening

Best Augmenting Agents for Side Effects
- Beta-blockers for peripheral autonomic side effects
- Dose reduction or switching to another agent may be more effective since most side effects cannot be improved with an augmenting agent

DOSING AND USE

Usual Dosage Range
- Narcolepsy: 5–60 mg/day (divided doses for tablet, once-daily morning dose for Spansule capsule)
- ADHD: 5–40 mg/day (divided doses for tablet, once-daily morning dose for Spansule capsule)

Dosage Forms
- Spansule capsule 5 mg, 10 mg, 15 mg
- Tablet 5 mg scored, 10 mg

How to Dose
- Narcolepsy (ages 12 and older): initial 10 mg/day; increase by 10 mg each week; give first dose on waking
- ADHD (ages 6 and older): initial 5–10 mg/day in 1–2 doses; increase by 5 mg each week; give first dose on waking
- Can give once-daily dosing with Spansule capsule or divided dosing with tablet (every 4–6 hours)

 Dosing Tips
- Clinical duration of action often differs from pharmacokinetic half-life
- ✻ Immediate release dextroamphetamine has 3–6 hour duration of clinical action
- ✻ Sustained release dextroamphetamine (Dexedrine spansule) has up to 8-hour duration of clinical action
- Tablets contain tartrazine, which may cause allergic reactions, particularly in patients allergic to aspirin
- Dexedrine spansules are controlled-release and should therefore not be chewed but rather should only be swallowed whole
- ✻ Controlled release delivery of dextroamphetamine may be sufficiently long in duration to allow elimination of

lunchtime dosing in many but not all patients

✱ This innovation can be an important practical element in stimulant utilization, eliminating the hassle and pragmatic difficulties of lunchtime dosing at school, including storage problems, potential diversion, and the need for a medical professional to supervise dosing away from home

- Avoid dosing late in the day because of the risk of insomnia

✱ May be possible to dose only during the school week for some ADHD patients

- Off-label uses are dosed the same as for ADHD

✱ May be able to give drug holidays over the summer in order to reassess therapeutic utility and effects on growth and to allow catch-up from any growth suppression as well as to assess any other side effects and the need to reinstitute stimulant treatment for the next school term

- Side effects are generally dose-related
- Taking with food may delay peak actions for 2–3 hours

Overdose

- Rarely fatal; panic, hyperreflexia, rhabdomyolysis, rapid respiration, confusion, coma, hallucination, convulsion, arrhythmia, change in blood pressure, circulatory collapse

Long-Term Use

- Often used long-term for ADHD when ongoing monitoring documents continued efficacy
- Dependence and/or abuse may develop
- Tolerance to therapeutic effects may develop in some patients
- Long-term stimulant use may be associated with growth suppression in children (controversial)
- Periodic monitoring of weight, blood pressure, CBC, platelet counts, and liver function may be prudent

Habit Forming

- High abuse potential, Schedule II drug
- Patients may develop tolerance, psychological dependence

How to Stop

- Taper to avoid withdrawal effects
- Withdrawal following chronic therapeutic use may unmask symptoms of the underlying disorder and may require follow-up and reinstitution of treatment
- Careful supervision is required during withdrawal from abusive use since severe depression may occur

Pharmacokinetics

- Half-life approximately 10–12 hours

 Drug Interactions

- May affect blood pressure and should be used cautiously with agents used to control blood pressure
- Gastrointestinal acidifying agents (guanethidine, reserpine, glutamic acid, ascorbic acid, fruit juices, etc.) and urinary acidifying agents (ammonium chloride, sodium phosphate, etc.) lower amphetamine plasma levels, so such agents can be useful to administer after an overdose but may also lower therapeutic efficacy of amphetamines
- Gastrointestinal alkalinizing agents (sodium bicarbonate, etc.) and urinary alkalinizing agents (acetazolamide, some thiazides) increase amphetamine plasma levels and potentiate amphetamine's actions
- Desipramine and protryptiline can cause striking and sustained increases in brain concentrations of d-amphetamine and may also add to d-amphetamine's cardiovascular effects
- Theoretically, other agents with norepinephrine reuptake blocking properties, such as venlafaxine, duloxetine, atomoxetine, milnacipran, and reboxetine, could also add to amphetamine's CNS and cardiovascular effects
- Amphetamines may counteract the sedative effects of antihistamines
- Haloperidol, chlorpromazine, and lithium may inhibit stimulatory effects of amphetamines
- Theoretically, atypical antipsychotics should also inhibit stimulatory effects of amphetamines
- Theoretically, amphetamines could inhibit the antipsychotic actions of antipsychotics

- Theoretically, amphetamines could inhibit the mood stabilizing actions of atypical antipsychotics in some patients
- Combinations of amphetamines with mood stabilizers (lithium, anticonvulsants, atypical antipsychotics) is generally something for experts only, when monitoring patients closely and when other options fail
- Absorption of amphetamines is delayed by phenobarbital, phenytoin, ethosuximide
- Amphetamines inhibit adrenergic blockers and enhance adrenergic effects of norepinephrine
- Amphetamines may antagonize hypotensive effects of veratrum alkaloids and other antihypertensives
- Amphetamines increase the analgesic effects of meperidine
- Amphetamines contribute to excessive CNS stimulation if used with large doses of propoxyphene
- Amphetamines can raise plasma corticosteroid levels
- MAOIs slow absorption of amphetamines and thus potentiate their actions, which can cause headache, hypertension, and rarely hypertensive crisis and malignant hyperthermia, sometimes with fatal results
- Use with MAOIs, including within 14 days of MAOI use, is not advised, but this can sometimes be considered by experts who monitor depressed patients closely when other treatment options for depression fail

 Other Warnings/ Precautions

- Use with caution in patients with any degree of hypertension, hyperthyroidism, or history of drug abuse
- Children who are not growing or gaining weight should stop treatment, at least temporarily
- May worsen motor and phonic tics
- May worsen symptoms of thought disorder and behavioral disturbance in psychotic patients
- Stimulants have a high potential for abuse and must be used with caution in anyone with a current or past history of substance abuse or alcoholism or in emotionally unstable patients
- Administration of stimulants for prolonged periods of time should be avoided

whenever possible or done only with close monitoring, as it may lead to marked tolerance and drug dependence, including psychological dependence with varying degrees of abnormal behavior
- Particular attention should be paid to the possibility of subjects obtaining stimulants for nontherapeutic use or distribution to others and the drugs should in general be prescribed sparingly with documentation of appropriate use
- Not an appropriate first-line treatment for depression or for normal fatigue
- May lower the seizure threshold
- Emergence or worsening of activation and agitation may represent the induction of a bipolar state, especially a mixed dysphoric bipolar II condition sometimes associated with suicidal ideation, and require the addition of a mood stabilizer and/or discontinuation of d-amphetamine

Do Not Use

- If patient has extreme anxiety or agitation
- If patient has motor tics or Tourette's sydrome or if there is a family history of Tourette's, unless administered by an expert in cases when the potential benefits for ADHD outweigh the risks of worsening tics
- Should generally not be administered with an MAOI, including within 14 days of MAOI use, except in heroic circumstances and by an expert
- If patient has arteriosclerosis, cardiovascular disease, or severe hypertension
- If patient has glaucoma
- If there is a proven allergy to any sympathomimetic agent

SPECIAL POPULATIONS

Renal Impairment
- No dose adjustment necessary

Hepatic Impairment
- Use with caution

Cardiac Impairment
- Use with caution, particularly in patients with recent myocardial infarction or other conditions that could be negatively affected by increased blood pressure

Elderly
• Some patients may tolerate lower doses better

 Children and Adolescents
• Safety and efficacy not established under age 3
• Use in young children should be reserved for the expert
• d-amphetamine may worsen symptoms of behavioral disturbance and thought disorder in psychotic children
• d-amphetamine has acute effects on growth hormone; long-term effects are unknown but weight and height should be monitored during long-term treatment
• Narcolepsy: ages 6–12: initial 5 mg/day; increase by 5 mg each week
• ADHD: ages 3–5: initial 2.5 mg/day; increase by 2.5 mg each week

 Pregnancy
• Risk Category C [some animal studies show adverse effects, no controlled studies in humans]
• There is a greater risk of premature birth and low birth weight in infants whose mothers take d-amphetamine during pregnancy
• Infants whose mothers take d-amphetamine during pregnancy may experience withdrawal symptoms
• Use in women of childbearing potential requires weighing potential benefits to the mother against potential risks to the fetus
✳ For ADHD patients, d-amphetamine should generally be discontinued before anticipated pregnancies

Breast Feeding
• Some drug is found in mother's breast milk
✳ Recommended either to discontinue drug or bottle feed
• If infant shows signs of irritability, drug may need to be discontinued

THE ART OF PSYCHOPHARMACOLOGY
Potential Advantages
• May work in ADHD patients unresponsive to other stimulants
• Established long-term efficacy of immediate release and spansule formulations

Potential Disadvantages
• Patients with current or past substance abuse
• Patients with current or past bipolar disorder or psychosis

Primary Target Symptoms
• Concentration, attention span
• Motor hyperactivity
• Impulsiveness
• Physical and mental fatigue
• Daytime sleepiness
• Depression

 Pearls
✳ May be useful for treatment of depressive symptoms in medically ill elderly patients
✳ May be useful for treatment of post-stroke depression
✳ A classical augmentation strategy for treatment-refractory depression
✳ Specifically, may be useful for treatment of cognitive dysfunction and fatigue as residual symptoms of major depressive disorder unresponsive to multiple prior treatments
✳ May also be useful for the treatment of cognitive impairment, depressive symptoms, and severe fatigue in patients with HIV infection and in cancer patients
• Can be used to potentiate opioid analgesia and reduce sedation, particularly in end-of-life management
• Unknown how d-amphetamine's mechanism of action differs from that of d,l-methylphenidate, but some patients respond to or tolerate d-amphetamine better than d,l-methylphenidate and vice versa
• Some patients may benefit from an occasional addition of 5–10 mg of immediate release d-amphetamine to their daily base of sustained release Dexedrine spansules

✳ Despite warnings, can be a useful adjunct to MAOIs for heroic treatment of highly refractory mood disorders when monitored with vigilance

✳ Can reverse sexual dysfunction caused by psychiatric illness and by some drugs such as SSRIs, including decreased libido, erectile dysfunction, delayed ejaculation, and anorgasmia

• Atypical antipsychotics may be useful in treating stimulant or psychotic consequences of overdose

• Taking with food may delay peak actions for 2–3 hours

• Half-life and duration of clinical action tend to be shorter in younger children

• Drug abuse may actually be lower in ADHD adolescents treated with stimulants than in ADHD adolescents who are not treated

 Suggested Reading

Fry JM. Treatment modalities for narcolepsy. Neurology. 1998;50(2 Suppl 1):S43–8.

Greenhill LL, Pliszka S, Dulcan MK, Bernet W, Arnold V, Beitchman J, Benson RS, Bukstein O, Kinlan J, McClellan J, Rue D, Shaw JA, Stock S. Practice parameter for the use of stimulant medications in the treatment of children, adolescents, and adults. J Am Acad Child Adolesc Psychiatry. 2002;41(2 Suppl):26S–49S.

Jadad AR, Boyle M, Cunningham C, Kim M, Schachar R. Treatment of attention-deficit/hyperactivity disorder. Evid Rep Technol Assess (Summ). 1999;(11):i–viii, 1–341.

Vinson DC. Therapy for attention-deficit hyperactivity disorder. Arch Fam Med. 1994;3:445–51.

Wender PH, Wolf LE, Wasserstein J. Adults with ADHD. An overview. Ann N Y Acad Sci. 2001;931:1–16.

DESIPRAMINE

THERAPEUTICS

Brands • Norpramin
see index for additional brand names

Generic? Yes

Class
• Tricyclic antidepressant (TCA)
• Predominantly a norepinephrine/ noradrenaline reuptake inhibitor

Commonly Prescribed For
(bold for FDA approved)
• **Depression**
• Anxiety
• Insomnia
• Neuropathic pain/chronic pain
• Treatment-resistant depression

How The Drug Works
• Boosts neurotransmitter norepinephrine/noradrenaline
• Blocks norepinephrine reuptake pump (norepinephrine transporter), presumably increasing noradrenergic neurotransmission
• Since dopamine is inactivated by norepinephrine reuptake in frontal cortex, which largely lacks dopamine transporters, desipramine can thus increase dopamine neurotransmission in this part of the brain
• A more potent inhibitor of norepinephrine reuptake pump than serotonin reuptake pump (serotonin transporter)
• At high doses may also boost neurotransmitter serotonin and presumably increase serotonergic neurotransmission

How Long Until It Works
• May have immediate effects in treating insomnia or anxiety
• Onset of therapeutic actions usually not immediate, but often delayed 2 to 4 weeks
• If it is not working within 6 to 8 weeks for depression, it may require a dosage increase or it may not work at all
• May continue to work for many years to prevent relapse of symptoms

If It Works
• The goal of treatment of depression is complete remission of current symptoms as well as prevention of future relapses
• The goal of treatment of chronic neuropathic pain is to reduce symptoms as much as possible, especially in combination with other treatments
• Treatment of depression most often reduces or even eliminates symptoms, but not a cure since symptoms can recur after medicine stopped
• Treatment of chronic neuropathic pain may reduce symptoms, but rarely eliminates them completely, and is not a cure since symptoms can recur after medicine is stopped
• Continue treatment of depression until all symptoms are gone (remission)
• Once symptoms of depression are gone, continue treating for 1 year for the first episode of depression
• For second and subsequent episodes of depression, treatment may need to be indefinite
• Use in anxiety disorders and chronic pain may also need to be indefinite, but long-term treatment is not well studied in these conditions

If It Doesn't Work
• Many depressed patients only have a partial response where some symptoms are improved but others persist (especially insomnia, fatigue, and problems concentrating)
• Other depressed patients may be nonresponders, sometimes called treatment-resistant or treatment-refractory
• Consider increasing dose, switching to another agent or adding an appropriate augmenting agent
• Consider psychotherapy
• Consider evaluation for another diagnosis or for a comorbid condition (e.g., medical illness, substance abuse, etc.)
• Some patients may experience apparent lack of consistent efficacy due to activation of latent or underlying bipolar disorder, and require antidepressant discontinuation and a switch to a mood stabilizer

Best Augmenting Combos for Partial Response or Treatment-Resistance

- Lithium, buspirone, thyroid hormone (for depression)
- Gabapentin, tiagabine, other anticonvulsants, even opiates if done by experts while monitoring carefully in difficult cases (for chronic pain)

Tests

❋ None for healthy individuals, although monitoring of plasma drug levels is available

❋ Since tricyclic and tetracyclic antidepressants are frequently associated with weight gain, before starting treatment, weigh all patients and determine if the patient is already overweight (BMI 25.0–29.9) or obese (BMI ≥30)

- Before giving a drug that can cause weight gain to an overweight or obese patient, consider determining whether the patient already has pre-diabetes (fasting plasma glucose 100–125 mg/dl), diabetes (fasting plasma glucose >126 mg/dl), or dyslipidemia (increased total cholesterol, LDL cholesterol and triglycerides; decreased HDL cholesterol), and treat or refer such patients for treatment, including nutrition and weight management, physical activity counseling, smoking cessation, and medical management

❋ Monitor weight and BMI during treatment

❋ While giving a drug to a patient who has gained >5% of initial weight, consider evaluating for the presence of pre-diabetes, diabetes, or dyslipidemia, or consider switching to a different antidepressant

- EKGs may be useful for selected patients (e.g., those with personal or family history of QTc prolongation; cardiac arrhythmia; recent myocardial infarction; uncompensated heart failure; or taking agents that prolong QTc interval such as pimozide, thioridazine, selected antiarrhythmics, moxifloxacin, sparfloxacin, etc.)
- Patients at risk for electrolyte disturbances (e.g., patients on diuretic therapy) should have baseline and periodic serum potassium and magnesium measurements

SIDE EFFECTS

How Drug Causes Side Effects

❋ Anticholinergic activity for desipramine may be somewhat less than for some other TCAs, yet can still explain the presence, if lower incidence, of sedative effects, dry mouth, constipation, and blurred vision

- Sedative effects and weight gain may be due to antihistamine properties
- Blockade of alpha adrenergic 1 receptors may explain dizziness, sedation, and hypotension
- Cardiac arrhythmias and seizures, especially in overdose, may be caused by blockade of ion channels

Notable Side Effects

- Blurred vision, constipation, urinary retention, increased appetite, dry mouth, nausea, diarrhea, heartburn, unusual taste in mouth, weight gain
- Fatigue, weakness, dizziness, sedation, headache, anxiety, nervousness, restlessness
- Sexual dysfunction, sweating

 Life Threatening or Dangerous Side Effects

- Paralytic ileus, hyperthermia (TCAs + anticholinergic agents)
- Lowered seizure threshold and rare seizures
- Orthostatic hypotension, sudden death, arrhythmias, tachycardia
- QTc prolongation
- Hepatic failure, extrapyramidal symptoms
- Increased intraocular pressure
- Blood dyscrasias
- Rare induction of mania and activation of suicidal ideation

Weight Gain

unusual   not unusual   **common**   problematic

- Many experience and/or can be significant in amount
- Can increase appetite and carbohydrate craving

Sedation

unusual   not unusual   **common**   problematic

- Many experience and/or can be significant in amount
- Tolerance to sedative effects may develop with long-term use

What To Do About Side Effects
- Wait
- Wait
- Wait
- Lower the dose
- Switch to an SSRI or newer antidepressant

Best Augmenting Agents for Side Effects
- Many side effects cannot be improved with an augmenting agent

DOSING AND USE

Usual Dosage Range
- 100–200 mg/day (for depression)
- 50–150 mg/day (for chronic pain)

Dosage Forms
- Tablets 10 mg, 25 mg, 50 mg, 75 mg, 100 mg, 150 mg

How to Dose
- Initial 25 mg/day at bedtime; increase by 25 mg every 3–7 days
- 75 mg/day once daily or in divided doses; gradually increase dose to achieve desired therapeutic effect; maximum dose 300 mg/day

 Dosing Tips
- If given in a single dose, should generally be administered at bedtime because of its sedative properties
- If given in split doses, largest dose should generally be given at bedtime because of its sedative properties
- If patients experience nightmares, split dose and do not give large dose at bedtime
- Patients treated for chronic pain may only require lower doses (e.g., 50–75 mg/day)
- Risk of seizure increases with dose
- ✷ Monitoring plasma levels of desipramine is recommended in patients who do not respond to the usual dose or whose treatment is regarded as urgent

- If intolerable anxiety, insomnia, agitation, akathisia, or activation occur either upon dosing initiation or discontinuation, consider the possibility of activated bipolar disorder, and switch to a mood stabilizer or an atypical antipsychotic

Overdose
- Death may occur; convulsions, cardiac dysrhythmias, severe hypotension, CNS depression, coma, changes in ECG

Long-Term Use
- Safe

Habit Forming
- No

How to Stop
- Taper to avoid withdrawal effects
- Even with gradual dose reduction some withdrawal symptoms may appear within the first 2 weeks
- Many patients tolerate 50% dose reduction for 3 days, then another 50% reduction for 3 days, then discontinuation
- If withdrawal symptoms emerge during discontinuation, raise dose to stop symptoms and then restart withdrawal much more slowly

Pharmacokinetics
- Substrate for CYP450 2D6 and 1A2
- Is the active metabolite of imipramine, formed by demethylation via CYP450 1A2
- Half-life approximately 24 hours

 Drug Interactions
- Tramadol increases the risk of seizures in patients taking TCAs
- Use of TCAs with anticholinergic drugs may result in paralytic ileus or hyperthermia
- Fluoxetine, paroxetine, bupropion, duloxetine, and other CYP450 2D6 inhibitors may increase TCA concentrations
- Cimetidine may increase plasma concentrations of TCAs and cause anticholinergic symptoms
- Phenothiazines or haloperidol may raise TCA blood concentrations
- May alter effects of antihypertensive drugs; may inhibit hypotensive effects of clonidine

- Use of TCAs with sympathomimetic agents may increase sympathetic activity
- Methylphenidate may inhibit metabolism of TCAs
- Activation and agitation, especially following switching or adding antidepressants, may represent the induction of a bipolar state, especially a mixed dysphoric bipolar II condition sometimes associated with suicidal ideation, and require the addition of lithium, a mood stabilizer or an atypical antipsychotic, and/or discontinuation of desipramine

 Other Warnings/ Precautions

- Add or initiate other antidepressants with caution for up to 2 weeks after discontinuing desipramine
- Generally, do not use with MAO inhibitors, including 14 days after MAOIs are stopped; do not start an MAOI until 2 weeks after discontinuing desipramine, but see Pearls
- Use with caution in patients with history of seizures, urinary retention, narrow angle-closure glaucoma, hyperthyroidism
- TCAs can increase QTc interval, especially at toxic doses, which can be attained not only by overdose but also by combining with drugs that inhibit TCA metabolism via CYP450 2D6, potentially causing torsade de pointes-type arrhythmia or sudden death
- Because TCAs can prolong QTc interval, use with caution in patients who have bradycardia or who are taking drugs that can induce bradycardia (e.g., beta blockers, calcium channel blockers, clonidine, digitalis)
- Because TCAs can prolong QTc interval, use with caution in patients who have hypokalemia and/or hypomagnesemia or who are taking drugs that can induce hypokalemia and/or magnesemia (e.g., diuretics, stimulant laxatives, intravenous amphotericin B, glucocorticoids, tetracosactide)

Do Not Use

- If patient is recovering from myocardial infarction
- If patient is taking agents capable of significantly prolonging QTc interval (e.g., pimozide, thioridazine, selected antiarrhythmics, moxifloxacin, sparfloxacin)
- If there is a history of QTc prolongation or cardiac arrhythmia, recent acute myocardial infarction, uncompensated heart failure
- If patient is taking drugs that inhibit TCA metabolism, including CYP450 2D6 inhibitors, except by an expert
- If there is reduced CYP450 2D6 function, such as patients who are poor 2D6 metabolizers, except by an expert and at low doses
- If there is a proven allergy to desipramine, imipramine, or lofepramine

Renal Impairment

- Use with caution; may need to lower dose
- May need to monitor plasma levels

Hepatic Impairment

- Use with caution; may need to lower dose
- May need to monitor plasma levels

Cardiac Impairment

- TCAs have been reported to cause arrhythmias, prolongation of conduction time, orthostatic hypotension, sinus tachycardia, and heart failure, especially in the diseased heart
- Myocardial infarction and stroke have been reported with TCAs
- TCAs produce QTc prolongation, which may be enhanced by the existence of bradycardia, hypokalemia, congenital or acquired long QTc interval, which should be evaluated prior to administering desipramine
- Use with caution if treating concomitantly with a medication likely to produce prolonged bradycardia, hypokalemia, slowing of intracardiac conduction, or prolongation of the QTc interval
- Avoid TCAs in patients with a known history of QTc prolongation, recent acute myocardial infarction, and uncompensated heart failure
- TCAs may cause a sustained increase in heart rate in patients with ischemic heart disease and may worsen (decrease) heart

rate variability, an independent risk of mortality in cardiac populations
• Since SSRIs may improve (increase) heart rate variability in patients following a myocardial infarct and may improve survival as well as mood in patients with acute angina or following a myocardial infarction, these are more appropriate agents for cardiac population than tricyclic/tetracyclic antidepressants
✳ Risk/benefit ratio may not justify use of TCAs in cardiac impairment

Elderly
• May be more sensitive to anticholinergic, cardiovascular, hypotensive, and sedative effects
• Initial dose 25–50 mg/day, raise to 100 mg/day; maximum 150 mg/day
• May be useful to monitor plasma levels in elderly patients

 Children and Adolescents
• Use with caution, observing for activation of known or unknown bipolar disorder and/or suicidal ideation, and strongly consider informing parents or guardian of this risk so they can help observe child or adolescent patients
• Not recommended for use under age 12
• Several studies show lack of efficacy of TCAs for depression
• May be used to treat enuresis or hyperactive/impulsive behaviors
• May reduce tic symptoms
• Some cases of sudden death have occurred in children taking TCAs
• Adolescents: initial dose 25–50 mg/day, increase to 100 mg/day; maximum dose 150 mg/day
• May be useful to monitor plasma levels in children and adolescents

 Pregnancy
• Risk Category C [some animal studies show adverse effects, no controlled studies in humans]
• Crosses the placenta
• Adverse effects have been reported in infants whose mothers took a TCA (lethargy, withdrawal symptoms, fetal malformations)

• Must weigh the risk of treatment (first trimester fetal development, third trimester newborn delivery) to the child against the risk of no treatment (recurrence of depression, maternal health, infant bonding) to the mother and child
• For many patients this may mean continuing treatment during pregnancy

Breast Feeding
• Some drug is found in mother's breast milk
✳ Recommended either to discontinue drug or bottle feed
• Immediate postpartum period is a high-risk time for depression, especially in women who have had prior depressive episodes, so drug may need to be reinstituted late in the third trimester or shortly after childbirth to prevent a recurrence during the postpartum period
• Must weigh benefits of breast feeding with risks and benefits of antidepressant treatment versus non-treatment to both the infant and the mother
• For many patients this may mean continuing treatment during breast feeding

THE ART OF PSYCHOPHARMACOLOGY

Potential Advantages
• Patients with insomnia
• Severe or treatment-resistant depression
• Patients for whom therapeutic drug monitoring is desirable

Potential Disadvantages
• Pediatric and geriatric patients
• Patients concerned with weight gain
• Cardiac patients

Primary Target Symptoms
• Depressed mood
• Chronic pain

 Pearls
• Tricyclic antidepressants are often a first-line treatment option for chronic pain
• Tricyclic antidepressants are no longer generally considered a first-line option for depression because of their side effect profile

- Tricyclic antidepressants continue to be useful for severe or treatment-resistant depression
- Noradrenergic reuptake inhibitors such as desipramine can be used as a second-line treatment for smoking cessation, cocaine dependence, and attention deficit disorder
- TCAs may aggravate psychotic symptoms
- Alcohol should be avoided because of additive CNS effects
- Underweight patients may be more susceptible to adverse cardiovascular effects
- Children, patients with inadequate hydration, and patients with cardiac disease may be more susceptible to TCA-induced cardiotoxicity than healthy adults
- For the expert only: although generally prohibited, a heroic but potentially dangerous treatment for severely treatment-resistant patients is to give a tricyclic/tetracyclic antidepressant other than clomipramine simultaneously with an MAO inhibitor for patients who fail to respond to numerous other antidepressants
- If this option is elected, start the MAOI with the tricyclic/tetracyclic antidepressant simultaneously at low doses after appropriate drug washout, then alternately increase doses of these agents every few days to a week as tolerated
- Although very strict dietary and concomitant drug restrictions must be observed to prevent hypertensive crises and serotonin syndrome, the most common side effects of MAOI/ tricyclic or tetracyclic combinations may be weight gain and orthostatic hypotension
- Patients on TCAs should be aware that they may experience symptoms such as photosensitivity or blue-green urine
- SSRIs may be more effective than TCAs in women, and TCAs may be more effective than SSRIs in men
- Not recommended for first-line use in children with ADHD because of the availability of safer treatments with better documented efficacy and because of desipramine's potential for sudden death in children

✻ Desipramine is one of the few TCAs where monitoring of plasma drug levels has been well studied

✻ Fewer anticholinergic side effects than some other TCAs

- Since tricyclic/tetracyclic antidepressants are substrates for CYP450 2D6, and 7% of the population (especially Caucasians) may have a genetic variant leading to reduced activity of 2D6, such patients may not safely tolerate normal doses of tricyclic/tetracyclic antidepressants and may require dose reduction
- Phenotypic testing may be necessary to detect this genetic variant prior to dosing with a tricyclic/tetracyclic antidepressant, especially in vulnerable populations such as children, elderly, cardiac populations, and those on concomitant medications
- Patients who seem to have extraordinarily severe side effects at normal or low doses may have this phenotypic CYP450 2D6 variant and require low doses or switching to another antidepressant not metabolized by 2D6

Suggested Reading

Anderson IM. Meta-analytical studies on new antidepressants. Br Med Bull 2001; 57:161–178.

Anderson IM. Selective serotonin reuptake inhibitors versus tricyclic antidepressants: a meta-analysis of efficacy and tolerability. J Aff Disorders 2000;58:19–36.

Janowsky DS, Byerley B. Desipramine: an overview. J Clin Psychiatry 1984;45:3–9.

Levin FR, Lehman AF. Meta-analysis of desipramine as an adjunct in the treatment of cocaine addiction. J Clin Psychopharmacol 1991;11:374–8.

DIAZEPAM

THERAPEUTICS

Brands
- Valium
- Diastat

see index for additional brand names

Generic? Yes (not Diastat)

Class
- Benzodiazepine (anxiolytic, muscle relaxant, anticonvulsant)

Commonly Prescribed For
(bold for FDA approved)
- **Anxiety disorder**
- **Symptoms of anxiety (short-term)**
- **Acute agitation, tremor, impending or acute delirium tremens and hallucinosis in acute alcohol withdrawal**
- **Skeletal muscle spasm due to reflex spasm to local pathology**
- **Spasticity caused by upper motor neuron disorder**
- **Athetosis**
- **Stiffman syndrome**
- **Convulsive disorder (adjunctive)**
- **Anxiety during endoscopic procedures (adjunctive) (injection only)**
- **Pre-operative anxiety (injection only)**
- **Anxiety relief prior to cardioversion (intravenous)**
- **Initial treatment of status epilepticus (injection only)**
- Insomnia

How The Drug Works
- Binds to benzodiazepine receptors at the GABA-A ligand-gated chloride channel complex
- Enhances the inhibitory effects of GABA
- Boosts chloride conductance through GABA-regulated channels
- Inhibits neuronal activity presumably in amygdala-centered fear circuits to provide therapeutic benefits in anxiety disorders
- Inhibiting actions in cerebral cortex may provide therapeutic benefits in seizure disorders
- Inhibitory actions in spinal cord may provide therapeutic benefits for muscle spasms

How Long Until It Works
- Some immediate relief with first dosing is common; can take several weeks with daily dosing for maximal therapeutic benefit

If It Works
- For short-term symptoms of anxiety or muscle spasms – after a few weeks, discontinue use or use on an "as-needed" basis
- Chronic muscle spasms may require chronic diazepam treatment
- For chronic anxiety disorders, the goal of treatment is complete remission of symptoms as well as prevention of future relapses
- For chronic anxiety disorders, treatment most often reduces or even eliminates symptoms, but not a cure since symptoms can recur after medicine stopped
- For long-term symptoms of anxiety, consider switching to an SSRI or SNRI for long term maintenance
- If long-term maintenance with a benzodiazepine is necessary, continue treatment for 6 months after symptoms resolve, and then taper dose slowly
- If symptoms reemerge, consider treatment with an SSRI or SNRI, or consider restarting the benzodiazepine; sometimes benzodiazepines have to be used in combination with SSRIs or SNRIs for best results

If It Doesn't Work
- Consider switching to another agent or adding an appropriate augmenting agent
- Consider psychotherapy, especially cognitive behavioral psychotherapy
- Consider presence of concomitant substance abuse
- Consider presence of diazepam abuse
- Consider another diagnosis, such as a comorbid medical condition

Best Augmenting Combos for Partial Response or Treatment-Resistance
- Benzodiazepines are frequently used as augmenting agents for antipsychotics and mood stabilizers in the treatment of psychotic and bipolar disorders
- Benzodiazepines are frequently used as augmenting agents for SSRIs and SNRIs in the treatment of anxiety disorders

- Not generally rational to combine with other benzodiazepines
- Caution if using as an anxiolytic concomitantly with other sedative hypnotics for sleep

Tests

- In patients with seizure disorders, concomitant medical illness, and/or those with multiple concomitant long-term medications, periodic liver tests and blood counts may be prudent

SIDE EFFECTS

How Drug Causes Side Effects

- Same mechanism for side effects as for therapeutic effects – namely due to excessive actions at benzodiazepine receptors
- Long-term adaptations in benzodiazepine receptors may explain the development of dependence, tolerance, and withdrawal
- Side effects are generally immediate, but immediate side effects often disappear in time

Notable Side Effects

❋ Sedation, fatigue, depression
❋ Dizziness, ataxia, slurred speech, weakness
❋ Forgetfulness, confusion
❋ Hyper-excitability, nervousness
❋ Pain at injection site
- Rare hallucinations, mania
- Rare hypotension
- Hypersalivation, dry mouth

 Life Threatening or Dangerous Side Effects

- Respiratory depression, especially when taken with CNS depressants in overdose
- Rare hepatic dysfunction, renal dysfunction, blood dyscrasias

Weight Gain

unusual / not unusual / common / problematic

- Reported but not expected

Sedation

unusual / not unusual / **common** / problematic

- Many experience and/or can be significant in amount
- Especially at initiation of treatment or when dose increases
- Tolerance often develops over time

What To Do About Side Effects

- Wait
- Wait
- Wait
- Lower the dose
- Take largest dose at bedtime to avoid sedative effects during the day
- Switch to another agent
- Administer flumazenil if side effects are severe or life-threatening

Best Augmenting Agents for Side Effects

- Many side effects cannot be improved with an augmenting agent

DOSING AND USE

Usual Dosage Range

- Oral: 4–40 mg/day in divided doses
- Intravenous (adults): 5 mg/minute
- Intravenous (children): 0.25 mg/kg/3 minutes

Dosage Forms

- Tablet 2 mg scored, 5 mg scored, 10 mg scored
- Liquid 5 mg/5 mL, concentrate 5 mg/mL
- Injection vial 5 mg/mL; 10 mL, boxes of 1; 2 mL boxes of 10
- Rectal gel 5 mg/mL; 2.5 mg, 5 mg, 10 mg, 15 mg, 20 mg

How to Dose

- Oral (anxiety, muscle spasm, seizure): 2–10 mg, 2–4 times/day
- Oral (alcohol withdrawal): Initial 10 mg, 3–4 times/day for 1 day; reduce to 5 mg, 3–4 times/day; continue treatment as needed
- Liquid formulation should be mixed with water or fruit juice, applesauce, or pudding
- Because of risk of respiratory depression, rectal diazepam treatment should not be

given more than once in 5 days or more than twice during a treatment course, especially for alcohol withdrawal or status epilepticus

 Dosing Tips

❋ Only benzodiazepine with a formulation specifically for rectal administration
❋ One of the few benzodiazepines available in an oral liquid formulation
❋ One of the few benzodiazepines available in an injectable formulation
• Diazepam injection is intended for acute use; patients who require long-term treatment should be switched to the oral formulation
• Use lowest possible effective dose for the shortest possible period of time (a benzodiazepine-sparing strategy)
• Assess need for continued treatment regularly
• Risk of dependence may increase with dose and duration of treatment
• For inter-dose symptoms of anxiety, can either increase dose or maintain same total daily dose but divide into more frequent doses
• Can also use an as-needed occasional "top up" dose for inter-dose anxiety
• Because some anxiety disorder patients and muscle spasm patients can require doses higher than 40 mg/day or more, the risk of dependence may be greater in these patients
• Frequency of dosing in practice is often greater than predicted from half-life, as duration of biological activity is often shorter than pharmacokinetic terminal half-life

Overdose
• Fatalities can occur; hypotension, tiredness, ataxia, confusion, coma

Long-Term Use
• Evidence of efficacy up to 16 weeks
• Risk of dependence, particularly for treatment periods longer than 12 weeks and especially in patients with past or current polysubstance abuse
• Not recommended for long-term treatment of seizure disorders

Habit Forming
• Diazepam is a Schedule IV drug
• Patients may develop dependence and/or tolerance with long-term use

How to Stop
• Patients with history of seizure may seize upon withdrawal, especially if withdrawal is abrupt
• Taper by 2 mg every 3 days to reduce chances of withdrawal effects
• For difficult to taper cases, consider reducing dose much more slowly after reaching 20 mg/day, perhaps by as little as 0.5–1 mg every week or less
• For other patients with severe problems discontinuing a benzodiazepine, dosing may need to be tapered over many months (i.e., reduce dose by 1% every 3 days by crushing tablet and suspending or dissolving in 100 ml of fruit juice and then disposing of 1 ml while drinking the rest; 3–7 days later, dispose of 2 ml, and so on). This is both a form of very slow biological tapering and a form of behavioral desensitization
• Be sure to differentiate reemergence of symptoms requiring reinstitution of treatment from withdrawal symptoms
• Benzodiazepine-dependent anxiety patients and insulin-dependent diabetics are not addicted to their medications. When benzodiazepine-dependent patients stop their medication, disease symptoms can reemerge, disease symptoms can worsen (rebound), and/or withdrawal symptoms can emerge

Pharmacokinetics
• Elimination half-life 20–50 hours

 Drug Interactions
• Increased depressive effects when taken with other CNS depressants
• Cimetidine may reduce the clearance and raise the levels of diazepam
• Flumazenil (used to reverse the effects of benzodiazepines) may precipitate seizures and should not be used in patients treated for seizure disorders with diazepam

Other Warnings/ Precautions

- Dosage changes should be made in collaboration with prescriber
- Use with caution in patients with pulmonary disease; rare reports of death after initiation of benzodiazepines in patients with severe pulmonary impairment
- History of drug or alcohol abuse often creates greater risk for dependency
- Some depressed patients may experience a worsening of suicidal ideation
- Some patients may exhibit abnormal thinking or behavioral changes similar to those caused by other CNS depressants (i.e., either depressant actions or disinhibiting actions)

Do Not Use

- If narrow angle-closure glaucoma
- If there is a proven allergy to diazepam or any benzodiazepine

SPECIAL POPULATIONS

Renal Impairment

- Initial 2–2.5 mg, 1–2 times/day; increase gradually as needed

Hepatic Impairment

- Initial 2–2.5 mg, 1–2 times/day; increase gradually as needed

Cardiac Impairment

- Benzodiazepines have been used to treat anxiety associated with acute myocardial infarction
- Diazepam may be used as an adjunct during cardiovascular emergencies

Elderly

- Initial 2–2.5 mg, 1–2 times/day; increase gradually as needed

 Children and Adolescents

- 6 months and up: Initial 1–2.5 mg, 3–4 times/day; increase gradually as needed
- Parenteral: 30 days or older
- Rectal: 2 years or older
- Long-term effects of diazepam in children/adolescents are unknown

- Should generally receive lower doses and be more closely monitored

 Pregnancy

- Risk Category D [positive evidence of risk to human fetus; potential benefits may still justify its use during pregnancy]
- Possible increased risk of birth defects when benzodiazepines taken during pregnancy
- Because of the potential risks, diazepam is not generally recommended as treatment for anxiety during pregnancy, especially during the first trimester
- Drug should be tapered if discontinued
- Infants whose mothers received a benzodiazepine late in pregnancy may experience withdrawal effects
- Neonatal flaccidity has been reported in infants whose mothers took a benzodiazepine during pregnancy
- Seizures, even mild seizures, may cause harm to the embryo/fetus

Breast Feeding

- Unknown if diazepam is secreted in human breast milk, but all psychotropics assumed to be secreted in breast milk
- ✱ Recommended either to discontinue drug or bottle feed
- Effects of benzodiazepines on nursing infants have been reported and include feeding difficulties, sedation, and weight loss

THE ART OF PSYCHOPHARMACOLOGY

Potential Advantages

- Rapid onset of action
- Availability of oral liquid, rectal, and injectable dosage formulations

Potential Disadvantages

- Euphoria may lead to abuse
- Abuse especially risky in past or present substance abusers
- Can be sedating at doses necessary to treat moderately severe anxiety disorders

Primary Target Symptoms

- Panic attacks
- Anxiety

- Incidence of seizures (adjunct)
- Muscle spasms

 Pearls

- Can be a useful adjunct to SSRIs and SNRIs in the treatment of numerous anxiety disorders, but not used as frequently as other benzodiazepines for this purpose
- Not effective for treating psychosis as a monotherapy, but can be used as an adjunct to antipsychotics
- Not effective for treating bipolar disorder as a monotherapy, but can be used as an adjunct to mood stabilizers and antipsychotics
- ✳ Diazepam is often the first choice benzodiazepine to treat status epilepticus, and is administered either intravenously or rectally
- Because diazepam suppresses stage 4 sleep, it may prevent night terrors in adults

- May both cause depression and treat depression in different patients
- Was once one of the most commonly prescribed drugs in the world and the most commonly prescribed benzodiazepine
- ✳ Remains a popular benzodiazepine for treating muscle spasms
- A commonly used benzodiazepine to treat sleep disorders
- ✳ Remains a popular benzodiazepine to treat acute alcohol withdrawal
- Not especially useful as an oral anticonvulsant
- ✳ Multiple dosage formulations (oral tablet, oral liquid, rectal gel, injectable) allow more flexibility of administration compared to most other benzodiazepines
- When using to treat insomnia, remember that insomnia may be a symptom of some other primary disorder itself, and thus warrant evaluation for comorbid psychiatric and/or medical conditions

 Suggested Reading

Ashton H. Guidelines for the rational use of benzodiazepines. When and what to use. Drugs 1994;48:25–40.

De Negri M, Baglietto MG. Treatment of status epilepticus in children. Paediatr Drugs 2001; 3:411–20.

Mandelli M, Tognoni G, Garattini S. Clinical pharmacokinetics of diazepam. Clin Pharmacokinet 1978;3:72–91.

Rey E. Treluver JM, Pons G. Pharmacokinetic optimization of benzodiazepine therapy for acute seizures. Focus on delivery routes. Clin Pharmacokinet 1999;36:409–24.

D,L-AMPHETAMINE

THERAPEUTICS

Brands
- Adderall
- Adderall XR

see index for additional brand names

Generic? No

 Class
- Stimulant

Commonly Prescribed For
(bold for FDA approved)
- **Attention deficit hyperactivity disorder in children**
- **Attention deficit hyperactivity disorder in adults (Adderall XR)**
- **Narcolepsy (Adderall)**
- Treatment-resistant depression

 How The Drug Works
- * Increases norepinephrine and especially dopamine actions by blocking their reuptake and facilitating their release
- Enhancement of dopamine and norepinephrine actions in certain brain regions (e.g., dorsolateral prefrontal cortex) may improve attention, concentration, executive function, and wakefulness
- Enhancement of dopamine actions in other brain regions (e.g., basal ganglia) may improve hyperactivity
- Enhancement of dopamine and norepinephrine in yet other brain regions (e.g., medial prefrontal cortex, hypothalamus) may improve depression, fatigue, and sleepiness

How Long Until It Works
- Some immediate effects can be seen with first dosing
- Can take several weeks to attain maximum therapeutic benefit

If It Works (for ADHD)
- The goal of treatment of ADHD is reduction of symptoms of inattentiveness, motor hyperactivity, and/or impulsiveness that disrupt social, school, and/or occupational functioning
- Continue treatment until all symptoms are under control or improvement is stable and then continue treatment indefinitely as long as improvement persists
- Reevaluate the need for treatment periodically
- Treatment for ADHD begun in childhood may need to be continued into adolescence and adulthood if continued benefit is documented

If It Doesn't Work (for ADHD)
- Consider adjusting dose or switching to another formulation of d,l-amphetamine or to another agent
- Consider behavioral therapy
- Consider the presence of noncompliance and counsel patient and parents
- Consider evaluation for another diagnosis or for a comorbid condition (e.g., bipolar disorder, substance abuse, medical illness, etc.)
- * Some ADHD patients and some depressed patients may experience lack of consistent efficacy due to activation of latent or underlying bipolar disorder, and require either augmenting with a mood stabilizer or switching to a mood stabilizer

 Best Augmenting Combos for Partial Response or Treatment-Resistance
- Best to attempt other monotherapies prior to augmenting
- For the expert, can combine immediate release formulation with a sustained release formulation of d,l-amphetamine for ADHD
- For the expert, can combine with modafinil or atomoxetine for ADHD
- For the expert, can occasionally combine with atypical antipsychotics in highly treatment-resistant cases of bipolar disorder or ADHD
- For the expert, can combine with antidepressants to boost antidepressant efficacy in highly treatment-resistant cases of depression while carefully monitoring patient

Tests
- Blood pressure should be monitored regularly
- In children, monitor weight and height

SIDE EFFECTS

How Drug Causes Side Effects
- Increases in norepinephrine peripherally can cause autonomic side effects, including tremor, tachycardia, hypertension, and cardiac arrhythmias
- Increases in norepinephrine and dopamine centrally can cause CNS side effects such as insomnia, agitation, psychosis and substance abuse

Notable Side Effects
* ✻ Insomnia, headache, exacerbation of tics, nervousness, irritability, overstimulation, tremor, dizziness
- Anorexia, nausea, dry mouth, constipation, diarrhea, weight loss
- Can temporarily slow normal growth in children (controversial)
- Sexual dysfunction long-term (impotence, libido changes) but can also improve sexual dysfunction short-term

 Life Threatening or Dangerous Side Effects
- Psychotic episodes, especially with parenteral abuse
- Seizures
- Palpitations, tachycardia, hypertension
- Rare activation of hypomania, mania, or suicidal ideation (controversial)

Weight Gain

unusual / not unusual / common / problematic
- Reported but not expected
- Some patients may experience weight loss

Sedation

unusual / not unusual / common / problematic
- Reported but not expected
- Activation much more common than sedation

What To Do About Side Effects
- Wait
- Adjust dose
- Switch to a long-acting stimulant
- Switch to another agent
- For insomnia, avoid dosing in afternoon/evening

Best Augmenting Agents for Side Effects
- Beta-blockers for peripheral autonomic side effects
- Dose reduction or switching to another agent may be more effective since most side effects cannot be improved with an augmenting agent

DOSING AND USE

Usual Dosage Range
- Narcolepsy: 5–60 mg/day in divided doses
- ADHD: 5–40 mg/day (divided doses for immediate release tablet, once-daily morning dose for extended release tablet)

Dosage Forms
- Immediate release tablet 5 mg double-scored, 7.5 mg double-scored, 10 mg double-scored, 12.5 mg double-scored, 15 mg double-scored, 20 mg double-scored, 30 mg double-scored
- Extended release tablet 5 mg, 10 mg, 15 mg, 20 mg, 25 mg, 30 mg

How to Dose
- Immediate release formulation in ADHD (ages 6 and older): initial 5 mg once or twice per day; can increase by 5 mg each week; maximum dose generally 40 mg/day; split daily dose with first dose on waking and every 4–6 hours thereafter
- Immediate release formulation in narcolepsy (ages 12 and older): initial 10 mg/day; increase by 10 mg each week; give first dose on waking and every 4–6 hours thereafter
- Extended release formulation in ADHD: initial 10 mg/day in the morning; can increase by 5–10 mg/day at weekly intervals; maximum dose generally 30 mg/day

 Dosing Tips
- Clinical duration of action often differs from pharmacokinetic half-life
* ✻ Immediate release d,l-amphetamine has 3–6 hour duration of clinical action
* ✻ Extended release d,l-amphetamine has up to 8-hour duration of clinical action

- Adderall XR is controlled-release and should therefore not be chewed but rather should only be swallowed whole
- ✳ Controlled release delivery of d,l-amphetamine is sufficiently long in duration to allow elimination of lunchtime dosing
- ✳ This innovation can be an important practical element in stimulant utilization, eliminating the hassle and pragmatic difficulties of lunchtime dosing at school, including storage problems, potential diversion, and the need for a medical professional to supervise dosing away from home
- Avoid dosing late in the day because of the risk of insomnia
- May be possible to dose only during the school week for some ADHD patients
- Off-label uses are dosed the same as for ADHD
- ✳ May be able to give drug holidays over the summer in order to reassess therapeutic utility and effects on growth and to allow catch-up from any growth suppression as well as to assess any other side effects and the need to reinstitute stimulant treatment for the next school term
- Side effects are generally dose-related
- Taking with food may delay peak actions for 2–3 hours

Overdose
- Rarely fatal; panic, hyperreflexia, rhabdomyolysis, rapid respiration, confusion, coma, hallucinations, convulsions, arrhythmia, change in blood pressure, circulatory collapse

Long-Term Use
- Often used long-term for ADHD when ongoing monitoring documents continued efficacy
- Dependence and/or abuse may develop
- Tolerance to therapeutic effects may develop in some patients
- Long-term stimulant use may be associated with growth suppression in children (controversial)
- Periodic monitoring of weight, blood pressure, CBC, platelet counts, and liver function may be prudent

Habit Forming
- High abuse potential, Schedule II drug
- Patients may develop tolerance, psychological dependence

How to Stop
- Taper to avoid withdrawal effects
- Withdrawal following chronic therapeutic use may unmask symptoms of the underlying disorder and may require follow-up and reinstitution of treatment
- Careful supervision is required during withdrawal from abusive use since severe depression may occur

Pharmacokinetics
- Adderall and Adderall XR are a mixture of d-amphetamine and l-amphetamine salts in the ratio of 3:1
- A single dose of Adderall XR 20 mg gives drug levels of both d-amphetamine and l-amphetamine comparable to Adderall immediate release 20 mg administered in 2 divided doses 4 hours apart
- In adults, half-life for d-amphetamine is 10 hours and for l-amphetamine is 13 hours
- For children ages 6–12, half-life for d-amphetamine is 9 hours and for l-amphetamine is 11 hours

 Drug Interactions
- May affect blood pressure and should be used cautiously with agents used to control blood pressure
- Gastrointestinal acidifying agents (guanethidine, reserpine, glutamic acid, ascorbic acid, fruit juices, etc.) and urinary acidifying agents (ammonium chloride, sodium phosphate, etc.) lower amphetamine plasma levels, so such agents can be useful to administer after an overdose but may also lower therapeutic efficacy of amphetamines
- Gastrointestinal alkalinizing agents (sodium bicarbonate, etc.) and urinary alkalinizing agents (acetazolamide, some thiazides) increase amphetamine plasma levels and potentiate amphetamine's actions
- Desipramine and protryptiline can cause striking and sustained increases in brain concentrations of amphetamine and may also add to amphetamine's cardiovascular effects

- Theoretically, other agents with norepinephrine reuptake blocking properties, such as venlafaxine, duloxetine, atomoxetine, milnacipran, and reboxetine, could also add to amphetamine's CNS and cardiovascular effects
- Amphetamines may counteract the sedative effects of antihistamines
- Haloperidol, chlorpromazine, and lithium may inhibit stimulatory effects of amphetamines
- Theoretically, atypical antipsychotics should also inhibit stimulatory effects of amphetamines
- Theoretically, amphetamines could inhibit the antipsychotic actions of antipsychotics
- Theoretically, amphetamines could inhibit the mood stabilizing actions of atypical antipsychotics in some patients
- Combinations of amphetamines with mood stabilizers (lithium, anticonvulsants, atypical antipsychotics) is generally something for experts only, when monitoring patients closely and when other options fail
- Absorption of amphetamine is delayed by phenobarbital, phenytoin, ethosuximide
- Amphetamines inhibit adrenergic blockers and enhance adrenergic effects of norepinephrine
- Amphetamines may antagonize hypotensive effects of veratrum alkaloids and other antihypertensives
- Amphetamines increase the analgesic effects of meperidine
- Amphetamines contribute to excessive CNS stimulation if used with large doses of propoxyphene
- Amphetamines can raise plasma corticosteroid levels
- MAOIs slow absorption of amphetamines and thus potentiate their actions, which can cause headache, hypertension, and rarely hypertensive crisis and malignant hyperthermia, sometimes with fatal results
- Use with MAOIs, including within 14 days of MAOI use, is not advised, but this can sometimes be considered by experts who monitor depressed patients closely when other treatment options for depression fail

 Other Warnings/ Precautions

- Use with caution in patients with any degree of hypertension, hyperthyroidism, or history of drug abuse
- Children who are not growing or gaining weight should stop treatment, at least temporarily
- May worsen motor and phonic tics
- May worsen symptoms of thought disorder and behavioral disturbance in psychotic patients
- Stimulants have a high potential for abuse and must be used with caution in anyone with a current or past history of substance abuse or alcoholism or in emotionally unstable patients
- Administration of stimulants for prolonged periods of time should be avoided whenever possible or done only with close monitoring, as it may lead to marked tolerance and drug dependence, including psychological dependence with varying degrees of abnormal behavior
- Particular attention should be paid to the possibility of subjects obtaining stimulants for nontherapeutic use or distribution to others and the drugs should in general be prescribed sparingly with documentation of appropriate use
- Not an appropriate first-line treatment for depression or for normal fatigue
- May lower the seizure threshold
- Emergence or worsening of activation and agitation may represent the induction of a bipolar state, especially a mixed dysphoric bipolar II condition sometimes associated with suicidal ideation, and require the addition of a mood stabilizer and/or discontinuation of d,l-amphetamine

Do Not Use

- If patient has extreme anxiety or agitation
- If patient has motor tics or Tourette's sydrome or if there is a family history of Tourette's, unless administered by an expert in cases when the potential benefits for ADHD outweigh the risks of worsening tics
- Should generally not be administered with an MAOI, including within 14 days of MAOI use, except in heroic circumstances and by an expert

- If patient has arteriosclerosis, cardiovascular disease, or severe hypertension
- If patient has glaucoma
- If there is a proven allergy to any sympathomimetic agent

SPECIAL POPULATIONS

Renal Impairment
- No dose adjustment necessary

Hepatic Impairment
- No dose adjustment necessary

Cardiac Impairment
- Use with caution, particularly in patients with recent myocardial infarction or other conditions that could be negatively affected by increased blood pressure

Elderly
- Some patients may tolerate lower doses better

 Children and Adolescents
- Safety and efficacy not established under age 3
- Use in young children should be reserved for the expert
- d,l-amphetamine may worsen symptoms of behavioral disturbance and thought disorder in psychotic children
- d,l-amphetamine has acute effects on growth hormone; long-term effects are unknown but weight and height should be monitored during long-term treatment
- ADHD: ages 3–5: initial 2.5 mg/day; can increase by 2.5 mg each week
- Narcolepsy: ages 6–12: initial 5 mg/day; increase by 5 mg each week

 Pregnancy
- Risk Category C [some animal studies show adverse effects, no controlled studies in humans]
- Infants whose mothers take d,l-amphetamine during pregnancy may experience withdrawal symptoms

- Use in women of childbearing potential requires weighing potential benefits to the mother against potential risks to the fetus
- ✳ For ADHD patients, d,l-amphetamine should generally be discontinued before anticipated pregnancies

Breast Feeding
- Some drug is found in mother's breast milk
- ✳ Recommended either to discontinue drug or bottle feed
- If infant shows signs of irritability, drug may need to be discontinued

THE ART OF PSYCHOPHARMACOLOGY

Potential Advantages
- May work in ADHD patients unresponsive to other stimulants, including pure d-amphetamine sulfate
- New sustained release option

Potential Disadvantages
- Patients with current or past substance abuse
- Patients with current or past bipolar disorder or psychosis

Primary Target Symptoms
- Concentration, attention span
- Motor hyperactivity
- Impulsiveness
- Physical and mental fatigue
- Daytime sleepiness
- Depression

 Pearls
- ✳ May be useful for treatment of depressive symptoms in medically ill elderly patients
- ✳ May be useful for treatment of post-stroke depression
- ✳ A classical augmentation strategy for treatment-refractory depression
- ✳ Specifically, may be useful for treatment of cognitive dysfunction and fatigue as residual symptoms of major depressive disorder unresponsive to multiple prior treatments
- ✳ May also be useful for the treatment of cognitive impairment, depressive symptoms, and severe fatigue in patients with HIV infection and in cancer patients

- Can be used to potentiate opioid analgesia and reduce sedation, particularly in end-of-life management
- ✽ Despite warnings, can be a useful adjunct to MAOIs for heroic treatment of highly refractory mood disorders when monitored with vigilance
- ✽ Can reverse sexual dysfunction caused by psychiatric illness and by some drugs such as SSRIs, including decreased libido, erectile dysfunction, delayed ejaculation, and anorgasmia
- Atypical antipsychotics may be useful in treating stimulant or psychotic consequences of overdose
- Taking with food may delay peak actions for 2–3 hours
- Half-life and duration of clinical action tend to be shorter in younger children
- Drug abuse may actually be lower in ADHD adolescents treated with stimulants than in ADHD adolescents who are not treated
- Unknown how d,l-amphetamine's mechanism of action differs from that of d,l-methylphenidate, but some patients respond to or tolerate d,l-amphetamine better than d,l-methylphenidate and vice versa
- ✽ Adderall and Adderall XR are a mixture of d-amphetamine and l-amphetamine salts in the ratio of 3:1
- ✽ Specifically, Adderall and Adderall XR combine 1 part dextro-amphetamine saccharate, 1 part dextro-amphetamine sulfate, 1 part d,l-amphetamine aspartate, and 1 part d,l-amphetamine sulfate
- ✽ This mixture of salts may have a different pharmacologic profile, including mechanism of therapeutic action and duration of action, compared to pure dextro-amphetamine, which is given as the sulfate salt
- ✽ Specifically, d-amphetamine may have more profound action on dopamine than norepinephrine whereas l-amphetamine may have a more balanced action on both dopamine and norepinephrine
- ✽ Theoretically, this could lead to relatively more noradrenergic actions of the Adderall mixture of amphetamine salts than that of pure dextro-amphetamine sulfate, but this is unproven and of no clear clinical significance
- Nevertheless, some patients may respond to or tolerate Adderall/Adderall XR differently than they do pure dextro-amphetamine sulfate
- Adderall XR capsules also contain 2 types of drug-containing beads designed to give a double-pulsed delivery of amphetamines to prolong their release

Suggested Reading

Fry JM. Treatment modalities for narcolepsy. Neurology 1998;50(2 Suppl 1):S43–8.

Greenhill LL, Pliszka S, Dulcan MK, Bernet W, Arnold V, Beitchman J, Benson RS, Bukstein O, Kinlan J, McClellan J, Rue D, Shaw JA, Stock S. Practice parameter for the use of stimulant medications in the treatment of children, adolescents, and adults. J Am Acad Child Adolesc Psychiatry 2002;41(2 Suppl):26S–49S.

Jadad AR, Boyle M, Cunningham C, Kim M, Schachar R. Treatment of attention-deficit/hyperactivity disorder. Evid Rep Technol Assess (Summ) 1999;(11):i–viii,1–341.

Vinson DC. Therapy for attention-deficit hyperactivity disorder. Arch Fam Med 1994;3:445–51.

Wender PH, Wolf LE, Wasserstein J. Adults with ADHD. An overview. Ann N Y Acad Sci 2001;931:1–16.

D,L-METHYLPHENIDATE

Brands
- Concerta
- Metadate CD
- Ritalin
- Ritalin LA

see index for additional brand names

Generic? Yes (for immediate release methylphenidate)

 Class
- Stimulant

Commonly Prescribed For
(bold for FDA approved)
- **Attention deficit hyperactivity disorder (ADHD)**
- **Narcolepsy (Metadate ER, Methylin ER, Ritalin, Ritalin SR)**
- Treatment-resistant depression

 How The Drug Works
- ✳ Increases norepinephrine and especially dopamine actions by blocking their reuptake and facilitating their release
- Enhancement of dopamine and norepinephrine actions in certain brain regions (e.g., dorsolateral prefrontal cortex) may improve attention, concentration, executive function, and wakefulness
- Enhancement of dopamine actions in other brain regions (e.g., basal ganglia) may improve hyperactivity
- Enhancement of dopamine and norepinephrine in yet other brain regions (e.g., medial prefrontal cortex, hypothalamus) may improve depression, fatigue, and sleepiness

How Long Until It Works
- Some immediate effects can be seen with first dosing
- Can take several weeks to attain maximum therapeutic benefit

If It Works (for ADHD)
- The goal of treatment of ADHD is reduction of symptoms of inattentiveness, motor hyperactivity, and/or impulsiveness that disrupt social, school, and/or occupational functioning

- Continue treatment until all symptoms are under control or improvement is stable and then continue treatment indefinitely as long as improvement persists
- Reevaluate the need for treatment periodically
- Treatment for ADHD begun in childhood may need to be continued into adolescence and adulthood if continued benefit is documented

If It Doesn't Work (for ADHD)
- Consider adjusting dose or switching to another formulation of d,l-methylphenidate or to another agent
- Consider behavioral therapy
- Consider the presence of noncompliance and counsel patient and parents
- Consider evaluation for another diagnosis or for a comorbid condition (e.g., bipolar disorder, substance abuse, medical illness, etc.)
- ✳ Some ADHD patients and some depressed patients may experience lack of consistent efficacy due to activation of latent or underlying bipolar disorder, and require either augmenting with a mood stabilizer or switching to a mood stabilizer

 Best Augmenting Combos for Partial Response or Treatment-Resistance
- ✳ Best to attempt other monotherapies prior to augmenting
- For the expert, can combine immediate release formulation with a sustained release formulation of d,l-methylphenidate for ADHD
- For the expert, can combine with modafinil or atomoxetine for ADHD
- For the expert, can occasionally combine with atypical antipsychotics in highly treatment-resistant cases of bipolar disorder or ADHD
- For the expert, can combine with antidepressants to boost antidepressant efficacy in highly treatment-resistant cases of depression while carefully monitoring patient

Tests
- Blood pressure should be monitored regularly
- In children, monitor weight and height

• Periodic complete blood cell and platelet counts may be considered during prolonged therapy (rare leukopenia and/or anemia)

SIDE EFFECTS

How Drug Causes Side Effects

• Increases in norepinephrine peripherally can cause autonomic side effects, including tremor, tachycardia, hypertension, and cardiac arrhythmias
• Increases in norepinephrine and dopamine centrally can cause CNS side effects such as insomnia, agitation, psychosis, and substance abuse

Notable Side Effects

✳ Insomnia, headache, exacerbation of tics, nervousness, irritability, overstimulation, tremor, dizziness
• Anorexia, nausea, abdominal pain, weight loss
• Can temporarily slow normal growth in children (controversial)
• Blurred vision

Life Threatening or Dangerous Side Effects

• Psychotic episodes, especially with parenteral abuse
• Seizures
• Palpitations, tachycardia, hypertension
• Rare neuroleptic malignant syndrome
• Rare activation of hypomania, mania, or suicidal ideation (controversial)

Weight Gain

unusual   not unusual   common   problematic

• Reported but not expected
• Some patients may experience weight loss

Sedation

unusual   not unusual   common   problematic

• Reported but not expected
• Activation much more common than sedation

What To Do About Side Effects

• Wait
• Adjust dose
• Switch to another formulation of d,l-methylphenidate
• Switch to another agent
• For insomnia, avoid dosing in afternoon/evening

Best Augmenting Agents for Side Effects

• Beta-blockers for peripheral autonomic side effects
• Dose reduction or switching to another agent may be more effective since most side effects cannot be improved with an augmenting agent

DOSING AND USE

Usual Dosage Range

• ADHD: up to 2 mg/kg/day in children 6 years and older, with a maximum daily dose of 60 mg/day; in adults usually 20–30 mg/day, but may use up to 40–60 mg/day
• Narcolepsy: 20–60 mg/day in 2–3 divided doses

Dosage Forms

• Immediate release tablets 5 mg, 10 mg, 20 mg (Ritalin, Methylin, generic methylphenidate)
• Older sustained release tablets 10 mg, 20 mg (Metadate ER, Methylin ER); 20 mg (Ritalin SR)
✳ Newer sustained release capsules 20 mg, 30 mg, 40 mg (Ritalin LA); 10 mg, 20 mg, 30 mg (Metadate CD)
✳ Newer sustained release tablets 18 mg, 27 mg, 36 mg, 54 mg (Concerta)

How to Dose

• Immediate release Ritalin, Methylin, and generic methylphenidate (2–4 hour duration of action)
  • ADHD: initial 5 mg in morning, 5 mg at lunch; can increase by 5–10 mg each week; maximum dose generally 60 mg/day
  • Narcolepsy: give each dose 30–45 minutes before meals; maximum dose generally 60 mg/day
• Older extended release Ritalin SR, Methylin SR, and Metadate ER
  • These formulations have a duration of action of approximately 4–6 hours;

therefore, these formulations may be used in place of immediate release formulations when the 4–6 hour dosage of these sustained release formulations corresponds to the titrated 4–6 hour dosage of the immediate release formulation
  • Average dose is 20–30 mg/day, usually in 2 divided doses
✳ Newer sustained release formulations for ADHD
  • Concerta (up to 12 hours duration of action): initial 18 mg/day in morning; can increase by 18 mg each week; maximum dose generally 54 mg/day
  • Ritalin LA and Metadate CD (up to 8 hours duration of action): initial 20 mg once daily; dosage may be adjusted in weekly 10 mg increments to a maximum of 60 mg/day taken in the morning

 Dosing Tips

• Clinical duration of action often differs from pharmacokinetic half-life
• Taking with food may delay peak actions for 2–3 hours
✳ Immediate release formulations (Ritalin, Methylin, generic methylphenidate) have 2–4 hour durations of clinical action
✳ Older sustained release formulations such as Methylin ER, Ritalin SR, Metadate ER, and generic methylphenidate sustained release all have approximately 4–6 hour durations of clinical action, which for most patients is generally not long enough for once daily dosing in the morning and thus generally requires lunchtime dosing at school
✳ The newer sustained release Metadate CD has an early peak and an 8-hour duration of action
✳ The newer sustained release Ritalin LA also has an early peak and an 8-hour duration of action, with 2 pulses (immediate and after 4 hours)
✳ The newer sustained release Concerta trilayer tablet has longest duration of action (12 hours)
• Sustained release formulations (especially Concerta, Metadate CD, and Ritalin LA) should not be chewed but rather should only be swallowed whole

✳ All 3 newer sustained release formulations have a sufficiently long duration of clinical action to eliminate the need for a lunchtime dosing if taken in the morning
✳ This innovation can be an important practical element in stimulant utilization, eliminating the hassle and pragmatic difficulties of lunchtime dosing at school, including storage problems, potential diversion, and the need for a medical professional to supervise dosing away from home
• Off-label uses are dosed the same as for ADHD
✳ May be possible to dose only during the school week for some ADHD patients
✳ May be able to give drug holidays over the summer in order to reassess therapeutic utility and effects on growth and to allow catch-up from any growth suppression as well as to assess any other side effects and the need to reinstitute stimulant treatment for the next school term
• Avoid dosing late in the day because of the risk of insomnia
• Concerta tablet does not change shape in the GI tract and generally should not be used in patients with gastrointestinal narrowing because of the risk of intestinal obstruction
• Side effects are generally dose-related

Overdose
• Vomiting, tremor, coma, convulsion, hyperreflexia, euphoria, confusion, hallucination, tachycardia, flushing, palpitations, sweating, hyperprexia, hypertension, arrhythmia, mydriasis

Long-Term Use
• Often used long-term for ADHD when ongoing monitoring documents continued efficacy
• Dependence and/or abuse may develop
• Tolerance to therapeutic effects may develop in some patients
• Long-term stimulant use may be associated with growth suppression in children (controversial)
• Periodic monitoring of weight, blood pressure, CBC, platelet counts, and liver function may be prudent

Habit Forming
- High abuse potential, Schedule II drug
- Patients may develop tolerance, psychological dependence

How to Stop
- Taper to avoid withdrawal effects
- Withdrawal following chronic therapeutic use may unmask symptoms of the underlying disorder and may require follow-up and reinstitution of treatment
- Careful supervision is required during withdrawal from abusive use since severe depression may occur

Pharmacokinetics
- Average half-life in adults is 3.5 hours (1.3–7.7 hours)
- Average half-life in children is 2.5 hours (1.5–5 hours)

 Drug Interactions
- May affect blood pressure and should be used cautiously with agents used to control blood pressure
- May inhibit metabolism of SSRIs, anticonvulsants (phenobarbital, phenytoin, primidone), tricyclic antidepressants, and coumarin anticoagulants, requiring downward dosage adjustments of these drugs
- Serious adverse effects may occur if combined with clonidine (controversial)
- Use with MAOIs, including within 14 days of MAOI use, is not advised, but this can sometimes be considered by experts who monitor depressed patients closely when other treatment options for depression fail
- CNS and cardiovascular actions of d,l-methylphenidate could theoretically be enhanced by combination with agents that block norepinephrine reuptake, such as the tricyclic antidepressants desipramine or protriptyline, venlafaxine, duloxetine, atomoxetine, milnacipran, and reboxetine
- Theoretically, antipsychotics should inhibit the stimulatory effects of d,l-methylphenidate
- Theoretically, d,l-methylphenidate could inhibit the antipsychotic actions of antipsychotics

- Theoretically, d,l-methylphenidate could inhibit the mood stabilizing actions of atypical antipsychotics in some patients
- Combination of d,l-methylphenidate with mood stabilizers (lithium, anticonvulsants, atypical antipsychotics) is generally something for experts only, when monitoring patients closely and when other options fail

 Other Warnings/ Precautions
- Use with caution in patients with any degree of hypertension, hyperthyroidism, or history of drug abuse
- Children who are not growing or gaining weight should stop treatment, at least temporarily
- May worsen motor and phonic tics
- May worsen symptoms of thought disorder and behavioral disturbance in psychotic patients
- Stimulants have a high potential for abuse and must be used with caution in anyone with a current or past history of substance abuse or alcoholism or in emotionally unstable patients
- Administration of stimulants for prolonged periods of time should be avoided whenever possible or done only with close monitoring, as it may lead to marked tolerance and drug dependence, including psychological dependence with varying degrees of abnormal behavior
- Particular attention should be paid to the possibility of subjects obtaining stimulants for nontherapeutic use or distribution to others and the drugs should in general be prescribed sparingly with documentation of appropriate use
- Not an appropriate first-line treatment for depression or for normal fatigue
- May lower the seizure threshold
- Emergence or worsening of activation and agitation may represent the induction of a bipolar state, especially a mixed dysphoric bipolar II condition sometimes associated with suicidal ideation, and require the addition of a mood stabilizer and/or discontinuation of d,l-methylphenidate

Do Not Use
- If patient has extreme anxiety or agitation

- If patient has motor tics or Tourette's sydrome or if there is a family history of Tourette's, unless administered by an expert in cases when the potential benefits for ADHD outweigh the risks of worsening tics
- If patient has glaucoma
- Should generally not be administered with an MAOI, including within 14 days of MAOI use, except in heroic circumstances and by an expert
- If there is a proven allergy to methylphenidate

Renal Impairment
- No dose adjustment necessary

Hepatic Impairment
- No dose adjustment necessary

Cardiac Impairment
- Use with caution, particularly in patients with recent myocardial infarction or other conditions that could be negatively affected by increased blood pressure

Elderly
- Some patients may tolerate lower doses better

Children and Adolescents
- Safety and efficacy not established under age 6
- Use in young children should be reserved for the expert
- Methylphenidate has acute effects on growth hormone; long-term effects are unknown but weight and height should be monitored during long-term treatment

Pregnancy
- Risk Category C [some animal studies show adverse effects, no controlled studies in humans]
- Infants whose mothers took methylphenidate during pregnancy may experience withdrawal symptoms

- Use in women of childbearing potential requires weighing potential benefits to the mother against potential risks to the fetus
- ✱ For ADHD patients, methylphenidate should generally be discontinued before anticipated pregnancies

Breast Feeding
- Unknown if methylphenidate is secreted in human breast milk, but all psychotropics assumed to be secreted in breast milk
- ✱ Recommended either to discontinue drug or bottle feed
- If infant shows signs of irritability, drug may need to be discontinued

Potential Advantages
- Established long-term efficacy as a first-line treatment for ADHD
- Multiple options for drug delivery, peak actions, and duration of action

Potential Disadvantages
- Patients with current or past substance abuse
- Patients with current or past bipolar disorder or psychosis

Primary Target Symptoms
- Concentration, attention span
- Motor hyperactivity
- Impulsiveness
- Physical and mental fatigue
- Daytime sleepiness
- Depression

Pearls
- ✱ May be useful for treatment of depressive symptoms in medically ill elderly patients
- ✱ May be useful for treatment of post-stroke depression
- ✱ A classical augmentation strategy for treatment-refractory depression
- ✱ Specifically, may be useful for treatment of cognitive dysfunction and fatigue as residual symptoms of major depressive disorder unresponsive to multiple prior treatments
- ✱ May also be useful for the treatment of cognitive impairment, depressive

symptoms, and severe fatigue in patients with HIV infection and in cancer patients
- Can be used to potentiate opioid analgesia and reduce sedation, particularly in end-of-life management
- Atypical antipsychotics may be useful in treating stimulant or psychotic consequences of overdose
- Unknown how methylphenidate's mechanism of action differs from that of amphetamine, but some patients respond to or tolerate methylphenidate better than amphetamine and vice versa
- Taking with food may delay peak actions for 2–3 hours
- Half-life and duration of clinical action tend to be shorter in younger children
- Drug abuse may actually be lower in ADHD adolescents treated with stimulants than in ADHD adolescents who are not treated
- Older sustained release technologies for methylphenidate were not significant advances over immediate release methylphenidate because they did not eliminate the need for lunchtime dosing or allow once daily administration
- ✱ Newer sustained release technologies are truly once a day dosing systems

✱ Metadate CD and Ritalin LA are somewhat similar to each other, both with an early peak and duration of action of about 8 hours
✱ Concerta has less of an early peak but a longer duration of action (up to 12 hours)
✱ Concerta trilayer tablet consists of 3 compartments (2 containing drug, 1 a "push" compartment) and an orifice at the head of the first drug compartment; water fills the push compartment and gradually pushes drug up and out of the tablet through the orifice
✱ Concerta may be preferable for those ADHD patients who work in the evening or do homework up to 12 hours after morning dosing
✱ Metadate CD and Ritalin LA may be preferable for those ADHD patients who lose their appetite for dinner or have insomnia with Concerta
- Some patients may benefit from an occasional addition of 5–10 mg of immediate release methylphenidate to their daily base of sustained release methylphenidate
- A transdermal methylphenidate patch is in development

Suggested Reading

Challman TD, Lipsky JJ. Methylphenidate: its pharmacology and uses. Mayo Clin Proc 2000;75:711–21.

Kimko HC, Cross JT, Abemethy DR. Pharmacokinetics and clinical effectiveness of methylphenidate. Clin Pharmacokinet 1999;37:457–70.

Wolraich ML, Greenhill LL, Pelham W, Swanson J, Wilens T, Palumbo D, Atkins M, McBurnett K, Bukstein O, August G. Randomized, controlled trial of oros methylphenidate once a day in children with attention-deficit/hyperactivity disorder. Pediatrics 2001;108:883–92.

D-METHYLPHENIDATE

THERAPEUTICS

Brands • Focalin
see index for additional brand names

Generic? No

 Class
• Stimulant

Commonly Prescribed For
(bold for FDA approved)
• **Attention deficit hyperactivity disorder (ADHD)**
• Narcolepsy
• Treatment-resistant depression

 How The Drug Works
* Increases norepinephrine and especially dopamine actions by blocking their reuptake and facilitating their release
• Enhancement of dopamine and norepinephrine actions in certain brain regions (e.g., dorsolateral prefrontal cortex) may improve attention, concentration, executive function, and wakefulness
• Enhancement of dopamine actions in other brain regions (e.g., basal ganglia) may improve hyperactivity
• Enhancement of dopamine and norepinephrine in yet other brain regions (e.g., medial prefrontal cortex, hypothalamus) may improve depression, fatigue, and sleepiness

How Long Until It Works
• Some immediate effects can be seen with first dosing
• Can take several weeks to attain maximum therapeutic benefit

If It Works (for ADHD)
• The goal of treatment of ADHD is reduction of symptoms of inattentiveness, motor hyperactivity, and/or impulsiveness that disrupt social, school, and/or occupational functioning
• Continue treatment until all symptoms are under control or improvement is stable and then continue treatment indefinitely as long as improvement persists
• Reevaluate the need for treatment periodically

• Treatment for ADHD begun in childhood may need to be continued into adolescence and adulthood if continued benefit is documented

If It Doesn't Work (for ADHD)
• Consider adjusting dose or switching to a formulation of d,l-methylphenidate or to another agent
• Consider behavioral therapy
• Consider the presence of noncompliance and counsel patient and parents
• Consider evaluation for another diagnosis or for a comorbid condition (e.g., bipolar disorder, substance abuse, medical illness, etc.)
* Some ADHD patients and some depressed patients may experience lack of consistent efficacy due to activation of latent or underlying bipolar disorder, and require either augmenting with a mood stabilizer or switching to a mood stabilizer

 Best Augmenting Combos for Partial Response or Treatment-Resistance
* Best to attempt other monotherapies prior to augmenting
• For the expert, can combine immediate release formulation of d-methylphenidate with a sustained release formulation of d,l-methylphenidate for ADHD
• For the expert, can combine with modafinil or atomoxetine for ADHD
• For the expert, can occasionally combine with atypical antipsychotics in highly treatment-resistant cases of bipolar disorder or ADHD
• For the expert, can combine with antidepressants to boost antidepressant efficacy in highly treatment-resistant cases of depression while carefully monitoring patient

Tests
• Blood pressure should be monitored regularly
• In children, monitor weight and height
• Periodic complete blood cell and platelet counts may be considered during prolonged therapy (rare leukopenia and/or anemia)

SIDE EFFECTS

How Drug Causes Side Effects
- Increases in norepinephrine peripherally can cause autonomic side effects, including tremor, tachycardia, hypertension, and cardiac arrhythmias
- Increases in norepinephrine and dopamine centrally can cause CNS side effects such as insomnia, agitation, psychosis, and substance abuse

Notable Side Effects
- ✳ Insomnia, headache, exacerbation of tics, nervousness, irritability, overstimulation, tremor, dizziness
- Anorexia, nausea, abdominal pain, weight loss
- Can temporarily slow normal growth in children (controversial)
- Blurred vision

Life Threatening or Dangerous Side Effects
- Psychotic episodes, especially with parenteral abuse
- Seizures
- Palpitations, tachycardia, hypertension
- Rare neuroleptic malignant syndrome
- Rare activation of hypomania, mania, or suicidal ideation (controversial)

Weight Gain

unusual / not unusual / common / problematic
- Reported but not expected
- Some patients may experience weight loss

Sedation

unusual / not unusual / common / problematic
- Reported but not expected
- Activation much more common than sedation

What To Do About Side Effects
- Wait
- Adjust dose
- Switch to a formulation of d,l-methylphenidate
- Switch to another agent
- For insomnia, avoid dosing in afternoon/evening

Best Augmenting Agents for Side Effects
- Beta-blockers for peripheral autonomic side effects
- Dose reduction or switching to another agent may be more effective since most side effects cannot be improved with an augmenting agent

DOSING AND USE

Usual Dosage Range
- 2.5–10 mg twice per day

Dosage Forms
- Tablet 2.5 mg, 5 mg, 10 mg

How to Dose
- Patients who are not taking racemic d,l-methylphenidate: initial 2.5 mg twice per day in 4-hour intervals; may adjust dose in weekly intervals by 2.5–5 mg/day; maximum dose generally 10 mg twice per day
- Patients currently taking racemic d,l-methylphenidate: initial dose should be half the current dose of racemic d,l-methylphenidate; maximum dose generally 10 mg twice per day

Dosing Tips
- ✳ d-methylphenidate is an immediate release formulation with the same onset of action and duration of action as immediate release racemic d,l-methylphenidate (i.e., 2–4 hours) but at half the dose
- Although d-methylphenidate is generally considered to be twice as potent as racemic d,l-methylphenidate, some studies suggest that the d-isomer is actually more than twice as effective as racemic d,l-methylphenidate
- Side effects are generally dose-related
- Off-label uses are dosed the same as for ADHD
- ✳ May be possible to dose only during the school week for some ADHD patients
- ✳ May be able to give drug holidays over the summer in order to reassess therapeutic utility and effects on growth and to allow catch-up from any growth suppression as well as to assess any other

side effects and the need to reinstitute stimulant treatment for the next school term
- Avoid dosing late in the day because of the risk of insomnia
- Taking with food may delay peak actions for 2–3 hours

Overdose
- Vomiting, tremor, coma, convulsion, hyperreflexia, euphoria, confusion, hallucination, tachycardia, flushing, palpitations, sweating, hyperpyrexia, hypertension, arrhythmia, mydriasis, agitation, delirium, headache

Long-Term Use
- Often used long-term for ADHD when ongoing monitoring documents continued efficacy
- Dependence and/or abuse may develop
- Tolerance to therapeutic effects may develop in some patients
- Long-term stimulant use may be associated with growth suppression in children (controversial)
- Periodic monitoring of weight, blood pressure, CBC, platelet counts, and liver function may be prudent

Habit Forming
- High abuse potential, Schedule II drug
- Patients may develop tolerance, psychological dependence

How to Stop
- Taper to avoid withdrawal effects
- Withdrawal following chronic therapeutic use may unmask symptoms of the underlying disorder and may require follow-up and reinstitution of treatment
- Careful supervision is required during withdrawal from abusive use since severe depression may occur

Pharmacokinetics
- *d-threo*-enantiomer of racemic d,l-methylphenidate
- Mean plasma elimination half-life approximately 2.2 hours (same as d,l-methylphenidate)
- Does not inhibit CYP450 enzymes

 Drug Interactions
- May affect blood pressure and should be used cautiously with agents used to control blood pressure
- May inhibit metabolism of SSRIs, anticonvulsants (phenobarbital, phenytoin, primidone), tricyclic antidepressants, and coumarin anticoagulants, requiring downward dosage adjustments of these drugs
- Serious adverse effects may occur if combined with clonidine (controversial)
- Use with MAOIs, including within 14 days of MAOI use, is not advised, but this can sometimes be considered by experts who monitor depressed patients closely when other treatment options for depression fail
- CNS and cardiovascular actions of d-methylphenidate could theoretically be enhanced by combination with agents that block norepinephrine reuptake, such as the tricyclic antidepressants desipramine or protriptyline, venlafaxine, duloxetine, atomoxetine, milnacipran, and reboxetine
- Theoretically, antipsychotics should inhibit the stimulatory effects of d-methylphenidate
- Theoretically, d-methylphenidate could inhibit the antipsychotic actions of antipsychotics
- Theoretically, d-methylphenidate could inhibit the mood stabilizing actions of atypical antipsychotics in some patients
- Combinations of d-methylphenidate with mood stabilizers (lithium, anticonvulsants, atypical antipsychotics) is generally something for experts only, when monitoring patients closely and when other options fail

 Other Warnings/ Precautions
- Use with caution in patients with any degree of hypertension, hyperthyroidism, or history of drug abuse
- Children who are not growing or gaining weight should stop treatment, at least temporarily
- May worsen motor and phonic tics
- May worsen symptoms of thought disorder and behavioral disturbance in psychotic patients

- Stimulants have a high potential for abuse and must be used with caution in anyone with a current or past history of substance abuse or alcoholism or in emotionally unstable patients
- Administration of stimulants for prolonged periods of time should be avoided whenever possible or done only with close monitoring, as it may lead to marked tolerance and drug dependence, including psychological dependence with varying degrees of abnormal behavior
- Particular attention should be paid to the possibility of subjects obtaining stimulants for nontherapeutic use or distribution to others and the drugs should in general be prescribed sparingly with documentation of appropriate use
- Not an appropriate first-line treatment for depression or for normal fatigue
- May lower the seizure threshold
- Emergence or worsening of activation and agitation may represent the induction of a bipolar state, especially a mixed dysphoric bipolar II condition sometimes associated with suicidal ideation, and require the addition of a mood stabilizer and/or discontinuation of d-methylphenidate

Do Not Use

- If patient has extreme anxiety or agitation
- If patient has motor tics or Tourette's sydrome or if there is a family history of Tourette's, unless administered by an expert in cases when the potential benefits for ADHD outweigh the risks of worsening tics
- If patient has glaucoma
- Should generally not be administered with an MAOI, including within 14 days of MAOI use, except in heroic circumstances and by an expert
- If there is a proven allergy to methylphenidate

Renal Impairment

- No dose adjustment necessary

Hepatic Impairment

- No dose adjustment necessary

Cardiac Impairment

- Use with caution, particularly in patients with recent myocardial infarction or other conditions that could be negatively affected by increased blood pressure

Elderly

- Some patients may tolerate lower doses better

 Children and Adolescents

- Safety and efficacy not established under age 6
- Use in young children should be reserved for the expert
- Methylphenidate has acute effects on growth hormone; long-term effects are unknown but weight and height should be monitored during long-term treatment

 Pregnancy

- Risk Category C [some animal studies show adverse effects, no controlled studies in humans]
- Infants whose mothers took methylphenidate during pregnancy may experience withdrawal symptoms
- Use in women of childbearing potential requires weighing potential benefits to the mother against potential risks to the fetus
- ✱ For ADHD patients, methylphenidate should generally be discontinued before anticipated pregnancies

Breast Feeding

- Unknown if methylphenidate is secreted in human breast milk, but all psychotropics assumed to be secreted in breast milk
- ✱ Recommended either to discontinue drug or bottle feed
- If infant shows signs of irritability, drug may need to be discontinued

THE ART OF PSYCHOPHARMACOLOGY

Potential Advantages

- The active d enantiomer of methylphenidate may be slightly more than twice as efficacious as racemic d,l-methylphenidate

Potential Disadvantages

- Patients with current or past substance abuse, bipolar disorder, or psychosis
- No controlled release formulations currently available

Primary Target Symptoms

- Concentration, attention span
- Motor hyperactivity
- Impulsiveness
- Physical and mental fatigue
- Daytime sleepiness
- Depression

 Pearls

✱ Unclear what its advantages are over immediate release racemic d,l-methylphenidate
- A controlled release formulation for once daily administration is in development
- May be useful for treatment of depressive symptoms in medically ill elderly patients
- May be useful for treatment of post-stroke depression
- A classical augmentation strategy for treatment-refractory depression

- Specifically, may be useful for treatment of cognitive dysfunction and fatigue as residual symptoms of major depressive disorder unresponsive to multiple prior treatments
- May also be useful for the treatment of cognitive impairment, depressive symptoms, and severe fatigue in patients with HIV infection and in cancer patients
- Can be used to potentiate opioid analgesia and reduce sedation, particularly in end-of-life management
- Atypical antipsychotics may be useful in treating stimulant or psychotic consequences of overdose
- Unknown how methylphenidate's mechanism of action differs from that of amphetamine, but some patients respond to or tolerate methylphenidate better than amphetamine, and vice versa
- Taking with food may delay peak actions for 2–3 hours
- Half-life and duration of clinical action tend to be shorter in younger children
- Drug abuse may actually be lower in ADHD adolescents treated with stimulants than in ADHD adolescents who are not treated

 Suggested Reading

Dexmethylphenidate—Novartis/Celgene. Focalin, D-MPH, D-methylphenidate hydrochloride, D-methylphenidate, dexmethylphenidate, dexmethylphenidate hydrochloride. Drugs R D. 2002;3(4):279–82.

Keating GM, Figgitt DP. Dexmethylphenidate. Drugs. 2002;62(13):1899–904.

DONEPEZIL

THERAPEUTICS

Brands • Aricept
• Memac
see index for additional brand names

Generic? No

Class
• Cholinesterase inhibitor (selective acetylcholinesterase inhibitor); cognitive enhancer

Commonly Prescribed For
(bold for FDA approved)
• **Alzheimer disease**
• Memory disorders in other conditions
• Mild cognitive impairment

How The Drug Works
✳ Reversibly but noncompetitively inhibits centrally-active acetylcholinesterase (AChE), making more acetylcholine available
• Increased availability of acetylcholine compensates in part for degenerating cholinergic neurons in neocortex that regulate memory
• Does not inhibit butyrylcholinesterase
• May release growth factors or interfere with amyloid deposition

How Long Until It Works
• May take up to 6 weeks before any improvement in baseline memory or behavior is evident
• May take months before any stabilization in degenerative course is evident

If It Works
• May improve symptoms and slow progression of disease, but does not reverse the degenerative process

If It Doesn't Work
• Consider adjusting dose, switching to a different cholinesterase inhibitor or adding an appropriate augmenting agent
• Reconsider diagnosis and rule out other conditions such as depression or a dementia other than Alzheimer disease

Best Augmenting Combos for Partial Response or Treatment-Resistance
✳ Atypical antipsychotics to reduce behavioral disturbances
✳ Antidepressants if concomitant depression, apathy, or lack of interest
✳ Memantine for moderate to severe Alzheimer disease
• Divalproex, carbamazepine, or oxcarbazepine for behavioral disturbances
• Not rational to combine with another cholinesterase inhibitor

Tests
• None for healthy individuals

SIDE EFFECTS

How Drug Causes Side Effects
• Peripheral inhibition of acetylcholinesterase can cause gastrointestinal side effects
• Central inhibition of acetylcholinesterase may contribute to nausea, vomiting, weight loss, and sleep disturbances

Notable Side Effects
✳ Nausea, diarrhea, vomiting, appetite loss, increased gastric acid secretion, weight loss
• Insomnia, dizziness
• Muscle cramps, fatigue, depression, abnormal dreams

Life Threatening or Dangerous Side Effects
• Rare seizures
• Rare syncope

Weight Gain

unusual   not unusual   common   problematic

• Reported but not expected
• Some patients may experience weight loss

Sedation

unusual   not unusual   common   problematic

• Reported but not expected

What To Do About Side Effects
• Wait
• Wait

- Wait
- Take in daytime to reduce insomnia
- Use slower dose titration
- Consider lowering dose, switching to a different agent or adding an appropriate augmenting agent

Best Augmenting Agents for Side Effects

- Hypnotics or trazodone may improve insomnia
- Many side effects cannot be improved with an augmenting agent

DOSING AND USE

Usual Dosage Range
- 5–10 mg at night

Dosage Forms
- Tablet 5 mg, 10 mg

How to Dose
- Initial 5 mg/day; may increase to 10 mg/day after 4–6 weeks

 Dosing Tips

* Only cholinesterase inhibitor with once daily dosing
- Side effects occur more frequently at 10 mg/day than at 5 mg/day
- Slower titration (e.g., 6 weeks to 10 mg/day) may reduce the risk of side effects
- Food does not affect the absorption of donepezil
- Probably best to utilize highest tolerated dose within the usual dosage range
- Some off-label uses for cognitive disturbances other than Alzheimer disease have anecdotally utilized doses higher than 10 mg/day
* When switching to another cholinesterase inhibitor, probably best to cross-titrate from one to the other to prevent precipitous decline in function if the patient washes out of one drug entirely

Overdose
- Can be lethal; nausea, vomiting, excess salivation, sweating, hypotension, bradycardia, collapse, convulsions, muscle weakness (weakness of respiratory muscles can lead to death)

Long-Term Use
- Drug may lose effectiveness in slowing degenerative course of Alzheimer disease after 6 months
- Can be effective in some patients for several years

Habit Forming
- No

How to Stop
- Taper to avoid withdrawal effects
- Discontinuation may lead to notable deterioration in memory and behavior, which may not be restored when drug is restarted or another cholinesterase inhibitor is initiated

Pharmacokinetics
- Metabolized by CYP450 2D6 and CYP450 3A4
- Elimination half-life approximately 70 hours

 Drug Interactions

- Donepezil may increase the effects of anesthetics and should be discontinued prior to surgery
- Inhibitors of CYP450 2D6 and CYP450 3A4 may inhibit donepezil metabolism and increase its plasma levels
- Inducers of CYP450 2D6 and CYP450 3A4 may increase clearance of donepezil and decrease its plasma levels
- Donepezil may interact with anticholinergic agents and the combination may decrease the efficacy of both
- May have synergistic effect if administered with cholinomimetics (e.g., bethanechol)
- Bradycardia may occur if combined with beta blockers
- Theoretically, could reduce the efficacy of levodopa in Parkinson's disease
- Not rational to combine with another cholinesterase inhibitor

 Other Warnings/ Precautions

- May exacerbate asthma or other pulmonary disease

- Increased gastric acid secretion may increase the risk of ulcers
- Bradycardia or heart block may occur in patients with or without cardiac impairment

Do Not Use
- If there is a proven allergy to donepezil

SPECIAL POPULATIONS

Renal Impairment
- Few data available but dose adjustment is most likely unnecessary

Hepatic Impairment
- Few data available; may need to lower dose

Cardiac Impairment
- Should be used with caution
- Syncopal episodes have been reported with the use of donepezil

Elderly
- Some patients may tolerate lower doses better

Children and Adolescents
- Safety and efficacy have not been established
- Preliminary reports of efficacy as an adjunct in ADHD (ages 8–17)

Pregnancy
- Risk Category C [some animal studies show adverse effects, no controlled studies in humans]
- ✳ Not recommended for use in pregnant women or women of childbearing potential

Breast Feeding
- Unknown if donepezil is secreted in human breast milk, but all psychotropics assumed to be secreted in breast milk
- ✳ Recommended either to discontinue drug or bottle feed
- Donepezil is not recommended for use in nursing women

THE ART OF PSYCHOPHARMACOLOGY

Potential Advantages
- Once a day dosing
- May be used in vascular dementia
- May work in some patients who do not respond to other cholinesterase inhibitors
- May work in some patients who do not tolerate other cholinesterase inhibitors

Potential Disadvantages
- Patients with insomnia

Primary Target Symptoms
- Memory loss in Alzheimer disease
- Behavioral symptoms in Alzheimer disease
- Memory loss in other dementias

Pearls
- Dramatic reversal of symptoms of Alzheimer disease is not generally seen with cholinesterase inhibitors
- Can lead to therapeutic nihilism among prescribers and lack of an appropriate trial of a cholinesterase inhibitor
- ✳ Perhaps only 50% of Alzheimer patients are diagnosed, and only 50% of those diagnosed are treated, and only 50% of those treated are given a cholinesterase inhibitor, and then only for 200 days in a disease that lasts 7–10 years
- Must evaluate lack of efficacy and loss of efficacy over months, not weeks
- ✳ Treats behavioral and psychological symptoms of Alzheimer dementia as well as cognitive symptoms (i.e., especially apathy, disinhibition, delusions, anxiety, cooperation, pacing)
- Patients who complain themselves of memory problems may have depression, whereas patients whose spouses or children complain of the patient's memory problems may have Alzheimer disease
- Treat the patient but ask the caregiver about efficacy
- What you see may depend upon how early you treat
- The first symptoms of Alzheimer disease are generally mood changes; thus, Alzheimer disease may initially be diagnosed as depression
- Women may experience cognitive symptoms in perimenopause as a result of

- hormonal changes that are not a sign of dementia or Alzheimer disease
- Aggressively treat concomitant symptoms with augmentation (e.g., atypical antipsychotics for agitation, antidepressants for depression)
- If treatment with antidepressants fails to improve apathy and depressed mood in the elderly, it is possible that this represents early Alzheimer disease and a cholinesterase inhibitor like donepezil may be helpful
- What to expect from a cholinesterase inhibitor:
  - Patients do not generally improve dramatically although this can be observed in a significant minority of patients
  - Onset of behavioral problems and nursing home placement can be delayed
  - Functional outcomes, including activities of daily living, can be preserved
  - Caregiver burden and stress can be reduced
- Delay in progression in Alzheimer disease is not evidence of disease-modifying actions of cholinesterase inhibition
- Cholinesterase inhibitors like donepezil depend upon the presence of intact targets for acetylcholine for maximum effectiveness and thus may be most effective in the early stages of Alzheimer disease
- The most prominent side effects of donepezil are gastrointestinal effects, which are usually mild and transient
- ✳ May cause more sleep disturbances than some other cholinesterase inhibitors
- For patients with intolerable side effects, generally allow a washout period with resolution of side effects prior to switching to another cholinesterase inhibitor
- Weight loss can be a problem in Alzheimer patients with debilitation and muscle wasting
- Women over 85, particularly with low body weights, may experience more adverse effects

- Use with caution in underweight or frail patients
- Cognitive improvement may be linked to substantial (>65%) inhibition of acetylcholinesterase
- Donepezil has greater action on CNS acetylcholinesterase than on peripheral acetylcholinesterase
- Some Alzheimer patients who fail to respond to donepezil may respond to another cholinesterase inhibitor
- Some Alzheimer patients who fail to respond to another cholinesterase inhibitor may respond when switched to donepezil
- To prevent potential clinical deterioration, generally switch from long-term treatment with one cholinesterase inhibitor to another without a washout period
- ✳ Donepezil may slow the progression of mild cognitive impairment to Alzheimer disease
- ✳ May be useful for dementia with Lewy bodies (DLB, constituted by early loss of attentiveness and visual perception with possible hallucinations, Parkinson-like movement problems, fluctuating cognition such as daytime drowsiness and lethargy, staring into space for long periods, episodes of disorganized speech)
- May decrease delusions, apathy, agitation, and hallucinations in dementia with Lewy bodies
- ✳ May be useful for vascular dementia (e.g., acute onset with slow stepwise progression that has plateaus, often with gait abnormalities, focal signs, imbalance, and urinary incontinence)
- May be helpful for dementia in Down's Syndrome
- Suggestions of utility in some cases of treatment-resistant bipolar disorder
- Theoretically, may be useful for ADHD, but not yet proven
- Theoretically, could be useful in any memory condition characterized by cholinergic deficiency (e.g., some cases of brain injury, cancer chemotherapy-induced cognitive changes, etc.)

Suggested Reading

Bentue-Ferrer D, Tribut O, Polard E, Allain H. Clinically significant drug interactions with cholinesterase inhibitors: a guide for neurologists. CNS Drugs 2003;17:947–63.

Birks, JS, Harvey R. Donepezil for dementia due to Alzheimer's disease. Cochrane Database Syst Rev 2003;CD001190.

Bonner LT, Peskind ER. Pharmacologic treatments of dementia. Med Clin North Am 2002;86:657–74.

Jones RW. Have cholinergic therapies reached their clinical boundary in Alzheimer's disease? Int J Geriatr Psychiatry 2003;18(Suppl 1): S7–S13.

Stahl SM. Cholinesterase inhibitors for Alzheimer's disease. Hosp Pract (Off Ed) 1998;33:131–6.

Stahl SM. The new cholinesterase inhibitors for Alzheimer's disease, part 1. J Clin Psychiatry 2000;61:710–11.

Stahl SM. The new cholinesterase inhibitors for Alzheimer's disease, part 2. J Clin Psychiatry 2000;61:813–14.

DOTHIEPIN

THERAPEUTICS

Brands • Prothiaden
see index for additional brand names

Generic? In United Kingdom

Class
• Tricyclic antidepressant (TCA)
• Serotonin and norepinephrine/
  noradrenaline reuptake inhibitor

Commonly Prescribed For
(bold for FDA approved)
• Major depressive disorder
• Anxiety
• Insomnia
• Neuropathic pain/chronic pain
• Treatment-resistant depression

How The Drug Works
• Boosts neurotransmitters serotonin and
  norepinephrine/noradrenaline
• Blocks serotonin reuptake pump (serotonin
  transporter), presumably increasing
  serotonergic neurotransmission
• Blocks norepinephrine reuptake pump
  (norepinephrine transporter), presumably
  increasing noradrenergic
  neurotransmission
• Presumably desensitizes both serotonin 1A
  receptors and beta adrenergic receptors
• Since dopamine is inactivated by
  norepinephrine reuptake in frontal cortex,
  which largely lacks dopamine transporters,
  dothiepin can increase dopamine
  neurotransmission in this part of the brain

How Long Until It Works
• May have immediate effects in treating
  insomnia or anxiety
• Onset of therapeutic actions usually not
  immediate, but often delayed 2 to 4 weeks
• If it is not working within 6 to 8 weeks for
  depression, it may require a dosage
  increase or it may not work at all
• May continue to work for many years to
  prevent relapse of symptoms

If It Works
• The goal of treatment of depression is
  complete remission of current symptoms
  as well as prevention of future relapses
• The goal of treatment of chronic
  neuropathic pain is to reduce symptoms as
  much as possible, especially in
  combination with other treatments
• Treatment of depression most often
  reduces or even eliminates symptoms, but
  not a cure since symptoms can recur after
  medicine stopped
• Treatment of chronic neuropathic pain may
  reduce symptoms, but rarely eliminates
  them completely, and is not a cure since
  symptoms can recur after medicine is
  stopped
• Continue treatment of depression until all
  symptoms are gone (remission)
• Once symptoms of depression are gone,
  continue treating for 1 year for the first
  episode of depression
• For second and subsequent episodes of
  depression, treatment may need to be
  indefinite
• Use in anxiety disorders and chronic pain
  may also need to be indefinite, but long-
  term treatment is not well studied in these
  conditions

If It Doesn't Work
• Many depressed patients only have a
  partial response where some symptoms
  are improved but others persist (especially
  insomnia, fatigue, and problems
  concentrating)
• Other depressed patients may be
  nonresponders, sometimes called
  treatment-resistant or treatment-refractory
• Consider increasing dose, switching to
  another agent or adding an appropriate
  augmenting agent
• Consider psychotherapy
• Consider evaluation for another diagnosis
  or for a comorbid condition (e.g, medical
  illness, substance abuse, etc.)
• Some patients may experience apparent
  lack of consistent efficacy due to activation
  of latent or underlying bipolar disorder, and
  require antidepressant discontinuation and
  a switch to a mood stabilizer

Best Augmenting Combos for Partial Response or Treatment-Resistance

- Lithium, buspirone, thyroid hormone (for depression)
- Gabapentin, tiagabine, other anticonvulsants, even opiates if done by experts while monitoring carefully in difficult cases (for chronic pain)

Tests

- None for healthy individuals
- ✳ Since tricyclic and tetracyclic antidepressants are frequently associated with weight gain, before starting treatment, weigh all patients and determine if the patient is already overweight (BMI 25.0–29.9) or obese (BMI ≥30)
- Before giving a drug that can cause weight gain to an overweight or obese patient, consider determining whether the patient already has pre-diabetes (fasting plasma glucose 100–125 mg/dl), diabetes (fasting plasma glucose >126 mg/dl), or dyslipidemia (increased total cholesterol, LDL cholesterol and triglycerides; decreased HDL cholesterol), and treat or refer such patients for treatment including nutrition and weight management, physical activity counseling, smoking cessation, and medical management
- ✳ Monitor weight and BMI during treatment
- ✳ While giving a drug to a patient who has gained >5% of initial weight, consider evaluating for the presence of pre-diabetes, diabetes, or dyslipidemia, or consider switching to a different antidepressant
- EKGs may be useful for selected patients (e.g., those with personal or family history of QTc prolongation; cardiac arrhythmia; recent myocardial infarction; uncompensated heart failure; or taking agents that prolong QTc interval such as pimozide, thioridazine, selected antiarrhythmics, moxifloxacin, sparfloxacin, etc.)
- Patients at risk for electrolyte disturbances (e.g., patients on diuretic therapy) should have baseline and periodic serum potassium and magnesium measurements

SIDE EFFECTS

How Drug Causes Side Effects

- Anticholinergic activity may explain sedative effects, dry mouth, constipation, and blurred vision
- Sedative effects and weight gain may be due to antihistamine properties
- Blockade of alpha adrenergic 1 receptors may explain dizziness, sedation, and hypotension
- Cardiac arrhythmias and seizures, especially in overdose, may be caused by blockade of ion channels

Notable Side Effects

- Blurred vision, constipation, urinary retention, increased appetite, dry mouth, nausea, diarrhea, heartburn, unusual taste in mouth, weight gain
- Fatigue, weakness, dizziness, sedation, headache, anxiety, nervousness, restlessness
- Sexual dysfunction, sweating

Life Threatening or Dangerous Side Effects

- Paralytic ileus, hyperthermia (TCAs + anticholinergic agents)
- Lowered seizure threshold and rare seizures
- Orthostatic hypotension, sudden death, arrhythmias, tachycardia
- QTc prolongation
- Hepatic failure, extrapyramidal symptoms
- Increased intraocular pressure
- Rare induction of mania and activation of suicidal ideation

Weight Gain

unusual   not unusual   **common**   problematic

- Many experience and/or can be significant in amount
- Can increase appetite and carbohydrate craving

Sedation

unusual   not unusual   **common**   problematic

- Many experience and/or can be significant in amount
- Tolerance to sedative effect may develop with long-term use

What To Do About Side Effects
• Wait
• Wait
• Wait
• Lower the dose
• Switch to an SSRI or newer antidepressant

Best Augmenting Agents for Side Effects
• Many side effects cannot be improved with an augmenting agent

---

DOSING AND USE

Usual Dosage Range
• 75–150 mg/day

Dosage Forms
• Capsule 25 mg
• Tablet 75 mg

How to Dose
• 75 mg/day once daily or in divided doses; gradually increase dose to achieve desired therapeutic effect; maximum dose 300 mg/day

 Dosing Tips
• If given in a single dose, should generally be administered at bedtime because of its sedative properties
• If given in split doses, largest dose should generally be given at bedtime because of its sedative properties
• If patients experience nightmares, split dose and do not give large dose at bedtime
• Patients treated for chronic pain may only require lower doses
• Risk of seizure increases with dose
• If intolerable anxiety, insomnia, agitation, akathisia, or activation occur either upon dosing initiation or discontinuation, consider the possibility of activated bipolar disorder, and switch to a mood stabilizer or an atypical antipsychotic

Overdose
• Death may occur; convulsions, cardiac dysrhythmias, severe hypotension, CNS depression, coma, changes in ECG

Long-Term Use
• Safe

Habit Forming
• No

How to Stop
• Taper to avoid withdrawal effects
• Even with gradual dose reduction some withdrawal symptoms may appear within the first 2 weeks
• Many patients tolerate 50% dose reduction for 3 days, then another 50% reduction for 3 days, then discontinuation
• If withdrawal symptoms emerge during discontinuation, raise dose to stop symptoms and then restart withdrawal much more slowly

Pharmacokinetics
• Substrate for CYP450 2D6
• Half-life approximately 14–40 hours

 Drug Interactions
• Tramadol increases the risk of seizures in patients taking TCAs
• Use of TCAs with anticholinergic drugs may result in paralytic ileus or hyperthermia
• Fluoxetine, paroxetine, bupropion, duloxetine, and other CYP450 2D6 inhibitors may increase TCA concentrations
• Cimetidine may increase plasma concentrations of TCAs and cause anticholinergic symptoms
• Phenothiazines or haloperidol may raise TCA blood concentrations
• May alter effects of antihypertensive drugs; may inhibit hypotensive effects of clonidine
• Use of TCAs with sympathomimetic agents may increase sympathetic activity
• Methylphenidate may inhibit metabolism of TCAs
• Activation and agitation, especially following switching or adding antidepressants, may represent the induction of a bipolar state, especially a mixed dysphoric bipolar II condition sometimes associated with suicidal ideation, and require the addition of lithium, a mood stabilizer or an atypical antipsychotic, and/or discontinuation of dothiepin

Other Warnings/ Precautions

- Add or initiate other antidepressants with caution for up to 2 weeks after discontinuing dothiepin
- Generally, do not use with MAO inhibitors, including 14 days after MAOIs are stopped; do not start an MAOI until 2 weeks after discontinuing dothiepin, but see Pearls
- Use with caution in patients with history of seizures, urinary retention, narrow angle-closure glaucoma, hyperthyroidism, and in patients recovering from myocardial infarction
- TCAs can increase QTc interval, especially at toxic doses, which can be attained not only by overdose but also by combining with drugs that inhibit TCA metabolism via CYP450 2D6, potentially causing torsade de pointes-type arrhythmia or sudden death
- Because TCAs can prolong QTc interval, use with caution in patients who have bradycardia or who are taking drugs that can induce bradycardia (e.g., beta blockers, calcium channel blockers, clonidine, digitalis)
- Because TCAs can prolong QTc interval, use with caution in patients who have hypokalemia and/or hypomagnesemia or who are taking drugs that can induce hypokalemia and/or magnesemia (e.g., diuretics, stimulant laxatives, intravenous amphotericin B, glucocorticoids, tetracosactide)

Do Not Use

- If patient is recovering from myocardial infarction
- If patient is taking agents capable of significantly prolonging QTc interval (e.g., pimozide, thioridazine, selected antiarrhythmics, moxifloxacin, sparfloxacin)
- If there is a history of QTc prolongation or cardiac arrhythmia, recent acute myocardial infarction, uncompensated heart failure
- If patient is taking drugs that inhibit TCA metabolism, including CYP450 2D6 inhibitors, except by an expert
- If there is reduced CYP450 2D6 function, such as patients who are poor 2D6 metabolizers, except by an expert and at low doses
- If there is a proven allergy to dothiepin

Renal Impairment

- Use with caution

Hepatic Impairment

- Use with caution

Cardiac Impairment

- TCAs have been reported to cause arrhythmias, prolongation of conduction time, orthostatic hypotension, sinus tachycardia, and heart failure, especially in the diseased heart
- Myocardial infarction and stroke have been reported with TCAs
- TCAs produce QTc prolongation, which may be enhanced by the existence of bradycardia, hypokalemia, congenital or acquired long QTc interval, which should be evaluated prior to administering dothiepin
- Use with caution if treating concomitantly with a medication likely to produce prolonged bradycardia, hypokalemia, slowing of intracardiac conduction, or prolongation of the QTc interval
- Avoid TCAs in patients with a known history of QTc prolongation, recent acute myocardial infarction, and uncompensated heart failure
- TCAs may cause a sustained increase in heart rate in patients with ischemic heart disease and may worsen (decrease) heart rate variability, an independent risk of mortality in cardiac populations
- Since SSRIs may improve (increase) heart rate variability in patients following a myocardial infarct and may improve survival as well as mood in patients with acute angina or following a myocardial infarction, these are more appropriate agents for cardiac population than tricyclic/tetracyclic antidepressants
- ✳ Risk/benefit ratio may not justify use of TCAs in cardiac impairment

Elderly
- May be more sensitive to anticholinergic, cardiovascular, hypotensive, and sedative effects

Children and Adolescents
- Use with caution, observing for activation of known or unknown bipolar disorder and/or suicidal ideation, and strongly consider informing parents or guardian of this risk so they can help observe child or adolescent patients
- Not recommended for use under age 18
- Several studies show lack of efficacy of TCAs for depression
- May be used to treat enuresis or hyperactive/impulsive behaviors
- Some cases of sudden death have occurred in children taking TCAs

Pregnancy
- Risk Category C [some animal studies show adverse effects, no controlled studies in humans]
- Crosses the placenta
- Adverse effects have been reported in infants whose mothers took a TCA (lethargy, withdrawal symptoms, fetal malformations)
- Not generally recommended for use during pregnancy, especially during first trimester
- Must weigh the risk of treatment (first trimester fetal development, third trimester newborn delivery) to the child against the risk of no treatment (recurrence of depression, maternal health, infant bonding) to the mother and child
- For many patients this may mean continuing treatment during pregnancy

Breast Feeding
- Some drug is found in mother's breast milk
- ✳ Recommended either to discontinue drug or bottle feed
- Immediate postpartum period is a high-risk time for depression, especially in women who have had prior depressive episodes, so drug may need to be reinstituted late in the third trimester or shortly after childbirth to prevent a recurrence during the postpartum period

- Must weigh benefits of breast feeding with risks and benefits of antidepressant treatment versus non-treatment to both the infant and the mother
- For many patients this may mean continuing treatment during breast feeding

THE ART OF PSYCHOPHARMACOLOGY

Potential Advantages
- Patients with insomnia
- Severe or treatment-resistant depression
- Anxious depression

Potential Disadvantages
- Pediatric and geriatric patients
- Patients concerned with weight gain
- Cardiac patients

Primary Target Symptoms
- Depressed mood
- Chronic pain

Pearls
- ✳ Close structural similarity to amitriptyline
- Tricyclic antidepressants are often a first-line treatment option for chronic pain
- Tricyclic antidepressants are no longer generally considered a first-line option for depression because of their side effect profile
- Tricyclic antidepressants continue to be useful for severe or treatment-resistant depression
- TCAs may aggravate psychotic symptoms
- Alcohol should be avoided because of additive CNS effects
- Underweight patients may be more susceptible to adverse cardiovascular effects
- Children, patients with inadequate hydration, and patients with cardiac disease may be more susceptible to TCA-induced cardiotoxicity than healthy adults
- For the expert only: a heroic treatment (but potentially dangerous) for severely treatment-resistant patients is to give simultaneously with monoamine oxidase inhibitors for patients who fail to respond to numerous other antidepressants, but generally recommend a different TCA than dothiepin for this use

• If this option is elected, start the MAOI with the tricyclic/tetracyclic antidepressant simultaneously at low doses after appropriate drug washout, then alternately increase doses of these agents every few days to a week as tolerated

• Although very strict dietary and concomitant drug restrictions must be observed to prevent hypertensive crises and serotonin syndrome, the most common side effects of MAOI and tricyclic/tetracyclic antidepressant combinations may be weight gain and orthostatic hypotension

• Patients on TCAs should be aware that they may experience symptoms such as photosensitivity or blue-green urine

• SSRIs may be more effective than TCAs in women, and TCAs may be more effective than SSRIs in men

• Since tricyclic/tetracyclic antidepressants are substrates for CYP450 2D6, and 7% of the population (especially Caucasians) may have a genetic variant leading to reduced activity of 2D6, such patients may not safely tolerate normal doses of tricyclic/tetracyclic antidepressants and may require dose reduction

• Phenotypic testing may be necessary to detect this genetic variant prior to dosing with a tricyclic/tetracyclic antidepressant, especially in vulnerable populations such as children, elderly, cardiac populations, and those on concomitant medications

• Patients who seem to have extraordinarily severe side effects at normal or low doses may have this phenotypic CYP450 2D6 variant and require low doses or switching to another antidepressant not metabolized by 2D6

 Suggested Reading

Anderson IM. Meta-analytical studies on new antidepressants. Br Med Bull. 2001; 57:161–178.

Anderson IM. Selective serotonin reuptake inhibitors versus tricyclic antidepressants: a meta-analysis of efficacy and tolerability. J Aff Disorders. 2000;58:19–36.

Donovan S, Dearden L, Richardson L. The tolerability of dothiepin: a review of clinical studies between 1963 and 1990 in over 13,000 depressed patients. Prog Neuropsychopharmacol Biol Psychiatry. 1994; 18:1143–62.

Lancaster SG, Gonzalez JP. Dothiepin. A review of its pharmacodynamic and pharmacokinetic properties, and therapeutic efficacy in depressive illness. Drugs. 1989; 38:123–47.

DOXEPIN

THERAPEUTICS

Brands • Sinequan
see index for additional brand names

Generic? Yes

Class

- Tricyclic antidepressant (TCA)
- Serotonin and norepinephrine/ noradrenaline reuptake inhibitor

Commonly Prescribed For
(bold for FDA approved)

- **Psychoneurotic patient with depression and/or anxiety**
- **Depression and/or anxiety associated with alcoholism**
- **Depression and/or anxiety associated with organic disease**
- **Psychotic depressive disorders with associated anxiety**
- **Involutional depression**
- **Manic-depressive disorder**
- ✱ Pruritus/itching (topical)
- Dermatitis, atopic (topical)
- Lichen simplex chronicus (topical)
- Anxiety
- Insomnia
- Neuropathic pain/chronic pain
- Treatment-resistant depression

How The Drug Works

- Boosts neurotransmitters serotonin and norepinephrine/noradrenaline
- Blocks serotonin reuptake pump (serotonin transporter), presumably increasing serotonergic neurotransmission
- Blocks norepinephrine reuptake pump (norepinephrine transporter), presumably increasing noradrenergic neurotransmission
- Presumably desensitizes both serotonin 1A receptors and beta adrenergic receptors
- Since dopamine is inactivated by norepinephrine reuptake in frontal cortex, which largely lacks dopamine transporters, doxepin can thus increase dopamine neurotransmission in this part of the brain
- May be effective in treating skin conditions because of its strong antihistamine properties

How Long Until It Works

- May have immediate effects in treating insomnia or anxiety
- Onset of therapeutic actions usually not immediate, but often delayed 2 to 4 weeks
- If it is not working within 6 to 8 weeks for depression, it may require a dosage increase or it may not work at all
- May continue to work for many years to prevent relapse of symptoms

If It Works

- The goal of treatment of depression is complete remission of current symptoms as well as prevention of future relapses
- The goal of treatment of chronic neuropathic pain is to reduce symptoms as much as possible, especially in combination with other treatments
- Treatment of depression most often reduces or even eliminates symptoms, but not a cure since symptoms can recur after medicine stopped
- Treatment of chronic neuropathic pain may reduce symptoms, but rarely eliminates them completely, and is not a cure since symptoms can recur after medicine is stopped
- Continue treatment of depression until all symptoms are gone (remission)
- Once symptoms of depression are gone, continue treating for 1 year for the first episode of depression
- For second and subsequent episodes of depression, treatment may need to be indefinite
- Use in anxiety disorders, chronic pain, and skin conditions may also need to be indefinite, but long-term treatment is not well studied in these conditions

If It Doesn't Work

- Many depressed patients only have a partial response where some symptoms are improved but others persist (especially insomnia, fatigue, and problems concentrating)
- Other depressed patients may be nonresponders, sometimes called treatment-resistant or treatment-refractory
- Consider increasing dose, switching to another agent or adding an appropriate augmenting agent
- Consider psychotherapy

- Consider evaluation for another diagnosis or for a comorbid condition (e.g., medical illness, substance abuse, etc.)
- Some patients may experience apparent lack of consistent efficacy due to activation of latent or underlying bipolar disorder, and require antidepressant discontinuation and a switch to a mood stabilizer

Best Augmenting Combos for Partial Response or Treatment-Resistance

- Lithium, buspirone, thyroid hormone (for depression)
- Gabapentin, tiagabine, other anticonvulsants, even opiates if done by experts while monitoring carefully in difficult cases (for chronic pain)

Tests

- None for healthy individuals
- ✱ Since tricyclic and tetracyclic antidepressants are frequently associated with weight gain, before starting treatment, weigh all patients and determine if the patient is already overweight (BMI 25.0–29.9) or obese (BMI ≥30)
- Before giving a drug that can cause weight gain to an overweight or obese patient, consider determining whether the patient already has pre-diabetes (fasting plasma glucose 100–125 mg/dl), diabetes (fasting plasma glucose >126 mg/dl), or dyslipidemia (increased total cholesterol, LDL cholesterol and triglycerides; decreased HDL cholesterol), and treat or refer such patients for treatment including nutrition and weight management, physical activity counseling, smoking cessation, and medical management
- ✱ Monitor weight and BMI during treatment
- ✱ While giving a drug to a patient who has gained >5% of initial weight, consider evaluating for the presence of pre-diabetes, diabetes, or dyslipidemia, or consider switching to a different antidepressant
- EKGs may be useful for selected patients (e.g., those with personal or family history of QTc prolongation; cardiac arrhythmia; recent myocardial infarction; uncompensated heart failure; or taking agents that prolong QTc interval such as pimozide, thioridazine, selected antiarrhythmics, moxifloxacin, sparfloxacin, etc.)

- Patients at risk for electrolyte disturbances (e.g., patients on diuretic therapy) should have baseline and periodic serum potassium and magnesium measurements

SIDE EFFECTS

How Drug Causes Side Effects

- Anticholinergic activity may explain sedative effects, dry mouth, constipation, and blurred vision
- Sedative effects and weight gain may be due to antihistamine properties
- Blockade of alpha adrenergic 1 receptors may explain dizziness, sedation, and hypotension
- Cardiac arrhythmias and seizures, especially in overdose, may be caused by blockade of ion channels

Notable Side Effects

- Blurred vision, constipation, urinary retention, increased appetite, dry mouth, nausea, diarrhea, heartburn, unusual taste in mouth, weight gain
- Fatigue, weakness, dizziness, sedation, headache, anxiety, nervousness, restlessness
- Sexual dysfunction, sweating
- Topical: burning, stinging, itching, or swelling at application site

Life Threatening or Dangerous Side Effects

- Paralytic ileus, hyperthermia (TCAs + anticholinergic agents)
- Lowered seizure threshold and rare seizures
- Orthostatic hypotension, sudden death, arrhythmias, tachycardia
- QTc prolongation
- Hepatic failure, extrapyramidal symptoms
- Increased intraocular pressure, increased psychotic symptoms
- Rare induction of mania and activation of suicidal ideation

Weight Gain

unusual   not unusual   common   problematic

- Many experience and/or can be significant in amount
- Can increase appetite and carbohydrate craving

Sedation

unusual   not unusual   **common**   problematic

- Many experience and/or can be significant in amount
- Tolerance to sedative effect may develop with long-term use

What To Do About Side Effects

- Wait
- Wait
- Wait
- Lower the dose
- Switch to an SSRI or newer antidepressant

Best Augmenting Agents for Side Effects

- Many side effects cannot be improved with an augmenting agent

---

DOSING AND USE

Usual Dosage Range

- 75–150 mg/day

Dosage Forms

- Capsule 10 mg, 25 mg, 50 mg, 75 mg, 100 mg, 150 mg
- Solution 10 mg/mL
- Topical 5%

How to Dose

- Initial 25 mg/day at bedtime; increase by 25 mg every 3–7 days
- 75 mg/day; increase gradually until desired efficacy is achieved; can be dosed once a day at bedtime or in divided doses; maximum dose 300 mg/day
- Topical: apply thin film 4 times a day (or every 3–4 hours while awake)

 Dosing Tips

- If given in a single dose, should generally be administered at bedtime because of its sedative properties
- If given in split doses, largest dose should generally be given at bedtime because of its sedative properties
- If patients experience nightmares, split dose and do not give large dose at bedtime
- Patients treated for chronic pain may only require lower doses

- Liquid formulation should be diluted with water or juice, excluding grape juice
- 150 mg capsule available only for maintenance use, not initial therapy
- * Topical administration is absorbed systematically and can cause the same systematic side effects as oral administration
- If intolerable anxiety, insomnia, agitation, akathisia, or activation occur either upon dosing initiation or discontinuation, consider the possibility of activated bipolar disorder, and switch to a mood stabilizer or an atypical antipsychotic

Overdose

- Death may occur; convulsions, cardiac dysrhythmias, severe hypotension, CNS depression, coma, changes in ECG

Long-Term Use

- Safe

Habit Forming

- No

How to Stop

- Taper to avoid withdrawal effects
- Even with gradual dose reduction some withdrawal symptoms may appear within the first 2 weeks
- Many patients tolerate 50% dose reduction for 3 days, then another 50% reduction for 3 days, then discontinuation
- If withdrawal symptoms emerge during discontinuation, raise dose to stop symptoms and then restart withdrawal much more slowly

Pharmacokinetics

- Substrate for CYP450 2D6
- Half-life approximately 8–24 hours

 Drug Interactions

- Tramadol increases the risk of seizures in patients taking TCAs
- Use of TCAs with anticholinergic drugs may result in paralytic ileus or hyperthermia
- Fluoxetine, paroxetine, bupropion, duloxetine, and other CYP450 2D6 inhibitors may increase TCA concentrations

- Cimetidine may increase plasma concentrations of TCAs and cause anticholinergic symptoms
- Phenothiazines or haloperidol may raise TCA blood concentrations
- May alter effects of antihypertensive drugs; may inhibit hypotensive effects of clonidine
- Use with sympathomimetic agents may increase sympathetic activity
- Methylphenidate may inhibit metabolism of TCAs
- Activation and agitation, especially following switching or adding antidepressants, may represent the induction of a bipolar state, especially a mixed dysphoric bipolar II condition sometimes associated with suicidal ideation, and require the addition of lithium, a mood stabilizer or an atypical antipsychotic, and/or discontinuation of doxepin

 Other Warnings/ Precautions

- Add or initiate other antidepressants with caution for up to 2 weeks after discontinuing doxepin
- Generally, do not use with MAO inhibitors, including 14 days after MAOIs are stopped; do not start an MAOI until 2 weeks after discontinuing doxepin, but see Pearls
- Use with caution in patients with history of seizures, urinary retention, narrow angle-closure glaucoma, hyperthyroidism
- TCAs can increase QTc interval, especially at toxic doses, which can be attained not only by overdose but also by combining with drugs that inhibit TCA metabolism via CYP450 2D6, potentially causing torsade de pointes-type arrhythmia or sudden death
- Because TCAs can prolong QTc interval, use with caution in patients who have bradycardia or who are taking drugs that can induce bradycardia (e.g., beta blockers, calcium channel blockers, clonidine, digitalis)
- Because TCAs can prolong QTc interval, use with caution in patients who have hypokalemia and/or hypomagnesemia or who are taking drugs that can induce hypokalemia and/or magnesemia (e.g., diuretics, stimulant laxatives, intravenous amphotericin B, glucocorticoids, tetracosactide)

Do Not Use

- If patient is recovering from myocardial infarction
- If patient is taking agents capable of significantly prolonging QTc interval (e.g., pimozide, thioridazine, selected antiarrhythmics, moxifloxacin, sparfloxacin)
- If there is a history of QTc prolongation or cardiac arrhythmia, recent acute myocardial infarction, uncompensated heart failure
- If patient is taking drugs that inhibit TCA metabolism, including CYP450 2D6 inhibitors, except by an expert
- If there is reduced CYP450 2D6 function, such as patients who are poor 2D6 metabolizers, except by an expert and at low doses
- If patient has narrow angle-closure glaucoma
- If there is a proven allergy to doxepin

Renal Impairment
- Use with caution

Hepatic Impairment
- Use with caution – may need lower than usual adult dose

Cardiac Impairment
- TCAs have been reported to cause arrhythmias, prolongation of conduction time, orthostatic hypotension, sinus tachycardia, and heart failure, especially in the diseased heart
- Myocardial infarction and stroke have been reported with TCAs
- TCAs produce QTc prolongation, which may be enhanced by the existence of bradycardia, hypokalemia, congenital or acquired long QTc interval, which should be evaluated prior to administering doxepin
- Use with caution if treating concomitantly with a medication likely to produce prolonged bradycardia, hypokalemia, slowing of intracardiac conduction, or prolongation of the QTc interval
- Avoid TCAs in patients with a known history of QTc prolongation, recent acute myocardial infarction, and uncompensated heart failure

- TCAs may cause a sustained increase in heart rate in patients with ischemic heart disease and may worsen (decrease) heart rate variability, an independent risk of mortality in cardiac populations
- Since SSRIs may improve (increase) heart rate variability in patients following a myocardial infarct and may improve survival as well as mood in patients with acute angina or following a myocardial infarction, these are more appropriate agents for cardiac population than tricyclic/tetracyclic antidepressants

✱ Risk/benefit ratio may not justify use of TCAs in cardiac impairment

Elderly
- May be more sensitive to anticholinergic, cardiovascular, hypotensive, and sedative effects

 Children and Adolescents
- Use with caution, observing for activation of known or unknown bipolar disorder and/or suicidal ideation, and strongly consider informing parents or guardian of this risk so they can help observe child or adolescent patients
- Not recommended for use under age 12
- Several studies show lack of efficacy of TCAs for depression
- May be used to treat enuresis or hyperactive/impulsive behaviors
- Some cases of sudden death have occurred in children taking TCAs
- Initial dose 25–50 mg/day; maximum 100 mg/day

 Pregnancy
- Risk Category C [some animal studies show adverse effects, no controlled studies in humans]
- Crosses the placenta
- Adverse effects have been reported in infants whose mothers took a TCA (lethargy, withdrawal symptoms, fetal malformations)
- Not generally recommended for use during pregnancy, especially during first trimester
- Must weigh the risk of treatment (first trimester fetal development, third trimester newborn delivery) to the child against the risk of no treatment (recurrence of depression, maternal health, infant bonding) to the mother and child
- For many patients this may mean continuing treatment during pregnancy

Breast Feeding
- Some drug is found in mother's breast milk
- Significant drug levels have been detected in some nursing infants

✱ Recommended either to discontinue drug or bottle feed
- Immediate postpartum period is a high-risk time for depression, especially in women who have had prior depressive episodes, so drug may need to be reinstituted late in the third trimester or shortly after childbirth to prevent a recurrence during the postpartum period
- Must weigh benefits of breast feeding with risks and benefits of antidepressant treatment versus non-treatment to both the infant and the mother
- For many patients this may mean continuing treatment during breast feeding

THE ART OF PSYCHOPHARMACOLOGY

Potential Advantages
- Patients with insomnia
- Severe or treatment-resistant depression
- Patients with neuro-dermatitis and itching

Potential Disadvantages
- Pediatric and geriatric patients
- Patients concerned with weight gain
- Cardiac patients

Primary Target Symptoms
- Depressed mood
- Anxiety
- Disturbed sleep, energy
- Somatic symptoms
- Itching skin

 Pearls
✱ Only TCA available in topical formulation
✱ Topical administration may reduce symptoms in patients with various neuro-dermatitis syndromes, especially itching
- Tricyclic antidepressants are often a first-line treatment option for chronic pain

- Tricyclic antidepressants are no longer generally considered a first-line option for depression because of their side effect profile
- Tricyclic antidepressants continue to be useful for severe or treatment-resistant depression
- TCAs may aggravate psychotic symptoms
- Alcohol should be avoided because of additive CNS effects
- Underweight patients may be more susceptible to adverse cardiovascular effects
- Children, patients with inadequate hydration, and patients with cardiac disease may be more susceptible to TCA-induced cardiotoxicity than healthy adults
- For the expert only: although generally prohibited, a heroic but potentially dangerous treatment for severely treatment-resistant patients is to give a tricyclic/tetracyclic antidepressant other than clomipramine simultaneously with an MAO inhibitor for patients who fail to respond to numerous other antidepressants
- If this option is elected, start the MAOI with the tricyclic/tetracyclic antidepressant simultaneously at low doses after appropriate drug washout, then alternately increase doses of these agents every few days to a week as tolerated
- Although very strict dietary and concomitant drug restrictions must be

observed to prevent hypertensive crises and serotonin syndrome, the most common side effects of MAOI/tricyclic or tetracyclic combinations may be weight gain and orthostatic hypotension
- Patients on TCAs should be aware that they may experience symptoms such as photosensitivity or blue-green urine
- SSRIs may be more effective than TCAs in women, and TCAs may be more effective than SSRIs in men
- Since tricyclic/tetracyclic antidepressants are substrates for CYP450 2D6, and 7% of the population (especially Caucasians) may have a genetic variant leading to reduced activity of 2D6, such patients may not safely tolerate normal doses of tricyclic/tetracyclic antidepressants and may require dose reduction
- Phenotypic testing may be necessary to detect this genetic variant prior to dosing with a tricyclic/tetracyclic antidepressant, especially in vulnerable populations such as children, elderly, cardiac populations, and those on concomitant medications
- Patients who seem to have extraordinarily severe side effects at normal or low doses may have this phenotypic CYP450 2D6 variant and require low doses or switching to another antidepressant not metabolized by 2D6

 Suggested Reading

Anderson IM. Meta-analytical studies on new antidepressants. Br Med Bull 2001; 57:161–178.

Anderson IM. Selective serotonin reuptake inhibitors versus tricyclic antidepressants: a meta-analysis of efficacy and tolerability. J Aff Disorders 2000;58:19–36.

Godfrey RG. A guide to the understanding and use of tricyclic antidepressants in the overall management of fibromyalgia and other chronic pain syndromes. Arch Intern Med 1996; 156:1047–52.

DULOXETINE

THERAPEUTICS

Brands • Cymbalta
see index for additional brand names

Generic? No

Class
• SNRI (dual serotonin and norepinephrine reuptake inhibitor); may be classified as an antidepressant, but it is not just an antidepressant

Commonly Prescribed For
(bold for FDA approved)
• **Major depressive disorder**
• Stress urinary incontinence
• Neuropathic pain/chronic pain
• Fibromyalgia
• Generalized anxiety disorder
• Other anxiety disorders

How The Drug Works
• Boosts neurotransmitters serotonin, norepinephrine/noradrenaline, and dopamine
• Blocks serotonin reuptake pump (serotonin transporter), presumably increasing serotonergic neurotransmission
• Blocks norepinephrine reuptake pump (norepinephrine transporter), presumably increasing noradrenergic neurotransmission
• Presumably desensitizes both serotonin 1A receptors and beta adrenergic receptors
• Since dopamine is inactivated by norepinephrine reuptake in frontal cortex, which largely lacks dopamine transporters, duloxetine can increase dopamine neurotransmission in this part of the brain
• Weakly blocks dopamine reuptake pump (dopamine transporter), and may increase dopamine neurotransmission

How Long Until It Works
• Onset of therapeutic actions usually not immediate, but often delayed 2 to 4 weeks
• If it is not working within 6 to 8 weeks for depression, it may require a dosage increase or it may not work at all
• May continue to work for many years to prevent relapse of symptoms

If It Works
• The goal of treatment of depression and anxiety disorders is complete remission of current symptoms as well as prevention of future relapses
• The goal of treatment of fibromyalgia and chronic neuropathic pain is to reduce symptoms as much as possible, especially in combination with other treatments
• Treatment of depression most often reduces or even eliminates symptoms, but is not a cure since symptoms can recur after medicine stopped
• Treatment of fibromyalgia and chronic neuropathic pain may reduce symptoms, but rarely eliminates them completely, and is not a cure since symptoms can recur after medicine is stopped
• Continue treatment of depression and anxiety disorders until all symptoms are gone (remission)
• Once symptoms of depression are gone, continue treating for 1 year for the first episode of depression
• For second and subsequent episodes of depression, treatment may need to be indefinite
• Use in fibromyalgia and chronic neuropathic pain may also need to be indefinite, but long-term treatment is not well studied in these conditions

If It Doesn't Work
• Many depressed patients only have a partial response where some symptoms are improved but others persist (especially insomnia, fatigue, and problems concentrating)
• Other patients may be nonresponders, sometimes called treatment-resistant or treatment-refractory
• Some patients who have an initial response may relapse even though they continue treatment, sometimes called "poop-out"
• Consider increasing dose, switching to another agent or adding an appropriate augmenting agent
• Consider psychotherapy
• Consider evaluation for another diagnosis or for a comorbid condition (e.g., medical illness, substance abuse, etc.)
• Some patients may experience apparent lack of consistent efficacy due to activation of latent or underlying bipolar disorder, and

require antidepressant discontinuation and a switch to a mood stabilizer

 Best Augmenting Combos for Partial Response or Treatment-Resistance

✱ Augmentation experience is limited compared to other antidepressants

✱ Adding other agents to duloxetine for treating depression could follow the same practice for augmenting SSRIs or other SNRIs if done by experts while monitoring carefully in difficult cases

- Although no controlled studies and little clinical experience, adding other agents for treating fibromyalgia and neuropathic pain could theoretically include gabapentin, pregabalin, and tiagabine, if done by experts while monitoring carefully in difficult cases
- Mirtazapine ("California rocket fuel"; a potentially powerful dual serotonin and norepinephrine combination, but observe for activation of bipolar disorder and suicidal ideation)
- Bupropion, reboxetine, nortriptyline, desipramine, maprotiline, atomoxetine (all potentially powerful enhancers of noradrenergic action, but observe for activation of bipolar disorder and suicidal ideation)
- Modafinil, especially for fatigue, sleepiness, and lack of concentration
- Mood stabilizers or atypical antipsychotics for bipolar depression, psychotic depression or treatment-resistant depression
- Benzodiazepines
- If all else fails for anxiety disorders, consider gabapentin or tiagabine
- Hypnotics or trazodone for insomnia
- Classically, lithium, buspirone, or thyroid hormone

Tests
- Check blood pressure before initiating treatment and regularly during treatment

SIDE EFFECTS

How Drug Causes Side Effects
- Theoretically due to increases in serotonin and norepinephrine concentrations at

receptors in parts of the brain and body other than those that cause therapeutic actions (e.g., unwanted actions of serotonin in sleep centers causing insomnia, unwanted actions of norepinephrine on acetylcholine release causing decreased appetite, increased blood pressure, urinary retention, etc.)
- Most side effects are immediate but often go away with time

Notable Side Effects
- Insomnia, sedation
- Nausea, diarrhea, decreased appetite
- Sexual dysfunction (men: abnormal ejaculation/orgasm, impotence, decreased libido; women: abnormal orgasm)
- Sweating
- Increase in blood pressure (up to 2 mm Hg)

 Life Threatening or Dangerous Side Effects
- Rare seizures
- Rare induction of hypomania and activation of suicidal ideation, suicide attempts, and completed suicide

Weight Gain

unusual   not unusual   common   problematic
- Reported but not expected

Sedation

unusual   not unusual   common   problematic
- Occurs in significant minority
- May also be activating in some patients

What To Do About Side Effects
- Wait
- Wait
- Wait
- Lower the dose
- In a few weeks, switch or add other drugs

Best Augmenting Agents for Side Effects
- For urinary hesitancy, give an alpha 1 blocker such as tamsulosin
- Often best to try another antidepressant monotherapy prior to resorting to augmentation strategies to treat side effects

- Trazodone or a hypnotic for insomnia
- Bupropion, sildenafil, vardenafil, or tadalafil for sexual dysfunction
- Benzodiazepines for jitteriness and anxiety, especially at initiation of treatment and especially for anxious patients
- Mirtazapine for insomnia, agitation, and gastrointestinal side effects
- Many side effects are dose-dependent (i.e., they increase as dose increases, or they reemerge until tolerance re-develops)
- Many side effects are time-dependent (i.e., they start immediately upon dosing and upon each dose increase, but go away with time)
- Activation and agitation may represent the induction of a bipolar state, especially a mixed dysphoric bipolar II condition sometimes associated with suicidal ideation, and require the addition of lithium, a mood stabilizer or an atypical antipsychotic, and/or discontinuation of duloxetine

DOSING AND USE

Usual Dosage Range
- 40–60 mg/day in 1–2 doses for depression
- 40 mg twice daily for stress urinary incontinence

Dosage Forms
- Capsule 20 mg, 30 mg, 60 mg

How to Dose
- Initial 40 mg/day in 1–2 doses; can increase to 60 mg/day if necessary; maximum dose generally 120 mg/day

 Dosing Tips
- Studies have not demonstrated increased efficacy beyond 60 mg/day
❋ Some patients may require up to or more than 120 mg/day, but clinical experience is quite limited with high dosing
- Dosing for neuropathic pain and fibromyalgia may be similar to that for depression but different from dosing for stress urinary incontinence, but clinical experience is still evolving

- Some studies suggest that both serotonin and norepinephrine reuptake blockade are present at 40–60 mg/day
- Do not chew or crush and do not sprinkle on food or mix with food, but rather always swallow whole to avoid affecting enteric coating

Overdose
- No fatalities have been reported

Long-Term Use
- Blood pressure should be monitored regularly

Habit Forming
- No

How to Stop
- Taper to avoid withdrawal effects (dizziness, nausea, vomiting, headache, paresthesias, irritability)
- Many patients tolerate 50% dose reduction for 3 days, then another 50% reduction for 3 days, then discontinuation
❋ If withdrawal symptoms emerge during discontinuation, raise dose to stop symptoms and then restart withdrawal much more slowly

Pharmacokinetics
- Elimination half-life approximately 12 hours
- Metabolized mainly by CYP450 2D6 and CYP450 1A2
- Inhibitor of CYP450 2D6 and CYP450 1A2
- Absorption may be delayed by up to 3 hours and clearance may be increased by one-third after an evening dose as compared to a morning dose

 Drug Interactions
- Can increase tricyclic antidepressant levels; use with caution with tricyclic antidepressants or when switching from a TCA to duloxetine
- Can cause a fatal "serotonin syndrome" when combined with MAO inhibitors, so do not use with MAO inhibitors or for at least 14 days after MAOIs are stopped
- Do not start an MAO inhibitor for at least 5 days after discontinuing duloxetine
- Inhibitors of CYP450 1A2, such as fluvoxamine, may increase plasma levels of

duloxetine and require a dosage reduction of duloxetine

- Cigarette smoking induces CYP450 1A2 and may reduce plasma levels of duloxetine, but dosage modifications are not recommended for smokers
- ✳ Inhibitors of CYP450 2D6, such as paroxetine, fluoxetine, and quinidine, may increase plasma levels of duloxetine and require a dosage reduction of duloxetine
- Via CYP450 1A2 inhibition, duloxetine could theoretically reduce clearance of theophylline and clozapine; however, studies of co-administration with theophylline did not demonstrate significant effects of duloxetine on theophylline pharmacokinetics
- Via CYP450 2D6 inhibition, duloxetine could theoretically interfere with the analgesic actions of codeine, and increase the plasma levels of some beta blockers and of atomoxetine
- Via CYP450 2D6 inhibition, duloxetine could theoretically increase concentrations of thioridazine and cause dangerous cardiac arrhythmias

 Other Warnings/ Precautions

- Use with caution in patients with history of seizures
- Use with caution in patients with bipolar disorder unless treated with concomitant mood stabilizing agent
- Monitor patients for activation of suicidal ideation, especially children and adolescents
- Duloxetine may increase blood pressure, so blood pressure should be monitored during treatment

Do Not Use

- If patient has uncontrolled narrow angle-closure glaucoma
- If patient has substantial alcohol use
- If patient is taking an MAO inhibitor
- If patient is taking thioridazine
- If there is a proven allergy to duloxetine

Renal Impairment

- Dose adjustment generally not necessary for mild impairment
- Not recommended for use in patients with end-stage renal disease

Hepatic Impairment

- Not recommended for use in patients with hepatic impairment

Cardiac Impairment

- Drug should be used with caution
- Duloxetine may raise blood pressure

Elderly

- Some patients may tolerate lower doses better

 Children and Adolescents

- Use with caution, observing for activation of known or unknown bipolar disorder and/or suicidal ideation, and strongly consider informing parents or guardian of this risk so they can help observe child or adolescent patients
- Not specifically approved, but can be used by experts

 Pregnancy

- Risk Category C [some animal studies show adverse effects, no controlled studies in humans]
- Not generally recommended for use during pregnancy, especially during first trimester
- Nonetheless, continuous treatment during pregnancy may be necessary and has not been proven to be harmful to the fetus
- Must weigh the risk of treatment (first trimester fetal development, third trimester newborn delivery) to the child against the risk of no treatment (recurrence of depression, maternal health, infant bonding) to the mother and child
- For many patients this may mean continuing treatment during pregnancy
- Neonates exposed to SSRIs or SNRIs late in the third trimester have developed complications requiring prolonged hospitalization, respiratory support, and tube feeding; reported symptoms are consistent with either a direct toxic effect

of SSRIs and SNRIs or, possibly, a drug discontinuation syndrome, and include respiratory distress, cyanosis, apnea, seizures, temperature instability, feeding difficulty, vomiting, hypoglycemia, hypotonia, hypertonia, hyperreflexia, tremor, jitteriness, irritability, and constant crying

Breast Feeding

- Unknown if duloxetine is secreted in human breast milk, but all psychotropics assumed to be secreted in breast milk
- If child becomes irritable or sedated, breast feeding or drug may need to be discontinued
- Immediate postpartum period is a high-risk time for depression, especially in women who have had prior depressive episodes, so drug may need to be reinstituted late in the third trimester or shortly after childbirth to prevent a recurrence during the postpartum period
- Must weigh benefits of breast feeding with risks and benefits of antidepressant treatment versus non-treatment to both the infant and the mother
- For many patients, this may mean continuing treatment during breast feeding

THE ART OF PSYCHOPHARMACOLOGY

Potential Advantages

- Patients with physical symptoms of depression
- Patients with retarded depression
- Patients with atypical depression
- Patients with depression may have higher remission rates on SNRIs than on SSRIs
- Depressed patients with somatic symptoms, fatigue, and pain
- Patients who do not respond or do not remit on treatment with SSRIs

Potential Disadvantages

- Patients with urologic disorders, prostate disorders (e.g., older men)
- Patients sensitive to nausea

Primary Target Symptoms

- Depressed mood
- Energy, motivation, and interest
- Sleep disturbance
- Physical symptoms
- Pain

 Pearls

✳ Duloxetine has well-documented efficacy for the physical symptoms of depression
- Duloxetine has only somewhat greater potency for serotonin reuptake blockade than for norepinephrine reuptake blockade, but this is of unclear clinical significance as a differentiator from other SNRIs
- No head-to-head studies, but may have less hypertension than venlafaxine XR
- Powerful pro-noradrenergic actions may occur at doses greater than 60 mg/day
- Not well-studied in ADHD or anxiety disorders, but may be effective
✳ Well-studied in stress urinary incontinence and approval for this use is expected
- Patients may have higher remission rate for depression on SNRIs than on SSRIs
- Add or switch to or from pro-noradrenergic agents (e.g., atomoxetine, reboxetine, other SNRIs, mirtazapine, maprotiline, nortriptyline, desipramine, bupropion) with caution
- Add or switch to or from CYP450 2D6 substrates with caution (e.g., atomoxetine, maprotiline, nortriptyline, desipramine)
- Mechanism of action as SNRI suggests it may be effective in some patients who fail to respond to SSRIs

Suggested Reading

Bymaster FP, Dreshfield-Ahmad LJ, Threlkeld PG, Shaw JL, Thompson L, Nelson DL, Hemrick-Luecke SK, Wong DT. Comparative affinity of duloxetine and venlafaxine for serotonin and norepinephrine transporters in vitro and in vivo, human serotonin receptor subtypes, and other neuronal receptors. Neuropsychopharmacology 2001; 25(6):871–80.

Detke MJ, Lu Y, Goldstein DJ, Hayes JR, Demitrack MA. Duloxetine, 60 mg once daily, for major depressive disorder: a randomized double-blind placebo-controlled trial. J Clin Psychiatry 2002;63(4):308–15.

Goldstein DJ, Mallinckrodt C, Lu Y, Demitrack MA. Duloxetine in the treatment of major depressive disorder: a double-blind clinical trial. J Clin Psychiatry 2002;63(3):225–31.

Karpa KD, Cavanaugh JE, Lakoski JM. Duloxetine pharmacology: profile of a dual monoamine modulator. CNS Drug Rev 2002;8(4):361–76.

Zinner NR. Duloxetine: a serotonin-noradrenaline re-uptake inhibitor for the treatment of stress urinary incontinence. Expert Opin Investig Drugs 2003; 12(9):1559–66.

ESCITALOPRAM

THERAPEUTICS

Brands • Lexapro
see index for additional brand names

Generic? Not in the U.S. or Europe

Class
- SSRI (selective serotonin reuptake inhibitor); often classified as an antidepressant, but it is not just an antidepressant

Commonly Prescribed For
(bold for FDA approved)
- **Major depressive disorder**
- **Generalized anxiety disorder**
- Panic disorder
- Obsessive-compulsive disorder (OCD)
- Posttraumatic stress disorder (PTSD)
- Social anxiety disorder (social phobia)
- Premenstrual dysphoric disorder (PMDD)

How The Drug Works
- Boosts neurotransmitter serotonin
- Blocks serotonin reuptake pump (serotonin transporter)
- Desensitizes serotonin receptors, especially serotonin 1A autoreceptors
- Presumably increases serotonergic neurotransmission

How Long Until It Works
- Onset of therapeutic actions usually not immediate, but often delayed 2 to 4 weeks
- If it is not working within 6 to 8 weeks, it may require a dosage increase or it may not work at all
- May continue to work for many years to prevent relapse of symptoms

If It Works
- The goal of treatment is complete remission of current symptoms as well as prevention of future relapses
- Treatment most often reduces or even eliminates symptoms, but not a cure since symptoms can recur after medicine stopped
- Continue treatment until all symptoms are gone (remission) or significantly reduced (e.g., OCD, PTSD)

- Once symptoms gone, continue treating for 1 year for the first episode of depression
- For second and subsequent episodes of depression, treatment may need to be indefinite
- Use in anxiety disorders may also need to be indefinite

If It Doesn't Work
- Many patients only have a partial response where some symptoms are improved but others persist (especially insomnia, fatigue, and problems concentrating in depression)
- Other patients may be nonresponders, sometimes called treatment-resistant or treatment-refractory
- Some patients who have an initial response may relapse even though they continue treatment, sometimes called "poop-out"
- Consider increasing dose, switching to another agent or adding an appropriate augmenting agent
- Consider psychotherapy
- Consider evaluation for another diagnosis or for a comorbid condition (e.g., medical illness, substance abuse, etc.)
- Some patients may experience apparent lack of consistent efficacy due to activation of latent or underlying bipolar disorder, and require antidepressant discontinuation and a switch to a mood stabilizer

Best Augmenting Combos for Partial Response or Treatment-Resistance

- Trazodone, especially for insomnia
- Bupropion, mirtazapine, reboxetine, or atomoxetine (use combinations of antidepressants with caution as this may activate bipolar disorder and suicidal ideation)
- Modafinil, especially for fatigue, sleepiness, and lack of concentration
- Mood stabilizers or atypical antipsychotics for bipolar depression, psychotic depression, treatment-resistant depression, or treatment-resistant anxiety disorders
- Benzodiazepines
- If all else fails for anxiety disorders, consider gabapentin or tiagabine
- Hypnotics for insomnia
- Classically, lithium, buspirone, or thyroid hormone

Tests
• None for healthy individuals

SIDE EFFECTS

How Drug Causes Side Effects
• Theoretically due to increases in serotonin concentrations at serotonin receptors in parts of the brain and body other than those that cause therapeutic actions (e.g., unwanted actions of serotonin in sleep centers causing insomnia, unwanted actions of serotonin in the gut causing diarrhea, etc.)
• Increasing serotonin can cause diminished dopamine release and might contribute to emotional flattening, cognitive slowing, and apathy in some patients
• Most side effects are immediate but often go away with time, in contrast to most therapeutic effects which are delayed and are enhanced over time
✱ As escitalopram has no known important secondary pharmacologic properties, its side effects are presumably all mediated by its serotonin reuptake blockade

Notable Side Effects
• Sexual dysfunction (men: delayed ejaculation, erectile dysfunction; men and women: decreased sexual desire, anorgasmia)
• Gastrointestinal (decreased appetite, nausea, diarrhea, constipation, dry mouth)
• Mostly central nervous system (insomnia but also sedation, agitation, tremors, headache, dizziness)
• Note: patients with diagnosed or undiagnosed bipolar or psychotic disorders may be more vulnerable to CNS-activating actions of SSRIs
• Autonomic (sweating)
• Bruising and rare bleeding
• Rare hyponatremia (mostly in elderly patients and generally reversible on discontinuation of escitalopram

Life Threatening or Dangerous Side Effects
• Rare seizures
• Rare induction of mania and activation of suicidal ideation

Weight Gain

unusual   not unusual   common   problematic
• Reported but not expected

Sedation

unusual   not unusual   common   problematic
• Reported but not expected

What To Do About Side Effects
• Wait
• Wait
• Wait
• In a few weeks, switch to another agent or add other drugs

Best Augmenting Agents for Side Effects
• Often best to try another SSRI or another antidepressant monotherapy prior to resorting to augmentation strategies to treat side effects
• Trazodone or a hypnotic for insomnia
• Bupropion, sildenafil, vardenafil, or tadalafil for sexual dysfunction
• Bupropion for emotional flattening, cognitive slowing, or apathy
• Mirtazapine for insomnia, agitation, and gastrointestinal side effects
• Benzodiazepines for jitteriness and anxiety, especially at initiation of treatment and especially for anxious patients
• Many side effects are dose-dependent (i.e., they increase as dose increases, or they reemerge until tolerance re-develops)
• Many side effects are time-dependent (i.e., they start immediately upon dosing and upon each dose increase, but go away with time)
• Activation and agitation may represent the induction of a bipolar state, especially a mixed dysphoric bipolar II condition sometimes associated with suicidal ideation, and require the addition of lithium, a mood stabilizer or an atypical antipsychotic, and/or discontinuation of escitalopram

DOSING AND USE

Usual Dosage Range
- 10–20 mg/day
- Oral solution 5 mg/5 mL

Dosage Forms
- Tablets 10 mg, 20 mg

How to Dose
- Initial 10 mg/day; increase to 20 mg/day if necessary; single dose administration, morning or evening

 Dosing Tips
- Given once daily, any time of day tolerated
- ✳ 10 mg of escitalopram may be comparable in efficacy to 40 mg of citalopram with fewer side effects
- Thus, give an adequate trial of 10 mg prior to giving 20 mg
- Some patients require dosing with 30 or 40 mg
- If intolerable anxiety, insomnia, agitation, akathisia, or activation occur either upon dosing initiation or discontinuation, consider the possibility of activated bipolar disorder and switch to a mood stabilizer or an atypical antipsychotic

Overdose
- Few reports of escitalopram overdose, but probably similar to citalopram overdose
- Rare fatalities have been reported in citalopram overdose, both in combination with other drugs and alone
- Symptoms associated with citalopram overdose include vomiting, sedation, heart rhythm disturbances, dizziness, sweating, nausea, tremor, and rarely amnesia, confusion, coma, convulsions

Long-Term Use
- Safe

Habit Forming
- No

How to Stop
- Taper not usually necessary
- However, tapering to avoid potential withdrawal reactions generally prudent

- Many patients tolerate 50% dose reduction for 3 days, then another 50% reduction for 3 days, then discontinuation
- If withdrawal symptoms emerge during discontinuation, raise dose to stop symptoms and then restart withdrawal much more slowly

Pharmacokinetics
- Mean terminal half-life 27–32 hours
- Steady-state plasma concentrations achieved within 1 week
- No significant actions on CYP450 enzymes

 Drug Interactions
- Tramadol increases the risk of seizures in patients taking an antidepressant
- Can cause a fatal "serotonin syndrome" when combined with MAO inhibitors, so do not use with MAO inhibitors or for at least 14 days after MAOIs are stopped
- Do not start an MAO inhibitor for at least 2 weeks after discontinuing escitalopram
- Could theoretically cause weakness, hyperreflexia, and incoordination when combined with sumatriptan or possibly other triptans, requiring careful monitoring of patient
- Few known adverse drug interactions

 Other Warnings/ Precautions
- Use with caution in patients with history of seizures
- Use with caution in patients with bipolar disorder unless treated with concomitant mood stabilizing agent
- Monitor patients for activation of suicidal ideation, especially children and adolescents

Do Not Use
- If patient is taking an MAO inhibitor
- If there is a proven allergy to escitalopram or citalopram

SPECIAL POPULATIONS

Renal Impairment
- Few data available for use in patients with renal impairment, but start with 10 mg/day

Hepatic Impairment
• Recommended dose 10 mg/day

Cardiac Impairment
• Not systematically evaluated in patients with cardiac impairment
• Preliminary data suggest that citalopram is safe in patients with cardiac impairment, suggesting that escitalopram is also safe
• Treating depression with SSRIs in patients with acute angina or following myocardial infarction may reduce cardiac events and improve survival as well as mood

Elderly
• Recommended dose 10 mg/day

Children and Adolescents
• Safety and efficacy have not been established
• Use with caution, observing for activation of known or unknown bipolar disorder and/or suicidal ideation, and strongly consider informing parents or guardian of this risk so they can help observe child or adolescent patients

Pregnancy
• Risk Category C [some animal studies show adverse effects, no controlled studies in humans]
• Not generally recommended for use during pregnancy, especially during first trimester
• Nonetheless, continuous treatment during pregnancy may be necessary and has not been proven to be harmful to the fetus
• At delivery there may be more bleeding in the mother and transient irritability or sedation in the newborn
• Must weigh the risk of treatment (first trimester fetal development, third trimester newborn delivery) to the child against the risk of no treatment (recurrence of depression, maternal health, infant bonding) to the mother and child
• For many patients, this may mean continuing treatment during pregnancy
• Neonates exposed to SSRIs or SNRIs late in the third trimester have developed complications requiring prolonged hospitalization, respiratory support, and tube feeding; reported symptoms are consistent with either a direct toxic effect of SSRIs and SNRIs or, possibly, a drug discontinuation syndrome, and include respiratory distress, cyanosis, apnea, seizures, temperature instability, feeding difficulty, vomiting, hypoglycemia, hypotonia, hypertonia, hyperreflexia, tremor, jitteriness, irritability, and constant crying

Breast Feeding
• Some drug is found in mother's breast milk
• Trace amounts may be present in nursing children whose mothers are on escitalopram
• If child becomes irritable or sedated, breast feeding or drug may need to be discontinued
• Immediate postpartum period is a high-risk time for depression, especially in women who have had prior depressive episodes, so drug may need to be reinstituted late in the third trimester or shortly after childbirth to prevent a recurrence during the postpartum period
• Must weigh benefits of breast feeding with risks and benefits of antidepressant treatment versus non-treatment to both the infant and the mother
• For many patients, this may mean continuing treatment during breast feeding

THE ART OF PSYCHOPHARMACOLOGY

Potential Advantages
• Patients taking concomitant medications (few drug interactions and fewer even than with citalopram)
• Patients requiring faster onset of action

Potential Disadvantages
• More expensive than citalopram in markets where citalopram is generic

Primary Target Symptoms
• Depressed mood
• Anxiety
• Panic attacks, avoidant behavior, re-experiencing, hyperarousal
• Sleep disturbance, both insomnia and hypersomnia

Pearls

❋ May be among the best-tolerated antidepressants
• May have less sexual dysfunction than some other SSRIs
• May be better tolerated than citalopram
• Can cause cognitive and affective "flattening"
❋ R-citalopram may interfere with the binding of S-citalopram at the serotonin transporter
❋ For this reason, S-citalopram may be more than twice as potent as R,S-citalopram (i.e., citalopram)
• Thus, 10 mg starting dose of S-citalopram may have the therapeutic efficacy of 40 mg of R,S-citalopram
• Thus, escitalopram may have faster onset and better efficacy with reduced side effects compared to R,S-citalopram
• Some data may actually suggest remission rates comparable to dual serotonin and norepinephrine reuptake inhibitors, but this is not proven
❋ Escitalopram is commonly used with augmenting agents, as it is the SSRI with the least interaction at either CYP450 2D6 or 3A4, therefore causing fewer pharmacokinetically-mediated drug interactions with augmenting agents than other SSRIs
• SSRIs may be less effective in women over 50, especially if they are not taking estrogen
• SSRIs may be useful for hot flushes in perimenopausal women
• Some postmenopausal women's depression will respond better to escitalopram plus estrogen augmentation than to escitalopram alone
• Nonresponse to escitalopram in elderly may require consideration of mild cognitive impairment or Alzheimer disease

Suggested Reading

Baldwin DS. Escitalopram: efficacy and tolerability in the treatment of depression. Hosp Med. 2002;63:668–71.

Burke WJ. Escitalopram. Expert Opin Investig Drugs. 2002;11(10):1477–86.

Edwards JG, Anderson I. Systematic review and guide to selection of selective serotonin reuptake inhibitors. Drugs. 1999;57:507–533.

Waugh J, Goa KL. Escitalopram : a review of its use in the management of major depressive and anxiety disorders. CNS Drugs. 2003;17:343–62.

ESTAZOLAM

THERAPEUTICS

Brands • ProSom
see index for additional brand names

Generic? Yes

Class
• Benzodiazepine (hypnotic)

Commonly Prescribed For
(bold for FDA approved)
• **Insomnia characterized by difficulty in falling asleep, frequent nocturnal awakenings, and/or early morning awakenings**

How The Drug Works
• Binds to benzodiazepine receptors at the GABA-A ligand-gated chloride channel complex
• Enhances the inhibitory effects of GABA
• Boosts chloride conductance through GABA-regulated channels
• Inhibitory actions in sleep centers may provide sedative hypnotic effects

How Long Until It Works
• Generally takes effect in less than an hour

If It Works
• Improves quality of sleep
• Effects on total wake-time and number of nighttime awakenings may be decreased over time

If It Doesn't Work
• If insomnia does not improve after 7–10 days, it may be a manifestation of a primary psychiatric or physical illness such as obstructive sleep apnea or restless leg syndrome, which requires independent evaluation
• Increase the dose
• Improve sleep hygiene
• Switch to another agent

Best Augmenting Combos for Partial Response or Treatment-Resistance
• Generally, best to switch to another agent
• Trazodone

• Agents with antihistamine actions (e.g., diphenhydramine, tricyclic antidepressants)

Tests
• In patients with seizure disorders, concomitant medical illness, and/or those with multiple concomitant long-term medications, periodic liver tests and blood counts may be prudent

SIDE EFFECTS

How Drug Causes Side Effects
• Same mechanism for side effects as for therapeutic effects – namely due to excessive actions at benzodiazepine receptors
• Actions at benzodiazepine receptors that carry over to next day can cause daytime sedation, amnesia, and ataxia
• Long-term adaptations in benzodiazepine receptors may explain the development of dependence, tolerance, and withdrawal

Notable Side Effects
✱ Sedation, fatigue, depression
✱ Dizziness, ataxia, slurred speech, weakness
✱ Forgetfulness, confusion
✱ Hyper-excitability, nervousness
• Rare hallucinations, mania
• Rare hypotension
• Hypersalivation, dry mouth
• Rebound insomnia when withdrawing from long-term treatment

Life Threatening or Dangerous Side Effects
• Respiratory depression, especially when taken with CNS depressants in overdose
• Rare hepatic dysfunction, renal dysfunction, blood dyscrasias

Weight Gain

unusual / not unusual / common / problematic

• Reported but not expected

Sedation

unusual / not unusual / **common** / problematic

• Many experience and/or can be significant in amount

What To Do About Side Effects

- Wait
- To avoid problems with memory, only take estazolam if planning to have a full night's sleep
- Lower the dose
- Switch to a shorter-acting sedative hypnotic
- Switch to a non-benzodiazepine hypnotic
- Administer flumazenil if side effects are severe or life-threatening

Best Augmenting Agents for Side Effects

- Many side effects cannot be improved with an augmenting agent

DOSING AND USE

Usual Dosage Range
- 1–2 mg/day at bedtime

Dosage Forms
- Tablet 1 mg scored, 2 mg scored

How to Dose
- Initial 1 mg/day at bedtime; increase to 2 mg/day at bedtime if ineffective

 Dosing Tips

- Use lowest possible effective dose and assess need for continued treatment regularly
- Estazolam should generally not be prescribed in quantities greater than a 1-month supply
- Patients with lower body weights may require lower doses
- Risk of dependence may increase with dose and duration of treatment

Overdose
- No death reported in monotherapy; sedation, slurred speech, poor coordination, confusion, coma, respiratory depression

Long-Term Use
- Not generally intended for long-term use
- Evidence of efficacy up to 12 weeks

Habit Forming
- Estazolam is a Schedule IV drug

- Some patients may develop dependence and/or tolerance; risk may be greater with higher doses
- History of drug addiction may increase risk of dependence

How to Stop
- If taken for more than a few weeks, taper to reduce chances of withdrawal effects
- Patients with seizure history may seize upon sudden withdrawal
- Rebound insomnia may occur the first 1–2 nights after stopping
- For patients with severe problems discontinuing a benzodiazepine, dosing may need to be tapered over many months (i.e., reduce dose by 1% every 3 days by crushing tablet and suspending or dissolving in 100 ml of fruit juice and then disposing of 1 ml while drinking the rest; 3–7 days later, dispose of 2 ml, and so on). This is both a form of very slow biological tapering and a form of behavioral desensitization

Pharmacokinetics
- Half-life 10–24 hours
- Inactive metabolites

 Drug Interactions

- Increased clearance and thus decreased estazolam levels in smokers
- Increased depressive effects when taken with other CNS depressants

 Other Warnings/ Precautions

- Insomnia may be a symptom of a primary disorder, rather than a primary disorder itself
- Some patients may exhibit abnormal thinking or behavioral changes similar to those caused by other CNS depressants (i.e., either depressant actions or disinhibiting actions)
- Some depressed patients may experience a worsening of suicidal ideation
- Use only with extreme caution in patients with impaired respiratory function or obstructive sleep apnea
- Estazolam should only be administered at bedtime

Do Not Use
- If patient is pregnant
- If patient has narrow angle-closure glaucoma
- If there is a proven allergy to estazolam or any benzodiazepine

Renal Impairment
- Drug should be used with caution

Hepatic Impairment
- Drug should be used with caution

Cardiac Impairment
- Benzodiazepines have been used to treat insomnia associated with acute myocardial infarction

Elderly
- No dose adjustment in healthy patients
- Debilitated patients: recommended initial dose of 0.5 mg/day

 Children and Adolescents
- Safety and efficacy have not been established
- Long-term effects of estazolam in children/adolescents are unknown
- Should generally receive lower doses and be more closely monitored

 Pregnancy
- Risk Category X [positive evidence of risk to human fetus; contraindicated for use in pregnancy]
- Infants whose mothers received a benzodiazepine late in pregnancy may experience withdrawal effects
- Neonatal flaccidity has been reported in infants whose mothers took a benzodiazepine during pregnancy

Breast Feeding
- Unknown if estazolam is secreted in human breast milk, but all psychotropics assumed to be secreted in breast milk
* Recommended either to discontinue drug or bottle feed
- Effects on infant have been observed and include feeding difficulties, sedation, and weight loss

 THE ART OF PSYCHOPHARMACOLOGY

Potential Advantages
- Transient insomnia

Potential Disadvantages
- Smokers (may need higher dose)

Primary Target Symptoms
- Time to sleep onset
- Total sleep time
- Nighttime awakenings

 Pearls
- If tolerance develops, it may result in increased anxiety during the day and/or increased wakefulness during the latter part of the night
- Best short-term use is for less than 10 consecutive days, and for less than half of the nights in a month
- Drug holidays may restore drug effectiveness if tolerance develops

Suggested Reading

Pierce MW, Shu VS. Efficacy of estazolam. The United States clinical experience. Am J Med 1990;88:6S–11S.

Pierce MW, Shu VS, Groves LJ. Safety of estazolam. The United States clinical experience. Am J Med 1990;88:12S–17S.

Vogel GW, Morris D. The effects of estazolam on sleep, performance, and memory: a long-term sleep laboratory study of elderly insomniacs. J Clin Pharmacol 1992; 32:647–51.

FLUMAZENIL

THERAPEUTICS

Brands
- Romazicon
- Anexate
- Lanexat

see index for additional brand names

Generic? No

Class
- Benzodiazepine receptor antagonist

Commonly Prescribed For
(bold for FDA approved)
- **Reversal of sedative effects of benzodiazepines after general anesthesia has been induced and/or maintained with benzodiazepines**
- **Reversal of sedative effects of benzodiazepines after sedation has been produced with benzodiazepines for diagnostic and therapeutic procedures**
- **Management of benzodiazepine overdose**
- **Reversal of conscious sedation induced with benzodiazepines (pediatric patients)**

How The Drug Works
- Blocks benzodiazepine receptors at GABA-A ligand-gated chloride channel complex, preventing benzodiazepines from binding there

How Long Until It Works
- Onset of action 1–2 minutes; peak effect 6–10 minutes

If It Works
* Reverses sedation and psychomotor retardation rapidly, but may not restore memory completely
* Patients treated for benzodiazepine overdose may experience CNS excitation
* Patients who receive flumazenil to reverse benzodiazepine effects should be monitored for up to 2 hours for resedation, respiratory depression, or other lingering benzodiazepine effects
- Flumazenil has not been shown to treat hypoventilation due to benzodiazepine treatment

If It Doesn't Work
- Sedation is most likely not due to a benzodiazepine, and treatment with flumazenil should be discontinued and other causes of sedation investigated

Best Augmenting Combos for Partial Response or Treatment-Resistance
- None – flumazenil is basically used as a monotherapy antidote to reverse the actions of benzodiazepines

Tests
- None for healthy individuals

SIDE EFFECTS

How Drug Causes Side Effects
- Blocks benzodiazepine receptors at GABA-A ligand-gated chloride channel complex, preventing benzodiazepines from binding there

Notable Side Effects
- May precipitate benzodiazepine withdrawal in patients dependent upon or tolerant to benzodiazepines
- Dizziness, injection site pain, sweating, headache, blurred vision

Life Threatening or Dangerous Side Effects
- Seizures
- Death (majority occurred in patients with severe underlying disease or who overdosed with non-benzodiazepines)
- Cardiac dysrhythmia

Weight Gain

- Reported but not expected

Sedation

- Reported but not expected
- Patients may experience resedation if the effects of flumazenil wear off before the effects of the benzodiazepine

What To Do About Side Effects
• Monitor patient
• Restrict ambulation because of dizziness, blurred vision, and possibility of resedation

Best Augmenting Agents for Side Effects
• None – augmenting agents are not appropriate to treat side effects associated with flumazenil use

DOSING AND USE

Usual Dosage Range
• 0.4–1 mg generally causes complete antagonism of therapeutic doses of benzodiazepines
• 1–3 mg generally reverses benzodiazepine overdose

Dosage Forms
• Intravenous 0.1 mg/mL – 5 mL multiple-use vial, 10 mL multiple-use vial

How to Dose
• Conscious sedation, general anesthesia: 0.2 mg (2 mL) over 15 seconds; can administer 0.2 mg again after 45 seconds; can administer 0.2 mg each additional 60 seconds; maximum 1 mg
• Benzodiazepine overdose: 0.2 mg over 30 seconds; can administer 0.3 mg over next 30 seconds; can administer 0.5 mg over 30 seconds after 1 minute; maximum 5 mg

 Dosing Tips
• May need to administer follow up doses to reverse actions of benzodiazepines that have a longer half-life than flumazenil (i.e., longer than 1 hour)

Overdose
• Anxiety, agitation, increased muscle tone, hyperesthesia, convulsions

Long-Term Use
• Not a long-term treatment

Habit Forming
• No

How to Stop
• N/A

Pharmacokinetics
• Terminal half-life 41–79 minutes

 Drug Interactions
• Food increases its clearance

 Other Warnings/ Precautions
• Flumazenil may induce seizures, particularly in patients tolerant to or dependent on benzodiazepines, or who have overdosed on cyclic antidepressants, received recent/repeated doses of parenteral benzodiazepines, or have jerking or convulsion during overdose
• Patients dependent on benzodiazepines or receiving benzodiazepines to suppress seizures in cyclic antidepressant overdose should receive the minimally effective dose of flumazenil
• Use with caution in patients with head injury
• Greater risk of resedation if administered to a patient who took a long-acting benzodiazepine or a large dose of a short-acting benzodiazepine
• Flumazenil may induce panic attacks in patients with panic disorder
• Use with caution in cases of mixed overdose because toxic effects of other drugs used in overdose (e.g., convulsions) may appear when the effects of the benzodiazepine are reversed

Do Not Use
• Should not be used until after effects of neuromuscular blockers have been reversed
• If benzodiazepine was prescribed to control a life-threatening condition (e.g., status epilepticus, intracranial pressure)
• If there is a high risk of seizure
• If patient exhibits signs of serious cyclic antidepressant overdose
• If there is a proven allergy to flumazenil or benzodiazepines

SPECIAL POPULATIONS

Renal Impairment
• Dosage adjustment may not be necessary

Hepatic Impairment
• Prolongation of half-life
• Moderate: clearance reduced by half
• Severe: clearance reduced by three-quarters

Cardiac Impairment
• Dosage adjustment may not be necessary

Elderly
• Dosage adjustment may not be necessary

Children and Adolescents
• More variability of pharmacokinetics than in adults
• Safety and efficacy established for reversal of conscious sedation for children over age 1
• Initial 0.01 mg/kg (up to 0.2 mg) over 15 seconds; same dosing pattern as adults; maximum 0.05 mg/kg or 1 mg
• Safety and efficacy for reversal of benzodiazepine overdose, general anesthesia induction or resuscitation of a newborn have not been established, but anecdotal data suggest similar safety and efficacy as for conscious sedation

Pregnancy
• Risk Category C [some animal studies show adverse effects, no controlled studies in humans]

• Not recommended to treat the effects of benzodiazepines during labor and delivery because the effects on the infant have not been studied

Breast Feeding
• Unknown if flumazenil is secreted in human breast milk, but all psychotropics assumed to be secreted in breast milk
• If treatment with flumazenil is necessary, it should be administered with caution

THE ART OF PSYCHOPHARMACOLOGY

Potential Advantages
• To reverse a low dose of a short-acting benzodiazepine

Potential Disadvantages
• May be too short-acting

Primary Target Symptoms
• Effects of benzodiazepines
• Sedative effects
• Recall and psychomotor impairments
• Ventilatory depression

Pearls
• Can precipitate benzodiazepine withdrawal seizures
✳ Can wear off before the benzodiazepine it is reversing
✳ Can precipitate anxiety or panic in conscious patients with anxiety disorders

---

Suggested Reading

Malizia AL, Nutt DJ. The effects of flumazenil in neuropsychiatric disorders. Clin Neuropharmacol 1995;18:215–32.

McCloy RF. Reversal of conscious sedation by flumazenil: current status and future prospects. Acta Anaesthesiol Scand Suppl 1995;108:35–42.

Weinbroum AA, Flaishon R, Sorkine P, Szold O, Rudick V. A risk-benefit assessment of flumazenil in the management of benzodiazepine overdose. Drug Saf 1997; 17:181–96.

Whitwam JG, Amrein R. Pharmacology of flumazenil. Acta Anaesthesiol Scand Suppl 1995;108:3–14.

Whitwam JG. Flumazenil and midazolam in anaesthesia. Acta Anaesthesiol Scand Suppl 1995;108:15–22.

FLUNITRAZEPAM

THERAPEUTICS

Brands • Rohypnol
see index for additional brand names

Generic? No

 Class
• Benzodiazepine (hypnotic)

Commonly Prescribed For
(bold for FDA approved)
• Short-term treatment of insomnia (severe, disabling)

 How The Drug Works
• Binds to benzodiazepine receptors at the GABA-A ligand-gated chloride channel complex
• Enhances the inhibitory effects of GABA
• Boosts chloride conductance through GABA-regulated channels
• Inhibitory actions in sleep centers may provide sedative hypnotic effects

How Long Until It Works
• Generally takes effect in less than an hour

If It Works
• Improves quality of sleep
• Effects on total wake-time and number of nighttime awakenings may be decreased over time

If It Doesn't Work
• If insomnia does not improve after 7–10 days, it may be a manifestation of a primary psychiatric or physical illness such as obstructive sleep apnea or restless leg syndrome, which requires independent evaluation
• Increase the dose
• Improve sleep hygiene
• Switch to another agent

 Best Augmenting Combos for Partial Response or Treatment-Resistance
• Generally, best to switch to another agent
• Trazodone
• Agents with antihistamine actions (e.g., diphenhydramine, tricyclic antidepressants)

Tests
• In patients with seizure disorders, concomitant medical illness, and/or those with multiple concomitant long-term medications, periodic liver tests and blood counts may be prudent

SIDE EFFECTS

How Drug Causes Side Effects
• Same mechanism for side effects as for therapeutic effects – namely due to excessive actions at benzodiazepine receptors
• Actions at benzodiazepine receptors that carry over to next day can cause daytime sedation, amnesia, and ataxia
• Long-term adaptations in benzodiazepine receptors may explain the development of dependence, tolerance, and withdrawal

Notable Side Effects
✳ Sedation, fatigue, depression
✳ Dizziness, ataxia, slurred speech, weakness
✳ Forgetfulness, confusion
✳ Hyper-excitability, nervousness
• Rare hallucinations, mania
• Rare hypotension
• Hypersalivation, dry mouth
• Rebound insomnia when withdrawing from long-term treatment

 Life Threatening or Dangerous Side Effects
• Respiratory depression, especially when taken with CNS depressants in overdose
• Rare hepatic dysfunction, renal dysfunction, blood dyscrasias

Weight Gain

unusual not unusual common problematic
• Reported but not expected

Sedation

unusual not unusual common problematic
• Many experience and/or can be significant in amount

What To Do About Side Effects

- Wait
- To avoid problems with memory, only take flunitrazepam if planning to have a full night's sleep
- Lower the dose
- Switch to a shorter-acting sedative hypnotic
- Switch to a non-benzodiazepine hypnotic
- Administer flumazenil if side effects are severe or life-threatening

Best Augmenting Agents for Side Effects

- Many side effects cannot be improved with an augmenting agent

DOSING AND USE

Usual Dosage Range

- 0.5–1 mg/day at bedtime

Dosage Forms

- Tablet 0.5 mg, 1 mg, 2 mg, 4 mg

How to Dose

- Initial 0.5–1 mg/day at bedtime; maximum generally 2 mg/day at bedtime

 Dosing Tips

- Use lowest possible effective dose and assess need for continued treatment regularly
- Flunitrazepam should generally not be prescribed in quantities greater than a 1-month supply
- Patients with lower body weights may require lower doses
- Risk of dependence may increase with dose and duration of treatment
- Use doses over 1 mg only in exceptional circumstances
- Patients who request or who require doses over 1 mg may be more likely to have present or past substance abuse
- Flunitrazepam is 10 times more potent than diazepam

Overdose

- Sedation, slurred speech, poor coordination, confusion, coma, respiratory depression

Long-Term Use

- Not generally intended for long-term use
- Use is not recommended to exceed 4 weeks

Habit Forming

- Some patients may develop dependence and/or tolerance; risk may be greater with higher doses
- History of drug addiction may increase risk of dependence
- Currently classified as Schedule III by the World Health Organization
- Currently classified as a Schedule IV drug in the U.S., but not legally available in the U.S.

How to Stop

- If taken for more than a few weeks, taper to reduce chances of withdrawal effects
- Patients with seizure history may seize upon sudden withdrawal
- Rebound insomnia may occur the first 1–2 nights after stopping
- For patients with severe problems discontinuing a benzodiazepine, dosing may need to be tapered over many months (i.e., reduce dose by 1% every 3 days by crushing tablet and suspending or dissolving in 100 ml of fruit juice and then disposing of 1 ml while drinking the rest; 3–7 days later, dispose of 2 ml, and so on). This is both a form of very slow biological tapering and a form of behavioral desensitization

Pharmacokinetics

- Elimination half-life 16–35 hours
- Half-life of active metabolite 23–33 hours

 Drug Interactions

- Increased depressive effects when taken with other CNS depressants
- Cisapride may hasten the absorption of flunitrazepam and thus cause a temporary increase in the sedative effects of flunitrazepam

 Other Warnings/ Precautions

- Insomnia may be a symptom of a primary disorder, rather than a primary disorder itself

- Some patients may exhibit abnormal thinking or behavioral changes similar to those caused by other CNS depressants (i.e., either depressant actions or disinhibiting actions)
- Some depressed patients may experience a worsening of suicidal ideation
- Use only with extreme caution in patients with impaired respiratory function or obstructive sleep apnea
- Flunitrazepam should only be administered at bedtime

Do Not Use
- If patient is pregnant
- If patient has severe chronic hypercapnia, myasthenia gravis, severe respiratory insufficiency, sleep apnea, or severe hepatic insufficiency
- In children
- If patient has narrow angle-closure glaucoma
- If there is a proven allergy to flunitrazepam or any benzodiazepine

SPECIAL POPULATIONS

Renal Impairment
- Drug should be used with caution

Hepatic Impairment
- Dose should be lowered
- Should not be used in patients with severe hepatic insufficiency, as it may precipitate encephalopathy

Cardiac Impairment
- Benzodiazepines have been used to treat insomnia associated with acute myocardial infarction

Elderly
- Initial starting dose 0.5 mg at bedtime; maximum generally 1 mg/day at bedtime
- Paradoxical reactions with restlessness and agitation are more likely to occur in the elderly

 Children and Adolescents
- Safety and efficacy have not been established

- Not recommended for use in children or adolescents
- Paradoxical reactions with restlessness and agitation are more likely to occur in children

 Pregnancy
- Positive evidence of risk to human fetus; contraindicated for use in pregnancy
- Infants whose mothers received a benzodiazepine late in pregnancy may experience withdrawal effects
- Neonatal flaccidity has been reported in infants whose mothers took a benzodiazepine during pregnancy

Breast Feeding
- Unknown if flunitrazepam is secreted in human breast milk, but all psychotropics assumed to be secreted in breast milk
* Recommended either to discontinue drug or bottle feed
- Effects on infant have been observed and include feeding difficulties, sedation, and weight loss

THE ART OF PSYCHOPHARMACOLOGY

Potential Advantages
- For severe, disabling insomnia unresponsive to other sedative hypnotics

Potential Disadvantages
- For those who need treatment for longer than a few weeks
- For those with current or past substance abuse

Primary Target Symptoms
- Time to sleep onset
- Total sleep time
- Nighttime awakenings

 Pearls
* Psychiatric symptoms and "paradoxical" reactions may be quite severe with flunitrazepam and may be more frequent than with other benzodiazepines
* "Paradoxical" reactions include symptoms such as restlessness, agitation, irritability, aggressiveness, delusions, rage,

nightmares, hallucinations, psychosis, inappropriate behavior, and other adverse behavioral effects
- Although legally available in Europe, Mexico, South America, and many other countries, it is not legally available in the U.S.
- Although currently classified as a Schedule IV drug, the U.S. drug enforcement agency is considering reclassifying it as Schedule I
- ✱ Has earned a reputation as a "date rape drug" in which sexual predators have allegedly slipped flunitrazepam into women's drinks to induce sexual relations
- ✱ Flunitrazepam, especially in combination with alcohol, is claimed to reduce the woman's judgment, inhibitions, or physical ability to resist sexual advances, as well as to reduce or eliminate her recall of the events
- ✱ Until 1999 was colorless, but a colorimetric compound is now added that turns the drug blue when added to a liquid, making it obvious that a drink was tampered with

- Illicit use since 1999 has fallen in part due to this additive
- Illicit use has also fallen in the U.S. due to the Drug-Induced Rape Prevention and Punishment act of 1996, making it punishable to commit a violent crime using a controlled substance such as flunitrazepam
- Street names for flunitrazepam, based in part upon its trade name of Rohypnol, manufacturer Roche, and the presence of RO-2 on the surface of the tablets, include "roofies", "ruffies", "roapies", "la roacha", "roach-2", "Mexican valium", "rope", "roache vitamins", and others
- If tolerance develops, it may result in increased anxiety during the day and/or increased wakefulness during the latter part of the night
- Best short-term use is for less than 10 consecutive days, and for less than half of the nights in a month
- Drug holidays may restore drug effectiveness if tolerance develops

Suggested Reading

Simmons MM, Cupp MJ. Use and abuse of flunitrazepam. Ann Pharmacother. 1998;32(1):117–9.

Woods JH, Winger G. Abuse liability of flunitrazepam. J Clin Psychopharmacol. 1997;17(3 Suppl 2):1S–57S.

FLUOXETINE

THERAPEUTICS

Brands • Prozac • Prozac weekly
 • Sarafem
see index for additional brand names

Generic? Yes

 Class
- SSRI (selective serotonin reuptake inhibitor); often classified as an antidepressant, but it is not just an antidepressant

Commonly Prescribed For
(bold for FDA approved)
- **Major depressive disorder**
- **Obsessive-compulsive disorder (OCD)**
- **Premenstrual dysphoric disorder (PMDD)**
- **Bulimia nervosa**
- **Panic disorder**
- **Bipolar depression [in combination with olanzapine (Symbyax)]**
- Social anxiety disorder (social phobia)
- Posttraumatic stress disorder (PTSD)

 How The Drug Works
- Boosts neurotransmitter serotonin
- Blocks serotonin reuptake pump (serotonin transporter)
- Desensitizes serotonin receptors, especially serotonin 1A receptors
- Presumably increases serotonergic neurotransmission
- ✱ Fluoxetine also has antagonist properties at 5HT2C receptors, which could increase norepinephrine and dopamine neurotransmission

How Long Until It Works
- ✱ Some patients may experience increased energy or activation early after initiation of treatment
- Onset of therapeutic actions usually not immediate, but often delayed 2 to 4 weeks
- If it is not working within 6 to 8 weeks, it may require a dosage increase or it may not work at all
- May continue to work for many years to prevent relapse of symptoms

If It Works
- The goal of treatment is complete remission of current symptoms as well as prevention of future relapses
- Treatment most often reduces or even eliminates symptoms, but not a cure since symptoms can recur after medicine stopped
- Continue treatment until all symptoms are gone (remission) or significantly reduced (e.g., OCD, PTSD)
- Once symptoms gone, continue treating for 1 year for the first episode of depression
- For second and subsequent episodes of depression, treatment may need to be indefinite
- For anxiety disorders and bulimia, treatment may also need to be indefinite

If It Doesn't Work
- Many patients only have a partial response where some symptoms are improved but others persist (especially insomnia, fatigue, and problems concentrating in depression)
- Other patients may be nonresponders, sometimes called treatment-resistant or treatment-refractory
- Some patients who have an initial response may relapse even though they continue treatment, sometimes called "poop-out"
- Consider increasing dose, switching to another agent or adding an appropriate augmenting agent
- Consider psychotherapy
- Consider evaluation for another diagnosis or for a comorbid condition (e.g., medical illness, substance abuse, etc.)
- Some patients may experience apparent lack of consistent efficacy due to activation of latent or underlying bipolar disorder, and require antidepressant discontinuation and a switch to a mood stabilizer

 Best Augmenting Combos for Partial Response or Treatment-Resistance
- Trazodone, especially for insomnia
- Bupropion, mirtazapine, reboxetine, or atomoxetine (add with caution and at lower doses since fluoxetine could theoretically raise atomoxetine levels); use combinations of antidepressants with caution as this may activate bipolar disorder and suicidal ideation

- Modafinil, especially for fatigue, sleepiness, and lack of concentration
- Mood stabilizers or atypical antipsychotics for bipolar depression, psychotic depression, treatment-resistant depression, or treatment-resistant anxiety disorders
* Fluoxetine has been specifically studied in combination with olanzapine (olanzapine-fluoxetine combination) with excellent results for bipolar depression, treatment-resistant unipolar depression, and psychotic depression
- Benzodiazepines
- If all else fails for anxiety disorders, consider gabapentin or tiagabine
- Hypnotics for insomnia
- Classically, lithium, buspirone, or thyroid hormone

Tests
- None for healthy individuals

SIDE EFFECTS

How Drug Causes Side Effects
- Theoretically due to increases in serotonin concentrations at serotonin receptors in parts of the brain and body other than those that cause therapeutic actions (e.g., unwanted actions of serotonin in sleep centers causing insomnia, unwanted actions of serotonin in the gut causing diarrhea, etc.)
- Increasing serotonin can cause diminished dopamine release and might contribute to emotional flattening, cognitive slowing, and apathy in some patients
- Most side effects are immediate but often go away with time, in contrast to most therapeutic effects which are delayed and are enhanced over time
* Fluoxetine's unique 5HT2C antagonist properties could contribute to agitation, anxiety, and undesirable activation, especially early in dosing

Notable Side Effects
- Sexual dysfunction (men: delayed ejaculation, erectile dysfunction; men and women: decreased sexual desire, anorgasmia)
- Gastrointestinal (decreased appetite, nausea, diarrhea, constipation, dry mouth)

- Mostly central nervous system (insomnia but also sedation, agitation, tremors, headache, dizziness)
- Note: patients with diagnosed or undiagnosed bipolar or psychotic disorders may be more vulnerable to CNS-activating actions of SSRIs
- Autonomic (sweating)
- Bruising and rare bleeding

 Life Threatening or Dangerous Side Effects
- Rare seizures
- Rare induction of mania and activation of suicidal ideation

Weight Gain

unusual   not unusual   common   problematic

- Reported but not expected
- Possible weight loss, especially short-term

Sedation

unusual   not unusual   common   problematic

- Reported but not expected

What To Do About Side Effects
- Wait
- Wait
- Wait
- If fluoxetine is activating, take in the morning to help reduce insomnia
- Reduce dose to 10 mg, and either stay at this dose if tolerated and effective, or consider increasing again to 20 mg or more if tolerated but not effective at 10 mg
- In a few weeks, switch or add other drugs

Best Augmenting Agents for Side Effects
- Often best to try another SSRI or another antidepressant monotherapy prior to resorting to augmentation strategies to treat side effects
- Trazodone or a hypnotic for insomnia
- Bupropion, sildenafil, vardenafil, or tadalafil for sexual dysfunction
- Bupropion for emotional flattening, cognitive slowing, or apathy
- Mirtazapine for insomnia, agitation, and gastrointestinal side effects

- Benzodiazepines for jitteriness and anxiety, especially at initiation of treatment and especially for anxious patients
- Many side effects are dose-dependent (i.e., they increase as dose increases, or they reemerge until tolerance re-develops)
- Many side effects are time-dependent (i.e., they start immediately upon dosing and upon each dose increase, but go away with time)
- Activation and agitation may represent the induction of a bipolar state, especially a mixed dysphoric bipolar II condition sometimes associated with suicidal ideation, and require the addition of lithium, a mood stabilizer or an atypical antipsychotic, and/or discontinuation of fluoxetine

DOSING AND USE

Usual Dosage Range
- 20–80 mg for depression and anxiety disorders
- 60–80 mg for bulimia

Dosage Forms
- Capsules 10 mg, 20 mg, 40 mg
- Tablet 10 mg
- Liquid 20 mg / 5 ml – 120 ml bottles
- Weekly capsule 90 mg

How to Dose
- Depression and OCD: Initial dose 20 mg/day in morning, usually wait a few weeks to assess drug effects before increasing dose; maximum dose generally 80 mg/day
- Bulimia: Initial dose 60 mg/day in morning; some patients may need to begin at lower dose and titrate over several days

 Dosing Tips
- The long half-lives of fluoxetine and its active metabolites mean that dose changes will not be fully reflected in plasma for several weeks, lengthening titration to final dose and extending withdrawal from treatment
- Give once daily, often in the mornings, but at any time of day tolerated

- Often available in capsules, not tablets, so unable to break capsules in half
- Occasional patients are dosed above 80 mg
- Liquid formulation easiest for doses below 10 mg when used for cases that are very intolerant to fluoxetine or for very slow up and down titration needs
- ✱ For some patients, weekly dosing with the weekly formulation may enhance compliance
- The more anxious and agitated the patient, the lower the starting dose, the slower the titration, and the more likely the need for a concomitant agent such as trazodone or a benzodiazepine
- If intolerable anxiety, insomnia, agitation, akathisia, or activation occur either upon dosing initiation or discontinuation, consider the possibility of activated bipolar disorder and switch to a mood stabilizer or an atypical antipsychotic

Overdose
- Rarely lethal in monotherapy overdose; respiratory depression especially with alcohol, ataxia, sedation, possible seizures

Long-Term Use
- Safe

Habit Forming
- No

How to Stop
- Taper rarely necessary since fluoxetine tapers itself after immediate discontinuation, due to the long half-life of fluoxetine and its active metabolites

Pharmacokinetics
- Active metabolite (norfluoxetine) has 2 week half-life
- Parent drug has 2–3 day half-life
- Inhibits CYP450 2D6
- Inhibits CYP450 3A4

 Drug Interactions
- Tramadol increases the risk of seizures in patients taking an antidepressant
- Can increase tricyclic antidepressant levels; use with caution with tricyclic antidepressants or when switching from a TCA to fluoxetine

- Can cause a fatal "serotonin syndrome" when combined with MAO inhibitors, so do not use with MAO inhibitors or for at least 14 days after MAOIs are stopped
- Do not start an MAO inhibitor for at least 5 weeks after discontinuing fluoxetine
- May displace highly protein bound drugs (e.g., warfarin)
- Can rarely cause weakness, hyperreflexia, and incoordination when combined with sumatriptan, or possibly with other triptans, requiring careful monitoring of patient
- Via CYP450 2D6 inhibition, could theoretically interfere with the analgesic actions of codeine, and increase the plasma levels of some beta blockers and of atomoxetine
- Via CYP450 2D6 inhibition, fluoxetine could theoretically increase concentrations of thioridazine and cause dangerous cardiac arrhythmias
- May reduce the clearance of diazepam or trazodone, thus increasing their levels
- Via CYP450 3A4 inhibition, may increase the levels of alprazolam, buspirone, and triazolam
- Via CYP450 3A4 inhibition, fluoxetine could theoretically increase concentrations of certain cholesterol lowering HMG CoA reductase inhibitors, especially simvastatin, atorvastatin, and lovastatin, but not pravastatin or fluvastatin, which would increase the risk of rhabdomyolysis; thus, coadministration of fluoxetine with certain HMG CoA reductase inhibitors should proceed with caution
- Via CYP450 3A4 inhibition, fluoxetine could theoretically increase the concentrations of pimozide, and cause QTc prolongation and dangerous cardiac arrhythmias

 Other Warnings/ Precautions

* Add or initiate other antidepressants with caution for up to 5 weeks after discontinuing fluoxetine
- Use with caution in patients with history of seizure
- Use with caution in patients with bipolar disorder unless treated with concomitant mood stabilizing agent

- Monitor patients for activation of suicidal ideation, especially children and adolescents

Do Not Use
- If patient is taking an MAO inhibitor
- If patient is taking thioridazine
- If patient is taking pimozide
- If there is a proven allergy to fluoxetine

Renal Impairment
- No dose adjustment
- Not removed by hemodialysis

Hepatic Impairment
- Lower dose or give less frequently, perhaps by half

Cardiac Impairment
- Preliminary research suggests that fluoxetine is safe in these patients
- Treating depression with SSRIs in patients with acute angina or following myocardial infarction may reduce cardiac events and improve survival as well as mood

Elderly
- Some patients may tolerate lower doses better

 Children and Adolescents
- Use with caution, observing for activation of known or unknown bipolar disorder and/or suicidal ideation, and strongly consider informing parents or guardian of this risk so they can help observe child or adolescent patients
- Approved for OCD and depression
- Adolescents often receive adult dose, but doses slightly lower for children
- Children taking fluoxetine may have slower growth; long-term effects are unknown

 Pregnancy
- Risk Category C [some animal studies show adverse effects, no controlled studies in humans]
- Not generally recommended for use during pregnancy, especially during first trimester

- Nonetheless, continuous treatment during pregnancy may be necessary and has not been proven to be harmful to the fetus
- Current patient registries of children whose mothers took fluoxetine during pregnancy do not show adverse consequences
- At delivery there may be more bleeding in the mother and transient irritability or sedation in the newborn
- Must weigh the risk of treatment (first trimester fetal development, third trimester newborn delivery) to the child against the risk of no treatment (recurrence of depression, maternal health, infant bonding) to the mother and child
- For many patients this may mean continuing treatment during pregnancy
- Neonates exposed to SSRIs or SNRIs late in the third trimester have developed complications requiring prolonged hospitalization, respiratory support, and tube feeding; reported symptoms are consistent with either a direct toxic effect of SSRIs and SNRIs or, possibly, a drug discontinuation syndrome, and include respiratory distress, cyanosis, apnea, seizures, temperature instability, feeding difficulty, vomiting, hypoglycemia, hypotonia, hypertonia, hyperreflexia, tremor, jitteriness, irritability, and constant crying

Breast Feeding

- Some drug is found in mother's breast milk
- Trace amounts may be present in nursing children whose mothers are on fluoxetine
- If child becomes irritable or sedated, breast feeding or drug may need to be discontinued
- Immediate postpartum period is a high-risk time for depression, especially in women who have had prior depressive episodes, so drug may need to be reinstituted late in the third trimester or shortly after childbirth to prevent a recurrence during the postpartum period
- Must weigh benefits of breast feeding with risks and benefits of antidepressant treatment versus non-treatment to both the infant and the mother
- For many patients this may mean continuing treatment during breast feeding

THE ART OF PSYCHOPHARMACOLOGY

Potential Advantages
- Patients with atypical depression (hypersomnia, increased appetite)
- Patients with fatigue and low energy
- Patients with comorbid eating and affective disorders
- Generic is less expensive than brand name where available
- Patients for whom weekly administration is desired
- Children with OCD or depression

Potential Disadvantages
- Patients with anorexia
- Initiating treatment in anxious, agitated patients
- Initiating treatment in severe insomnia

Primary Target Symptoms
- Depressed mood
- Energy, motivation, and interest
- Anxiety (eventually, but can actually increase anxiety, especially short-term)
- Sleep disturbance, both insomnia and hypersomnia (eventually, but may actually cause insomnia, especially short-term)

 Pearls

* May be a first-line choice for atypical depression (e.g., hypersomnia, hyperphagia, low energy, mood reactivity)
- Consider avoiding in agitated insomniacs
- Can cause cognitive and affective "flattening"
- Not as well tolerated as some other SSRIs for panic disorder and other anxiety disorders, especially when dosing is initiated, unless given with co-therapies such as benzodiazepines or trazodone
- Long half-life; even longer lasting active metabolite
* Actions at 5HT2C receptors may explain its activating properties
* Actions at 5HT2C receptors may explain in part fluoxetine's efficacy in combination with olanzapine for bipolar depression and treatment-resistant depression, since both agents have this property
- For sexual dysfunction, can augment with bupropion, sildenafil, vardenafil, or tadalafil, or switch to a non-SSRI such as bupropion or mirtazapine

- Mood disorders can be associated with eating disorders (especially in adolescent females) and be treated successfully with fluoxetine
- SSRIs may be less effective in women over 50, especially if they are not taking estrogen
- SSRIs may be useful for hot flushes in perimenopausal women
- Some postmenopausal women's depression will respond better to fluoxetine plus estrogen augmentation than to fluoxetine alone

- Nonresponse to fluoxetine in elderly may require consideration of mild cognitive impairment or Alzheimer disease
- SSRIs may not cause as many patients to attain remission of depression as some other classes of antidepressants (e.g., SNRIs)
- A single pill containing both fluoxetine and olanzapine is available for combination treatment of bipolar depression, psychotic depression, and treatment-resistant unipolar depression

 Suggested Reading

Anderson IM. Selective serotonin reuptake inhibitors versus tricyclic antidepressants: a meta-analysis of efficacy and tolerability. Journal of Affective Disorders. 2000;58:19–36.

Beasley CM Jr, Koke SC, Nilsson ME, Gonzales JS. Adverse events and treatment discontinuations in clinical trials of fluoxetine in major depressive disorder: an updated meta-analysis. Clinical Therapeutics. 2000;22:1319–1330.

Calil HM. Fluoxetine: a suitable long-term treatment. J Clin Psychiatry. 2001;62 (suppl 22):24–9.

Edwards JG, Anderson I. Systematic review and guide to selection of selective serotonin reuptake inhibitors. Drugs. 1999;57:507–533.

Wagstaff AJ, Goa KL. Once-weekly fluoxetine. Drugs. 2001;61:2221–8.

FLUPENTHIXOL

THERAPEUTICS

Brands • Depixol
see index for additional brand names

Generic? No

 Class
• Conventional antipsychotic (neuroleptic, thioxanthene, dopamine 2 antagonist)

Commonly Prescribed For
(bold for FDA approved)
• Schizophrenia
• Depression (low dose)
• Other psychotic disorders
• Bipolar disorder

 How The Drug Works
• Blocks dopamine 2 receptors, reducing positive symptoms of psychosis

How Long Until It Works
• With injection, psychotic symptoms can improve within a few days, but it may take 1–2 weeks for notable improvement
• With oral formulation, psychotic symptoms can improve within 1 week, but it may take several weeks for full effect on behavior

If It Works
• Most often reduces positive symptoms in schizophrenia but does not eliminate them
• Most schizophrenic patients do not have a total remission of symptoms but rather a reduction of symptoms by about a third
• Continue treatment in schizophrenia until reaching a plateau of improvement
• After reaching a satisfactory plateau, continue treatment for at least a year after first episode of psychosis in schizophrenia
• For second and subsequent episodes of psychosis in schizophrenia, treatment may need to be indefinite
• Reduces symptoms of acute psychotic mania but not proven as a mood stabilizer or as an effective maintenance treatment in bipolar disorder
• After reducing acute psychotic symptoms in mania, switch to a mood stabilizer and/or an atypical antipsychotic for mood stabilization and maintenance

If It Doesn't Work
• Consider trying one of the first-line atypical antipsychotics (risperidone, olanzapine, quetiapine, ziprasidone, aripiprazole, amisulpride)
• Consider trying another conventional antipsychotic
• If 2 or more antipsychotic monotherapies do not work, consider clozapine

 Best Augmenting Combos for Partial Response or Treatment-Resistance
• Augmentation of conventional antipsychotics has not been systematically studied
• Addition of a mood stabilizing anticonvulsant such as valproate, carbamazepine, or lamotrigine may be helpful in both schizophrenia and bipolar mania
• Augmentation with lithium in bipolar mania may be helpful
• Addition of a benzodiazepine, especially short-term for agitation

Tests
✱ Since conventional antipsychotics are frequently associated with weight gain, before starting treatment, weigh all patients and determine if the patient is already overweight (BMI 25.0–29.9) or obese (BMI ≥30)
• Before giving a drug that can cause weight gain to an overweight or obese patient, consider determining whether the patient already has pre-diabetes (fasting plasma glucose 100–125 mg/dl), diabetes (fasting plasma glucose >126 mg/dl), or dyslipidemia (increased total cholesterol, LDL cholesterol and triglycerides; decreased HDL cholesterol), and treat or refer such patients for treatment, including nutrition and weight management, physical activity counseling, smoking cessation, and medical management
✱ Monitor weight and BMI during treatment
✱ While giving a drug to a patient who has gained >5% of initial weight, consider evaluating for the presence of pre-diabetes, diabetes, or dyslipidemia, or consider switching to a different antipsychotic
• Monitoring elevated prolactin levels of dubious clinical benefit

SIDE EFFECTS

How Drug Causes Side Effects
- By blocking dopamine 2 receptors in the striatum, it can cause motor side effects
- By blocking dopamine 2 receptors in the pituitary, it can cause elevations in prolactin
- By blocking dopamine 2 receptors excessively in the mesocortical and mesolimbic dopamine pathways, especially at high doses, it can cause worsening of negative and cognitive symptoms (neuroleptic-induced deficit syndrome)
- Anticholinergic actions may cause sedation, blurred vision, constipation, dry mouth
- Antihistaminic actions may cause sedation, weight gain
- By blocking alpha 1 adrenergic receptors, it can cause dizziness, sedation, and hypotension
- Mechanism of weight gain and any possible increased incidence of diabetes or dyslipidemia with conventional antipsychotics is unknown

Notable Side Effects
- ✳ Neuroleptic-induced deficit syndrome
- ✳ Extrapyramidal symptoms (more common at start of treatment), Parkinsonism
- ✳ Insomnia, restlessness, agitation, sedation
- ✳ Tardive dyskinesia (risk increases with duration of treatment and with dose)
- ✳ Galactorrhea, amenorrhea
- Tachycardia
- Weight gain
- Hypomania
- Rare eosinophilia

Life Threatening or Dangerous Side Effects
- Rare neuroleptic malignant syndrome
- Rare seizures
- Rare jaundice, leucopenia

Weight Gain

- Many experience and/or can be significant in amount

Sedation

- Occurs in significant minority

What To Do About Side Effects
- Wait
- Wait
- Wait
- For motor symptoms, add an anticholinergic agent
- Reduce the dose
- For sedation, give at night
- Switch to an atypical antipsychotic
- Weight loss, exercise programs, and medical management for high BMIs, diabetes, dyslipidemia

Best Augmenting Agents for Side Effects
- Benztropine or trihexyphenidyl for motor side effects
- Sometimes amantadine can be helpful for motor side effects
- Benzodiazepines may be helpful for akathisia
- Many side effects cannot be improved with an augmenting agent

DOSING AND USE

Usual Dosage Range
- Oral 3–6 mg/day in divided doses
- Intramuscular 40–120 mg every 1–4 weeks

Dosage Forms
- Tablet 0.5 mg, 3 mg
- Injection 20 mg/mL, 100 mg/mL

How to Dose
- Oral: initial 1 mg 3 times a day; increase by 1 mg every 2–3 days; maximum generally 18 mg/day
- Intramuscular: initial dose 20 mg for patients who have not been exposed to long-acting depot antipsychotics, 40 mg for patients who have previously demonstrated tolerance to long-acting depot antipsychotics; after 4–10 days can give additional 20 mg dose; maximum 200 mg every 1–4 weeks

Dosing Tips

- The peak of action for the decanoate is usually 7–10 days, and doses generally have to be administered every 2–3 weeks
- May have more activating effects at low doses, which can sometimes be useful as a second-line, short-term treatment of depression
- Some evidence that flupenthixol may improve anxiety and depression at low doses

Overdose

- Agitation, confusion, sedation, extrapyramidal symptoms, respiratory collapse, circulatory collapse

Long-Term Use

- Safe

Habit Forming

- No

How to Stop

- Slow down-titration of oral formulation (over 6 to 8 weeks), especially when simultaneously beginning a new antipsychotic while switching (i.e., cross-titration)
- Rapid oral discontinuation may lead to rebound psychosis and worsening of symptoms
- If antiparkinson agents are being used, they should be continued for a few weeks after flupenthixol is discontinued

Pharmacokinetics

- Oral: maximum plasma concentrations within 3 to 8 hours
- Intramuscular: rate-limiting half-life approximately 8 days with single dose, approximately 17 days with multiple doses

Drug Interactions

- May decrease the effects of levodopa, dopamine agonists
- May increase the effects of antihypertensive drugs except for guanethidine, whose antihypertensive actions flupenthixol may antagonize
- CNS effects may be increased if used with other CNS depressants

- Combined use with epinephrine may lower blood pressure
- Ritonavir may increase plasma levels of flupenthixol
- May increase carbamazepine plasma levels
- Some patients taking a neuroleptic and lithium have developed an encephalopathic syndrome similar to neuroleptic malignant syndrome

Other Warnings/ Precautions

- If signs of neuroleptic malignant syndrome develop, treatment should be immediately discontinued
- Use cautiously in patients with alcohol withdrawal or convulsive disorders because of possible lowering of seizure threshold
- In epileptic patients, dose 10–20 mg every 15 days for intramuscular formulation
- Use with caution if at all in patients with Parkinson's disease, severe arteriosclerosis, or Lewy Body dementia
- Possible antiemetic effect of flupenthixol may mask signs of other disorders or overdose; suppression of cough reflex may cause asphyxia
- Avoid extreme heat exposure
- Do not use epinephrine in event of overdose as interaction with some pressor agents may lower blood pressure

Do Not Use

- If patient is taking a large concomitant dose of a sedative hypnotic
- If patient has CNS depression
- If patient is comatose or if there is brain damage
- If there is blood dyscrasia
- In patient has phaeochromocytoma
- If patient has liver damage
- If patient has a severe cardiovascular disorder
- If patient has renal insufficiency
- If patient has cerebrovascular insufficiency
- If there is a proven allergy to flupenthixol

Renal Impairment

- Oral: recommended to take half or less of usual adult dose

• Intramuscular: recommended dose schedule generally 10–20 mg every 15 days

Hepatic Impairment

• Use with caution
• Oral: recommended to take half or less of usual adult dose

Cardiac Impairment

• Use with caution
• Oral: recommended to take half or less of usual adult dose

Elderly

• Intramuscular: recommended initial dose generally 5 mg; recommended dose schedule generally 10–20 mg every 15 days
• Oral: recommended to take half or less of usual adult dose

Children and Adolescents

• Not recommended for use in children

Pregnancy

• Not recommended for use during pregnancy
• Reports of extrapyramidal symptoms, jaundice, hyperreflexia, hyporeflexia in infants whose mothers took a conventional antipsychotic during pregnancy
• Psychotic symptoms may worsen during pregnancy and some form of treatment may be necessary
• Atypical antipsychotics may be preferable to conventional antipsychotics or anticonvulsant mood stabilizers if treatment is required during pregnancy

Breast Feeding

• Some drug is found in mother's breast milk
✳ Recommended either to discontinue drug or bottle feed

THE ART OF PSYCHOPHARMACOLOGY

Potential Advantages
• Non-compliant patients

Potential Disadvantages
• Children
• Elderly
• Patients with tardive dyskinesia

Primary Target Symptoms
• Positive symptoms of psychosis
• Negative symptoms of psychosis
• Aggressive symptoms

Pearls
• May activate manic patients
• Less sedation and orthostatic hypotension but more extrapyramidal symptoms than some other conventional antipsychotics
• Patients have very similar antipsychotic responses to any conventional antipsychotic, which is different from atypical antipsychotics where antipsychotic responses of individual patients can occasionally vary greatly from one atypical antipsychotic to another
• Patients with inadequate responses to atypical antipsychotics may benefit from a trial of augmentation with a conventional antipsychotic such as flupenthixol or from switching to a conventional antipsychotic such as flupenthixol
• However, long-term polypharmacy with a combination of a conventional antipsychotic such as flupenthixol with an atypical antipsychotic may combine their side effects without clearly augmenting the efficacy of either
• Although a frequent practice by some prescribers, adding 2 conventional antipsychotics together has little rationale and may reduce tolerability without clearly enhancing efficacy

Suggested Reading

Gerlach J. Depot neuroleptics in relapse prevention: advantages and disadvantages. Int Clin Psychopharmacol 1995; 9 Suppl 5: 17–20.

Quraishi S, David A. Depot flupenthixol decanoate for schizophrenia or other similar psychotic disorders. Cochrane Database Syst Rev 2000; (2): CD001470.

Soyka M, De Vry J. Flupenthixol as a potential pharmacotreatment of alcohol and cocaine abuse/dependence. Eur Neuropsychopharmacol 2000; 10 (5): 325–32.

FLUPHENAZINE

Brands • Prolixin
see index for additional brand names

Generic? Yes

 Class

• Conventional antipsychotic (neuroleptic, phenothiazine, dopamine 2 antagonist)

Commonly Prescribed For
(bold for FDA approved)
• **Psychotic disorders**
• Bipolar disorder

 How The Drug Works

• Blocks dopamine 2 receptors, reducing positive symptoms of psychosis

How Long Until It Works

• Psychotic symptoms can improve within 1 week, but it may take several weeks for full effect on behavior

If It Works

• Most often reduces positive symptoms in schizophrenia but does not eliminate them
• Most schizophrenic patients do not have a total remission of symptoms but rather a reduction of symptoms by about a third
• Continue treatment in schizophrenia until reaching a plateau of improvement
• After reaching a satisfactory plateau, continue treatment for at least a year after first episode of psychosis in schizophrenia
• For second and subsequent episodes of psychosis in schizophrenia, treatment may need to be indefinite
• Reduces symptoms of acute psychotic mania but not proven as a mood stabilizer or as an effective maintenance treatment in bipolar disorder
• After reducing acute psychotic symptoms in mania, switch to a mood stabilizer and/or an atypical antipsychotic for mood stabilization and maintenance

If It Doesn't Work

• Consider trying one of the first-line atypical antipsychotics (risperidone, olanzapine, quetiapine, ziprasidone, aripiprazole, amisulpride)

• Consider trying another conventional antipsychotic
• If 2 or more antipsychotic monotherapies do not work, consider clozapine

 Best Augmenting Combos for Partial Response or Treatment-Resistance

• Augmentation of conventional antipsychotics has not been systematically studied
• Addition of a mood stabilizing anticonvulsant such as valproate, carbamazepine, or lamotrigine may be helpful in both schizophrenia and bipolar mania
• Augmentation with lithium in bipolar mania may be helpful
• Addition of a benzodiazepine, especially short-term for agitation

Tests

✳ Since conventional antipsychotics are frequently associated with weight gain, before starting treatment, weigh all patients and determine if the patient is already overweight (BMI 25.0–29.9) or obese (BMI ≥30)
• Before giving a drug that can cause weight gain to an overweight or obese patient, consider determining whether the patient already has pre-diabetes (fasting plasma glucose 100–125 mg/dl), diabetes (fasting plasma glucose >126 mg/dl), or dyslipidemia (increased total cholesterol, LDL cholesterol and triglycerides; decreased HDL cholesterol), and treat or refer such patients for treatment, including nutrition and weight management, physical activity counseling, smoking cessation, and medical management
✳ Monitor weight and BMI during treatment
✳ While giving a drug to a patient who has gained >5% of initial weight, consider evaluating for the presence of pre-diabetes, diabetes, or dyslipidemia, or consider switching to a different antipsychotic
• Should check blood pressure in the elderly before starting and for the first few weeks of treatment
• Monitoring elevated prolactin levels of dubious clinical benefit
• Phenothiazines may cause false-positive phenylketonuria results

SIDE EFFECTS

How Drug Causes Side Effects
- By blocking dopamine 2 receptors in the striatum, it can cause motor side effects
- By blocking dopamine 2 receptors in the pituitary, it can cause elevations in prolactin
- By blocking dopamine 2 receptors excessively in the mesocortical and mesolimbic dopamine pathways, especially at high doses, it can cause worsening of negative and cognitive symptoms (neuroleptic-induced deficit syndrome)
- Anticholinergic actions may cause sedation, blurred vision, constipation, dry mouth
- Antihistaminic actions may cause sedation, weight gain
- By blocking alpha 1 adrenergic receptors, it can cause dizziness, sedation, and hypotension
- Mechanism of weight gain and any possible increased incidence of diabetes or dyslipidemia with conventional antipsychotics is unknown

Notable Side Effects
- ✳ Neuroleptic-induced deficit syndrome
- ✳ Akathisia
- ✳ Priapism
- ✳ Extrapyramidal symptoms, Parkinsonism, tardive dyskinesia, tardive dystonia
- ✳ Galactorrhea, amenorrhea
- Dizziness, sedation
- Dry mouth, constipation, urinary retention, blurred vision
- Decreased sweating, depression
- Sexual dysfunction
- Hypotension, tachycardia, syncope
- Weight gain

Life Threatening or Dangerous Side Effects
- Rare neuroleptic malignant syndrome
- Rare jaundice, agranulocytosis
- Rare seizures

Weight Gain

unusual   not unusual   common   problematic

- Occurs in significant minority

Sedation

unusual   not unusual   common   problematic

- Occurs in significant minority

What To Do About Side Effects
- Wait
- Wait
- Wait
- For motor symptoms, add an anticholinergic agent
- Reduce the dose
- For sedation, take at night
- Switch to an atypical antipsychotic
- Weight loss, exercise programs, and medical management for high BMIs, diabetes, dyslipidemia

Best Augmenting Agents for Side Effects
- Benztropine or trihexyphenidyl for motor side effects
- Sometimes amantadine can be helpful for motor side effects
- Benzodiazepines may be helpful for akathisia
- Many side effects cannot be improved with an augmenting agent

DOSING AND USE

Usual Dosage Range
- Oral: 1–20 mg/day maintenance
- Intramuscular: generally 1/3 to 1/2 the oral dose
- Decanoate for intramuscular or subcutaneous administration: 12.5 mg/0.5 mL – 50 mg/2 mL

Dosage Forms
- Tablet 1 mg, 2.5 mg scored, 5 mg scored, 10 mg scored
- Decanoate for long-acting intramuscular or subcutaneous administration 25 mg/mL
- Injection for acute intramuscular administration 2.5 mg/mL
- Elixir 2.5 mg/5 mL
- Concentrate 5 mg/mL

How to Dose
- Oral: initial 0.5–10 mg/day in divided doses; maximum 40 mg/day
- Intramuscular (short-acting): initial 1.25 mg; 2.5–10 mg/day can be given in divided doses every 6–8 hours; maximum dose generally 10 mg/day

• Decanoate (long-acting): initial 12.5–25 mg (0.5 to 1 mL); subsequent doses and intervals determined in accordance with the patient's response; generally no more than 50 mg/2 mL given at intervals not longer than 4 weeks

Dosing Tips

• Patients receiving atypical antipsychotics may occasionally require a "top up" of a conventional antipsychotic to control aggression or violent behavior
• Fluphenazine tablets 2.5 mg, 5 mg, and 10 mg contain tartrazine, which can cause allergic reactions, especially in patients sensitive to aspirin
• Oral solution should not be mixed with drinks containing caffeine, tannic acid (tea), or pectinates (apple juice)
• 12.5 mg/0.5 mL of the long-acting decanoate may be comparable to 10 mg of oral fluphenazine
• Onset of action of decanoate at 24–72 hours after injection with significant antipsychotic actions within 48–96 hours

Overdose

• Extrapyramidal symptoms, coma, hypotension, sedation, seizures, respiratory depression

Long-Term Use

• Some side effects may be irreversible (e.g., tardive dyskinesia)

Habit Forming

• No

How to Stop

• Slow down-titration of oral formulation (over 6 to 8 weeks), especially when simultaneously beginning a new antipsychotic while switching (i.e., cross-titration)
• Rapid oral discontinuation may lead to rebound psychosis and worsening of symptoms
• If antiparkinson agents are being used, they should be continued for a few weeks after fluphenazine is discontinued

Pharmacokinetics

• Mean half-life of oral formulation approximately 15 hours

• Mean half-life of intramuscular formulation approximately 6.8–9.6 days

Drug Interactions

• May decrease the effects of levodopa, dopamine agonists
• May increase the effects of antihypertensive drugs except for guanethidine, whose antihypertensive actions fluphenazine may antagonize
• Additive effects may occur if used with CNS depressants
• Additive anticholinergic effects may occur if used with atropine or related compounds
• Alcohol and diuretics may increase the risk of hypotension
• Some patients taking a neuroleptic and lithium have developed an encephalopathic syndrome similar to neuroleptic malignant syndrome
• Combined use with epinephrine may lower blood pressure

⚠ Other Warnings/ Precautions

• If signs of neuroleptic malignant syndrome develop, treatment should be immediately discontinued
• Use cautiously in patients with alcohol withdrawal or convulsive disorders because of possible lowering of seizure threshold
• Avoid undue exposure to sunlight
• Use cautiously in patients with respiratory disorders
• Avoid extreme heat exposure
• Antiemetic effect can mask signs of other disorders or overdose
• Do not use epinephrine in event of overdose as interaction with some pressor agents may lower blood pressure
• Use only with caution if at all in Parkinson's disease or Lewy Body dementia

Do Not Use

• If patient is in a comatose state or has CNS depression
• If patient is taking cabergoline, pergolide, or metrizamide
• If there is a proven allergy to fluphenazine
• If there is a known sensitivity to any phenothiazine

FLUPHENAZINE (continued)

Renal Impairment
• Use with caution; titration should be slower

Hepatic Impairment
• Use with caution; titration should be slower

Cardiac Impairment
• Cardiovascular toxicity can occur, especially orthostatic hypotension

Elderly
• Titration should be slower; lower initial dose (1–2.5 mg/day)
• Elderly patients may be more susceptible to adverse effects

 Children and Adolescents
• Safety and efficacy not established
• Decanoate and enanthate injectable formulations are contraindicated under age 12
• Generally consider second-line after atypical antipsychotics

 Pregnancy
• Risk Category C [some animal studies show adverse effects, no controlled studies in humans]
• Reports of extrapyramidal symptoms, jaundice, hyperreflexia, hyporeflexia in infants whose mothers took a phenothiazine during pregnancy
• Fluphenazine should only be used during pregnancy if clearly indicated
• Psychotic symptoms may worsen during pregnancy and some form of treatment may be necessary
• Atypical antipsychotics may be preferable to conventional antipsychotics or anticonvulsant mood stabilizers if treatment is required during pregnancy

Breast Feeding
• Some drug is found in mother's breast milk
• Effects on infant have been observed (dystonia, tardive dyskinesia, sedation)
✱ Recommended either to discontinue drug or bottle feed

Potential Advantages
• Intramuscular formulation for emergency use

Potential Disadvantages
• Patients with tardive dyskinesia
• Children
• Elderly

Primary Target Symptoms
• Positive symptoms of psychosis
• Motor and autonomic hyperactivity
• Violent or aggressive behavior

 Pearls
• Fluphenazine is a high potency phenothiazine
• Less risk of sedation and orthostatic hypotension but greater risk of extrapyramidal symptoms than with low potency phenothiazines
• Conventional antipsychotics are much less expensive than atypical antipsychotics
• Not shown to be effective for behavioral problems in mental retardation
• Patients have very similar antipsychotic responses to any conventional antipsychotic, which is different from atypical antipsychotics where antipsychotic responses of individual patients can occasionally vary greatly from one atypical antipsychotic to another
• Patients with inadequate responses to atypical antipsychotics may benefit from a trial of augmentation with a conventional antipsychotic such as fluphenazine or from switching to a conventional antipsychotic such as fluphenazine
• However, long-term polypharmacy with a combination of a conventional antipsychotic such as fluphenazine with an atypical antipsychotic may combine their side effects without clearly augmenting the efficacy of either
• Although a frequent practice by some prescribers, adding 2 conventional antipsychotics together has little rationale and may reduce tolerability without clearly enhancing efficacy

Suggested Reading

Adams CE, Eisenbruch M. Depot fluphenazine for schizophrenia. Cochrane Database Syst Rev 2000; (2): CD000307.

King DJ. Drug treatment of the negative symptoms of schizophrenia. Eur Neuropsychopharmacol 1998; 8 (1): 33–42.

Milton GV, Jann MW. Emergency treatment of psychotic symptoms. Pharmacokinetic considerations for antipsychotic drugs. Clin Pharmacokinet 1995; 28 (6): 494–504.

FLURAZEPAM

THERAPEUTICS

Brands • Dalmane
see index for additional brand names

Generic? Yes

Class
• Benzodiazepine (hypnotic)

Commonly Prescribed For
(bold for FDA approved)
• **Insomnia characterized by difficulty in falling asleep, frequent nocturnal awakenings, and/or early morning awakening**
• **Recurring insomnia or poor sleeping habits**
• **Acute or chronic medical situations requiring restful sleep**

 How The Drug Works
• Binds to benzodiazepine receptors at the GABA-A ligand-gated chloride channel complex
• Enhances the inhibitory effects of GABA
• Boosts chloride conductance through GABA-regulated channels
• Inhibitory actions in sleep centers may provide sedative hypnotic effects

How Long Until It Works
• Generally takes effect in less than an hour

If It Works
• Improves quality of sleep
• Effects on total wake-time and number of nighttime awakenings may be decreased over time

If It Doesn't Work
• If insomnia does not improve after 7–10 days, it may be a manifestation of a primary psychiatric or physical illness such as obstructive sleep apnea or restless leg syndrome, which requires independent evaluation
• Increase the dose
• Improve sleep hygiene
• Switch to another agent

 Best Augmenting Combos for Partial Response or Treatment-Resistance
• Generally, best to switch to another agent
• Trazodone
• Agents with antihistamine actions (e.g., diphenhydramine, tricyclic antidepressants)

Tests
• In patients with seizure disorders, concomitant medical illness, and/or those with multiple concomitant long-term medications, periodic liver tests and blood counts may be prudent

SIDE EFFECTS

How Drug Causes Side Effects
• Same mechanism for side effects as for therapeutic effects – namely due to excessive actions at benzodiazepine receptors
• Actions at benzodiazepine receptors that carry over to the next day can cause daytime sedation, amnesia, and ataxia
• Long-term adaptations in benzodiazepine receptors may explain the development of dependence, tolerance, and withdrawal

Notable Side Effects
✳ Sedation, fatigue, depression
✳ Dizziness, ataxia, slurred speech, weakness
✳ Forgetfulness, confusion
✳ Hyper-excitability, nervousness
• Rare hallucinations, mania
• Rare hypotension
• Hypersalivation, dry mouth
• Rebound insomnia when withdrawing from long-term treatment

 Life Threatening or Dangerous Side Effects
• Respiratory depression, especially when taken with CNS depressants in overdose
• Rare hepatic dysfunction, renal dysfunction, blood dyscrasias

Weight Gain

 unusual not unusual  common   problematic
• Reported but not expected

Sedation

unusual   not unusual   **common**   problematic

- Many experience and/or can be significant in amount

What To Do About Side Effects

- Wait
- To avoid problems with memory, only take flurazepam if planning to have a full night's sleep
- Lower the dose
- Switch to a shorter-acting sedative hypnotic
- Switch to a non-benzodiazepine hypnotic
- Administer flumazenil if side effects are severe or life-threatening

Best Augmenting Agents for Side Effects

- Many side effects cannot be improved with an augmenting agent

DOSING AND USE

Usual Dosage Range

- 15–30 mg/day at bedtime for 7–10 days

Dosage Forms

- Capsule 15 mg, 30 mg

How to Dose

- 15 mg/day at bedtime; may increase to 30 mg/day at bedtime if ineffective

 Dosing Tips

✱ Because flurazepam tends to accumulate over time, perhaps not the best hypnotic for chronic nightly use
- Use lowest possible effective dose and assess need for continued treatment regularly
- Flurazepam should generally not be prescribed in quantities greater than a 1-month supply
- Patients with lower body weights may require lower doses
- Risk of dependence may increase with dose and duration of treatment

Overdose

- No death reported in monotherapy; sedation, slurred speech, poor coordination, confusion, coma, respiratory depression

Long-Term Use

- Not generally intended for long-term use
✱ Because of its relatively longer half-life, flurazepam may cause some daytime sedation and/or impaired motor/cognitive function, and may do so progressively over time

Habit Forming

- Flurazepam is a Schedule IV drug
- Some patients may develop dependence and/or tolerance; risk may be greater with higher doses
- History of drug addiction may increase risk of dependence

How to Stop

- If taken for more than a few weeks, taper to reduce chances of withdrawal effects
- Patients with seizure history may seize upon sudden withdrawal
- Rebound insomnia may occur the first 1–2 nights after stopping
- For patients with severe problems discontinuing a benzodiazepine, dosing may need to be tapered over many months (i.e., reduce dose by 1% every 3 days by crushing tablet and suspending or dissolving in 100 ml of fruit juice and then disposing of 1 ml while drinking the rest; 3–7 days later, dispose of 2 ml, and so on). This is both a form of very slow biological tapering and a form of behavioral desensitization

Pharmacokinetics

- Elimination half-life approximately 24–100 hours
- Active metabolites

 Drug Interactions

- Cimetidine may decrease flurazepam clearance and thus raise flurazepam levels
- Flurazepam and kava combined use may affect clearance of either drug
- Increased depressive effects when taken with other CNS depressants

Other Warnings/ Precautions

- Insomnia may be a symptom of a primary disorder, rather than a primary disorder itself
- Some patients may exhibit abnormal thinking or behavioral changes similar to those caused by other CNS depressants (i.e., either depressant actions or disinhibiting actions)
- Some depressed patients may experience a worsening of suicidal ideation
- Use only with extreme caution in patients with impaired respiratory function or obstructive sleep apnea
- Flurazepam should only be administered at bedtime

Do Not Use

- If patient is pregnant
- If patient has narrow angle-closure glaucoma
- If there is a proven allergy to flurazepam or any benzodiazepine

Renal Impairment

- Recommended dose: 15 mg/day

Hepatic Impairment

- Recommended dose: 15 mg/day

Cardiac Impairment

- Benzodiazepines have been used to treat insomnia associated with acute myocardial infarction

Elderly

- Recommended dose: 15 mg/day

 Children and Adolescents

- Safety and efficacy have not been established
- Long-term effects of flurazepam in children/adolescents are unknown
- Should generally receive lower doses and be more closely monitored

 Pregnancy

- Risk Category X [positive evidence of risk to human fetus; contraindicated for use in pregnancy]
- Infants whose mothers received a benzodiazepine late in pregnancy may experience withdrawal effects
- Neonatal flaccidity has been reported in infants whose mothers took a benzodiazepine during pregnancy

Breast Feeding

- Unknown if flurazepam is secreted in human breast milk, but all psychotropics assumed to be secreted in breast milk
- ✳ Recommended either to discontinue drug or bottle feed
- Effects on infant have been observed and include feeding difficulties, sedation, and weight loss

Potential Advantages

- Transient insomnia

Potential Disadvantages

- Chronic nightly insomnia

Primary Target Symptoms

- Time to sleep onset
- Total sleep time
- Nighttime awakenings

 Pearls

- ✳ Flurazepam has a longer half-life than some other sedative hypnotics, so it may be less likely to cause rebound insomnia on discontinuation
- Flurazepam may not be as effective on the first night as it is on subsequent nights
- Was once one of the most widely used hypnotics
- ✳ Long-term accumulation of flurazepam and its active metabolites may cause insidious onset of confusion or falls, especially in the elderly

Suggested Reading

Greenblatt DJ. Pharmacology of benzodiazepine hypnotics. J Clin Psychiatry 1992;53 (Suppl):7–13.

Hilbert JM, Battista D. Quazepam and flurazepam: differential pharmacokinetic and pharmacodynamic characteristics. J Clin Psychiatry 1991;52(Suppl):21–6.

Johnson LC, Chernik DA, Sateia MJ. Sleep, performance, and plasma levels in chronic insomniacs during 14-day use of flurazepam and midazolam: an introduction. J Clin Psychopharmacol 1990;10(4 Suppl):5S–9S.

Roth T, Roehrs TA. A review of the safety profiles of benzodiazepine hypnotics. J Clin Psychiatry 1991;52(Suppl):38–41.

FLUVOXAMINE

THERAPEUTICS

Brands • Luvox
see index for additional brand names

Generic? Yes

Class
- SSRI (selective serotonin reuptake inhibitor); often classified as an antidepressant, but it is not just an antidepressant

Commonly Prescribed For
(bold for FDA approved)
- **Obsessive-compulsive disorder (OCD)**
- Depression
- Panic disorder
- Generalized anxiety disorder (GAD)
- Social anxiety disorder (social phobia)
- Posttraumatic stress disorder (PTSD)

How The Drug Works
- Boosts neurotransmitter serotonin
- Blocks serotonin reuptake pump (serotonin transporter)
- Desensitizes serotonin receptors, especially serotonin 1A receptors
- Presumably increases serotonergic neurotransmission
- ✱ Fluvoxamine also has antagonist properties at sigma 1 receptors

How Long Until It Works
- ✱ Some patients may experience relief of insomnia or anxiety early after initiation of treatment
- Onset of therapeutic actions usually not immediate, but often delayed 2 to 4 weeks
- If it is not working within 6 to 8 weeks, it may require a dosage increase or it may not work at all
- May continue to work for many years to prevent relapse of symptoms

If It Works
- The goal of treatment is complete remission of current symptoms as well as prevention of future relapses
- Treatment most often reduces or even eliminates symptoms, but not a cure since symptoms can recur after medicine stopped
- Continue treatment until all symptoms are gone (remission) or significantly reduced (e.g., OCD)
- Once symptoms gone, continue treating for 1 year for the first episode of depression
- For second and subsequent episodes of depression, treatment may need to be indefinite
- Use in anxiety disorders may also need to be indefinite

If It Doesn't Work
- Many patients only have a partial response where some symptoms are improved but others persist (especially insomnia, fatigue, and problems concentrating in depression)
- Other patients may be nonresponders, sometimes called treatment-resistant or treatment-refractory
- Some patients who have an initial response may relapse even though they continue treatment, sometimes called "poop-out"
- Consider increasing dose, switching to another agent or adding an appropriate augmenting agent
- Consider psychotherapy
- Consider evaluation for another diagnosis or for a comorbid condition (e.g., medical illness, substance abuse, etc.)
- Some patients may experience apparent lack of consistent efficacy due to activation of latent or underlying bipolar disorder, and require antidepressant discontinuation and a switch to a mood stabilizer

Best Augmenting Combos for Partial Response or Treatment-Resistance

- For the expert, consider cautious addition of clomipramine for treatment-resistant OCD
- Trazodone, especially for insomnia
- Bupropion, mirtazapine, reboxetine, or atomoxetine (use combinations of antidepressants with caution as this may activate bipolar disorder and suicidal ideation)
- Modafinil, especially for fatigue, sleepiness, and lack of concentration
- Mood stabilizers or atypical antipsychotics for bipolar depression, psychotic depression, treatment-resistant depression, or treatment-resistant anxiety disorders
- Benzodiazepines

- If all else fails for anxiety disorders, consider gabapentin or tiagabine
- Hypnotics for insomnia
- Classically, lithium, buspirone, or thyroid hormone
- In Europe and Japan, augmentation is more commonly administered for the treatment of depression and anxiety disorders, especially with benzodiazepines and lithium
- In the US, augmentation is more commonly administered for the treatment of OCD, especially with atypical antipsychotics, buspirone, or even clomipramine; clomipramine should be added with caution and at low doses as fluvoxamine can alter clomipramine metabolism and raise its levels

Tests
- None for healthy individuals

SIDE EFFECTS

How Drug Causes Side Effects
- Theoretically due to increases in serotonin concentrations at serotonin receptors in parts of the brain and body other than those that cause therapeutic actions (e.g., unwanted actions of serotonin in sleep centers causing insomnia, unwanted actions of serotonin in the gut causing diarrhea, etc.)
- Increasing serotonin can cause diminished dopamine release and might contribute to emotional flattening, cognitive slowing, and apathy in some patients
- Most side effects are immediate but often go away with time, in contrast to most therapeutic effects which are delayed and are enhanced over time
- ✳ Fluvoxamine's sigma 1 antagonist properties may contribute to sedation and fatigue in some patients

Notable Side Effects
- Sexual dysfunction (men: delayed ejaculation, erectile dysfunction; men and women: decreased sexual desire, anorgasmia)
- Gastrointestinal (decreased appetite, nausea, diarrhea, constipation, dry mouth)

- Mostly central nervous system (insomnia but also sedation, agitation, tremors, headache, dizziness)
- Note: patients with diagnosed or undiagnosed bipolar or psychotic disorders may be more vulnerable to CNS-activating actions of SSRIs
- Autonomic (sweating)
- Bruising and rare bleeding
- Rare hyponatremia

 Life Threatening or Dangerous Side Effects
- Rare seizures
- Rare induction of mania and activation of suicidal ideation

Weight Gain

unusual   not unusual   common   problematic
- Reported but not expected
- Patients may actually experience weight loss

Sedation

unusual   not unusual   common   problematic
- Many experience and/or can be significant in amount

What To Do About Side Effects
- Wait
- Wait
- Wait
- If fluvoxamine is sedating, take at night to reduce drowsiness
- Reduce dose
- In a few weeks, switch or add other drugs

Best Augmenting Agents for Side Effects
- Often best to try another SSRI or another antidepressant monotherapy prior to resorting to augmentation strategies to treat side effects
- Trazodone or a hypnotic for insomnia
- Bupropion, sildenafil, vardenafil, or tadalafil for sexual dysfunction
- Bupropion for emotional flattening, cognitive slowing, or apathy
- Mirtazapine for insomnia, agitation, and gastrointestinal side effects

- Benzodiazepines for jitteriness and anxiety, especially at initiation of treatment and especially for anxious patients
- Many side effects are dose-dependent (i.e., they increase as dose increases, or they reemerge until tolerance re-develops)
- Many side effects are time-dependent (i.e., they start immediately upon dosing and upon each dose increase, but go away with time)
- Activation and agitation may represent the induction of a bipolar state, especially a mixed dysphoric bipolar II condition sometimes associated with suicidal ideation, and require the addition of lithium, a mood stabilizer or an atypical antipsychotic, and/or discontinuation of fluvoxamine

DOSING AND USE

Usual Dosage Range
- 100–300 mg/day for OCD
- 100–200 mg/day for depression

Dosage Forms
- Tablets 25 mg, 50 mg scored, 100 mg scored

How to Dose
- Initial 50 mg/day; increase by 50 mg/day in 4–7 days; usually wait a few weeks to assess drug effects before increasing dose further, but can increase by 50 mg/day every 4–7 days until desired efficacy is reached; maximum 300 mg/day
- Doses below 100 mg/day usually given as a single dose at bedtime; doses above 100 mg/day can be divided into two doses to enhance tolerability, with the larger dose administered at night, but can also be given as a single dose at bedtime

 Dosing Tips
- 50 mg and 100 mg tablets are scored, so to save costs, give 25 mg as half of 50 mg tablet, and give 50 mg as half of 100 mg tablet
- To improve tolerability, dosing can either be given once a day, usually all at night, or split either symmetrically or

asymmetrically, usually with more of the dose given at night
- Some patients take more than 300 mg/day
- If intolerable anxiety, insomnia, agitation, akathisia, or activation occur either upon dosing initiation or discontinuation, consider the possibility of activated bipolar disorder and switch to a mood stabilizer or an atypical antipsychotic

Overdose
- Rare fatalities have been reported, both in combination with other drugs and alone; sedation, dizziness, vomiting, diarrhea, irregular heartbeat, seizures, coma, breathing difficulty

Long-Term Use
- Safe

Habit Forming
- No

How to Stop
- Taper to avoid withdrawal effects (dizziness, nausea, stomach cramps, sweating, tingling, dysesthesias)
- Many patients tolerate 50% dose reduction for 3 days, then another 50% reduction for 3 days, then discontinuation
- If withdrawal symptoms emerge during discontinuation, raise dose to stop symptoms and then restart withdrawal much more slowly

Pharmacokinetics
- Parent drug has 9–28 hour half-life
- Inhibits CYP450 3A4
- Inhibits CYP450 1A2
- Inhibits CYP450 2C9/2C19

 Drug Interactions
- Tramadol increases the risk of seizures in patients taking an antidepressant
- Can increase tricyclic antidepressant levels; use with caution with tricyclic antidepressants
- Can cause a fatal "serotonin syndrome" when combined with MAO inhibitors, so do not use with MAO inhibitors or for at least 14 days after MAOIs are stopped
- Do not start an MAO inhibitor for at least 2 weeks after discontinuing fluvoxamine

- May displace highly protein bound drugs (e.g., warfarin)
- Can rarely cause weakness, hyperreflexia, and incoordination when combined with sumatriptan or possibly with other triptans, requiring careful monitoring of patient
- Via CYP450 1A2 inhibition, fluvoxamine may reduce clearance of theophylline and clozapine, thus raising their levels and requiring their dosing to be lowered
- Fluvoxamine administered with either caffeine or theophylline can thus cause jitteriness, excessive stimulation, or rarely seizures, so concomitant use should proceed cautiously
- Metabolism of fluvoxamine may be enhanced in smokers and thus its levels lowered, requiring higher dosing
- Via CYP450 3A4 inhibition, fluvoxamine may reduce clearance of carbamazepine and benzodiazepines such as alprazolam and triazolam, and thus require dosage reduction
- Via CYP450 3A4 inhibition, fluvoxamine could theoretically increase concentrations of certain cholesterol lowering HMG CoA reductase inhibitors, especially simvastatin, atorvastatin, and lovastatin, but not pravastatin or fluvastatin, which would increase the risk of rhabdomyolysis; thus, coadministration of fluvoxamine with certain HMG CoA reductase inhibitors should proceed with caution
- Via CYP450 3A4 inhibition, fluvoxamine could theoretically increase the concentrations of pimozide, and cause QTc prolongation and dangerous cardiac arrhythmias

⚠ Other Warnings/ Precautions

- Add or initiate other antidepressants with caution for up to two weeks after discontinuing fluvoxamine
- Use with caution in patients with history of seizure
- Use with caution in patients with bipolar disorder unless treated with concomitant mood stabilizing agent
- May cause photosensitivity
- Monitor patients for activation of suicidal ideation, especially children and adolescents

Do Not Use

- If patient is taking an MAO inhibitor
- If patient is taking thioridazine or pimozide
- If there is a proven allergy to fluvoxamine

SPECIAL POPULATIONS

Renal Impairment

- No dose adjustment

Hepatic Impairment

- Lower dose or give less frequently, perhaps by half; use slower titration

Cardiac Impairment

- Preliminary research suggests that fluvoxamine is safe in these patients
- Treating depression with SSRIs in patients with acute angina or following myocardial infarction may reduce cardiac events and improve survival as well as mood

Elderly

- May require lower initial dose and slower titration

Children and Adolescents

- Approved for ages 8–17 for OCD
- 8–17: initial 25 mg/day at bedtime; increase by 25 mg/day every 4–7 days; maximum 200 mg/day; doses above 50 mg/day should be divided into 2 doses with the larger dose administered at bedtime
- Preliminary evidence suggests efficacy for other anxiety disorders and depression in children and adolescents
- Use with caution, observing for activation of known or unknown bipolar disorder and/or suicidal ideation, and strongly consider informing parents or guardian of this risk so they can help observe child or adolescent patients

Pregnancy

- Risk Category C [some animal studies show adverse effects, no controlled studies in humans]
- Not generally recommended for use during pregnancy, especially during first trimester

- Nonetheless, continuous treatment during pregnancy may be necessary and has not been proven to be harmful to the fetus
- At delivery there may be more bleeding in the mother and transient irritability or sedation in the newborn
- Must weigh the risk of treatment (first trimester fetal development, third trimester newborn delivery) to the child against the risk of no treatment (recurrence of depression, maternal health, infant bonding) to the mother and child
- For many patients this may mean continuing treatment during pregnancy
- Neonates exposed to SSRIs or SNRIs late in the third trimester have developed complications requiring prolonged hospitalization, respiratory support, and tube feeding; reported symptoms are consistent with either a direct toxic effect of SSRIs and SNRIs or, possibly, a drug discontinuation syndrome, and include respiratory distress, cyanosis, apnea, seizures, temperature instability, feeding difficulty, vomiting, hypoglycemia, hypotonia, hypertonia, hyperreflexia, tremor, jitteriness, irritability, and constant crying

Breast Feeding

- Some drug is found in mother's breast milk
- Trace amounts may be present in nursing children whose mothers are on fluvoxamine
- If child becomes irritable or sedated, breast feeding or drug may need to be discontinued
- Immediate postpartum period is a high-risk time for depression, especially in women who have had prior depressive episodes, so drug may need to be reinstituted late in the third trimester or shortly after childbirth to prevent a recurrence during the postpartum period
- Must weigh benefits of breast feeding with risks and benefits of antidepressant treatment versus non-treatment to both the infant and the mother
- For many patients this may mean continuing treatment during breast feeding

THE ART OF PSYCHOPHARMACOLOGY

Potential Advantages
- Patients with mixed anxiety/depression
- Generic is less expensive than brand name where available

Potential Disadvantages
- Patients with irritable bowel or multiple gastrointestinal complaints
- Can require dose titration and twice daily dosing

Primary Target Symptoms
- Depressed mood
- Anxiety

 Pearls

✳ Often a preferred treatment of anxious depression as well as major depressive disorder comorbid with anxiety disorders
- Some withdrawal effects, especially gastrointestinal effects
- May have lower incidence of sexual dysfunction than other SSRIs
- Preliminary research suggests that fluvoxamine is efficacious in obsessive-compulsive symptoms in schizophrenia when combined with antipsychotics
- Not FDA approved for depression, but used widely for depression in many countries
- SSRIs may be less effective in women over 50, especially if they are not taking estrogen
- SSRIs may be useful for hot flushes in perimenopausal women

✳ Actions at sigma 1 receptors may explain in part fluvoxamine's sometimes rapid onset effects in anxiety disorders and insomnia

✳ Actions at sigma 1 receptors may explain potential advantages of fluvoxamine for psychotic depression and delusional depression

✳ For treatment-resistant OCD, consider cautious combination of fluvoxamine and clomipramine by an expert
- Normally, clomipramine (CMI), a potent serotonin reuptake blocker, at steady state is metabolized extensively to its active metabolite desmethyl-clomipramine (de-CMI), a potent noradrenergic reuptake blocker

- Thus, at steady state, plasma drug activity is generally more noradrenergic (with higher de-CMI levels) than serotonergic (with lower parent CMI levels)
- Addition of a CYP450 1A2 inhibitor, fluvoxamine, blocks this conversion and results in higher CMI levels than de-CMI levels
- Thus, addition of the SSRI fluvoxamine to CMI in treatment-resistant OCD can

powerfully enhance serotonergic activity, not only due to the inherent serotonergic activity of fluvoxamine, but also due to a favorable pharmacokinetic interaction inhibiting CYP450 1A2 and thus converting CMI's metabolism to a more powerful serotonergic portfolio of parent drug

Suggested Reading

Cheer SM, Figgitt DP. Spotlight on fluvoxamine in anxiety disorders in children and adolescents. CNS Drugs. 2002;16:139–44.

Edwards JG, Anderson I. Systematic review and guide to selection of selective serotonin reuptake inhibitors. Drugs. 1999;57:507–533.

Figgitt DP, McClellan KJ. Fluvoxamine. An updated review of its use in the management of adults with anxiety disorders. Drugs. 2000;60:925–954.

Pigott TA, Seay SM. A review of the efficacy of selective serotonin reuptake inhibitors in obsessive-compulsive disorder. Journal of Clinical Psychiatry. 1999;60:101–106.

Wares MR. Fluvoxamine: a review of the controlled trials in depression. Journal of Clinical Psychiatry. 1997;58(suppl 5):15–23.

GABAPENTIN

THERAPEUTICS

Brands • Neurontin
see index for additional brand names

Generic? Not in U.S. or Europe

Class

• Anticonvulsant, antineuralgic for chronic pain, alpha 2 delta ligand at voltage-sensitive calcium channels

Commonly Prescribed For
(bold for FDA approved)

• **Partial seizures with or without secondary generalization (adjunctive)**
• **Postherpetic neuralgia**
• Neuropathic pain/chronic pain
• Anxiety (adjunctive)
• Bipolar disorder (adjunctive)

How The Drug Works

• Is a leucine analogue and is transported both into the blood from the gut and also across the blood-brain barrier into the brain from the blood by the system L transport system
✳ Binds to the alpha 2 delta subunit of voltage-sensitive calcium channels
• This closes N and P/Q presynaptic calcium channels, diminishing excessive neuronal activity and neurotransmitter release
• Although structurally related to gamma-aminobutyric acid (GABA), no known direct actions on GABA or its receptors

How Long Until It Works

• Should reduce seizures by 2 weeks
• Should also reduce pain in postherpetic neuralgia by 2 weeks; some patients respond earlier
• May reduce pain in other neuropathic pain syndromes within a few weeks
• If it is not reducing pain within 6–8 weeks, it may require a dosage increase or it may not work at all
• May reduce anxiety in a variety of disorders within a few weeks
• Not yet clear if it has mood stabilizing effects in bipolar disorder or antineuralgic actions in chronic neuropathic pain, but some patients may respond and if so, would be expected to show clinical effects

starting by 2 weeks although it may take several weeks to months to optimize

If It Works

• The goal of treatment is complete remission of symptoms (e.g., seizures)
• The goal of treatment of chronic neuropathic pain is to reduce symptoms as much as possible, especially in combination with other treatments
• Treatment of chronic neuropathic pain most often reduces but does not eliminate symptoms and is not a cure since symptoms usually recur after medicine stopped
• Continue treatment until all symptoms are gone or until improvement is stable and then continue treating indefinitely as long as improvement persists

If It Doesn't Work (for neuropathic pain or bipolar disorder)

✳ May only be effective in a subset of bipolar patients, in some patients who fail to respond to other mood stabilizers, or it may not work at all
• Many patients only have a partial response where some symptoms are improved but others persist or continue to wax and wane without stabilization of pain or mood
• Other patients may be nonresponders, sometimes called treatment-resistant or treatment-refractory
• Consider increasing dose, switching to another agent or adding an appropriate augmenting agent
• Consider biofeedback or hypnosis for pain
• Consider the presence of noncompliance and counsel patient
• Switch to another agent with fewer side effects
• Consider evaluation for another diagnosis or for a comorbid condition (e.g., medical illness, substance abuse, etc.)

Best Augmenting Combos for Partial Response or Treatment-Resistance

✳ Gabapentin is itself an augmenting agent to numerous other anticonvulsants in treating epilepsy; and to lithium, atypical antipsychotics and other anticonvulsants in the treatment of bipolar disorder
• For postherpetic neuralgia, gabapentin can decrease concomitant opiate use

✳ For neuropathic pain, gabapentin can augment tricyclic antidepressants and SNRIs as well as tiagabine, other anticonvulsants and even opiates if done by experts while carefully monitoring in difficult cases
• For anxiety, gabapentin is a second-line treatment to augment SSRIs, SNRIs, or benzodiazepines

Tests
• None for healthy individuals
• False positive readings with the Ames N-Multistix SG® dipstick test for urinary protein have been reported when gabapentin was administered with other anticonvulsants

SIDE EFFECTS

How Drug Causes Side Effects
• CNS side effects may be due to excessive blockade of voltage-sensitive calcium channels

Notable Side Effects
✳ Sedation, dizziness, ataxia, fatigue, nystagmus, tremor
• Vomiting, dyspepsia, diarrhea, dry mouth, constipation, weight gain
• Blurred vision
• Peripheral edema
• Additional effects in children under age 12: hostility, emotional lability, hyperkinesia, thought disorder, weight gain

 Life Threatening or Dangerous Side Effects
• Sudden unexplained deaths have occurred in epilepsy (unknown if related to gabapentin use)

Weight Gain

unusual — **not unusual** — common — problematic
• Occurs in significant minority

Sedation

unusual — not unusual — **common** — problematic
• Many experience and/or can be significant in amount

• Dose-related; can be problematic at high doses
• Can wear off with time, but may not wear off at high doses

What To Do About Side Effects
• Wait
• Wait
• Wait
• Take more of the dose at night to reduce daytime sedation
• Lower the dose
• Switch to another agent

Best Augmenting Agents for Side Effects
• Many side effects cannot be improved with an augmenting agent

DOSING AND USE

Usual Dosage Range
• 900–1800 mg/day in 3 divided doses

Dosage Forms
• Capsule 100 mg, 300 mg, 400 mg
• Tablet 600 mg, 800 mg
• Liquid 250 mg/5 mL – 470 mL bottle

How to Dose
• Postherpetic neuralgia: 300 mg on day 1; on day 2 increase to 600 mg in 2 doses; on day 3 increase to 900 mg in 3 doses; maximum dose generally 1800 mg/day in 3 doses
• Seizures (ages 12 and older): Initial 900 mg/day in 3 doses; recommended dose generally 1800 mg/day in 3 doses; maximum dose generally 3600 mg/day; time between any 2 doses should usually not exceed 12 hours
• Seizures (under age 13): see Children and Adolescents

 Dosing Tips
• Gabapentin should not be taken until 2 hours after administration of an antacid
• If gabapentin is added to a second anticonvulsant, the titration period should be at least a week to improve tolerance to sedation

- Some patients need to take gabapentin only twice daily in order to experience adequate symptomatic relief for pain or anxiety
- At the high end of the dosing range, tolerability may be enhanced by splitting dose into more than 3 divided doses
- For intolerable sedation, can give most of the dose at night and less during the day
- To improve slow-wave sleep, may only need to take gabapentin at bedtime

Overdose
- No fatalities; slurred speech, sedation, double vision, diarrhea

Long-Term Use
- Safe

Habit Forming
- No

How to Stop
- Taper over a minimum of 1 week
- Epilepsy patients may seize upon withdrawal, especially if withdrawal is abrupt
- ✳ Rapid discontinuation may increase the risk of relapse in bipolar disorder
- Discontinuation symptoms uncommon

Pharmacokinetics
- Gabapentin is not metabolized but excreted intact renally
- Not protein bound
- Elimination half-life approximately 5–7 hours

 Drug Interactions
- Antacids may <u>reduce</u> the bioavailability of gabapentin, so gabapentin should be administered approximately 2 hours before antacid medication
- Naproxen may <u>increase</u> absorption of gabapentin
- Morphine and hydrocodone may <u>increase</u> plasma AUC (area under the curve) values of gabapentin and thus gabapentin plasma levels over time

 Other Warnings/ Precautions
- Depressive effects may be increased by other CNS depressants (alcohol, MAOIs, other anticonvulsants, etc.)
- Dizziness and sedation could increase the chances of accidental injury (falls) in the elderly
- Pancreatic acinar adenocarcinomas have developed in male rats that were given gabapentin, but clinical significance is unknown
- Development of new tumors or worsening of tumors has occurred in humans taking gabapentin; it is unknown whether gabapentin affected the development or worsening of tumors

Do Not Use
- If there is a proven allergy to gabapentin or pregabalin

Renal Impairment
- Gabapentin is renally excreted, so the dose may need to be lowered
- Dosing can be adjusted according to creatinine clearance, such that patients with clearance below 16 mL/min should receive 100–300 mg/day in 1 dose, patients with clearance between 16–29 mL/min should receive 200–700 mg/day in 1 dose, and patients with clearance between 30–59 mL/min should receive 400–1400 mg/day in 2 doses
- Can be removed by hemodialysis; patients receiving hemodialysis may require supplemental doses of gabapentin
- Use in renal impairment has not been studied in children under age 12

Hepatic Impairment
- No available data but not metabolized by the liver and clinical experience suggests normal dosing

Cardiac Impairment
- No specific recommendations

Elderly
- Some patients may tolerate lower doses better

Children and Adolescents

- Approved for use starting at age 3 as adjunct treatment for partial seizures
- Ages 5–12: initial 10–15 mg/kg/day in 3 doses; titrate over 3 days to 25–35 mg/kg/day given in 3 doses; maximum dose generally 50 mg/kg/day; time between any 2 doses should usually not exceed 12 hours
- Ages 3–4: initial 10–15 mg/kg/day in 3 doses; titrate over 3 days to 40 mg/kg/day; maximum dose generally 50 mg/kg/day; time between any 2 doses should usually not exceed 12 hours

Pregnancy

- Risk category C [some animal studies show adverse effects, no controlled studies in humans]
- Use in women of childbearing potential requires weighing potential benefits to the mother against the risks to the fetus
- Taper drug if discontinuing
- Seizures, even mild seizures, may cause harm to the embryo/fetus
- ✻ Lack of convincing efficacy for treatment of bipolar disorder or psychosis suggests risk/benefit ratio is in favor of discontinuing gabapentin during pregnancy for these indications
- ✻ For bipolar patients, gabapentin should generally be discontinued before anticipated pregnancies
- ✻ For bipolar patients, given the risk of relapse in the postpartum period, mood stabilizer treatment, especially with agents with better evidence of efficacy than gabapentin, should generally be restarted immediately after delivery if patient is unmedicated during pregnancy
- ✻ Atypical antipsychotics may be preferable to gabapentin if treatment of bipolar disorder is required during pregnancy
- Bipolar symptoms may recur or worsen during pregnancy and some form of treatment may be necessary

Breast Feeding

- Some drug is found in mother's breast milk

- ✻ Recommended either to discontinue drug or bottle feed
- If drug is continued while breast feeding, infant should be monitored for possible adverse effects
- If infant becomes irritable or sedated, breast feeding or drug may need to be discontinued
- ✻ Bipolar disorder may recur during the postpartum period, particularly if there is a history of prior postpartum episodes of either depression or psychosis
- ✻ Relapse rates may be lower in women who receive prophylactic treatment for postpartum episodes of bipolar disorder
- Atypical antipsychotics and anticonvulsants such as valproate may be safer and more effective than gabapentin during the postpartum period when treating a nursing mother with bipolar disorder

THE ART OF PSYCHOPHARMACOLOGY

Potential Advantages
- Chronic neuropathic pain
- Has relatively mild side effect profile
- Has few pharmacokinetic drug interactions
- Treatment-resistant bipolar disorder

Potential Disadvantages
- Usually requires 3 times a day dosing
- Poor documentation of efficacy for many off-label uses, especially bipolar disorder

Primary Target Symptoms
- Seizures
- Pain
- Anxiety

Pearls
- Gabapentin is generally well-tolerated, with only mild adverse effects
- Well-studied in epilepsy and postherpetic neuralgia
- ✻ Most use is off-label
- ✻ Off-label use for first-line treatment of neuropathic pain may be justified
- ✻ Off-label use for second-line treatment of anxiety may be justified
- ✻ Off-label use as an adjunct for bipolar disorder may not be justified

- Elderly patients may be more susceptible to adverse effects

✳ Misperceptions about gabapentin's efficacy in bipolar disorder have led to its use in more patients than other agents with proven efficacy, such as lamotrigine

✳ Off-label use as an adjunct for schizophrenia may not be justified

• May be useful for some patients in alcohol withdrawal

✳ One of the few agents that enhances slow-wave delta sleep, which may be helpful in chronic neuropathic pain syndromes

✳ May be a useful adjunct for fibromyalgia

• Drug absorption and clinical efficacy may not necessarily be proportionately increased at high doses, and thus response to high doses may not be consistent

Suggested Reading

Backonja NM. Use of anticonvulsants for treatment of neuropathic pain. Neurology 2002;59(Suppl 2):S14–7.

MacDonald KJ, Young LT. Newer antiepileptic drugs in bipolar disorder. CNS Drugs 2002;16:549–62.

Marson AG, Kadir ZA, Hutton JL, Chadwick DW. Gabapentin for drug-resistant partial epilepsy. Cochrane Database Syst Rev. 2000;(2):CD001415.

Rose MA, Kam PC. Gabapentin: pharmacology and its use in pain management. Anaesthesia. 2002;57:451–62.

Stahl SM. Anticonvulsants and the relief of chronic pain: pregabalin and gabapentin as alpha(2)delta ligands at voltage-gated calcium channels. J Clin Psychiatry. 2004;65:596–7.

Stahl SM. Anticonvulsants as anxiolytics, part 2: Pregabalin and gabapentin as alpha(2)delta ligands at voltage-gated calcium channels. J Clin Psychiatry. 2004;65:460–1.

GALANTAMINE

THERAPEUTICS

Brands • Reminyl
see index for additional brand names

Generic? No

Class
• Cholinesterase inhibitor
(acetylcholinesterase inhibitor); also an
allosteric nicotinic cholinergic modulator;
cognitive enhancer

Commonly Prescribed For
(bold for FDA approved)
• **Alzheimer disease**
• Memory disturbances in other dementias
• Memory disturbances in other conditions
• Mild cognitive impairment

How The Drug Works
❋ Reversibly and competitively inhibits
centrally-active acetylcholinesterase
(AChE), making more acetylcholine
available
• Increased availability of acetylcholine
compensates in part for degenerating
cholinergic neurons in neocortex that
regulate memory
❋ Modulates nicotinic receptors, which
enhances actions of acetylcholine
• Nicotinic modulation may also enhance the
actions of other neurotransmitters by
increasing the release of dopamine,
norepinephrine, serotonin, GABA, and
glutamate
• Does not inhibit butyrylcholinesterase
• May release growth factors or interfere
with amyloid deposition

How Long Until It Works
• May take up to 6 weeks before any
improvement in baseline memory or
behavior is evident
• May take months before any stabilization in
degenerative course is evident

If It Works
• May improve symptoms and slow
progression of disease, but does not
reverse the degenerative process

If It Doesn't Work
• Consider adjusting dose, switching to a
different cholinesterase inhibitor or adding
an appropriate augmenting agent
• Reconsider diagnosis and rule out other
conditions such as depression or a
dementia other than Alzheimer disease

Best Augmenting Combos for Partial Response or Treatment-Resistance
❋ Atypical antipsychotics to reduce
behavioral disturbances
❋ Antidepressants if concomitant
depression, apathy, or lack of interest
❋ Memantine for moderate to severe
Alzheimer disease
• Divalproex, carbamazepine, or
oxcarbazepine for behavioral disturbances
• Not rational to combine with another
cholinesterase inhibitor

Tests
• None for healthy individuals

SIDE EFFECTS

How Drug Causes Side Effects
• Peripheral inhibition of acetylcholinesterase
can cause gastrointestinal side effects
• Central inhibition of acetylcholinesterase
may contribute to nausea, vomiting, weight
loss, and sleep disturbances

Notable Side Effects
❋ Nausea, diarrhea, vomiting, appetite loss,
increased gastric acid secretion, weight
loss
• Headache, dizziness
• Fatigue, depression

Life Threatening or Dangerous Side Effects
• Rare seizures
• Rare syncope

Weight Gain

unusual / not unusual / common / problematic

• Reported but not expected
• Some patients may experience weight loss

Sedation

unusual   not unusual   common   problematic

• Reported but not expected

What To Do About Side Effects
• Wait
• Wait
• Wait
• Use slower dose titration
• Consider lowering dose, switching to a different agent or adding an appropriate augmenting agent

Best Augmenting Agents for Side Effects
• Many side effects cannot be improved with an augmenting agent

DOSING AND USE

Usual Dosage Range
• 16–24 mg/day

Dosage Forms
• Tablet 4 mg, 8 mg, 12 mg
• Liquid 4 mg/mL – 100 mL bottle

How to Dose
• Initial 8 mg twice daily; after 4 weeks may increase dose to 16 mg twice daily; maximum dose generally 32 mg/day

 Dosing Tips
• Gastrointestinal side effects may be reduced if drug is administered with food
• Gastrointestinal side effects may also be reduced if dose is titrated slowly
• Probably best to utilize highest tolerated dose within the usual dosing range
✱ When switching to another cholinesterase inhibitor, probably best to cross-titrate from one to the other to prevent precipitous decline in function if the patient washes out of one drug entirely

Overdose
• Can be lethal; nausea, vomiting, excess salivation, sweating, hypotension, bradycardia, collapse, convulsions, muscle weakness (weakness of respiratory muscles can lead to death)

Long-Term Use
• Drug may lose effectiveness in slowing degenerative course of Alzheimer disease after 6 months
• Can be effective in some patients for several years

Habit Forming
• No

How to Stop
• Taper not necessary
• Discontinuation may lead to notable deterioration in memory and behavior, which may not be restored when drug is restarted or another cholinesterase inhibitor is initiated

Pharmacokinetics
• Terminal elimination half-life approximately 7 hours
• Metabolized by CYP450 2D6 and 3A4

 Drug Interactions
• Galantamine may increase the effects of anesthetics and should be discontinued prior to surgery
• Inhibitors of CYP450 2D6 and CYP450 3A4 may inhibit galantamine metabolism and raise galantamine plasma levels
• Galantamine may interact with anticholinergic agents and the combination may decrease the efficacy of both
• Cimetidine may increase bioavailability of galantamine
• May have synergistic effect if administered with cholinomimetics (e.g., bethanechol)
• Bradycardia may occur if combined with beta blockers
• Theoretically, could reduce the efficacy of levodopa in Parkinson's disease
• Not rational to combine with another cholinesterase inhibitor

 Other Warnings/ Precautions
• May exacerbate asthma or other pulmonary disease
• Increased gastric acid secretion may increase the risk of ulcers
• Bradycardia or heart block may occur in patients with or without cardiac impairment

Do Not Use
• If there is a proven allergy to galantamine

Renal Impairment
• Should be used with caution
• Not recommended for use in patients with severe renal impairment

Hepatic Impairment
• Should be used with caution
• Reduction of clearance may increase with the degree of hepatic impairment
• Not recommended for use in patients with severe hepatic impairment

Cardiac Impairment
• Should be used with caution
• Syncopal episodes have been reported with the use of galantamine

Elderly
• Clearance is reduced in elderly patients

 Children and Adolescents
• Safety and efficacy have not been established

 Pregnancy
• Risk Category B [animal studies do not show adverse effects, no controlled studies in humans]
✱ Not recommended for use in pregnant women or in women of childbearing potential

Breast Feeding
• Unknown if galantamine is secreted in human breast milk, but all psychotropics assumed to be secreted in breast milk
✱ Recommended either to discontinue drug or bottle feed
• Galantamine is not recommended for use in nursing women

Potential Advantages
• Alzheimer disease with cerebrovascular disease
• Theoretically, nicotinic modulation may provide added therapeutic benefits for memory and behavior in some Alzheimer patients
• Theoretically, nicotinic modulation may also provide efficacy for cognitive disorders other than Alzheimer disease

Potential Disadvantages
• Patients who have difficulty taking a medication twice daily

Primary Target Symptoms
• Memory loss in Alzheimer disease
• Behavioral symptoms in Alzheimer disease
• Memory loss in other dementias

 Pearls
• Dramatic reversal of symptoms of Alzheimer disease is not generally seen with cholinesterase inhibitors
• Can lead to therapeutic nihilism among prescribers and lack of an appropriate trial of a cholinesterase inhibitor
✱ Perhaps only 50% of Alzheimer patients are diagnosed, and only 50% of those diagnosed are treated, and only 50% of those treated are given a cholinesterase inhibitor, and then only for 200 days in a disease that lasts 7–10 years
• Must evaluate lack of efficacy and loss of efficacy over months, not weeks
✱ Treats behavioral and psychological symptoms of Alzheimer dementia as well as cognitive symptoms (i.e., especially apathy, disinhibition, delusions, anxiety, cooperation, pacing)
• Patients who complain themselves of memory problems may have depression, whereas patients whose spouses or children complain of the patient's memory problems may have Alzheimer disease
• Treat the patient but ask the caregiver about efficacy
• What you see may depend upon how early you treat
• The first symptoms of Alzheimer disease are generally mood changes; thus,

Alzheimer disease may initially be diagnosed as depression

- Women may experience cognitive symptoms in perimenopause as a result of hormonal changes that are not a sign of dementia or Alzheimer disease
- Aggressively treat concomitant symptoms with augmentation (e.g., atypical antipsychotics for agitation, antidepressants for depression)
- If treatment with antidepressants fails to improve apathy and depressed mood in the elderly, it is possible that this represents early Alzheimer disease and a cholinesterase inhibitor like galantamine may be helpful
- What to expect from a cholinesterase inhibitor:
  - Patients do not generally improve dramatically although this can be observed in a significant minority of patients
  - Onset of behavioral problems and nursing home placement can be delayed
  - Functional outcomes, including activities of daily living, can be preserved
  - Caregiver burden and stress can be reduced
- Delay in progression in Alzheimer disease is not evidence of disease-modifying actions of cholinesterase inhibition
- Cholinesterase inhibitors like galantamine depend upon the presence of intact targets for acetylcholine for maximum effectiveness and thus may be most effective in the early stages of Alzheimer disease
- The most prominent side effects of galantamine are gastrointestinal effects, which are usually mild and transient
- For patients with intolerable side effects, generally allow a washout period with resolution of side effects prior to switching to another cholinesterase inhibitor
- Weight loss can be a problem in Alzheimer patients with debilitation and muscle wasting
- Women over 85, particularly with low body weights, may experience more adverse effects
- Use with caution in underweight or frail patients
- Cognitive improvement may be linked to substantial (>65%) inhibition of acetylcholinesterase
- ✳ Galantamine is a natural product present in daffodils and snowdrops

- ✳ Novel dual action uniquely combines acetylcholinesterase inhibition with allosteric nicotine modulation
- ✳ Novel dual action should theoretically enhance cholinergic actions but incremental clinical benefits have been difficult to demonstrate
- ✳ Actions at nicotinic receptors enhance not only the release of acetylcholine but also that of other neurotransmitters, which may boost attention and improve behaviors caused by deficiencies in those neurotransmitters in Alzheimer disease
- Some Alzheimer patients who fail to respond to another cholinesterase inhibitor may respond when switched to galantamine
- Some Alzheimer patients who fail to respond to galantamine may respond to another cholinesterase inhibitor
- To prevent potential clinical deterioration, generally switch from long-term treatment with one cholinesterase inhibitor to another without a washout period
- ✳ Galantamine may slow the progression of mild cognitive impairment to Alzheimer disease
- ✳ May be useful for dementia with Lewy bodies (DLB, constituted by early loss of attentiveness and visual perception with possible hallucinations, Parkinson-like movement problems, fluctuating cognition such as daytime drowsiness and lethargy, staring into space for long periods, episodes of disorganized speech)
- May decrease delusions, apathy, agitation, and hallucinations in dementia with Lewy bodies
- ✳ May be useful for vascular dementia (e.g., acute onset with slow stepwise progression that has plateaus, often with gait abnormalities, focal signs, imbalance, and urinary incontinence)
- May be helpful for dementia in Down's Syndrome
- Suggestions of utility in some cases of treatment-resistant bipolar disorder
- Theoretically, may be useful for ADHD, but not yet proven
- Theoretically, could be useful in any memory condition characterized by cholinergic deficiency (e.g., some cases of brain injury, cancer chemotherapy-induced cognitive changes, etc.)

Suggested Reading

Bentue-Ferrer D, Tribut O, Polard E, Allain H. Clinically significant drug interactions with cholinesterase inhibitors: a guide for neurologists. CNS Drugs 2003;17:947–63.

Bonner LT, Peskind ER. Pharmacologic treatments of dementia. Med Clin North Am 2002;86:657–74.

Coyle J, Kershaw P. Galantamine, a cholinesterase inhibitor that allosterically modulates nicotinic receptors: effects on the course of Alzheimer's disease. Biol Psychiatry 2001;49:289–99.

Jones RW. Have cholinergic therapies reached their clinical boundary in Alzheimer's disease? Int J Geriatr Psychiatry 2003;18(Suppl 1): S7–S13.

Olin J, Schneider L. Galantamine for Alzheimer's disease. Cochrane Database Syst Rev 2002;(3):CD001747.

Stahl SM. Cholinesterase inhibitors for Alzheimer's disease. Hosp Pract (Off Ed) 1998;33:131–6.

Stahl SM. The new cholinesterase inhibitors for Alzheimer's disease, part 1. J Clin Psychiatry 2000;61:710–11.

Stahl SM. The new cholinesterase inhibitors for Alzheimer's disease, part 2. J Clin Psychiatry 2000;61:813–14.

HALOPERIDOL

THERAPEUTICS

Brands • Haldol
see index for additional brand names

Generic? Yes

Class
• Conventional antipsychotic (neuroleptic, butyrophenone, dopamine 2 antagonist)

Commonly Prescribed For
(bold for FDA approved)
• **Manifestations of psychotic disorders (oral, immediate release injection)**
• **Tics and vocal utterances in Tourette's Disorder (oral, immediate release injection)**
• **Second-line treatment of severe behavior problems in children of combative, explosive hyperexcitability (oral, immediate release injection)**
• **Second-line short-term treatment of hyperactive children (oral, immediate release injection)**
• **Treatment of schizophrenic patients who require prolonged parenteral antipsychotic therapy (depot intramuscular decanoate)**
• Bipolar disorder
• Behavioral disturbances in dementias

How The Drug Works
• Blocks dopamine 2 receptors, reducing positive symptoms of psychosis and possibly combative, explosive, and hyperactive behaviors
• Blocks dopamine 2 receptors in the nigrostriatal pathway, improving tics and other symptoms in Tourette's syndrome

How Long Until It Works
• Psychotic symptoms can improve within 1 week, but it may take several weeks for full effect on behavior

If It Works
• Most often reduces positive symptoms in schizophrenia but does not eliminate them
• Most schizophrenic patients do not have a total remission of symptoms but rather a reduction of symptoms by about a third

• Continue treatment in schizophrenia until reaching a plateau of improvement
• After reaching a satisfactory plateau, continue treatment for at least a year after first episode of psychosis in schizophrenia
• For second and subsequent episodes of psychosis in schizophrenia, treatment may need to be indefinite
• Reduces symptoms of acute psychotic mania but not proven as a mood stabilizer or as an effective maintenance treatment in bipolar disorder
• After reducing acute psychotic symptoms in mania, switch to a mood stabilizer and/or an atypical antipsychotic for mood stabilization and maintenance

If It Doesn't Work
• Consider trying one of the first-line atypical antipsychotics (risperidone, olanzapine, quetiapine, ziprasidone, aripiprazole, amisulpride)
• Consider trying another conventional antipsychotic
• If 2 or more antipsychotic monotherapies do not work, consider clozapine

Best Augmenting Combos for Partial Response or Treatment-Resistance
• Augmentation of conventional antipsychotics has not been systematically studied
• Addition of a mood stabilizing anticonvulsant such as valproate, carbamazepine, or lamotrigine may be helpful in both schizophrenia and bipolar mania
• Augmentation with lithium in bipolar mania may be helpful
• Addition of a benzodiazepine, especially short-term for agitation

Tests
✳ Since conventional antipsychotics are frequently associated with weight gain, before starting treatment, weigh all patients and determine if the patient is already overweight (BMI 25.0–29.9) or obese (BMI ≥30)
• Before giving a drug that can cause weight gain to an overweight or obese patient, consider determining whether the patient already has pre-diabetes (fasting plasma glucose 100–125 mg/dl), diabetes (fasting

plasma glucose >126 mg/dl), or dyslipidemia (increased total cholesterol, LDL cholesterol and triglycerides; decreased HDL cholesterol), and treat or refer such patients for treatment, including nutrition and weight management, physical activity counseling, smoking cessation, and medical management

✳ Monitor weight and BMI during treatment
✳ While giving a drug to a patient who has gained >5% of initial weight, consider evaluating for the presence of pre-diabetes, diabetes, or dyslipidemia, or consider switching to a different antipsychotic
• Should check blood pressure in the elderly before starting and for the first few weeks of treatment
• Monitoring elevated prolactin levels of dubious clinical benefit

SIDE EFFECTS

How Drug Causes Side Effects

• By blocking dopamine 2 receptors in the striatum, it can cause motor side effects
• By blocking dopamine 2 receptors in the pituitary, it can cause elevations in prolactin
• By blocking dopamine 2 receptors excessively in the mesocortical and mesolimbic dopamine pathways, especially at high doses, it can cause worsening of negative and cognitive symptoms (neuroleptic-induced deficit syndrome)
• By blocking alpha 1 adrenergic receptors, it can cause dizziness, sedation, and hypotension
• Mechanism of weight gain and any possible increased incidence of diabetes or dyslipidemia with conventional antipsychotics is unknown

Notable Side Effects

✳ Neuroleptic-induced deficit syndrome
✳ Akathisia
✳ Extrapyramidal symptoms, Parkinsonism, tardive dyskinesia, tardive dystonia
✳ Galactorrhea, amenorrhea
• Dizziness, sedation
• Dry mouth, constipation, urinary retention, blurred vision
• Decreased sweating
• Hypotension, tachycardia, hypertension
• Weight gain

Life Threatening or Dangerous Side Effects

• Rare neuroleptic malignant syndrome
• Rare seizures
• Rare jaundice, agranulocytosis, leukopenia

Weight Gain

unusual | not unusual | common | problematic

• Occurs in significant minority

Sedation

unusual | not unusual | common | problematic

• Sedation is usually transient

What To Do About Side Effects

• Wait
• Wait
• Wait
• For motor symptoms, add an anticholinergic agent
• Reduce the dose
• For sedation, give at night
• Switch to an atypical antipsychotic
• Weight loss, exercise programs, and medical management for high BMIs, diabetes, dyslipidemia

Best Augmenting Agents for Side Effects

• Benztropine or trihexyphenidyl for motor side effects
• Sometimes amantadine can be helpful for motor side effects
• Benzodiazepines may be helpful for akathisia
• Many side effects cannot be improved with an augmenting agent

DOSING AND USE

Usual Dosage Range

• 1–40 mg/day orally
• Immediate release injection 2–5 mg each dose
• Decanoate injection 10–20 times the previous daily dose of oral antipsychotic

Dosage Forms
- Tablet 0.5 mg scored, 1 mg scored, 2 mg scored, 5 mg scored, 10 mg scored, 20 mg scored
- Concentrate 2 mg/mL
- Solution 1 mg/mL
- Injection 5 mg/mL (immediate release)
- Decanoate injection 50 mg haloperidol as 70.5 mg/mL haloperidol decanoate, 100 mg haloperidol as 141.04 mg/mL haloperidol decanoate

How to Dose
- Oral: initial 1–15 mg/day; can give once daily or in divided doses at the beginning of treatment during rapid dose escalation; increase as needed; can be dosed up to 100 mg/day; safety not established for doses over 100 mg/day
- Immediate release injection: initial dose 2–5 mg; subsequent doses may be given as often as every hour; patient should be switched to oral administration as soon as possible
- Decanoate injection: initial dose 10–15 times the previous oral dose for patients maintained on low antipsychotic doses (e.g., up to equivalent of 10 mg/day oral haloperidol); initial dose may be as high as 20 times the previous oral dose for patients maintained on higher antipsychotic doses; maximum dose 100 mg, if higher than 100 mg dose is required the remainder can be administered 3–7 days later; administer total dose every 4 weeks

 Dosing Tips
- Haloperidol is frequently dosed too high
- Some studies suggest that patients who respond well to low doses of haloperidol (e.g., approximately 2 mg/day) may have efficacy similar to atypical antipsychotics for both positive and negative symptoms of schizophrenia
- Higher doses may actually induce or worsen negative symptoms of schizophrenia
- Low doses, however, may not have beneficial actions on cognitive and affective symptoms in schizophrenia
- One of the only antipsychotics with a depot formulation lasting for up to a month

Overdose
- Fatalities have been reported; extrapyramidal symptoms, hypotension, sedation, respiratory depression, shock-like state

Long-Term Use
- Often used for long-term maintenance
- Some side effects may be irreversible (e.g., tardive dyskinesia)

Habit Forming
- No

How to Stop
- Slow down-titration of oral formulation (over 6 to 8 weeks), especially when simultaneously beginning a new antipsychotic while switching (i.e., cross-titration)
- Rapid oral discontinuation may lead to rebound psychosis and worsening of symptoms
- If antiparkinson agents are being used, they should be continued for a few weeks after haloperidol is discontinued

Pharmacokinetics
- Decanoate half-life approximately 3 weeks
- Oral half-life approximately 12–38 hours

 Drug Interactions
- May decrease the effects of levodopa, dopamine agonists
- May increase the effects of antihypertensive drugs except for guanethidine, whose antihypertensive actions haloperidol may antagonize
- Additive effects may occur if used with CNS depressants; dose of other agent should be reduced
- Some pressor agents (e.g., epinephrine) may interact with haloperidol to lower blood pressure
- Haloperidol and anticholinergic agents together may increase intraocular pressure
- Reduces effects of anticoagulants
- Plasma levels of haloperidol may be lowered by rifampin
- Some patients taking haloperidol and lithium have developed an encephalopathic syndrome similar to neuroleptic malignant syndrome

• May enhance effects of antihypertensive drugs

 Other Warnings/ Precautions

• If signs of neuroleptic malignant syndrome develop, treatment should be immediately discontinued
• Use with caution in patients with respiratory disorders
• Avoid extreme heat exposure
• If haloperidol is used to treat mania, patients may experience a rapid switch to depression
• Patients with thyrotoxicosis may experience neurotoxicity
• Use only with caution if at all in Parkison's disease on Lewy Body dementia

Do Not Use

• If patient is in comatose state or has CNS depression
• If patient has Parkinson's disease
• If there is a proven allergy to haloperidol

SPECIAL POPULATIONS

Renal Impairment
• Use with caution

Hepatic Impairment
• Use with caution

Cardiac Impairment
• Use with caution because of risk of orthostatic hypertension

Elderly
• Lower doses should be used and patient should be monitored closely
• Elderly may be more susceptible to respiratory side effects and hypotension

 Children and Adolescents

• Safety and efficacy have not been established; not intended for use under age 3
• Oral: initial 0.5 mg/day; target dose 0.05–0.15 mg/kg/day for psychotic disorders; 0.05–0.075 mg/kg/day for nonpsychotic disorders
• Generally consider second-line after atypical antipsychotics

 Pregnancy

• Risk Category C [some animal studies show adverse effects, no controlled studies in humans]
• Reports of extrapyramidal symptoms, jaundice, hyperreflexia, hyporeflexia in infants whose mothers took a conventional antipsychotic during pregnancy
• Reports of limb deformity in infants whose mothers took haloperidol during pregnancy
• Haloperidol should generally not be used during the first trimester
• Haloperidol should only be used during pregnancy if clearly needed
• Psychotic symptoms may worsen during pregnancy and some form of treatment may be necessary
• Atypical antipsychotics may be preferable to conventional antipsychotics or anticonvulsant mood stabilizers if treatment is required during pregnancy

Breast Feeding

• Some drug is found in mother's breast milk
✳ Recommended either to discontinue drug or bottle feed

THE ART OF PSYCHOPHARMACOLOGY

Potential Advantages
• Intramuscular formulation for emergency use
• Depot formulation for noncompliance
• Low dose responders may have comparable positive and negative symptom efficacy to atypical antipsychotics
• Low cost, effective treatment

Potential Disadvantages
• Patients with tardive dyskinesia or who wish to avoid tardive dyskinesia and extrapyramidal symptoms
• Vulnerable populations such as children or elderly
• Patients with notable cognitive or mood symptoms

Primary Target Symptoms
• Positive symptoms of psychosis
• Violent or aggressive behavior

Pearls

- Prior to the introduction of atypical antipsychotics, haloperidol was one of the most preferred antipsychotics
- Haloperidol may still be a useful antipsychotic, especially at low doses for those patients who require management with a conventional antipsychotic or who cannot afford an atypical antipsychotic
- Low doses may not induce negative symptoms, but high doses may
- Not clearly effective for improving cognitive or affective symptoms of schizophrenia
- May be effective for bipolar maintenance, but there may be more tardive dyskinesia when affective disorders are treated with a conventional antipsychotic long-term
- Less sedating than many other conventional antipsychotics, especially "low potency" phenothiazines
- Haloperidol's long-acting intramuscular formulation lasts up to 4 weeks, whereas some other long-acting intramuscular antipsychotics may only last up to 2 weeks
- Decanoate administration is intended for patients with chronic schizophrenia who have been stabilized on oral antipsychotic medication
- Patients have very similar antipsychotic responses to any conventional antipsychotic, which is different from atypical antipsychotics where antipsychotic responses of individual patients can occasionally vary greatly from one atypical antipsychotic to another
- Conventional antipsychotics are much less expensive than atypical antipsychotics
- Patients receiving atypical antipsychotics may occasionally require a "top up" of a conventional antipsychotic such as haloperidol to control aggression or violent behavior
- Patients with inadequate responses to atypical antipsychotics may benefit from a trial of augmentation with a conventional antipsychotic such as haloperidol or from switching to a conventional antipsychotic such as haloperidol
- However, long-term polypharmacy with a combination of a conventional antipsychotic such as haloperidol with an atypical antipsychotic may combine their side effects without clearly augmenting the efficacy of either
- Although a frequent practice by some prescribers, adding 2 conventional antipsychotics together has little rationale and may reduce tolerability without clearly enhancing efficacy

Suggested Reading

Csernansky JG, Mahmoud R, Brenner R, Risperidone-USA-79 Study Group. A comparison of risperidone and haloperidol for the prevention of relapse in patients with schizophrenia. N Engl J Med 2002;346:16–22.

Davis JM, Chen N, Glick ID. A meta-analysis of the efficacy of second-generation antipsychotics. Arch Gen Psychiatry 2003;60:553–64.

Geddes J, Freemantle N, Harrison P, Bebbington P. Atypical antipsychotics in the treatment of schizophrenia: systematic overview and meta-regression analysis. BMJ 2000;321:1371–6.

Joy CB, Adams CE, Lawrie SM. Haloperidol versus placebo for schizophrenia. Cochrane Database Syst Rev 2001;(2):CD003082.

Kudo S, Ishizaki T. Pharmacokinetics of haloperidol: an update. Clin Pharmacokinet 1999;37:435–56.

Quraishi S ,David A. Depot haloperidol decanoate for schizophrenia. Cochrane Database Syst Rev 2000;(2):CD001361.

HYDROXYZINE

THERAPEUTICS

Brands • Atarax
• Marax
• Vistaril
see index for additional brand names

Generic? Yes

 Class
• Antihistamine (anxiolytic, hypnotic, antiemetic)

Commonly Prescribed For
(bold for FDA approved)
• **Anxiety and tension associated with psychoneurosis**
• **Adjunct in organic disease states in which anxiety is manifested**
• **Pruritus due to allergic conditions**
• **Histamine-mediated pruritus**
• **Premedication sedation**
• **Sedation following general anesthesia**
• **Acute disturbance/hysteria (injection)**
• **Anxiety withdrawal symptoms in alcoholics or patients with delirium tremens (injection)**
• **Adjunct in pre/postoperative and pre/postpartum patients to allay anxiety, control emesis, and reduce narcotic dose (injection)**
• **Nausea and vomiting (injection)**
• Insomnia

 How The Drug Works
• Blocks histamine 1 receptors

How Long Until It Works
• 15–20 minutes (oral administration)
• Some immediate relief with first dosing is common; can take several weeks with daily dosing for maximal therapeutic benefit in chronic conditions

If It Works
• For short-term symptoms of anxiety – after a few weeks, discontinue use or use on an "as-needed" basis
• For chronic anxiety disorders, the goal of treatment is complete remission of symptoms as well as prevention of future relapses
• For chronic anxiety disorders, treatment most often reduces or even eliminates symptoms, but not a cure since symptoms can recur after medicine stopped
• For long-term symptoms of anxiety, consider switching to an SSRI or SNRI for long-term maintenance
• If long-term maintenance is necessary, continue treatment for 6 months after symptoms resolve, and then taper dose slowly
• If symptoms reemerge, consider treatment with an SSRI or SNRI, or consider restarting hydroxyzine

If It Doesn't Work
• Consider switching to another agent or adding an appropriate augmenting agent

 Best Augmenting Combos for Partial Response or Treatment-Resistance
• Hydroxyzine can be used as an adjunct to SSRIs or SNRIs in treating anxiety disorders

Tests
• None for healthy individuals
• Hydroxyzine may cause falsely elevated urinary concentrations of 17-hydroxycorticosteroids in certain lab tests (e.g., Porter-Silber reaction, Glenn-Nelson method)

SIDE EFFECTS

How Drug Causes Side Effects
• Blocking histamine 1 receptors can cause sedation

Notable Side Effects
• Dry mouth, sedation, tremor

 Life Threatening or Dangerous Side Effects
• Rare convulsions (generally at high doses)
• Rare cardiac arrest, death (intramuscular formulation combined with CNS depressants)
• Bronchodilation
• Respiratory depression

Weight Gain

unusual not unusual common problematic

• Reported but not expected

Sedation

unusual not unusual **common** problematic

• Many experience and/or can be significant in amount
• Sedation is usually transient

What To Do About Side Effects
• Wait
• Wait
• Wait
• Switch to another agent

Best Augmenting Agents for Side Effects
• Many side effects cannot be improved with an augmenting agent

---

DOSING AND USE

Usual Dosage Range
• Anxiety: 50–100 mg 4 times a day
• Sedative: 50–100 mg oral, 25–100 mg intramuscular injection
• Pruritus: 75 mg/day divided into 3–4 doses

Dosage Forms
• Tablet 10 mg, 25 mg, 50 mg, 100 mg
• Capsule 25 mg, 50 mg, 100 mg
• Oral Liquid 10 mg/5 mL, 25 mg/5 mL
• Intramuscular 25 mg/mL, 50 mg/mL, 100 mg/2 mL

How to Dose
• Oral dosing does not require titration
• Emergency intramuscular injection: Initial 50–100 mg, repeat every 4–6 hours as needed
• Hydroxyzine intramuscular injection should not be given in the lower or mid-third of the arm and should only be given in the deltoid area if it is well-developed
• In adults, hydroxyzine intramuscular injections may be given in the upper outer quadrant of the buttock or in the mid-lateral thigh

 Dosing Tips
• Hydroxyzine may be administered intramuscularly initially, but should be changed to oral administration as soon as possible
• Tolerance usually develops to sedation, allowing higher dosing over time

Overdose
• Sedation, hypotension

Long-Term Use
• Evidence of efficacy for up to 16 weeks

Habit Forming
• No

How to Stop
• Taper generally not necessary

Pharmacokinetics
• Rapidly absorbed from gastrointestinal tract
• Mean elimination half-life approximately 20 hours

 Drug Interactions
• If hydroxyzine is taken in conjunction with another CNS depressant, the dose of the CNS depressant should be reduced by half
• If hydroxyzine is used pre- or post-operatively, the dose of narcotic can be reduced
• If anticholinergic agents are used with hydroxyzine, the anticholinergic effects may be enhanced
• Hydroxyzine may reverse the vasopressor effect of epinephrine; patients requiring a vasopressor agent should use norepinephrine or metaraminol instead

 Other Warnings/ Precautions
• Hydroxyzine should not be administered subcutaneously, intra-arterially, or intravenously

Do Not Use
• If patient is in early stages of pregnancy
• If there is a proven allergy to hydroxyzine

SPECIAL POPULATIONS

Renal Impairment
• Dosage adjustment may not be necessary

Hepatic Impairment
• Dosage adjustment may not be necessary

Cardiac Impairment
• Hydroxyzine may be used to treat anxiety associated with cardiac impairment

Elderly
• Some patients may tolerate lower doses better
• Elderly patients may be more sensitive to sedative and anticholinergic effects

 Children and Adolescents
• Anxiety, pruritus (6 and older): 50–100 mg/day in divided doses
• Anxiety, pruritus (under 6): 50 mg/day in divided doses
• Sedative: 0.6 mg/kg oral, 0.5 mg/lb intramuscular injection
• Small children should not receive hydroxyzine by intramuscular injection in the periphery of the upper quadrant of the buttock unless absolutely necessary because of risk of damage to the sciatic nerve
• Hyperactive children should be monitored for paradoxical effects

 Pregnancy
✳ Hydroxyzine is contraindicated in early pregnancy
• Hydroxyzine intramuscular injection can be used prepartum, reducing narcotic requirements by up to 50%

Breast Feeding
• Unknown if hydroxyzine is secreted in human breast milk, but all psychotropics assumed to be secreted in breast milk
✳ Recommended either to discontinue drug or bottle feed

THE ART OF PSYCHOPHARMACOLOGY

Potential Advantages
• Has multiple formulations, including oral capsules, tablets, and liquid, as well as injectable
• No abuse liability, dependence, or withdrawal

Potential Disadvantages
• Patients with severe anxiety disorders

Primary Target Symptoms
• Anxiety
• Skeletal muscle tension
• Itching
• Nausea, vomiting

 Pearls
✳ A preferred anxiolytic for patients with dermatitis or skin symptoms such as pruritis
• Anxiolytic actions may be proportional to sedating actions
• Hydroxyzine tablets are made with 1,1,1-trichloroethane, which destroys ozone
• Hydroxyzine by intramuscular injection may be used to treat agitation during alcohol withdrawal
• Hydroxyzine may not be as effective as benzodiazepines or newer agents in the management of anxiety

 Suggested Reading

Diehn F, Tefferi A. Pruritus in polycythaemia vera: prevalence, laboratory correlates and management. Br J Haematol 2001;115:619–21.

Ferreri M, Hantouche EG. Recent clinical trials of hydroxyzine in generalized anxiety disorder. Acta Psychiatr Scand Suppl 1998;393:102–8.

Paton DM, Webster DR. Clinical pharmacokinetics of H1-receptor antagonists (the antihistamines). Clin Pharmacokinet 1985;10:477–97.

IMIPRAMINE

THERAPEUTICS

Brands • Tofranil
see index for additional brand names

Generic? Yes

Class
• Tricyclic antidepressant (TCA)
• Serotonin and norepinephrine/
  noradrenaline reuptake inhibitor

Commonly Prescribed For
(bold for FDA approved)
• **Depression**
✱ Enuresis
• Anxiety
• Insomnia
• Neuropathic pain/chronic pain
• Treatment-resistant depression
• Cataplexy syndrome

How The Drug Works
• Boosts neurotransmitters serotonin and
  norepinephrine/noradrenaline
• Blocks serotonin reuptake pump (serotonin
  transporter), presumably increasing
  serotonergic neurotransmission
• Blocks norepinephrine reuptake pump
  (norepinephrine transporter), presumably
  increasing noradrenergic
  neurotransmission
• Presumably desensitizes both serotonin 1A
  receptors and beta adrenergic receptors
• Since dopamine is inactivated by
  norepinephrine reuptake in frontal cortex,
  which largely lacks dopamine transporters,
  imipramine can increase dopamine
  neurotransmission in this part of the brain
• May be effective in treating enuresis
  because of its anticholinergic properties

How Long Until It Works
• May have immediate effects in treating
  insomnia or anxiety
• Onset of therapeutic actions usually not
  immediate, but often delayed 2 to 4 weeks
• If it is not working within 6 to 8 weeks for
  depression, it may require a dosage
  increase or it may not work at all
• May continue to work for many years to
  prevent relapse of symptoms

If It Works
• The goal of treatment of depression is
  complete remission of current symptoms
  as well as prevention of future relapses
• The goal of treatment of chronic
  neuropathic pain is to reduce symptoms as
  much as possible, especially in
  combination with other treatments
• Treatment of depression most often
  reduces or even eliminates symptoms, but
  not a cure since symptoms can recur after
  medicine stopped
• Treatment of chronic neuropathic pain may
  reduce symptoms, but rarely eliminates
  them completely, and is not a cure since
  symptoms can recur after medicine is
  stopped
• Continue treatment of depression until all
  symptoms are gone (remission)
• Once symptoms of depression are gone,
  continue treating for 1 year for the first
  episode of depression
• For second and subsequent episodes of
  depression, treatment may need to be
  indefinite
• Use in anxiety disorders and chronic pain
  may also need to be indefinite, but long-
  term treatment is not well studied in these
  conditions

If It Doesn't Work
• Many depressed patients only have a
  partial response where some symptoms
  are improved but others persist (especially
  insomnia, fatigue, and problems
  concentrating)
• Other depressed patients may be
  nonresponders, sometimes called
  treatment-resistant or treatment-refractory
• Consider increasing dose, switching to
  another agent or adding an appropriate
  augmenting agent
• Consider psychotherapy
• Consider evaluation for another diagnosis
  or for a comorbid condition (e.g., medical
  illness, substance abuse, etc.)
• Some patients may experience apparent
  lack of consistent efficacy due to activation
  of latent or underlying bipolar disorder, and
  require antidepressant discontinuation and
  a switch to a mood stabilizer

Best Augmenting Combos for Partial Response or Treatment-Resistance

- Lithium, buspirone, thyroid hormone (for depression)
- Gabapentin, tiagabine, other anticonvulsants, even opiates if done by experts while monitoring carefully in difficult cases (for chronic pain)

Tests

- None for healthy individuals
- ✳ Since tricyclic and tetracyclic antidepressants are frequently associated with weight gain, before starting treatment, weigh all patients and determine if the patient is already overweight (BMI 25.0–29.9) or obese (BMI ≥30)
- Before giving a drug that can cause weight gain to an overweight or obese patient, consider determining whether the patient already has pre-diabetes (fasting plasma glucose 100–125 mg/dl), diabetes (fasting plasma glucose >126 mg/dl), or dyslipidemia (increased total cholesterol, LDL cholesterol and triglycerides; decreased HDL cholesterol), and treat or refer such patients for treatment, including nutrition and weight management, physical activity counseling, smoking cessation, and medical management
- ✳ Monitor weight and BMI during treatment
- ✳ While giving a drug to a patient who has gained >5% of initial weight, consider evaluating for the presence of pre-diabetes, diabetes, or dyslipidemia, or consider switching to a different antidepressant
- EKGs may be useful for selected patients (e.g., those with personal or family history of QTc prolongation; cardiac arrhythmia; recent myocardial infarction; uncompensated heart failure; or taking agents that prolong QTc interval such as pimozide, thioridazine, selected antiarrhythmics, moxifloxacin, sparfloxacin, etc.)
- Patients at risk for electrolyte disturbances (e.g., patients on diuretic therapy) should have baseline and periodic serum potassium and magnesium measurements

SIDE EFFECTS

How Drug Causes Side Effects

- Anticholinergic activity may explain sedative effects, dry mouth, constipation, and blurred vision
- Sedative effects and weight gain may be due to antihistamine properties
- Blockade of alpha adrenergic 1 receptors may explain dizziness, sedation, and hypotension
- Cardiac arrhythmias and seizures, especially in overdose, may be caused by blockade of ion channels

Notable Side Effects

- Blurred vision, constipation, urinary retention, increased appetite, dry mouth, nausea, diarrhea, heartburn, unusual taste in mouth, weight gain
- Fatigue, weakness, dizziness, sedation, headache, anxiety, nervousness, restlessness
- Sexual dysfunction, sweating

Life Threatening or Dangerous Side Effects

- Paralytic ileus, hyperthermia (TCAs + anticholinergic agents)
- Lowered seizure threshold and rare seizures
- Orthostatic hypotension, sudden death, arrhythmias, tachycardia
- QTc prolongation
- Hepatic failure, extrapyramidal symptoms
- Increased intraocular pressure, increased psychotic symptoms
- Rare induction of mania and activation of suicidal ideation

Weight Gain

unusual   not unusual   **common**   problematic

- Many experience and/or can be significant in amount
- Can increase appetite and carbohydrate craving

Sedation

unusual   not unusual   **common**   problematic

- Many experience and/or can be significant in amount
- Tolerance to sedative effects may develop with long-term use

What To Do About Side Effects
- Wait
- Wait
- Wait
- Lower the dose
- Switch to an SSRI or newer antidepressant

Best Augmenting Agents for Side Effects
- Many side effects cannot be improved with an augmenting agent

DOSING AND USE

Usual Dosage Range
- 50–150 mg/day

Dosage Forms
- Capsule 75 mg, 100 mg, 125 mg, 150 mg
- Tablet 10 mg, 25 mg, 50 mg

How to Dose
- Initial 25 mg/day at bedtime; increase by 25 mg every 3–7 days
- 75–100 mg/day once daily or in divided doses; gradually increase daily dose to achieve desired therapeutic effects; dose at bedtime for daytime sedation and in morning for insomnia; maximum dose 300 mg/day

 Dosing Tips
- If given in a single dose, should generally be administered at bedtime because of its sedative properties
- If given in split doses, largest dose should generally be given at bedtime because of its sedative properties
- If patients experience nightmares, split dose and do not give large dose at bedtime
- Patients treated for chronic pain may only require lower doses
- Tofranil-PM(r) (imipramine pamoate) 100- and 125-mg capsules contain the dye tartrazine (FD&C yellow No. 5), which may cause allergic reactions in some patients; this reaction is more likely in patients with sensitivity to aspirin
- If intolerable anxiety, insomnia, agitation, akathisia, or activation occur either upon dosing initiation or discontinuation, consider the possibility of activated bipolar disorder, and switch to a mood stabilizer or an atypical antipsychotic

Overdose
- Death may occur; convulsions, cardiac dysrhythmias, severe hypotension, CNS depression, coma, changes in ECG

Long-Term Use
- Safe

Habit Forming
- No

How to Stop
- Taper to avoid withdrawal effects
- Even with gradual dose reduction some withdrawal symptoms may appear within the first 2 weeks
- Many patients tolerate 50% dose reduction for 3 days, then another 50% reduction for 3 days, then discontinuation
- If withdrawal symptoms emerge during discontinuation, raise dose to stop symptoms and then restart withdrawal much more slowly

Pharmacokinetics
- Substrate for CYP450 2D6 and 1A2
- Metabolized to an active metabolite, desipramine, a predominantly norepinephrine reuptake inhibitor, by demethylation via CYP450 1A2

 Drug Interactions
- Tramadol increases the risk of seizures in patients taking TCAs
- Use of TCAs with anticholinergic drugs may result in paralytic ileus or hyperthermia
- Fluoxetine, paroxetine, bupropion, duloxetine, and other CYP450 2D6 inhibitors may increase TCA concentrations
- Fluvoxamine, a CYP450 1A2 inhibitor, can decrease the conversion of imipramine to desmethylimipramine (desipramine) and increase imipramine plasma concentrations
- Cimetidine may increase plasma concentrations of TCAs and cause anticholinergic symptoms
- Phenothiazines or haloperidol may raise TCA blood concentrations
- May alter effects of antihypertensive drugs; may inhibit hypotensive effects of clonidine

IMIPRAMINE (continued)

- Use with sympathomimetic agents may increase sympathetic activity
- Methylphenidate may inhibit metabolism of TCAs
- Activation and agitation, especially following switching or adding antidepressants, may represent the induction of a bipolar state, especially a mixed dysphoric bipolar II condition sometimes associated with suicidal ideation, and require the addition of lithium, a mood stabilizer or an atypical antipsychotic, and/or discontinuation of imipramine

 Other Warnings/ Precautions

- Add or initiate other antidepressants with caution for up to 2 weeks after discontinuing imipramine
- Generally, do not use with MAO inhibitors, including 14 days after MAOIs are stopped; do not start an MAOI until 2 weeks after discontinuing imipramine, but see Pearls
- Use with caution in patients with history of seizure, urinary retention, narrow angle-closure glaucoma, hyperthyroidism
- TCAs can increase QTc interval, especially at toxic doses, which can be attained not only by overdose but also by combining with drugs that inhibit its metabolism via CYP450 2D6, potentially causing torsade de pointes-type arrhythmia or sudden death
- Because TCAs can prolong QTc interval, use with caution in patients who have bradycardia or who are taking drugs that can induce bradycardia (e.g., beta blockers, calcium channel blockers, clonidine, digitalis)
- Because TCAs can prolong QTc interval, use with caution in patients who have hypokalemia and/or hypomagnesemia or who are taking drugs that can induce hypokalemia and/or magnesemia (e.g., diuretics, stimulant laxatives, intravenous amphotericin B, glucocorticoids, tetracosactide)

Do Not Use

- If patient is recovering from myocardial infarction
- If patient is taking agents capable of significantly prolonging QTc interval (e.g., pimozide, thioridazine, selected antiarrhythmics, moxifloxacin, sparfloxacin)
- If there is a history of QTc prolongation or cardiac arrhythmia, recent acute myocardial infarction, uncompensated heart failure
- If patient is taking drugs that inhibit TCA metabolism, including CYP450 2D6 inhibitors, except by an expert
- If there is reduced CYP450 2D6 function, such as patients who are poor 2D6 metabolizers, except by an expert and at low doses
- If there is a proven allergy to imipramine, desipramine, or lofepramine

SPECIAL POPULATIONS

Renal Impairment

- Cautious use; may need lower dose

Hepatic Impairment

- Cautious use; may need lower dose

Cardiac Impairment

- TCAs have been reported to cause arrhythmias, prolongation of conduction time, orthostatic hypotension, sinus tachycardia, and heart failure, especially in the diseased heart
- Myocardial infarction and stroke have been reported with TCAs
- TCAs produce QTc prolongation, which may be enhanced by the existence of bradycardia, hypokalemia, congenital or acquired long QTc interval, which should be evaluated prior to administering imipramine
- Use with caution if treating concomitantly with a medication likely to produce prolonged bradycardia, hypokalemia, slowing of intracardiac conduction, or prolongation of the QTc interval
- Avoid TCAs in patients with a known history of QTc prolongation, recent acute myocardial infarction, and uncompensated heart failure
- TCAs may cause a sustained increase in heart rate in patients with ischemic heart disease and may worsen (decrease) heart rate variability, an independent risk of mortality in cardiac populations

- Since SSRIs may improve (increase) heart rate variability in patients following a myocardial infarct and may improve survival as well as mood in patients with acute angina or following a myocardial infarction, these are more appropriate agents for cardiac population than tricyclic/tetracyclic antidepressants
- ❋ Risk/benefit ratio may not justify use of TCAs in cardiac impairment

Elderly
- May be more sensitive to anticholinergic, cardiovascular, hypotensive, and sedative effects
- Initial 30–40 mg/day; maximum dose 100 mg/day

 Children and Adolescents
- Use with caution, observing for activation of known or unknown bipolar disorder and/or suicidal ideation, and strongly consider informing parents or guardian of this risk so they can help observe child or adolescent patients
- Used age 6 and older for enuresis; age 12 and older for other disorders
- Several studies show lack of efficacy of TCAs for depression
- May be used to treat hyperactive/impulsive behaviors
- Some cases of sudden death have occurred in children taking TCAs
- Adolescents: initial 30–40 mg/day; maximum 100 mg/day
- Children: initial 1.5 mg/kg/day; maximum 5 mg/kg/day
- Functional enuresis: 50 mg/day (age 6–12) or 75 mg/day (over 12)

 Pregnancy
- Risk Category D [positive evidence of risk to human fetus; potential benefits may still justify its use during pregnancy]
- Crosses the placenta
- Should be used only if potential benefits outweigh potential risks
- Adverse effects have been reported in infants whose mothers took a TCA (lethargy, withdrawal symptoms, fetal malformations)

- Evaluate for treatment with an antidepressant with a better risk/benefit ratio

Breast Feeding
- Some drug is found in mother's breast milk
- ❋ Recommended either to discontinue drug or bottle feed
- Immediate postpartum period is a high-risk time for depression, especially in women who have had prior depressive episodes, so drug may need to be reinstituted late in the third trimester or shortly after childbirth to prevent a recurrence during the postpartum period
- Must weigh benefits of breast feeding with risks and benefits of antidepressant treatment versus non-treatment to both the infant and the mother
- For many patients this may mean continuing treatment during breast feeding

THE ART OF PSYCHOPHARMACOLOGY

Potential Advantages
- Patients with insomnia
- Severe or treatment-resistant depression
- Patients with enuresis

Potential Disadvantages
- Pediatric and geriatric patients
- Patients concerned with weight gain
- Cardiac patients

Primary Target Symptoms
- Depressed mood
- Chronic pain

 Pearls
- Was once one of the most widely prescribed agents for depression
- ❋ Probably the most preferred TCA for treating enuresis in children
- ❋ Preference of some prescribers for imipramine over other TCAs for the treatment of enuresis is based more upon art and anecdote and empiric clinical experience than comparative clinical trials with other TCAs
- Tricyclic antidepressants are no longer generally considered a first-line treatment option for depression because of their side effect profile

- TCAs may aggravate psychotic symptoms
- Alcohol should be avoided because of additive CNS effects
- Underweight patients may be more susceptible to adverse cardiovascular effects
- Children, patients with inadequate hydration, and patients with cardiac disease may be more susceptible to TCA-induced cardiotoxicity than healthy adults
- For the expert only: although generally prohibited, a heroic but potentially dangerous treatment for severely treatment-resistant patients is to give a tricyclic/tetracyclic antidepressant other than clomipramine simultaneously with an MAO inhibitor for patients who fail to respond to numerous other antidepressants
- If this option is elected, start the MAOI with the tricyclic/tetracyclic antidepressant simultaneously at low doses after appropriate drug washout, then alternately increase doses of these agents every few days to a week as tolerated
- Although very strict dietary and concomitant drug restrictions must be observed to prevent hypertensive crises and serotonin syndrome, the most common side effects of MAOI/tricyclic or tetracyclic combinations may be weight gain and orthostatic hypotension
- Patients on TCAs should be aware that they may experience symptoms such as photosensitivity or blue-green urine
- SSRIs may be more effective than TCAs in women, and TCAs may be more effective than SSRIs in men
- Since tricyclic/tetracyclic antidepressants are substrates for CYP450 2D6, and 7% of the population (especially Caucasians) may have a genetic variant leading to reduced activity of 2D6, such patients may not safely tolerate normal doses of tricyclic/tetracyclic antidepressants and may require dose reduction
- Phenotypic testing may be necessary to detect this genetic variant prior to dosing with a tricyclic/tetracyclic antidepressant, especially in vulnerable populations such as children, elderly, cardiac populations, and those on concomitant medications
- Patients who seem to have extraordinarily severe side effects at normal or low doses may have this phenotypic CYP450 2D6 variant and require low doses or switching to another antidepressant not metabolized by 2D6

 Suggested Reading

Anderson IM. Meta-analytical studies on new antidepressants. Br Med Bull 2001; 57:161–178.

Anderson IM. Selective serotonin reuptake inhibitors versus tricyclic antidepressants: a meta-analysis of efficacy and tolerability. J Aff Disorders 2000;58:19–36.

Preskorn SH. Comparison of the tolerability of bupropion, fluoxetine, imipramine, nefazodone, paroxetine, sertraline, and venlafaxine. J Clin Psychiatry 1995;56(Suppl 6):12–21.

Workman EA, Short DD. Atypical antidepressants versus imipramine in the treatment of major depression: a meta-analysis. J Clin Psychiatry 1993;54:5–12.

ISOCARBOXAZID

THERAPEUTICS

Brands • Marplan
see index for additional brand names

Generic? Not in U.S.

Class
• Monoamine oxidase inhibitor (MAOI)

Commonly Prescribed For
(bold for FDA approved)
• **Depression**
• Treatment-resistant depression
• Treatment-resistant panic disorder
• Treatment-resistant social anxiety disorder

How The Drug Works
• Irreversibly blocks monoamine oxidase (MAO) from breaking down norepinephrine, serotonin, and dopamine
• This presumably boosts noradrenergic, serotonergic, and dopaminergic neurotransmission

How Long Until It Works
• Onset of therapeutic actions usually not immediate, but often delayed 2 to 4 weeks
• If it is not working within 6 to 8 weeks, it may require a dosage increase or it may not work at all
• May continue to work for many years to prevent relapse of symptoms

If It Works
• The goal of treatment is complete remission of current symptoms as well as prevention of future relapses
• Treatment most often reduces or even eliminates symptoms, but not a cure since symptoms can recur after medicine stopped
• Continue treatment until all symptoms are gone (remission)
• Once symptoms gone, continue treating for 1 year for the first episode of depression
• For second and subsequent episodes of depression, treatment may need to be indefinite
• Use in anxiety disorders may also need to be indefinite

If It Doesn't Work
• Many patients only have a partial response where some symptoms are improved but others persist (especially insomnia, fatigue, and problems concentrating)
• Other patients may be nonresponders, sometimes called treatment-resistant or treatment-refractory
• Some patients who have an initial response may relapse even though they continue treatment, sometimes called "poop-out"
• Consider increasing dose, switching to another agent or adding an appropriate augmenting agent
• Consider psychotherapy
• Consider evaluation for another diagnosis or for a comorbid condition (e.g., medical illness, substance abuse, etc.)
• Some patients may experience apparent lack of consistent efficacy due to activation of latent or underlying bipolar disorder, and require antidepressant discontinuation and a switch to a mood stabilizer

Best Augmenting Combos for Partial Response or Treatment-Resistance
✳ Augmentation of MAOIs has not been systematically studied, and this is something for the expert, to be done with caution and with careful monitoring
✳ A stimulant such as d-amphetamine or methylphenidate (with caution; may activate bipolar disorder and suicidal ideation; may elevate blood pressure)
• Lithium
• Mood stabilizing anticonvulsants
• Atypical antipsychotics (with special caution for those agents with monoamine reuptake blocking properties, such as ziprasidone and zotepine)

Tests
• Patients should be monitored for changes in blood pressure
• Patients receiving high doses or long-term treatment should have hepatic function evaluated periodically
✳ Since MAO inhibitors are frequently associated with weight gain, before starting treatment, weigh all patients and determine if the patient is already overweight (BMI 25.0–29.9) or obese (BMI ≥30)

- Before giving a drug that can cause weight gain to an overweight or obese patient, consider determining whether the patient already has pre-diabetes (fasting plasma glucose 100–125 mg/dl), diabetes (fasting plasma glucose >126 mg/dl), or dyslipidemia (increased total cholesterol, LDL cholesterol and triglycerides; decreased HDL cholesterol), and treat or refer such patients for treatment, including nutrition and weight management, physical activity counseling, smoking cessation, and medical management
* Monitor weight and BMI during treatment
* While giving a drug to a patient who has gained >5% of initial weight, consider evaluating for the presence of pre-diabetes, diabetes, or dyslipidemia, or consider switching to a different antidepressant

SIDE EFFECTS

How Drug Causes Side Effects

- Theoretically due to increases in monoamines in parts of the brain and body and at receptors other than those that cause therapeutic actions (e.g., unwanted actions of serotonin in sleep centers causing insomnia, unwanted actions of norepinephrine on vascular smooth muscle causing hypertension, etc.)
- Side effects are generally immediate, but immediate side effects often disappear in time

Notable Side Effects

- Dizziness, sedation, headache, sleep disturbances, fatigue, weakness, tremor, movement problems, blurred vision, increased sweating
- Constipation, dry mouth, nausea, change in appetite, weight gain
- Sexual dysfunction
- Orthostatic hypotension (dose-related); syncope may develop at high doses

Life Threatening or Dangerous Side Effects

- Hypertensive crisis (especially when MAOIs are used with certain tyramine-containing foods or prohibited drugs)
- Induction of mania and activation of suicidal ideation

- Seizures
- Hepatotoxicity

Weight Gain

unusual   not unusual   **common**   problematic

- Many experience and/or can be significant in amount

Sedation

unusual   not unusual   **common**   problematic

- Many experience and/or can be significant in amount
- Can also cause activation

What To Do About Side Effects

- Wait
- Wait
- Wait
- Lower the dose
- Take at night if daytime sedation
- Switch after appropriate washout to an SSRI or newer antidepressant

Best Augmenting Agents for Side Effects

- Trazodone (with caution) for insomnia
- Benzodiazepines for insomnia
* Single oral or sublingual dose of a calcium channel blocker (e.g., nifedipine) for urgent treatment of hypertension due to drug interaction or dietary tyramine
- Many side effects cannot be improved with an augmenting agent

DOSING AND USE

Usual Dosage Range

- 40–60 mg/day

Dosage Forms

- Tablet 10 mg

How to Dose

- Initial 10 mg twice a day; increase by 10 mg/day every 2–4 days; dosed 2–4 times/day; maximum dose 60 mg/day

Dosing Tips

- Orthostatic hypotension, especially at high doses, may require splitting into 3 or 4 daily doses
- Patients receiving high doses may need to be evaluated periodically for effects on the liver
- Little evidence to support efficacy of isocarboxazid at doses below 30 mg/day

Overdose

- Dizziness, sedation, ataxia, headache, insomnia, restlessness, anxiety, irritability; cardiovascular effects, confusion, respiratory depression, or coma may also occur

Long-Term Use

- May require periodic evaluation of hepatic function
- MAOIs may lose some efficacy long-term

Habit Forming

- Some patients have developed dependence to MAOIs

How to Stop

- Generally no need to taper, as drug wears off slowly over 2–3 weeks

Pharmacokinetics

- Clinical duration of action may be up to 21 days due to irreversible enzyme inhibition

Drug Interactions

- Tramadol may increase the risk of seizures in patients taking an MAO inhibitor
- Can cause a fatal "serotonin syndrome" when combined with drugs that block serotonin reuptake (e.g., SSRIs, SNRIs, sibutramine, tramadol, etc.), so do not use with a serotonin reuptake inhibitor or for up to 5 weeks after stopping the serotonin reuptake inhibitor
- Hypertensive crisis with headache, intracranial bleeding, and death may result from combining MAO inhibitors with sympathomimetic drugs (e.g., amphetamines, methylphenidate, cocaine, dopamine, epinephrine, norepinephrine, and related compounds methyldopa,

levodopa, L-tryptophan, L-tyrosine, and phenylalanine)
- Excitation, seizures, delirium, hyperpyrexia, circulatory collapse, coma, and death may result from combining MAO inhibitors with mepiridine or dextromethorphan
- Do not combine with another MAO inhibitor, alcohol, buspirone, bupropion, or guanethidine
- Adverse drug reactions can results from combining MAO inhibitors with tricyclic/tetracyclic antidepressants and related compounds, including carbamazepine, cyclobenzaprine, and mirtazapine, and should be avoided except by experts to treat difficult cases (see Pearls)
- MAO inhibitors in combination with spinal anesthesia may cause combined hypotensive effects
- Combination of MAOIs and CNS depressants may enhance sedation and hypotension

Other Warnings/ Precautions

- Use requires low tyramine diet
- Patients taking MAO inhibitors should avoid high protein food that has undergone protein breakdown by aging, fermentation, pickling, smoking, or bacterial contamination
- Patients taking MAO inhibitors should avoid cheeses (especially aged varieties), pickled herring, beer, wine, liver, yeast extract, dry sausage, hard salami, pepperoni, Lebanon bologna, pods of broad beans (fava beans), yogurt, and excessive use of caffeine and chocolate
- Patient and prescriber must be vigilant to potential interactions with any drug, including antihypertensives and over-the-counter cough/cold preparations
- Over-the-counter medications to avoid include cough and cold preparations, including those containing dextromethorphan, nasal decongestants (tablets, drops, or spray), hay-fever medications, sinus medications, asthma inhalant medications, anti-appetite medications, weight reducing preparations, "pep" pills

- Use cautiously in patients receiving reserpine, anesthetics, disulfiram, metrizamide, anticholinergic agents
- Isocarboxazid is not recommended for use in patients who cannot be monitored closely
- Monitor patients for activation of suicidal ideation, especially children and adolescents

Do Not Use

- If patient is taking meperidine (pethidine)
- If patient is taking a sympathomimetic agent or taking guanethidine
- If patient is taking another MAOI
- If patient is taking any agent that can inhibit serotonin reuptake (e.g., SSRIs, sibutramine, tramadol, milnacipran, duloxetine, venlafaxine, clomipramine, etc.)
- If patient is taking diuretics, dextromethorphan, buspirone, bupropion
- If patient has pheochromocytoma
- If patient has cardiovascular or cerebrovascular disease
- If patient has frequent or severe headaches
- If patient is undergoing elective surgery and requires general anesthesia
- If patient has a history of liver disease or abnormal liver function tests
- If patient is taking a prohibited drug
- If patient is not compliant with a low-tyramine diet
- If there is a proven allergy to isocarboxazid

SPECIAL POPULATIONS

Renal Impairment

- Use with caution – drug may accumulate in plasma
- May require lower than usual adult dose

Hepatic Impairment

- Not for use in hepatic impairment

Cardiac Impairment

- Contraindicated in patients with congestive heart failure or hypertension
- Any other cardiac impairment may require lower than usual adult dose
- Patients with angina pectoris or coronary artery disease should limit their exertion

Elderly

- Initial dose lower than usual adult dose

- Elderly patients may have greater sensitivity to adverse effects

Children and Adolescents

- Not recommended for use under age 16
- Use with caution, observing for activation of known or unknown bipolar disorder and/or suicidal ideation, and strongly consider informing parents or guardian of this risk so they can help observe child or adolescent patients

Pregnancy

- Risk Category C [some animal studies show adverse effects, no controlled studies in humans]
- Not generally recommended for use during pregnancy, especially during first trimester
- Should evaluate patient for treatment with an antidepressant with a better risk/benefit ratio

Breast Feeding

- Some drug is found in mother's breast milk
- Immediate postpartum period is a high-risk time for depression, especially in women who have had prior depressive episodes, so drug may need to be reinstituted late in the third trimester or shortly after childbirth to prevent a recurrence during the postpartum period
- Should evaluate patient for treatment with an antidepressant with a better risk/benefit ratio

THE ART OF PSYCHOPHARMACOLOGY

Potential Advantages

- Atypical depression
- Severe depression
- Treatment-resistant depression or anxiety disorders

Potential Disadvantages

- Requires compliance to dietary restrictions, concomitant drug restrictions
- Patients with cardiac problems or hypertension
- Multiple daily doses

Primary Target Symptoms

- Depressed mood
- Somatic symptoms
- Sleep and eating disturbances
- Psychomotor retardation
- Morbid preoccupation

 Pearls

- MAOIs are generally reserved for second-line use after SSRIs, SNRIs, and combinations of newer antidepressants have failed
- Despite little utilization, some patients respond to isocarboxazid who do not respond to other antidepressants including other MAOIs
- Patient should be advised not to take any prescription or over-the-counter drugs without consulting their doctor because of possible drug interactions with the MAOI
- Headache is often the first symptom of hypertensive crisis
- Foods generally to avoid as they are usually high in tyramine content: dry sausage, pickled herring, liver, broad bean pods, sauerkraut, cheese, yogurt, alcoholic beverages, nonalcoholic beer and wine, chocolate, caffeine, meat and fish
- The rigid dietary restrictions may reduce compliance
- Mood disorders can be associated with eating disorders (especially in adolescent females), and isocarboxazid can be used to treat both depression and bulimia
- MAOIs are a viable second-line treatment option in depression, but are not frequently used
- ✱ Myths about the danger of dietary tyramine can be exaggerated, but prohibitions against concomitant drugs often not followed closely enough
- Orthostatic hypotension, insomnia, and sexual dysfunction are often the most troublesome common side effects
- ✱ MAOIs should be for the expert, especially if combining with agents of potential risk (e.g., stimulants, trazodone, TCAs)
- ✱ MAOIs should not be neglected as therapeutic agents for the treatment-resistant
- Although generally prohibited, a heroic but potentially dangerous treatment for severely treatment-resistant patients is for an expert to give a tricyclic/tetracyclic antidepressant other than clomipramine simultaneously with an MAO inhibitor for patients who fail to respond to numerous other antidepressants
- Use of MAOIs with clomipramine is always prohibited because of the risk of serotonin syndrome and death
- Amoxapine may be the preferred trycyclic/tetracyclic antidepressant to combine with an MAOI in heroic cases due to its theoretically protective 5HT2A antagonist properties
- If this option is elected, start the MAOI with the tricyclic/tetracyclic antidepressant simultaneously at low doses after appropriate drug washout, then alternately increase doses of these agents every few days to a week as tolerated
- Although very strict dietary and concomitant drug restrictions must be observed to prevent hypertensive crises and serotonin syndrome, the most common side effects of MAOI and tricyclic/tetracyclic combinations may be weight gain and orthostatic hypotension

 Suggested Reading

Kennedy SH. Continuation and maintenance treatments in major depression: the neglected role of monoamine oxidase inhibitors. J Psychiatry Neurosci 1997;22:127–31.

Lippman SB, Nash K. Monoamine oxidase inhibitor update. Potential adverse food and drug interactions. Drug Saf 1990;5:195–204.

Larsen JK, Rafaelsen OJ. Long-term treatment of depression with isocarboxazide. Acta Psychiatr Scand 1980;62(5):456–63.

LAMOTRIGINE

THERAPEUTICS

Brands
- Lamictal
- Labileno
- Lamictin

see index for additional brand names

Generic? No

 Class
- Anticonvulsant, mood stabilizer, voltage-sensitive sodium channel antagonist

Commonly Prescribed For
(bold for FDA approved)
- **Maintenance treatment of bipolar I disorder**
- **Partial seizures (adjunctive; adults and children over age 2)**
- **Generalized seizures of Lennox-Gastaut syndrome (adjunctive; adults and children over age 2)**
- **Conversion to monotherapy in adults with partial seizures who are receiving treatment with a single enzyme-inducing antiepileptic drug**
- Bipolar depression
- Bipolar mania (adjunctive and second-line)
- Psychosis, schizophrenia (adjunctive)
- Neuropathic pain/chronic pain

 How The Drug Works
- ✳ Acts as a use-dependent blocker of voltage-sensitive sodium channels
- ✳ Interacts with the open channel conformation of voltage-sensitive sodium channels
- ✳ Interacts at a specific site of the alpha pore-forming subunit of voltage-sensitive sodium channels
- Inhibits release of glutamate

How Long Until It Works
- May take several weeks to improve bipolar depression
- May take several weeks to months to optimize an effect on mood stabilization
- Should reduce seizures by 2 weeks

If It Works
- The goal of treatment is complete remission of symptoms (e.g., seizures, depression, pain)

- Continue treatment until all symptoms are gone or until improvement is stable and then continue treating indefinitely as long as improvement persists
- Continue treatment indefinitely to avoid recurrence of mania, depression, and/or seizures
- Treatment of chronic neuropathic pain may reduce but does not eliminate pain symptoms and is not a cure since pain usually recurs after medicine stopped

If It Doesn't Work (for bipolar disorder)
- ✳ Many patients only have a partial response where some symptoms are improved but others persist or continue to wax and wane without stabilization of mood
- Other patients may be nonresponders, sometimes called treatment-resistant or treatment-refractory
- Consider increasing dose, switching to another agent or adding an appropriate augmenting agent
- Consider adding psychotherapy
- Consider biofeedback or hypnosis for pain
- Consider the presence of noncompliance and counsel patient
- Switch to another mood stabilizer with fewer side effects
- Consider evaluation for another diagnosis or for a comorbid condition (e.g., medical illness, substance abuse, etc.)

 Best Augmenting Combos for Partial Response or Treatment-Resistance (for bipolar disorder)
- Lithium
- Atypical antipsychotics (especially risperidone, olanzapine, quetiapine, ziprasidone, and aripiprazole)
- ✳ Valproate (with caution and at half dose of lamotrigine in the presence of valproate, because valproate can double lamotrigine levels)
- ✳ Antidepressants (with caution because antidepressants can destabilize mood in some patients, including induction of rapid cycling or suicidal ideation; in particular consider bupropion; also SSRIs, SNRIs, others; generally avoid TCAs, MAOIs)

Tests
- Because lamotrigine binds to melanin-containing tissues, opthalmological checks may be considered

---

SIDE EFFECTS

How Drug Causes Side Effects
- CNS side effects theoretically due to excessive actions at voltage-sensitive sodium channels
- Rash hypothetically an allergic reaction

Notable Side Effects
- ✱ Benign rash (approximately 10%)
- Sedation, blurred or double vision, dizziness, ataxia, headache, tremor, insomnia, poor coordination, fatigue
- Nausea, vomiting, dyspepsia, abdominal pain, constipation, rhinitis
- Additional effects in pediatric patients: infection, flu syndrome, pharyngitis, asthenia

Life Threatening or Dangerous Side Effects
- ✱ Rare serious rash (risk may be greater in pediatric patients but still rare)
- Rare multi-organ failure associated with Stevens Johnson syndrome, toxic epidermal necrolysis or drug hypersensitivity syndrome
- Rare blood dyscrasias
- Rare sudden unexplained deaths have occurred in epilepsy (unknown if related to lamotrigine use)

Weight Gain

unusual / not unusual / common / problematic

- Reported but not expected

Sedation

unusual / not unusual / common / problematic

- Reported but not expected
- Dose-related
- Can wear off with time

What To Do About Side Effects
- Wait
- Take at night to reduce daytime sedation

- ✱ If patient develops signs of a rash with benign characteristics (i.e., a rash that peaks within days, settles in 10–14 days, is spotty, nonconfluent, nontender, has no systemic features, and laboratory tests are normal):
  - Reduce lamotrigine dose or stop dosage increase
  - Warn patient to stop drug and contact physician if rash worsens or new symptoms emerge
  - Prescribe antihistamine and/or topical corticosteroid for pruritis
  - Monitor patient closely
- ✱ If patient develops signs of a rash with serious characteristics (i.e., a rash that is confluent and widespread, or purpuric or tender; with any prominent involvement of neck or upper trunk; any involvement of eyes, lips, mouth, etc.; any associated fever, malaise, pharyngitis, anorexia, or lymphadenopathy; abnormal laboratory tests for complete blood count, liver function, urea, creatinine):
  - Stop lamotrigine (and valproate if administered)
  - Monitor and investigate organ involvement (hepatic, renal, hematologic)
  - Patient may require hospitalization

Best Augmenting Agents for Side Effects
- Antihistamines and/or topical corticosteroid for rash, pruritis
- Many side effects cannot be improved with an augmenting agent

---

DOSING AND USE

Usual Dosage Range
- Monotherapy for bipolar disorder: 100–200 mg/day
- Adjunctive treatment for bipolar disorder: 100 mg/day in combination with valproate; 400 mg/day in combination with enzyme-inducing antiepileptic drugs such as carbamazepine, phenobarbital, phenytoin, and primidone
- Monotherapy for seizures: 300–500 mg/day in 2 doses
- Adjunctive treatment for seizures: 100–400 mg/day for regimens containing

valproate; 100–200 mg/day for valproate alone; 300–500 mg/day in 2 doses for regimens not containing valproate

Dosage Forms
- Tablet 25 mg scored, 100 mg scored, 150 mg scored, 200 mg scored
- Chewable tablet 2 mg, 5 mg, 25 mg

How to Dose
✳ Bipolar disorder (monotherapy): for the first 2 weeks administer 25 mg/day; at week 3 increase to 50 mg/day; at week 5 increase to 100 mg/day; at week 6 increase to 200 mg/day; maximum dose generally 200 mg/day
✳ Bipolar disorder (adjunct to valproate): for the first 2 weeks administer 25 mg every other day; at week 3 increase to 25 mg/day; at week 5 increase to 50 mg/day; at week 6 increase to 100 mg/day; maximum dose generally 100 mg/day
- Bipolar disorder (adjunct to enzyme-inducing antiepileptic drugs): for the first 2 weeks administer 50 mg/day; at week 3 increase to 100 mg/day in divided doses; starting at week 5 increase by 100 mg/day each week; maximum dose generally 400 mg/day in divided doses
- When lamotrigine is added to epilepsy treatment that includes valproate (ages 12 and older): for the first 2 weeks administer 25 mg every other day; at week 3 increase to 25 mg/day; every 1–2 weeks can increase by 25–50 mg/day; usual maintenance dose 100–400 mg/day in 1–2 doses or 100–200 mg/day if lamotrigine is added to valproate alone
- When lamotrigine is added to epilepsy treatment that does not include valproate (ages 12 and older): for the first 2 weeks administer 50 mg/day; at week 3 increase to 100 mg/day in 2 doses; every 1–2 weeks can increase by 100 mg/day; usual maintenance dose 300–500 mg/day in 2 doses
- When converting from a single enzyme-inducing antiepileptic drug to lamotrigine monotherapy for epilepsy: titrate as described above to 500 mg/day in 2 doses while maintaining dose of previous medication; decrease first drug in 20% decrements each week over the next 4 weeks

- Seizures (under age 12): see Children and Adolescents

 Dosing Tips

✳ Very slow dose titration may reduce the incidence of skin rash
- Therefore, dose should not be titrated faster than recommended because of possible risk of increased side effects, including rash
- If patient stops taking lamotrigine for 5 days or more it may be necessary to restart the drug with the initial dose titration, as rashes have been reported on re-exposure
- Advise patient to avoid new medications, foods, or products during the first 3 months of lamotrigine treatment in order to decrease the risk of unrelated rash; patient should also not start lamotrigine within 2 weeks of a viral infection, rash, or vaccination
✳ If lamotrigine is added to patients taking valproate, remember that valproate inhibits lamotrigine metabolism and therefore titration rate and ultimate dose of lamotrigine should be reduced by 50% to reduce the risk of rash
✳ Thus, if concomitant valproate is discontinued after lamotrigine dose is stabilized, then the lamotrigine dose should be cautiously doubled over at least 2 weeks in equal increments each week following discontinuation of valproate
- Also, if concomitant enzyme-inducing antiepileptic drugs such as carbamazepine, phenobarbital, phenytoin, and primidone are discontinued after lamotrigine dose is stabilized, then the lamotrigine dose should be maintained for 1 week following discontinuation of the other drug and then reduced by half over 2 weeks in equal decrements each week
- Chewable dispersible tablets should only be administered as whole tablets; dose should be rounded down to the nearest whole tablet
- Chewable dispersible tablets can be dispersed by adding the tablet to liquid (enough to cover the drug); after approximately 1 minute the solution should be stirred and then consumed immediately in its entirety

Overdose

- Some fatalities have occurred; ataxia, nystagmus, seizures, coma, intraventricular conduction delay

Long-Term Use

- Safe
- Because lamotrigine binds to melanin-containing tissues, opthalmological checks may be considered

Habit Forming

- No

How to Stop

- Taper
- ✳ Rapid discontinuation can increase the risk of relapse in bipolar disorder
- Patients with epilepsy may seize upon withdrawal, especially if withdrawal is abrupt
- Discontinuation symptoms uncommon

Pharmacokinetics

- Elimination half-life in healthy volunteers approximately 33 hours after a single dose of lamotrigine
- Elimination half-life in patients receiving concomitant valproate treatment approximately 59 hours after a single dose of lamotrigine
- Elimination half-life in patients receiving concomitant enzyme-inducing antiepileptic drugs (such as carbamazepine, phenobarbital, phenytoin, and primidone) approximately 14 hours after a single dose of lamotrigine
- Metabolized in the liver but not through the CYP450 enzyme system
- Inactive metabolite
- Renally excreted
- Lamotrigine inhibits dihydrofolate reductase and may therefore reduce folate concentrations

 Drug Interactions

- ✳ Valproate increases plasma concentrations and half-life of lamotrigine, requiring lower doses of lamotrigine (half or less)
- ✳ Use of lamotrigine with valproate may be associated with an increased incidence of rash

- Enzyme-inducing antiepileptic drugs (e.g., carbamazepine, phenobarbital, phenytoin, primidone) may increase the clearance of lamotrigine and lower its plasma levels
- Oral contraceptives may decrease plasma levels of lamotrigine
- No likely pharmacokinetic interactions of lamotrigine with lithium, atypical antipsychotics, or antidepressants

 Other Warnings/ Precautions

- ✳ Life-threatening rashes have developed in association with lamotrigine use; lamotrigine should generally be discontinued at the first sign of serious rash
- ✳ Risk of rash may be increased with higher doses, faster dose escalation, concomitant use of valproate, or in children under age 12
- Patient should be instructed to report any symptoms of hypersensitivity immediately (fever; flu-like symptoms; rash; blisters on skin or in eyes, mouth, ears, nose, or genital areas; swelling of eyelids, conjunctivitis, lymphadenopathy)
- Depressive effects may be increased by other CNS depressants (alcohol, MAOIs, other anticonvulsants, etc.)
- A small number of people may experience a worsening of seizures
- May cause photosensitivity
- Lamotrigine binds to tissue that contains melanin, so for long-term treatment ophthalmological checks may be considered

Do Not Use

- If there is a proven allergy to lamotrigine

Renal Impairment

- Lamotrigine is renally excreted, so the dose may need to be lowered
- Can be removed by hemodialysis; patients receiving hemodialysis may require supplemental doses of lamotrigine

Hepatic Impairment

- Dose may need to be reduced and titration may need to be slower, perhaps by 50% in patients with moderate impairment and 75% in patients with severe impairment

Cardiac Impairment
• Drug should be used with caution

Elderly
• Some patients may tolerate lower doses better
• Elderly patients may be more susceptible to adverse effects

Children and Adolescents
• Ages 2 and older: approved as add-on for Lennox-Gastaut syndrome
• Ages 2 and older: approved as add-on for partial seizures
• No other use of lamotrigine is approved for patients under 16 years of age
✻ Risk of rash is increased in pediatric patients, especially in children under 12 and in children taking valproate
• When lamotrigine is added to treatment that includes valproate (ages 2–12): for the first 2 weeks administer 0.15 mg/kg/day in 1–2 doses rounded down to the nearest whole tablet; at week 3 increase to 0.3 mg/kg/day in 1–2 doses rounded down to the nearest whole tablet; every 1–2 weeks can increase by 0.3 mg/kg/day rounded down to the nearest whole tablet; usual maintenance dose 1–5 mg/kg/day in 1–2 doses (maximum generally 200 mg/day) or 1–3 mg/kg/day in 1–2 doses if lamotrigine is added to valproate alone
• When lamotrigine is added to treatment that does not include valproate (ages 2–12): for the first 2 weeks administer 0.6 mg/kg/day in 2 doses rounded down to the nearest whole tablet; at week 3 increase to 1.2 mg/kg/day in 2 doses rounded down to the nearest whole tablet; every 1–2 weeks can increase by 1.2 mg/kg/day rounded down to the nearest whole tablet; usual maintenance dose 5–15 mg/kg/day in 2 doses (maximum dose generally 400 mg/day)
• Clearance of lamotrigine may be influenced by weight, such that patients weighing less than 30 kg may require an increase of up to 50% for maintenance doses

Pregnancy
• Risk category C [some animal studies show adverse effects, no controlled studies in humans]
• Use in women of childbearing potential requires weighing potential benefits to the mother against the risks to the fetus
✻ If treatment with lamotrigine is continued, plasma concentrations of lamotrigine may be reduced during pregnancy, possibly requiring increased doses with dose reduction following delivery
• Taper drug if discontinuing
• Seizures, even mild seizures, may cause harm to the embryo/fetus
• Recurrent bipolar illness during pregnancy can be quite disruptive
✻ For bipolar patients, lamotrigine should generally be discontinued before anticipated pregnancies
✻ For bipolar patients in whom treatment is discontinued, given the risk of relapse in the postpartum period, lamotrigine should generally be restarted immediately after delivery
✻ Atypical antipsychotics may be preferable to lithium or anticonvulsants such as lamotrigine if treatment of bipolar disorder is required during pregnancy, but lamotrigine may be preferable to other anticonvulsants such as valproate if anticonvulsant treatment is required during pregnancy
• Bipolar symptoms may recur or worsen during pregnancy and some form of treatment may be necessary

Breast Feeding
• Some drug is found in mother's breast milk
✻ Generally recommended either to discontinue drug or bottle feed
• If drug is continued while breast feeding, infant should be monitored for possible adverse effects
• If infant shows signs of irritability or sedation, drug may need to be discontinued
✻ Bipolar disorder may recur during the postpartum period, particularly if there is a history of prior postpartum episodes of either depression or psychosis

* Relapse rates may be lower in women who receive prophylactic treatment for postpartum episodes of bipolar disorder
* Atypical antipsychotics and anticonvulsants such as valproate may be preferable to lithium or lamotrigine during the postpartum period when breast feeding

THE ART OF PSYCHOPHARMACOLOGY

Potential Advantages
* Depressive stages of bipolar disorder (bipolar depression)
* To prevent recurrences of both depression and mania in bipolar disorder

Potential Disadvantages
* May not be as effective in the manic stage of bipolar disorder

Primary Target Symptoms
* Incidence of seizures
* Unstable mood, especially depression, in bipolar disorder
* Pain

 Pearls

* Lamotrigine is a first-line treatment option that may be best for patients with bipolar depression
* Seems to be more effective in treating depressive episodes than manic episodes in bipolar disorder (treats from below better than it treats from above)
* Seems to be effective in preventing both manic relapses as well as depressive relapses (stabilizes both from above and from below) although it may be even better for preventing depressive relapses than for preventing manic relapses
* Despite convincing evidence of efficacy in bipolar disorder, is often used far less frequently than anticonvulsants without convincing evidence of efficacy in bipolar disorder (e.g., gabapentin or topiramate)
* Low levels of use may be based upon exaggerated fears of skin rashes or lack of knowledge about how to manage skin rashes if they occur
* May actually be one of the best tolerated mood stabilizers with little weight gain or sedation

* Actual risk of serious skin rash comparable to agents erroneously considered "safer" including carbamazepine, phenytoin, and phenobarbital
* Rashes are common even in placebo-treated patients in clinical trials of bipolar patients (5–10%) due to non-drug related causes including eczema, irritant, and allergic contact dermatitis, such as poison ivy and insect bite reactions
* To manage rashes in bipolar patients receiving lamotrigine, realize that rashes that occur within the first 5 days or after 8–12 weeks of treatment are rarely drug-related, and learn the clinical distinctions between a benign rash and a serious rash (see What to Do About Side Effects above)
* Rash, including serious rash, appears riskiest in patients with epilepsy, in younger children, in those who are receiving concomitant valproate, and/or in those receiving rapid lamotrigine titration and/or high dosing
* Risk of serious rash is less than 1% and has been declining since slower titration, lower dosing, adjustments to use of concomitant valproate administration, and limitations on use in children under 12 have been implemented
* Incidence of serious rash is very low (approaching zero) in recent studies of bipolar patients
* Benign rashes related to lamotrigine may affect up to 10% of patients and resolve rapidly with drug discontinuation
* Given the limited treatment options for bipolar depression, patients with benign rashes can even be re-challenged with lamotrigine 5–12 mg/day with very slow titration after risk-benefit analysis if they are informed, reliable, closely monitored, and warned to stop lamotrigine and contact their physician if signs of hypersensitivity occur
* Only a third of bipolar patients experience adequate relief with a monotherapy, so most patients need multiple medications for best control
* Lamotrigine is useful in combination with atypical antipsychotics and/or lithium for acute mania
* Usefulness for bipolar disorder in combination with anticonvulsants other than valproate is not well demonstrated;

such combinations can be expensive and are possibly ineffective or even irrational
• May be useful as an adjunct to atypical antipsychotics for rapid onset of action in schizophrenia

• Early studies suggest possible utility for patients with neuropathic pain such as diabetic peripheral neuropathy, HIV-associated neuropathy, and other pain conditions including migraine

Suggested Reading

Calabrese JR, Vieta E, Shelton MD. Latest maintenance data on lamotrigine in bipolar disorder. Eur Neuropsychopharmacol. 2003;13(Suppl 2):S57–66.

Calabrese JR, Sullivan JR, Bowden CL, Suppes T, Goldberg JF, Sachs GS, Shelton MD, Goodwin FK, Frye MA, Kusumakar V. Rash in multicenter trials of lamotrigine in mood disorders: clinical relevance and management. J Clin Psychiatry. 2002;63:1012–1019

Culy CR, Goa KL. Lamotrigine. A review of its use in childhood epilepsy. Paediatr Drugs. 2000; 2: 299–330.

Green B. Lamotrigine in mood disorders. Curr Med Res Opin. 2003;19:272–7.

LEVETIRACETAM

THERAPEUTICS

Brands • Keppra
see index for additional brand names

Generic? Not in U.S.

 Class
• Anticonvulsant, synaptic vesicle protein SV2A modulator

Commonly Prescribed For
(bold for FDA approved)
• **Adjunct therapy for partial seizures in adults with epilepsy**
• Neuropathic pain/chronic pain
• Mania

 How The Drug Works
✱ Binds to synaptic vesicle protein SV2A, which is involved in synaptic vesicle exocytosis
• No apparent effects on GABA neurotransmission or inhibition of voltage-sensitive sodium channels or voltage-sensitive calcium channels

How Long Until It Works
• Should reduce seizures by 2 weeks
• Not yet clear if it has mood stabilizing effects in bipolar disorder or antineuralgic actions in chronic neuropathic pain, but some patients may respond and if so, would be expected to show clinical effects starting by 2 weeks although it may take several weeks to months to optimize clinical effects

If It Works
• The goal of treatment is complete remission of symptoms (e.g., seizures, mania, pain)
• The goal of treatment of chronic neuropathic pain is to reduce symptoms as much as possible, especially in combination with other treatments
• Treatment of chronic neuropathic pain most often reduces but does not eliminate symptoms and is not a cure since symptoms usually recur after medicine stopped
• Continue treatment until all symptoms are gone or until mood is stable and then continue treating indefinitely as long as improvement persists
• Continue treatment indefinitely to avoid recurrence of seizures, mania, and pain

If It Doesn't Work (for bipolar disorder or neuropathic pain)
✱ May only be effective in a subset of bipolar patients, in some patients who fail to respond to other mood stabilizers, or it may not work at all
• Many patients only have a partial response where some symptoms are improved but others persist or continue to wax and wane without stabilization of pain or mood
• Other patients may be nonresponders, sometimes called treatment-resistant or treatment-refractory
• Consider increasing dose or switching to another agent with better demonstrated efficacy in bipolar disorder or neuropathic pain

 Best Augmenting Combos for Partial Response or Treatment-Resistance
• Levetiracetam is itself a second-line augmenting agent to numerous other anticonvulsants, lithium, and atypical antipsychotics for bipolar disorder and to gabapentin, tiagabine, other anticonvulsants, SNRIs, and tricyclic antidepressants for neuropathic pain

Tests
• None for healthy individuals

SIDE EFFECTS

How Drug Causes Side Effects
• CNS side effects may be due to excessive actions on SV2A synaptic vesicle proteins or to actions on various voltage-sensitive ion channels

Notable Side Effects
✱ Sedation, dizziness, ataxia, asthenia
• Hematologic abnormalities (decrease in red blood cell count and hemoglobin)

Life Threatening or Dangerous Side Effects

- Activation of suicidal ideation and acts (rare)

Weight Gain

unusual · not unusual · common · problematic

- Reported but not expected

Sedation

unusual · not unusual · **common** · problematic

- Many experience and/or can be significant in amount

What To Do About Side Effects

- Wait
- Wait
- Wait
- Take more of the dose at night to reduce daytime sedation
- Lower the dose
- Switch to another agent

Best Augmenting Agents for Side Effects

- Many side effects cannot be improved with an augmenting agent

DOSING AND USE

Usual Dosage Range

- 1000–3000 mg/day in 2 doses

Dosage Forms

- Tablet 250 mg, 500 mg, 750 mg
- Oral solution 100 mg/mL

How to Dose

- Initial 1000 mg/day in 2 divided doses; after 2 weeks can increase by 1000 mg/day every 2 weeks; maximum dose generally 3000 mg/day

 Dosing Tips

- For intolerable sedation, can give most of the dose at night and less during the day
- Some patients may tolerate and respond to doses greater than 3000 mg/day

Overdose

- No fatalities; sedation, agitation, aggression, respiratory depression, coma

Long-Term Use

- Safe

Habit Forming

- No

How to Stop

- Taper
- Epilepsy patients may seize upon withdrawal, especially if withdrawal is abrupt
- ✳ Rapid discontinuation can increase the risk of relapse in bipolar disorder
- Discontinuation symptoms uncommon

Pharmacokinetics

- Elimination half-life approximately 6–8 hours
- Inactive metabolites
- Not metabolized by CYP450 enzymes
- Does not inhibit/induce CYP450 enzymes
- Renally excreted

 Drug Interactions

- Because levetiracetam is not metabolized by CYP450 enzymes and does not inhibit or induce CYP450 enzymes, it is unlikely to have significant pharmacokinetic drug interactions

 Other Warnings/ Precautions

- Depressive effects may be increased by other CNS depressants (alcohol, MAOIs, other anticonvulsants, etc.)

Do Not Use

- If there is a proven allergy to levetiracetam

SPECIAL POPULATIONS

Renal Impairment

- Recommended dose for patients with mild impairment may be between 500 mg and 1500 mg twice a day
- Recommended dose for patients with moderate impairment may be between 250 mg and 750 mg twice a day

- Recommended dose for patients with severe impairment may be between 250 mg and 500 mg twice a day
- Patients on dialysis may require doses between 500 mg and 1000 mg once a day, with a supplemental dose of 250–500 mg following dialysis

Hepatic Impairment
- Dose adjustment usually not necessary

Cardiac Impairment
- No specific recommendations

Elderly
- Some patients may tolerate lower doses better
- Elderly patients may be more susceptible to adverse effects

 ## Children and Adolescents
- Safety and efficacy not established under age 16
- Children may require higher doses than adults; dosing should be adjusted according to weight

 ## Pregnancy
- Risk category C [some animal studies show adverse effects, no controlled studies in humans]
- Use in women of childbearing potential requires weighing potential benefits to the mother against the risks to the fetus
- Taper drug if discontinuing
- Seizures, even mild seizures, may cause harm to the embryo/fetus
- Lack of convincing efficacy for treatment of bipolar disorder or chronic neuropathic pain suggests risk/benefit ratio is in favor of discontinuing levetiracetam during pregnancy for these indications
- ✳ For bipolar patients, given the risk of relapse in the postpartum period, mood stabilizer treatment, especially with agents with better evidence of efficacy than levetiracetam, should generally be restarted immediately after delivery if patient is unmedicated during pregnancy
- ✳ For bipolar patients, levetiracetam should generally be discontinued before anticipated pregnancies

- ✳ Atypical antipsychotics may be preferable to levetiracetam if treatment of bipolar disorder is required during pregnancy
- Bipolar symptoms may recur or worsen during pregnancy and some form of treatment may be necessary

Breast Feeding
- Some drug is found in mother's breast milk
- ✳ Recommended either to discontinue drug or bottle feed
- If drug is continued while breast feeding, infant should be monitored for possible adverse effects
- If infant becomes irritable or sedated, breast feeding or drug may need to be discontinued
- ✳ Bipolar disorder may recur during the postpartum period, particularly if there is a history of prior postpartum episodes of either depression or psychosis
- ✳ Relapse rates may be lower in women who receive prophylactic treatment for postpartum episodes of bipolar disorder
- Atypical antipsychotics and anticonvulsants such as valproate may be safer than levetiracetam during the postpartum period when breast feeding

THE ART OF PSYCHOPHARMACOLOGY

Potential Advantages
- Patients on concomitant drugs (lack of drug interactions)
- Treatment-refractory bipolar disorder
- Treatment-refractory neuropathic pain

Potential Disadvantages
- Patients noncompliant with twice daily dosing
- Efficacy for bipolar disorder or neuropathic pain not well documented

Primary Target Symptoms
- Seizures
- Pain
- Mania

 ### Pearls
- Well studied in epilepsy
- ✳ Off-label use second-line and as an augmenting agent may be justified for

bipolar disorder and neuropathic pain unresponsive to other treatments

✳ Unique mechanism of action suggests utility where other anticonvulsants fail to work

✳ Unique mechanism of action as modulator of synaptic vesicle release

suggests theoretical utility for clinical conditions that are hypothetically linked to excessively activated neuronal circuits, such as anxiety disorders and neuropathic pain as well as epilepsy

Suggested Reading

Ben-Menachem E. Levetiracetam: treatment in epilepsy. Expert Opin Pharmacother. 2003;4(11):2079–88.

French J. Use of levetiracetam in special populations. Epilepsia. 2001;42 Suppl 4:40–3.

Leppik IE. Three new drugs for epilepsy: levetiracetam, oxcarbazepine, and zonisamide. J Child Neurol. 2002;17 Suppl 1:S53–7.

Lynch BA, Lambeng N, Nocka K, Kensel-Hammes P, Bajjalieh SM, Matagne A, Fuks B.. The synaptic vesicle protein SV2A is the binding site for the antiepileptic drug levetiracetam. Proc Natl Acad Sci U S A. 2004;101:9861–6.

Pinto A, Sander JW. Levetiracetam: a new therapeutic option for refractory epilepsy. Int J Clin Pract. 2003;57(7):616–21.

LITHIUM

THERAPEUTICS

Brands
- Eskalith
- Eskalith CR
- Lithobid slow release tablets
- Lithostat tablets
- Lithium carbonate tablets
- Lithium citrate syrup

see index for additional brand names

Generic? Yes

Class
- Mood stabilizer

Commonly Prescribed For
(bold for FDA approved)
- **Manic episodes of manic depressive illness**
- **Maintenance treatment for manic depressive patients with a history of mania**
- Bipolar depression
- Major depressive disorder (adjunctive)
- Vascular headache
- Neutropenia

How The Drug Works
- Unknown and complex
- Alters sodium transport across cell membranes in nerve and muscle cells
- Alters metabolism of neurotransmitters including catecholamines and serotonin
- ✳ May alter intracellular signaling through actions on second messenger systems
- Specifically, inhibits inositol monophosphatase, possibly affecting neurotransmission via phosphatidyl inositol second messenger system
- Also reduces protein kinase C activity, possibly affecting genomic expression associated with neurotransmission
- Increases cytoprotective proteins, activates signaling cascade utilized by endogenous growth factors, and increases gray matter content, possibly by activating neurogenesis and enhancing trophic actions that maintain synapses

How Long Until It Works
- 1–3 weeks

If It Works
- The goal of treatment is complete remission of symptoms (i.e., mania and/or depression)
- Continue treatment until all symptoms are gone or until improvement is stable and then continue treating indefinitely as long as improvement persists
- Continue treatment indefinitely to avoid recurrence of mania or depression

If It Doesn't Work
- ✳ Many patients only have a partial response where some symptoms are improved but others persist or continue to wax and wane without stabilization of mood
- Other patients may be nonresponders, sometimes called treatment-resistant or treatment-refractory
- Consider checking plasma drug level, increasing dose, switching to another agent or adding an appropriate augmenting agent
- Consider adding psychotherapy
- Consider the presence of noncompliance and counsel patient
- Switch to another mood stabilizer with fewer side effects
- Consider evaluation for another diagnosis or for a comorbid condition (e.g., medical illness, substance abuse, etc.)

Best Augmenting Combos for Partial Response or Treatment-Resistance

- Valproate
- Atypical antipsychotics (especially risperidone, olanzapine, quetiapine, ziprasidone, and aripiprazole)
- Lamotrigine
- ✳ Antidepressants (with caution because antidepressants can destabilize mood in some patients, including induction of rapid cycling or suicidal ideation; in particular consider bupropion; also SSRIs, SNRIs, others; generally avoid TCAs, MAOIs)

Tests
- ✳ Before initiating treatment, kidney function tests (including creatinine and urine specific gravity) and thyroid function tests; electrocardiogram for patients over 50
- Repeat kidney function tests 1–2 times/year

* Frequent tests to monitor trough lithium plasma levels (should generally be between 1.0 and 1.5 mEq/L for acute treatment, 0.6 and 1.2 mEq/l for chronic treatment)
* Since lithium is frequently associated with weight gain, before starting treatment, weigh all patients and determine if the patient is already overweight (BMI 25.0–29.9) or obese (BMI ≥30)
• Before giving a drug that can cause weight gain to an overweight or obese patient, consider determining whether the patient already has pre-diabetes (fasting plasma glucose 100–125 mg/dl), diabetes (fasting plasma glucose >126 mg/dl), or dyslipidemia (increased total cholesterol, LDL cholesterol and triglycerides; decreased HDL cholesterol), and treat or refer such patients for treatment, including nutrition and weight management, physical activity counseling, smoking cessation, and medical management
* Monitor weight and BMI during treatment
* While giving a drug to a patient who has gained >5% of initial weight, consider evaluating for the presence of pre-diabetes, diabetes, or dyslipidemia, or consider switching to a different agent

---

SIDE EFFECTS

How Drug Causes Side Effects
• Unknown and complex
• CNS side effects theoretically due to excessive actions at the same or similar sites that mediate its therapeutic actions
• Some renal side effects theoretically due to lithium's actions on ion transport

Notable Side Effects
* Ataxia, dysarthria, delirium, tremor, memory problems
* Polyuria, polydipsia (nephrogenic diabetes insipidus)
* Diarrhea, nausea
* Weight gain
• Euthyroid goiter or hypothyroid goiter, possibly with increased TSH and reduced thyroxine levels
• Acne, rash, alopecia
• Leukocytosis

 ### Life Threatening or Dangerous Side Effects
• Lithium toxicity
• Renal impairment (interstitial nephritis)
• Nephrogenic diabetes insipidus
• Arrhythmia, cardiovascular changes, sick sinus syndrome, bradycardia, hypotension
• T wave flattening and inversion
• Rare pseudotumor cerebri
• Rare seizures

Weight Gain

unusual   not unusual   common   problematic
• Many experience and/or can be significant in amount
• Can become a health problem in some
• May be associated with increased appetite

Sedation

unusual   not unusual   common   problematic
• Many experience and/or can be significant in amount
• May wear off with time

What To Do About Side Effects
• Wait
• Wait
• Wait
• Lower the dose
* Take entire dose at night as long as efficacy persists all day long with this administration
* Change to a different lithium preparation (e.g., controlled release)
* Reduce dosing from 3 times/day to 2 times/day
• If signs of lithium toxicity occur, discontinue immediately
• For stomach upset, take with food
• For tremor, avoid caffeine
• Switch to another agent

Best Augmenting Agents for Side Effects
* Propranolol 20–30 mg 2–3 times/day may reduce tremor
• For the expert, cautious addition of a diuretic (e.g., chlorothiazide 50 mg/day) while reducing lithium dose by 50% and monitoring plasma lithium levels may

reduce polydipsia and polyuria that does not go away with time alone
- Many side effects cannot be improved with an augmenting agent

DOSING AND USE

Usual Dosage Range
- 1800 mg/day in divided doses (acute)
- 900–1200 mg/day in divided doses (maintenance)
- Liquid: 10 mL three times/day (acute mania); 5 mL 3–4 times/day (long-term)

Dosage Forms
- Tablet 300 mg (slow release), 450 mg (controlled release)
- Capsule 150 mg, 300 mg, 600 mg
- Liquid 8 mEq/5 mL

How to Dose
- Start 300 mg 2–3 times/day and adjust dosage upward as indicated by plasma lithium levels

 Dosing Tips

* Sustained release formulation may reduce gastric irritation, lower peak lithium plasma levels, and diminish peak dose side effects (i.e., side effects occurring 1–2 hours after each dose of standard lithium carbonate may be improved by sustained release formulation)
- Lithium sulfate and other dosage strengths for lithium are available in Europe
- Check therapeutic blood levels as "trough" levels about 12 hours after the last dose
- After stabilization, some patients may do best with a once daily dose at night
- Responses in acute mania may take 7–14 days even with adequate plasma lithium levels
* Some patients apparently respond to doses as low as 300 mg twice a day, even with plasma lithium levels below 0.5 mEq/L
- Use the lowest dose of lithium associated with adequate therapeutic response
- Lower doses and lower plasma lithium levels (<0.6 mEq/L) are often adequate and advisable in the elderly
* Rapid discontinuation increases the risk of relapse, so lithium may need to be

tapered slowly over 3 months if it is to be discontinued after long-term maintenance

Overdose
- Fatalities have occurred; tremor, dysarthria, delirium, coma, seizures, autonomic instability

Long-Term Use
- Indicated for long-term prevention of relapse
- May cause reduced kidney function
- Requires regular therapeutic monitoring of lithium levels as well as of kidney function and thyroid function

Habit Forming
- No

How to Stop
- Taper gradually over 3 months to avoid relapse
- Rapid discontinuation increases the risk of relapse
- Discontinuation symptoms uncommon

Pharmacokinetics
- Half life 18–30 hours

 Drug Interactions

* Non-steroidal anti-inflammatory agents, including ibuprofen and selective Cox-2 inhibitors (cyclo-oxygenase 2), can increase plasma lithium concentrations; add with caution to patients stabilized on lithium
* Diuretics, especially thiazides, can increase plasma lithium concentrations; add with caution to patients stabilized on lithium
- Angiotensin-converting enzyme inhibitors can increase plasma lithium concentrations; add with caution to patients stabilized on lithium
- Metronidazole can lead to lithium toxicity through decreased renal clearance
- Acetazolamide, alkalizing agents, xanthine preparations, and urea may lower lithium plasma concentrations
- Methyldopa, carbamazepine, and phenytoin may interact with lithium to increase its toxicity

• Use lithium cautiously with calcium channel blockers, which may also increase lithium toxicity
• Use of lithium with an SSRI may raise risk of dizziness, confusion, diarrhea, agitation, tremor
• Some patients taking haloperidol and lithium have developed an encephalopathic syndrome similar to neuroleptic malignant syndrome
• Lithium may prolong effects of neuromuscular blocking agents
• No likely pharmacokinetic interactions of lithium with mood stabilizing anticonvulsants or atypical antipsychotics

 Other Warnings/ Precautions

✼ Toxic levels are near therapeutic levels; signs of toxicity include tremor, ataxia, diarrhea, vomiting, sedation
• Monitor for dehydration; lower dose if patient exhibits signs of infection, excessive sweating, diarrhea
• Closely monitor patients with thyroid disorders

Do Not Use

• If patient has severe kidney disease
• If patient has severe cardiovascular disease
• If patient has severe dehydration
• If patient has sodium depletion
• If there is a proven allergy to lithium

SPECIAL POPULATIONS

Renal Impairment
• Not recommended for use in patients with severe impairment

Hepatic Impairment
• No special indications

Cardiac Impairment
• Not recommended for use in patients with severe impairment

Elderly
• Likely that elderly patients will require lower doses to achieve therapeutic serum levels
• Elderly patients may be more sensitive to adverse effects

✼ Neurotoxicity, including delirium and other mental status changes, may occur even at therapeutic doses in elderly and organically compromised patients
• Lower doses and lower plasma lithium levels (<0.6 mEg/L) are often adequate and advisable in the elderly

 Children and Adolescents

• Safety and efficacy not established under age 12
• Use only with caution
• Younger children tend to have more frequent and severe side effects
• Children should be monitored more frequently

 Pregnancy

• Risk category D [positive evidence of risk to human fetus; potential benefits may still justify its use during pregnancy]
✼ Evidence of increased risk of major birth defects (perhaps 2–3 times the general population), but probably lower than with some other mood stabilizers (e.g., valproate)
• Evidence of increase in cardiac anomalies (especially Ebstein's anomaly) in infants whose mothers took lithium during pregnancy
• Lithium administration during delivery may be associated with hypotonia in the infant
• Use in women of childbearing potential requires weighing potential benefits to the mother against the risks to the fetus
• Taper drug if discontinuing
✼ For bipolar patients, lithium should generally be discontinued before anticipated pregnancies
• Recurrent bipolar illness during pregnancy can be quite disruptive
✼ For bipolar patients, given the risk of relapse in the postpartum period, lithium should generally be restarted immediately after delivery, but this generally means no breast feeding
✼ Atypical antipsychotics may be preferable to lithium or anticonvulsants if treatment of bipolar disorder is required during pregnancy

- Bipolar symptoms may recur or worsen during pregnancy and some form of treatment may be necessary

Breast Feeding
- Some drug is found in mother's breast milk, possibly at full therapeutic levels since lithium is soluble in breast milk
- ✳ Recommended either to discontinue drug or bottle feed
- ✳ Bipolar disorder may recur during the postpartum period, particularly if there is a history of prior postpartum episodes of either depression or psychosis
- ✳ Relapse rates may be lower in women who receive prophylactic treatment for postpartum episodes of bipolar disorder
- Atypical antipsychotics and anticonvulsants such as valproate may be safer than lithium during the postpartum period when breast feeding

THE ART OF PSYCHOPHARMACOLOGY

Potential Advantages
- Euphoric mania
- Treatment-resistant depression
- Reduces suicide risk
- Works well in combination with atypical antipsychotics and/or mood stabilizing anticonvulsants such as valproate

Potential Disadvantages
- Dysphoric mania
- Mixed mania, rapid-cycling mania
- Depressed phase of bipolar disorder
- Patients unable to tolerate weight gain, sedation, gastrointestinal effects, renal effects, and other side effects

Primary Target Symptoms
- Unstable mood
- Mania

 Pearls

- ✳ Lithium was the original mood stabilizer and is still a first-line treatment option but may be underutilized since it is an older agent and is less promoted for use in bipolar disorder than newer agents
- ✳ May be best for euphoric mania; patients with rapid-cycling and mixed state types of

bipolar disorder generally do less well on lithium
- ✳ Seems to be more effective in treating manic episodes than depressive episodes in bipolar disorder (treats from above better than it treats from below)
- ✳ May also be more effective in preventing manic relapses than in preventing depressive episodes (stabilizes from above better than it stabilizes from below)
- ✳ May decrease suicide and suicide attempts not only in bipolar I disorder but also in bipolar II disorder and in unipolar depression
- ✳ Due to its narrow therapeutic index, lithium's toxic side effects occur at doses close to its therapeutic effects
- Close therapeutic monitoring of plasma drug levels is required during lithium treatment; lithium is the first psychiatric drug that required blood level monitoring
- Probably less effective than atypical antipsychotics for severe, excited, disturbed, hyperactive, or psychotic patients with mania
- Due to delayed onset of action, lithium monotherapy may not be the first choice in acute mania, but rather may be used as an adjunct to atypical antipsychotics, benzodiazepines, and/or valproate loading
- After acute symptoms of mania are controlled, some patients can be maintained on lithium monotherapy
- However, only a third of bipolar patients experience adequate relief with a monotherapy, so most patients need multiple medications for best control
- Lithium is not a convincing augmentation agent to atypical antipsychotics for the treatment of schizophrenia
- Lithium is one of the most useful adjunctive agents to augment antidepressants for treatment-resistant unipolar depression
- Lithium may be useful for a number of patients with episodic, recurrent symptoms with or without affective illness, including episodic rage, anger or violence, and self-destructive behavior; such symptoms may be associated with psychotic or nonpsychotic illnesses, personality disorders, organic disorders, or mental retardation

- Lithium is better tolerated during acute manic phases than when manic symptoms have abated
- Adverse effects generally increase in incidence and severity as lithium serum levels increase
- Although not recommended for use in patients with severe renal or cardiovascular disease, dehydration, or sodium depletion, lithium can be administered cautiously in a hospital setting to such patients, with lithium serum levels determined daily
- Lithium-induced weight gain may be more common in women than in men

Suggested Reading

Delva NJ, Hawken ER. Preventing lithium intoxication. Guide for physicians. Can Fam Physician. 2001;47:1595–600.

Goodwin FK. Rationale for using lithium in combination with other mood stabilizers in the management of bipolar disorder. J Clin Psychiatry. 2003;64(Suppl 5):18–24.

Goodwin GM, Geddes GR. Latest maintenance data on lithium in bipolar disorder. Eur Neuropsychopharmacol. 2003;13(Suppl 2):S51–5.

Maj M. The effect of lithium in bipolar disorder: a review of recent research evidence. Bipolar Disord. 2003;5:180–8.

Tueth MJ, Murphy TK, Evans DL. Special considerations: use of lithium in children, adolescents, and elderly populations. J Clin Psychiatry. 1998;59 (Suppl 6):66–73.

LOFEPRAMINE

Brands • Deprimyl
• Gamanil
see index for additional brand names

Generic? Yes

Class
• Tricyclic antidepressant (TCA)
• Predominantly a norepinephrine/
noradrenaline reuptake inhibitor

Commonly Prescribed For
(bold for FDA approved)
• Major depressive disorder
• Anxiety
• Insomnia
• Neuropathic pain/chronic pain
• Treatment-resistant depression

How The Drug Works
• Boosts neurotransmitter
norepinephrine/noradrenaline
• Blocks norepinephrine reuptake pump
(norepinephrine transporter), presumably
increasing noradrenergic
neurotransmission
• Since dopamine is inactivated by
norepinephrine reuptake in frontal cortex,
which largely lacks dopamine transporters,
lofepramine can increase dopamine
neurotransmission in this part of the brain
• A more potent inhibitor of norepinephrine
reuptake pump than serotonin reuptake
pump (serotonin transporter)
• At high doses may also boost
neurotransmitter serotonin and presumably
increase serotonergic neurotransmission

How Long Until It Works
• May have immediate effects in treating
insomnia or anxiety
• Onset of therapeutic actions usually not
immediate, but often delayed 2 to 4 weeks
• If it is not working within 6 to 8 weeks for
depression, it may require a dosage
increase or it may not work at all
• May continue to work for many years to
prevent relapse of symptoms

If It Works
• The goal of treatment of depression is
complete remission of current symptoms
as well as prevention of future relapses
• The goal of treatment of chronic
neuropathic pain is to reduce symptoms as
much as possible, especially in
combination with other treatments
• Treatment of depression most often
reduces or even eliminates symptoms, but
not a cure since symptoms can recur after
medicine stopped
• Treatment of chronic neuropathic pain may
reduce symptoms, but rarely eliminates
them completely, and is not a cure since
symptoms can recur after medicine is
stopped
• Continue treatment of depression until all
symptoms are gone (remission)
• Once symptoms of depression are gone,
continue treating for 1 year for the first
episode of depression
• For second and subsequent episodes of
depression, treatment may need to be
indefinite
• Use in anxiety disorders and chronic pain
may also need to be indefinite, but long-
term treatment is not well studied in these
conditions

If It Doesn't Work
• Many depressed patients only have a
partial response where some symptoms
are improved but others persist (especially
insomnia, fatigue, and problems
concentrating)
• Other depressed patients may be
nonresponders, sometimes called
treatment-resistant or treatment-refractory
• Consider increasing dose, switching to
another agent or adding an appropriate
augmenting agent
• Consider psychotherapy
• Consider evaluation for another diagnosis
or for a comorbid condition (e.g, medical
illness, substance abuse, etc.)
• Some patients may experience apparent
lack of consistent efficacy due to activation
of latent or underlying bipolar disorder, and
require antidepressant discontinuation and
a switch to a mood stabilizer

Best Augmenting Combos for Partial Response or Treatment-Resistance

- Lithium, buspirone, thyroid hormone (for depression)
- Gabapentin, tiagabine, other anticonvulsants, even opiates if done by experts while monitoring carefully in difficult cases (for chronic pain)

Tests

- None for healthy individuals
- ✳ Since tricyclic and tetracyclic antidepressants are frequently associated with weight gain, before starting treatment, weigh all patients and determine if the patient is already overweight (BMI 25.0–29.9) or obese (BMI ≥30)
- Before giving a drug that can cause weight gain to an overweight or obese patient, consider determining whether the patient already has pre-diabetes (fasting plasma glucose 100–125 mg/dl), diabetes (fasting plasma glucose >126 mg/dl), or dyslipidemia (increased total cholesterol, LDL cholesterol and triglycerides; decreased HDL cholesterol), and treat or refer such patients for treatment, including nutrition and weight management, physical activity counseling, smoking cessation, and medical management
- ✳ Monitor weight and BMI during treatment
- ✳ While giving a drug to a patient who has gained >5% of initial weight, consider evaluating for the presence of pre-diabetes, diabetes, or dyslipidemia, or consider switching to a different antidepressant
- EKGs may be useful for selected patients (e.g., those with personal or family history of QTc prolongation; cardiac arrhythmia; recent myocardial infarction; uncompensated heart failure; or taking agents that prolong QTc interval such as pimozide, thioridazine, selected antiarrhythmics, moxifloxacin, sparfloxacin, etc.)
- Patients at risk for electrolyte disturbances (e.g., patients on diuretic therapy) should have baseline and periodic serum potassium and magnesium measurements

SIDE EFFECTS

How Drug Causes Side Effects

- Anticholinergic activity may explain sedative effects, dry mouth, constipation, and blurred vision
- Sedative effects and weight gain may be due to antihistamine properties
- Blockade of alpha adrenergic 1 receptors may explain dizziness, sedation, and hypotension
- Cardiac arrhythmias and seizures, especially in overdose, may be caused by blockade of ion channels

Notable Side Effects

- Blurred vision, constipation, urinary retention, increased appetite, dry mouth, nausea, diarrhea, heartburn, unusual taste in mouth, weight gain
- Fatigue, weakness, dizziness, sedation, headache, anxiety, nervousness, restlessness
- Sexual dysfunction, sweating

Life Threatening or Dangerous Side Effects

- Paralytic ileus, hyperthermia (TCAs + anticholinergic agents)
- Lowered seizure threshold and rare seizures
- Orthostatic hypotension, sudden death, arrhythmias, tachycardia
- QTc prolongation
- Hepatic failure, extrapyramidal symptoms
- Increased intraocular pressure
- Rare induction of mania and activation of suicidal ideation

Weight Gain

unusual   not unusual   common   problematic

- Many experience and/or can be significant in amount
- Can increase appetite and carbohydrate craving

Sedation

unusual   not unusual   common   problematic

- Many experience and/or can be significant in amount
- Tolerance to sedative effect may develop with long-term use

What To Do About Side Effects
- Wait
- Wait
- Wait
- Lower the dose
- Switch to an SSRI or newer antidepressant

Best Augmenting Agents for Side Effects
- Many side effects cannot be improved with an augmenting agent

DOSING AND USE

Usual Dosage Range
- 140–210 mg/day

Dosage Forms
- Tablet 70 mg multiscored
- Liquid 70 mg/5mL

How to Dose
- Initial 70 mg/day once daily or in divided doses; gradually increase daily dose to achieve desired therapeutic effects; dose at bedtime for daytime sedation and in morning for insomnia; maximum dose 280 mg/day for inpatients, 210 mg/day for outpatients

 Dosing Tips
- If given in a single dose, should generally be administered at bedtime because of its sedative properties
- If given in split doses, largest dose should generally be given at bedtime because of its sedative properties
- If patients experience nightmares, split dose and do not give large dose at bedtime
- Unusual dose compared to most TCAs
- Patients treated for chronic pain may only require lower doses
- If intolerable anxiety, insomnia, agitation, akathisia, or activation occur either upon dosing initiation or discontinuation, consider the possibility of activated bipolar disorder, and switch to a mood stabilizer or an atypical antipsychotic

Overdose
- Death may occur; convulsions, cardiac dysrhythmias, severe hypotension, CNS depression, coma, changes in ECG

Long-Term Use
- Safe

Habit Forming
- No

How to Stop
- Taper to avoid withdrawal effects
- Even with gradual dose reduction some withdrawal symptoms may appear within the first 2 weeks
- Many patients tolerate 50% dose reduction for 3 days, then another 50% reduction for 3 days, then discontinuation
- If withdrawal symptoms emerge during discontinuation, raise dose to stop symptoms and then restart withdrawal much more slowly

Pharmacokinetics
- Substrate for CYP450 2D6
- Half-life of parent compound approximately 1.5–6 hours
- ✳ Major metabolite is the antidepressant desipramine, with a half-life of approximately 24 hours

 Drug Interactions
- Tramadol increases the risk of seizures in patients taking TCAs
- Use of TCAs with anticholinergic drugs may result in paralytic ileus or hyperthermia
- Fluoxetine, paroxetine, bupropion, duloxetine, and other CYP450 2D6 inhibitors may increase TCA concentrations
- Cimetidine may increase plasma concentrations of TCAs and cause anticholinergic symptoms
- Phenothiazines or haloperidol may raise TCA blood concentrations
- May alter effects of antihypertensive drugs; may inhibit hypotensive effects of clonidine
- Use with sympathomimetic agents may increase sympathetic activity
- Methylphenidate may inhibit metabolism of TCAs
- Activation and agitation, especially following switching or adding

antidepressants, may represent the induction of a bipolar state, especially a mixed dysphoric bipolar II condition sometimes associated with suicidal ideation, and require the addition of lithium, a mood stabilizer or an atypical antipsychotic, and/or discontinuation of lofepramine

 Other Warnings/ Precautions

- Add or initiate other antidepressants with caution for up to 2 weeks after discontinuing lofepramine
- Generally, do not use with MAO inhibitors, including 14 days after MAOIs are stopped; do not start an MAOI until 2 weeks after discontinuing lofepramine, but see Pearls
- Use with caution in patients with history of seizure, urinary retention, narrow angle-closure glaucoma, hyperthyroidism
- TCAs can increase QTc interval, especially at toxic doses, which can be attained not only by overdose but also by combining with drugs that inhibit its metabolism via CYP450 2D6, potentially causing torsade de pointes-type arrhythmia or sudden death
- Because TCAs can prolong QTc interval, use with caution in patients who have bradycardia or who are taking drugs that can induce bradycardia (e.g., beta blockers, calcium channel blockers, clonidine, digitalis)
- Because TCAs can prolong QTc interval, use with caution in patients who have hypokalemia and/or hypomagnesemia or who are taking drugs that can induce hypokalemia and/or magnesemia (e.g., diuretics, stimulant laxatives, intravenous amphotericin B, glucocorticoids, tetracosactide)

Do Not Use

- If patient is recovering from myocardial infarction
- If patient is taking agents capable of significantly prolonging QTc interval (e.g., pimozide, thioridazine, selected antiarrhythmics, moxifloxacin, sparfloxacin)
- If there is a history of QTc prolongation or cardiac arrhythmia, recent acute

myocardial infarction, uncompensated heart failure
- If patient is taking drugs that inhibit TCA metabolism, including CYP450 2D6 inhibitors, except by an expert
- If there is reduced CYP450 2D6 function, such as patients who are poor 2D6 metabolizers, except by an expert and at low doses
- If there is a proven allergy to lofepramine, desipramine, or imipramine

SPECIAL POPULATIONS

Renal Impairment
- Use with caution

Hepatic Impairment
- Use with caution

Cardiac Impairment

- TCAs have been reported to cause arrhythmias, prolongation of conduction time, orthostatic hypotension, sinus tachycardia, and heart failure, especially in the diseased heart
- Myocardial infarction and stroke have been reported with TCAs
- TCAs produce QTc prolongation, which may be enhanced by the existence of bradycardia, hypokalemia, congenital or acquired long QTc interval, which should be evaluated prior to administering lofepramine
- Use with caution if treating concomitantly with a medication likely to produce prolonged bradycardia, hypokalemia, slowing of intracardiac conduction, or prolongation of the QTc interval
- Avoid TCAs in patients with a known history of QTc prolongation, recent acute myocardial infarction, and uncompensated heart failure
- TCAs may cause a sustained increase in heart rate in patients with ischemic heart disease and may worsen (decrease) heart rate variability, an independent risk of mortality in cardiac populations
- Since SSRIs may improve (increase) heart rate variability in patients following a myocardial infarct and may improve survival as well as mood in patients with acute angina or following a myocardial infarction, these are more appropriate

agents for cardiac population than tricyclic/tetracyclic antidepressants

✳ Risk/benefit ratio may not justify use of TCAs in cardiac impairment

Elderly

- May be more sensitive to anticholinergic, cardiovascular, hypotensive, and sedative effects

 Children and Adolescents

- Use with caution, observing for activation of known or unknown bipolar disorder and/or suicidal ideation, and strongly consider informing parents or guardian of this risk so they can help observe child or adolescent patients
- Not recommended for use under age 18
- Several studies show lack of efficacy of TCAs for depression
- May be used to treat enuresis or hyperactive/impulsive behaviors
- Some cases of sudden death have occurred in children taking TCAs

 Pregnancy

- Risk Category C [some animal studies show adverse effects, no controlled studies in humans]
- Crosses the placenta
- Adverse effects have been reported in infants whose mothers took a TCA (lethargy, withdrawal symptoms, fetal malformations)
- Not generally recommended for use during pregnancy, especially during first trimester
- Must weigh the risk of treatment (first trimester fetal development, third trimester newborn delivery) to the child against the risk of no treatment (recurrence of depression, maternal health, infant bonding) to the mother and child
- For many patients this may mean continuing treatment during pregnancy

Breast Feeding

- Some drug is found in mother's breast milk
- ✳ Recommended either to discontinue drug or bottle feed
- Immediate postpartum period is a high-risk time for depression, especially in women who have had prior depressive episodes, so drug may need to be reinstituted late in the third trimester or shortly after childbirth to prevent a recurrence during the postpartum period
- Must weigh benefits of breast feeding with risks and benefits of antidepressant treatment versus non-treatment to both the infant and the mother
- For many patients this may mean continuing treatment during breast feeding

THE ART OF PSYCHOPHARMACOLOGY

Potential Advantages

- Patients with insomnia
- Severe or treatment-resistant depression
- Anxious depression

Potential Disadvantages

- Pediatric and geriatric patients
- Patients concerned with weight gain
- Cardiac patients

Primary Target Symptoms

- Depressed mood

 Pearls

- Tricyclic antidepressants are often a first-line treatment option for chronic pain
- Tricyclic antidepressants are no longer generally considered a first-line option for depression because of their side effect profile
- Tricyclic antidepressants continue to be useful for severe or treatment-resistant depression
- Noradrenergic reuptake inhibitors such as lofepramine can be used as a second-line treatment for smoking cessation, cocaine dependence, and attention deficit disorder
- ✳ Lofepramine is a short acting prodrug of the TCA desipramine
- ✳ Fewer anticholinergic side effects, particularly sedation, than some other tricyclics
- Once a popular TCA in the UK, but not widely marketed throughout the world
- TCAs may aggravate psychotic symptoms
- Alcohol should be avoided because of additive CNS effects

- Underweight patients may be more susceptible to adverse cardiovascular effects
- Children, patients with inadequate hydration, and patients with cardiac disease may be more susceptible to TCA-induced cardiotoxicity than healthy adults
- For the expert only: although generally prohibited, a heroic treatment (but potentially dangerous) for severely treatment-resistant patients is to give a tricyclic/tetracyclic antidepressant other than clomipramine simultaneously with an MAO inhibitor for patients who fail to respond to numerous other antidepressants
- If this option is elected, start the MAOI with the tricyclic/tetracyclic antidepressant simultaneously at low doses after appropriate drug washout, then alternately increase doses of these agents every few days to a week as tolerated
- Although very strict dietary and concomitant drug restrictions must be observed to prevent hypertensive crises and serotonin syndrome, the most common side effects of MAOI/tricyclic or tetracyclic combinations may be weight gain and orthostatic hypotension
- Patients on TCAs should be aware that they may experience symptoms such as photosensitivity or blue-green urine
- SSRIs may be more effective than TCAs in women, and TCAs may be more effective than SSRIs in men
- Since tricyclic/tetracyclic antidepressants are substrates for CYP450 2D6, and 7% of the population (especially Caucasians) may have a genetic variant leading to reduced activity of 2D6, such patients may not safely tolerate normal doses of tricyclic/tetracyclic antidepressants and may require dose reduction
- Phenotypic testing may be necessary to detect this genetic variant prior to dosing with a tricyclic/tetracyclic antidepressant, especially in vulnerable populations such as children, elderly, cardiac populations, and those on concomitant medications
- Patients who seem to have extraordinarily severe side effects at normal or low doses may have this phenotypic CYP450 2D6 variant and require low doses or switching to another antidepressant not metabolized by 2D6

 Suggested Reading

Anderson IM. Meta-analytical studies on new antidepressants. Br Med Bull. 2001; 57:161–178.

Anderson IM. Selective serotonin reuptake inhibitors versus tricyclic antidepressants: a meta-analysis of efficacy and tolerability. J Aff Disorders. 2000;58:19–36.

Kerihuel JC, Dreyfus JF. Meta-analyses of the efficacy and tolerability of the tricyclic antidepressant lofepramine. J Int Med Res. 1991;19:183–201.

Lancaster SG, Gonzales JP. Lofepramine. A review of its pharmacodynamic and pharmacokinetic properties, and therapeutic efficacy in depressive illness. Drugs. 1989; 37:123–40.

LOFLAZEPATE

THERAPEUTICS

Brands • Meilax
see index for additional brand names

Generic? No

Class
• Benzodiazepine (anxiolytic)

Commonly Prescribed For
(bold for FDA approved)
• Anxiety, tension, depression, or sleep disorder in patients with neurosis
• Anxiety, tension, depression, or sleep disorder in patients with psychosomatic disease

 How The Drug Works
• Binds to benzodiazepine receptors at the GABA-A ligand-gated chloride channel complex
• Enhances the inhibitory effects of GABA
• Boosts chloride conductance through GABA-regulated channels
• Inhibits neuronal activity presumably in amygdala-centered fear circuits to provide therapeutic benefits in anxiety disorders

How Long Until It Works
• Some immediate relief with first dosing is common; can take several weeks with daily dosing for maximal therapeutic benefit

If It Works
• For short-term symptoms of anxiety – after a few weeks, discontinue use or use on an "as-needed" basis
• For chronic anxiety disorders, the goal of treatment is complete remission of symptoms as well as prevention of future relapses
• For chronic anxiety disorders, treatment most often reduces or even eliminates symptoms, but not a cure since symptoms can recur after medicine stopped
• For long-term symptoms of anxiety, consider switching to an SSRI or SNRI for long-term maintenance
• If long-term maintenance with a benzodiazepine is necessary, continue treatment for 6 months after symptoms resolve, and then taper dose slowly

• If symptoms reemerge, consider treatment with an SSRI or SNRI, or consider restarting the benzodiazepine; sometimes benzodiazepines have to be used in combination with SSRIs or SNRIs for best results

If It Doesn't Work
• Consider switching to another agent or adding an appropriate augmenting agent
• Consider psychotherapy, especially cognitive behavioral psychotherapy
• Consider presence of concomitant substance abuse
• Consider presence of loflazepate abuse
• Consider another diagnosis, such as a comorbid medical condition

 Best Augmenting Combos for Partial Response or Treatment-Resistance
• Benzodiazepines are frequently used as augmenting agents for antipsychotics and mood stabilizers in the treatment of psychotic and bipolar disorders
• Benzodiazepines are frequently used as augmenting agents for SSRIs and SNRIs in the treatment of anxiety disorders
• Not generally rational to combine with other benzodiazepines
• Caution if using as an anxiolytic concomitantly with other sedative hypnotics for sleep

Tests
• In patients with seizure disorders, concomitant medical illness, and/or those with multiple concomitant long-term medications, periodic liver tests and blood counts may be prudent

SIDE EFFECTS

How Drug Causes Side Effects
• Same mechanism for side effects as for therapeutic effects – namely due to excessive actions at benzodiazepine receptors
• Long-term adaptations in benzodiazepine receptors may explain the development of dependence, tolerance, and withdrawal
• Side effects are generally immediate, but immediate side effects often disappear in time

Notable Side Effects

* ✳ Sedation, fatigue, depression
* ✳ Dizziness, ataxia, slurred speech, weakness
* ✳ Forgetfulness, confusion
* ✳ Hyper-excitability, nervousness
* Rare hallucinations, mania
* Rare hypotension
* Hypersalivation, dry mouth

 Life Threatening or Dangerous Side Effects

* Respiratory depression, especially when taken with CNS depressants in overdose
* Rare hepatic dysfunction, renal dysfunction, blood dyscrasias

Weight Gain

unusual   not unusual   common   problematic

* Reported but not expected

Sedation

unusual   not unusual   common   problematic

* Occurs in significant minority
* Especially at initiation of treatment or when dose increases
* Tolerance often develops over time

What To Do About Side Effects

* Wait
* Wait
* Wait
* Lower the dose
* Take largest dose at bedtime to avoid sedative effects during the day
* Switch to another agent
* Administer flumazenil if side effects are severe or life-threatening

Best Augmenting Agents for Side Effects

* Many side effects cannot be improved with an augmenting agent

---

DOSING AND USE

Usual Dosage Range

* 1mg once or twice a day

Dosage Forms

* Tablet 1 mg, 2 mg

How to Dose

* Start at 1 mg, increase to 1mg twice/day or 2 mg once a day in a few days if necessary

 Dosing Tips

* ✳ Because of its long half-life, patients who require chronic treatment may need dose reduction after a few weeks due to drug accumulation
* ✳ Because of its long half-life, once daily dosing is the most frequent dosing generally necessary
* ✳ Because of its long half-life, some patients may have sustained benefits even if dosing is intermittently skipped on some days
* Use lowest possible effective dose for the shortest possible period of time (a benzodiazepine-sparing strategy)
* Assess need for continued treatment regularly
* Risk of dependence may increase with dose and duration of treatment
* For inter-dose symptoms of anxiety, can either increase dose or maintain same total daily dose but divide into more frequent doses
* Can also use an as-needed occasional "top up" dose for inter-dose anxiety
* Because panic disorder can require doses higher than 2 mg/day, the risk of dependence may be greater in these patients
* Some severely ill patients may require more than 2 mg/day
* Frequency of dosing in practice is often greater than predicted from half-life, as duration of biological activity is often shorter than pharmacokinetic terminal half-life, which is why once daily dosing is usually the favored option despite the long half-life

Overdose

* Sedation, confusion, poor coordination, diminished reflexes, coma

Long-Term Use

* Risk of dependence, particularly for treatment periods longer than 12 weeks and especially in patients with past or current polysubstance abuse

Habit Forming
- Patients may develop dependence and/or tolerance with long-term use

How to Stop
- Patients with history of seizures may seize upon withdrawal, especially if withdrawal is abrupt
- Taper by 0.5 mg every 3–7 days to reduce chances of withdrawal effects
- For difficult to taper cases, consider reducing dose much more slowly after reaching 3 mg/day, perhaps by as little as 0.25 mg every 7–10 days or slower
- For other patients with severe problems discontinuing a benzodiazepine, dosing may need to be tapered over many months (i.e., reduce dose by 1% every 3 days by crushing tablet and suspending or dissolving in 100 ml of fruit juice and then disposing of 1 ml while drinking the rest; 3–7 days later, dispose of 2 ml, and so on). This is both a form of very slow biological tapering and a form of behavioral desensitization
- Be sure to differentiate reemergence of symptoms requiring reinstitution of treatment from withdrawal symptoms
- Benzodiazepine-dependent anxiety patients and insulin-dependent diabetics are not addicted to their medications. When benzodiazepine-dependent patients stop their medication, disease symptoms can reemerge, disease symptoms can worsen (rebound), and/or withdrawal symptoms can emerge

Pharmacokinetics
- Elimination half-life approximately 122 hours (ultra-long half-life)

 Drug Interactions
- Increased depressive effects when taken with other CNS depressants
- Cimetidine raises loflazepate plasma levels
- Rapid dose reduction or discontinuation of loflazepate during concomitant use with tetracyclic antidepressants such as maprotiline may result in convulsive seizures, possibly due to the loss of anticonvulsant actions that suppress the pro-convulsant actions of tetracyclic antidepressants

 Other Warnings/ Precautions
- Dosage changes should be made in collaboration with prescriber
- Use with caution in patients with pulmonary disease; rare reports of death after initiation of benzodiazepines in patients with severe pulmonary impairment
- History of drug or alcohol abuse often creates greater risk for dependency
- Hypomania and mania have occurred in depressed patients taking loflazepate
- Use only with extreme caution if patient has obstructive sleep apnea
- Some depressed patients may experience a worsening of suicidal ideation
- Some patients may exhibit abnormal thinking or behavioral changes similar to those caused by other CNS depressants (i.e., either depressant actions or disinhibiting actions)

Do Not Use
- If patient has narrow angle-closure glaucoma
- If patient has myasthenia gravis
- If there is a proven allergy to loflazepate or any benzodiazepine

SPECIAL POPULATIONS

Renal Impairment
- Drug should be used with caution

Hepatic Impairment
- Drug should be used with caution

Cardiac Impairment
- Benzodiazepines have been used to treat anxiety associated with acute myocardial infarction

Elderly
- Drug should be used with caution
- Should begin with lower starting dose

 Children and Adolescents
- Safety and efficacy have not been established
- Benzodiazepines are often used in children and adolescents, especially short-term and at the lower end of the dosing scale

- Long-term effects of loflazepate in children/adolescents are unknown
- Should generally receive lower doses and be more closely monitored

Pregnancy

- Possible increased risk of birth defects when benzodiazepines taken during pregnancy
- Because of the potential risks, loflazepate is not generally recommended as treatment for anxiety during pregnancy, especially during the first trimester
- Drug should be tapered if discontinued
- Infants whose mothers received a benzodiazepine late in pregnancy may experience withdrawal effects
- Neonatal flaccidity has been reported in infants whose mothers took a benzodiazepine during pregnancy
- Seizures, even mild seizures, may cause harm to the embryo/fetus

Breast Feeding

- Some drug is found in mother's breast milk
- ✱ Recommended either to discontinue drug or bottle feed
- Effects on infant have been observed and include feeding difficulties, sedation, and weight loss

THE ART OF PSYCHOPHARMACOLOGY

Potential Advantages

- Patients who have inter-dose anxiety on shorter-acting benzodiazepines
- Patients who wish to take drug only once daily
- Patients who occasionally forget to take their dose

Potential Disadvantages

- Drug may accumulate in long-term users and require dosage reduction

Primary Target Symptoms

- Anxiety
- Tension

Pearls

- ✱ Is the only "ultra-long half-life" benzodiazepine with a half-life much longer than 24 hours
- ✱ Less inter-dose anxiety than other benzodiazepines
- ✱ Long half-life could theoretically reduce abuse and withdrawal symptoms
- Is a very useful adjunct to SSRIs and SNRIs in the treatment of numerous anxiety disorders
- Not effective for treating psychosis as a monotherapy, but can be used as an adjunct to antipsychotics
- Not effective for treating bipolar disorder as a monotherapy, but can be used as an adjunct to mood stabilizers and antipsychotics
- May both cause depression and treat depression in different patients
- Risk of seizure is greatest during the first 3 days after discontinuation of loflazepate, especially in those with prior seizures, head injuries or withdrawal from drugs of abuse
- Clinical duration of action may be shorter than plasma half-life, leading to dosing more frequently than 2–3 times daily in some patients
- When using to treat insomnia, remember that insomnia may be a symptom of some other primary disorder itself, and thus warrant evaluation for comorbid psychiatric and/or medical conditions

Suggested Reading

Ba BB, Iliadis A, Cano JP. Pharmacokinetic modeling of ethyl loflazepate (Victan) and its main active metabolites. Ann Biomed Eng. 1989;17(6):633–46.

Chambon JP, Perio A, Demarne H, Hallot A, Dantzer R, Roncucci R, Biziere K. Ethyl loflazepate: a prodrug from the benzodiazepine series designed to dissociate anxiolytic and sedative activities. Arzneimittelforschung. 1985;35(10):1573–7.

Murasaki M, Mori A, Noguchi T, Hada Y, Hasegawa K, Jinbo S, Kamijima K. Comparison of therapeutic efficacy of neuroses between CM6912 (ethyl loflazepate) and diazepam in a double-blind trial. Prog Neuropsychopharmacol Biol Psychiatry. 1989;13(1–2):145–54.

LORAZEPAM

THERAPEUTICS

Brands • Ativan
see index for additional brand names

Generic? Yes

Class
• Benzodiazepine (anxiolytic, anticonvulsant)

Commonly Prescribed For
(bold for FDA approved)
• **Anxiety disorder (oral)**
• **Anxiety associated with depressive symptoms (oral)**
• **Initial treatment of status epilepticus (injection)**
• **Preanesthetic (injection)**
• Insomnia
• Muscle spasm
• Alcohol withdrawal psychosis
• Headache
• Panic disorder
• Acute mania (adjunctive)
• Acute psychosis (adjunctive)

How The Drug Works
• Binds to benzodiazepine receptors at the GABA-A ligand-gated chloride channel complex
• Enhances the inhibitory effects of GABA
• Boosts chloride conductance through GABA-regulated channels
• Inhibits neuronal activity presumably in amygdala-centered fear circuits to provide therapeutic benefits in anxiety disorders
• Inhibitory actions in cerebral cortex may provide therapeutic benefits in seizure disorders

How Long Until It Works
• Some immediate relief with first dosing is common; can take several weeks for maximal therapeutic benefit with daily dosing

If It Works
• For short-term symptoms of anxiety – after a few weeks, discontinue use or use on an "as-needed" basis
• For chronic anxiety disorders, the goal of treatment is complete remission of symptoms as well as prevention of future relapses
• For chronic anxiety disorders, treatment most often reduces or even eliminates symptoms, but not a cure since symptoms can recur after medicine stopped
• For long-term symptoms of anxiety, consider switching to an SSRI or SNRI for long-term maintenance
• If long-term maintenance with a benzodiazepine is necessary, continue treatment for 6 months after symptoms resolve, and then taper dose slowly
• If symptoms reemerge, consider treatment with an SSRI or SNRI, or consider restarting the benzodiazepine; sometimes benzodiazepines have to be used in combination with SSRIs or SNRIs for best results

If It Doesn't Work
• Consider switching to another agent or adding an appropriate augmenting agent
• Consider psychotherapy, especially cognitive behavioral psychotherapy
• Consider presence of concomitant substance abuse
• Consider presence of lorazepam abuse
• Consider another diagnosis such as a comorbid medical condition

Best Augmenting Combos for Partial Response or Treatment-Resistance
• Benzodiazepines are frequently used as augmenting agents for antipsychotics and mood stabilizers in the treatment of psychotic and bipolar disorders
• Benzodiazepines are frequently used as augmenting agents for SSRIs and SNRIs in the treatment of anxiety disorders
• Not generally rational to combine with other benzodiazepines
• Caution if using as an anxiolytic concomitantly with other sedative hypnotics for sleep

Tests
• In patients with seizure disorders, concomitant medical illness, and/or those with multiple concomitant long-term medications, periodic liver tests and blood counts may be prudent

SIDE EFFECTS

How Drug Causes Side Effects
- Same mechanism for side effects as for therapeutic effects – namely due to excessive actions at benzodiazepine receptors
- Long-term adaptations in benzodiazepine receptors may explain the development of dependence, tolerance, and withdrawal
- Side effects are generally immediate, but immediate side effects often disappear in time

Notable Side Effects
* Sedation, fatigue, depression
* Dizziness, ataxia, slurred speech, weakness
* Forgetfulness, confusion
* Hyper-excitability, nervousness
* Pain at injection site
- Rare hallucinations, mania
- Rare hypotension
- Hypersalivation, dry mouth

Life Threatening or Dangerous Side Effects
- Respiratory depression, especially when taken with CNS depressants in overdose
- Rare hepatic dysfunction, renal dysfunction, blood dyscrasias

Weight Gain

unusual   not unusual   common   problematic

- Reported but not expected

Sedation

unusual   not unusual   **common**   problematic

- Many experience and/or can be significant in amount
- Especially at initiation of treatment or when dose increases
- Tolerance often develops over time

What To Do About Side Effects
- Wait
- Wait
- Wait
- Lower the dose
- Take largest dose at bedtime to avoid sedative effects during the day
- Switch to another agent

- Administer flumazenil if side effects are severe or life-threatening

Best Augmenting Agents for Side Effects
- Many side effects cannot be improved with an augmenting agent

DOSING AND USE

Usual Dosage Range
- Oral: 2–6 mg/day in divided doses, largest dose at bedtime
- Injection: 4 mg administered slowly

Dosage Forms
- Tablet 0.5 mg, 1 mg, 2 mg
- Liquid 0.5 mg/5mL, 2 mg/mL
- Injection 1 mg/0.5mL, 2 mg/mL, 4 mg/mL

How to Dose
- Oral: Initial 2–3 mg/day in 2–3 doses; increase as needed, starting with evening dose; maximum generally 10 mg/day
- Injection: Initial 4 mg administered slowly; after 10–15 minutes may administer again
- Take liquid formulation with water, soda, applesauce or pudding

Dosing Tips
* One of the few benzodiazepines available in an oral liquid formulation
* One of the few benzodiazepines available in an injectable formulation
- Lorazepam injection is intended for acute use; patients who require long-term treatment should be switched to the oral formulation
- Use lowest possible effective dose for the shortest possible period of time (a benzodiazepine-sparing strategy)
- Assess need for continued treatment regularly
- Risk of dependence may increase with dose and duration of treatment
- For inter-dose symptoms of anxiety, can either increase dose or maintain same total daily dose but divide into more frequent doses
- Can also use an as-needed occasional "top up" dose for inter-dose anxiety

- Because panic disorder can require doses higher than 6 mg/day, the risk of dependence may be greater in these patients
- Some severely ill patients may require 10 mg/day or more
- Frequency of dosing in practice is often greater than predicted from half-life, as duration of biological activity is often shorter than pharmacokinetic terminal half-life

Overdose
- Fatalities can occur; hypotension, tiredness, ataxia, confusion, coma

Long-Term Use
- Evidence of efficacy up to 16 weeks
- Risk of dependence, particularly for treatment periods longer than 12 weeks and especially in patients with past or current polysubstance abuse

Habit Forming
- Lorazepam is a Schedule IV drug
- Patients may develop dependence and/or tolerance with long-term use

How to Stop
- Patients with history of seizure may seize upon withdrawal, especially if withdrawal is abrupt
- Taper by 0.5 mg every 3 days to reduce chances of withdrawal effects
- For difficult to taper cases, consider reducing dose much more slowly once reaching 3 mg/day, perhaps by as little as 0.25 mg per week or less
- For other patients with severe problems discontinuing a benzodiazepine, dosing may need to be tapered over many months (i.e., reduce dose by 1% every 3 days by crushing tablet and suspending or dissolving in 100 ml of fruit juice and then disposing of 1 ml while drinking the rest; 3–7 days later, dispose of 2 ml, and so on). This is both a form of very slow biological tapering and a form of behavioral desensitization
- Be sure to differentiate reemergence of symptoms requiring reinstitution of treatment from withdrawal symptoms
- Benzodiazepine-dependent anxiety patients and insulin-dependent diabetics are not addicted to their medications. When benzodiazepine-dependent patients stop their medication, disease symptoms can reemerge, disease symptoms can worsen (rebound), and/or withdrawal symptoms can emerge

Pharmacokinetics
- Elimination half-life 10–20 hours
- No active metabolites

 Drug Interactions
- Increased depressive effects when taken with other CNS depressants
- Valproate and probenecid may reduce clearance and raise plasma concentrations of lorazepam
- Oral contraceptives may increase clearance and lower plasma concentrations of lorazepam
- Flumazenil (used to reverse the effects of benzodiazepines) may precipitate seizures and should not be used in patients treated for seizure disorders with lorazepam

 Other Warnings/ Precautions
- Dosage changes should be made in collaboration with prescriber
- Use with caution in patients with pulmonary disease; rare reports of death after initiation of benzodiazepines in patients with severe pulmonary impairment
- History of drug or alcohol abuse often creates greater risk for dependency
- Use oral formulation only with extreme caution if patient has obstructive sleep apnea; injection is contraindicated in patients with sleep apnea
- Some depressed patients may experience a worsening of suicidal ideation
- Some patients may exhibit abnormal thinking or behavioral changes similar to those caused by other CNS depressants (i.e., either depressant actions or disinhibiting actions)

Do Not Use
- If patient has narrow angle-closure glaucoma
- If patient has sleep apnea (injection)
- Must not be given intra-arterially because it may cause arteriospasm and result in gangrene

• If there is a proven allergy to lorazepam or any benzodiazepine

SPECIAL POPULATIONS

Renal Impairment
• 1–2 mg/day in 2–3 doses

Hepatic Impairment
• 1–2 mg/day in 2–3 doses
• Because of its short half-life and inactive metabolites, lorazepam may be a preferred benzodiazepine in some patients with liver disease

Cardiac Impairment
• Benzodiazepines have been used to treat anxiety associated with acute myocardial infarction
• Lorazepam may be used as an adjunct to control drug-induced cardiovascular emergencies

Elderly
• 1–2 mg/day in 2–3 doses
• May be more sensitive to sedative or respiratory effects

Children and Adolescents
• Oral: safety and efficacy not established under age 12
• Injection: safety and efficacy not established under age 18
• Long-term effects of lorazepam in children/adolescents are unknown
• Should generally receive lower doses and be more closely monitored

Pregnancy
• Risk Category D [positive evidence of risk to human fetus; potential benefits may still justify its use]
• Possible increased risk of birth defects when benzodiazepines taken during pregnancy
• Because of the potential risks, lorazepam is not generally recommended as treatment for anxiety during pregnancy, especially during the first trimester
• Drug should be tapered if discontinued

• Infants whose mothers received a benzodiazepine late in pregnancy may experience withdrawal effects
• Neonatal flaccidity has been reported in infants whose mothers took a benzodiazepine during pregnancy
• Seizures, even mild seizures, may cause harm to the embryo/fetus

Breast Feeding
• Some drug is found in mother's breast milk
✳ Recommended either to discontinue drug or bottle feed
• Effects on infant have been observed and include feeding difficulties, sedation, and weight loss

THE ART OF PSYCHOPHARMACOLOGY

Potential Advantages
• Rapid onset of action
• Availability of oral liquid as well as injectable dosage formulations

Potential Disadvantages
• Euphoria may lead to abuse
• Abuse especially risky in past or present substance abusers
• Possibly more sedation than some other benzodiazepines commonly used to treat anxiety

Primary Target Symptoms
• Panic attacks
• Anxiety
• Muscle spasms
• Incidence of seizures (adjunct)

Pearls
✳ One of the most popular and useful benzodiazepines for treatment of agitation associated with psychosis, bipolar disorder, and other disorders, especially in the inpatient setting; this is due in part to useful sedative properties and flexibility of administration with oral tablets, oral liquid, or injectable formulations, which is often useful in treating uncooperative patients
• Is a very useful adjunct to SSRIs and SNRIs in the treatment of numerous anxiety disorders

- Not effective for treating psychosis as a monotherapy, but can be used as an adjunct to antipsychotics
- Not effective for treating bipolar disorder as a monotherapy, but can be used as an adjunct to mood stabilizers and antipsychotics
- Because of its short half-life and inactive metabolites, lorazepam may be preferred over some benzodiazepines for patients with liver disease
* Lorazepam may be preferred over other benzodiazepines for the treatment of delirium

* Lorazepam is often used to induce pre-operative anterograde amnesia to assist in anesthesiology
- May both cause depression and treat depression in different patients
- Clinical duration of action may be shorter than plasma half-life, leading to dosing more frequently than 2–3 times daily in some patients
- When using to treat insomnia, remember that insomnia may be a symptom of some other primary disorder itself, and thus warrant evaluation for comorbid psychiatric and/or medical conditions

 Suggested Reading

Bonnet MH, Arand DL. The use of lorazepam TID for chronic insomnia. Int Clin Psychopharmacol 1999;14:81–9.

Greenblatt DJ. Clinical pharmacokinetics of oxazepam and lorazepam. Clin Pharmacokinet 1981;6:89–105.

Starreveld E, Starreveld AA. Status epilepticus. Current concepts and management. Can Fam Physician 2000;46:1817–23.

Wagner BK, O'Hara DA, Hammond JS. Drugs for amnesia in the ICU. Am J Crit Care 1997; 6:192–201.

LOXAPINE

THERAPEUTICS

Brands • Loxitane
see index for additional brand names

Generic? Yes

 Class

• Conventional antipsychotic (neuroleptic, dopamine 2 antagonist, serotonin dopamine antagonist)

Commonly Prescribed For
(bold for FDA approved)
• **Schizophrenia**
• Other psychotic disorders
• Bipolar disorder

 How The Drug Works

• Blocks dopamine 2 receptors, reducing positive symptoms of psychosis
✳ Although classified as a conventional antipsychotic, loxapine is a potent serotonin 2A antagonist
• Serotonin 2A antagonist properties might be relevant at low doses, but generally are overwhelmed by high dosing

How Long Until It Works

• Psychotic symptoms can improve within 1 week, but it may take several weeks for full effect on behavior

If It Works

• Most often reduces positive symptoms in schizophrenia but does not eliminate them
• Most schizophrenic patients do not have a total remission of symptoms but rather a reduction of symptoms by about a third
• Continue treatment in schizophrenia until reaching a plateau of improvement
• After reaching a satisfactory plateau, continue treatment for at least a year after first episode of psychosis in schizophrenia
• For second and subsequent episodes of psychosis in schizophrenia, treatment may need to be indefinite
• Reduces symptoms of acute psychotic mania but not proven as a mood stabilizer or as an effective maintenance treatment in bipolar disorder
• After reducing acute psychotic symptoms in mania, switch to a mood stabilizer

and/or an atypical antipsychotic for mood stabilization and maintenance

If It Doesn't Work

• Consider trying one of the first-line atypical antipsychotics (risperidone, olanzapine, quetiapine, ziprasidone, aripiprazole, amisulpride)
• Consider trying another conventional antipsychotic
• If 2 or more antipsychotic monotherapies do not work, consider clozapine

 Best Augmenting Combos for Partial Response or Treatment-Resistance

• Augmentation of conventional antipsychotics has not been systematically studied
• Addition of a mood stabilizing anticonvulsant such as valproate, carbamazepine, or lamotrigine may be helpful in both schizophrenia and bipolar mania
• Augmentation with lithium in bipolar mania may be helpful
• Addition of a benzodiazepine, especially short-term for agitation

Tests

✳ Since conventional antipsychotics are frequently associated with weight gain, before starting treatment, weigh all patients and determine if the patient is already overweight (BMI 25.0–29.9) or obese (BMI ≥30)
• Before giving a drug that can cause weight gain to an overweight or obese patient, consider determining whether the patient already has pre-diabetes (fasting plasma glucose 100–125 mg/dl), diabetes (fasting plasma glucose >126 mg/dl), or dyslipidemia (increased total cholesterol, LDL cholesterol and triglycerides; decreased HDL cholesterol), and treat or refer such patients for treatment, including nutrition and weight management, physical activity counseling, smoking cessation, and medical management
✳ Monitor weight and BMI during treatment
✳ While giving a drug to a patient who has gained >5% of initial weight, consider evaluating for the presence of pre-diabetes, diabetes, or dyslipidemia, or consider switching to a different antipsychotic

• Should check blood pressure in the elderly before starting and for the first few weeks of treatment
• Monitoring elevated prolactin levels of dubious clinical benefit

SIDE EFFECTS

How Drug Causes Side Effects
• By blocking dopamine 2 receptors in the striatum, it can cause motor side effects
• By blocking dopamine 2 receptors in the pituitary, it can cause elevations in prolactin
• By blocking dopamine 2 receptors excessively in the mesocortical and mesolimbic dopamine pathways, especially at high doses, it can cause worsening of negative and cognitive symptoms (neuroleptic-induced deficit syndrome)
• Anticholinergic actions may cause sedation, blurred vision, constipation, dry mouth
• Antihistaminic actions may cause sedation, weight gain
• By blocking alpha 1 adrenergic receptors, it can cause dizziness, sedation, and hypotension
• Mechanism of weight gain and any possible increased incidence of diabetes or dyslipidemia with conventional antipsychotics is unknown

Notable Side Effects
✳ Neuroleptic-induced deficit syndrome
✳ Akathisia
✳ Extrapyramidal symptoms, Parkinsonism, tardive dyskinesia
✳ Galactorrhea, amenorrhea
• Sedation
• Dry mouth, constipation, vision disturbance, urninary retention
• Hypotension, tachycardia

 Life Threatening or Dangerous Side Effects
• Rare neuroleptic malignant syndrome
• Rare agranulocytosis
• Rare hepatocellular injury
• Rare seizures

Weight Gain

unusual — not unusual — common — problematic
• Reported but not expected

Sedation

unusual — not unusual — common — problematic
• Many experience and/or can be significant in amount
• Sedation is usually transient
• Sedation is usually dose-dependent and may not be experienced at low doses where loxapine may function as an atypical antipsychotic (e.g., <50 mg/day; especially 5–25 mg/day)

What To Do About Side Effects
• Wait
• Wait
• Wait
• For motor symptoms, add an anticholinergic agent
• Reduce the dose
• For sedation, give at night
• Switch to an atypical antipsychotic
• Weight loss, exercise programs, and medical management for high BMIs, diabetes, dyslipidemia

Best Augmenting Agents for Side Effects
• Benztropine or trihexyphenidyl for motor side effects
• Sometimes amantadine can be helpful for motor side effects
• Benzodiazepines may be helpful for akathisia
• Many side effects cannot be improved with an augmenting agent

DOSING AND USE

Usual Dosage Range
• 60–100 mg/day in divided doses

Dosage Forms
• Capsule 6.8 mg loxapine succinate equivalent to 5 mg loxapine, 13.6 mg loxapine succinate equivalent to 10 mg loxapine, 34.0 mg loxapine succinate equivalent to 25 mg loxapine, 68.1 mg

loxapine succinate equivalent to 50 mg loxapine
- Oral liquid 25 mg/mL
- Injection 50 mg/mL

How to Dose
- Initial 20 mg/day in 2 doses; titrate over 7–10 days to 60–100 mg/day in 2–4 doses; maximum generally 250 mg/day
- Take liquid formulation in orange or grapefruit juice

 Dosing Tips
- Has conventional antipsychotic properties at originally recommended doses (i.e., starting at 10 mg twice a day, maintenance 60–100 mg/day, maximum 250 mg/day given in 2 divided doses)
- ✳ Binding studies, PET studies, and anecdotal clinical observations suggest that loxapine may be atypical at lower doses (perhaps 5–30 mg/day) but further studies needed
- Anecdotal evidence that many patients can be maintained at 20–60 mg/day as monotherapy
- To augment partial responders to an atypical antipsychotic, consider doses of loxapine as low as 5–60 mg/day, but use full doses if necessary
- No formal studies, but some patients may do well on once-daily dosing, especially at night, rather than twice-daily dosing
- Available as 5 mg and 10 mg capsules for low dose use and as 25 mg and 50 mg capsules for routine use
- Available as a liquid dosage formulation
- Available for acute intramuscular administration (50 mg/ml)
- Intramuscular loxapine may have faster onset of action and superior efficacy for agitated/excited and aggressive behavior in some patients than intramuscular haloperidol
- In the acute situation, give 25–50 mg intramuscularly (0.5–1.0 ml of 50 mg/ml solution) with onset of action within 60 minutes
- When initiating therapy with an atypical antipsychotic in an acute situation, consider short-term intramuscular loxapine to "lead in" to orally administered atypical; e.g., initiate oral dosing of an atypical

antipsychotic with 25–50 mg loxapine 2–3 times a day intramuscularly to achieve antipsychotic effects without extrapyramidal symptoms and sedation
- When using loxapine to "top-up" previously stabilized patients now decompensating, may use loxapine as single 25–50 mg doses as needed intramuscularly or as oral liquid or tablets
- Patients receiving atypical antipsychotics may occasionally require a "top up" of a conventional antipsychotic to control aggression or violent behavior

Overdose
- Deaths have occurred; extrapyramidal symptoms, CNS depression, cardiovascular effects, hypotension, seizures, respiratory depression, renal failure, coma

Long-Term Use
- Some side effects may be irreversible (e.g., tardive dyskinesia)

Habit Forming
- No

How to Stop
- Slow down-titration of oral formulation (over 6 to 8 weeks), especially when simultaneously beginning a new antipsychotic while switching (i.e., cross-titration)
- Rapid oral discontinuation may lead to rebound psychosis and worsening of symptoms
- If antiparkinson agents are being used, they should be continued for a few weeks after loxapine is discontinued

Pharmacokinetics
- Half-life approximately 4 hours for oral formulation
- Half-life approximately 12 hours for intramuscular formulation
- Multiple active metabolites with longer half-lives than parent drug
- ✳ N-desmethyl loxapine is amoxapine, an antidepressant
- 8-hydroxyloxapine and 7-hydroxyloxapine are also serotonin-dopamine antagonists
- 8-hydroxyamoxapine and 7-hydroxyamoxapine are also serotonin-dopamine antagonists

Drug Interactions

- Respiratory depression may occur when loxapine is combined with lorazepam
- Additive effects may occur if used with CNS depressants
- May decrease the effects of levodopa, dopamine agonists
- Some patients taking a neuroleptic and lithium have developed an encephalopathic syndrome similar to neuroleptic malignant syndrome
- Combined use with epinephrine may lower blood pressure
- May increase the effects of antihypertensive drugs except for guanethidine, whose antihypertensive actions loxapine may antagonize

⚠ Other Warnings/ Precautions

- If signs of neuroleptic malignant syndrome develop, treatment should be immediately discontinued
- Use cautiously in patients with alcohol withdrawal or convulsive disorders because of possible lowering of seizure threshold
- Antiemetic effect can mask signs of other disorders or overdose
- Do not use epinephrine in event of overdose, as interaction with some pressor agents may lower blood pressure
- Use cautiously in patients with glaucoma, urinary retention
- Observe for signs of ocular toxicity (pigmentary retinopathy, lenticular pigmentation)
- Avoid extreme heat exposure
- Use only with caution if at all in Parkinson's disease or Lewy Body dementia

Do Not Use

- If patient is in a comatose state or has CNS depression
- If there is a proven allergy to loxapine
- If there is a known sensitivity to any dibenzoxazepine

Renal Impairment
- Use with caution

Hepatic Impairment
- Use with caution

Cardiac Impairment
- Use with caution

Elderly
- Some patients may tolerate lower doses better

Children and Adolescents
- Safety and efficacy not established
- Generally, consider second-line after atypical antipsychotics

Pregnancy
- Renal papillary abnormalities have been seen in rats during pregnancy
- No studies in pregnant women
- Psychotic symptoms may worsen during pregnancy and some form of treatment may be necessary
- Atypical antipsychotics may be preferable to conventional antipsychotics or anticonvulsant mood stabilizers if treatment is required during pregnancy

Breast Feeding
- Unknown if loxapine is secreted in human breast milk, but all psychotropics assumed to be secreted in breast milk
- ✳ Recommended either to discontinue drug or bottle feed

Potential Advantages
- Intramuscular formulation for emergency use

Potential Disadvantages
- Patients with tardive dyskinesia

Primary Target Symptoms
- Positive symptoms of psychosis
- Motor and autonomic hyperactivity
- Violent or aggressive behavior

Pearls

✳ Recently discovered to be a serotonin dopamine antagonist (binding studies and PET scans)

✳ Active metabolites are also serotonin dopamine antagonists with longer half-lives than parent drug, thus possibly allowing once-daily treatment

✳ One active metabolite is an antidepressant (amoxapine, also known as N-desmethyl-loxapine)

• Theoretically, loxapine should have antidepressant actions, especially at high doses, but no controlled studies

• Theoretically, loxapine may have advantages for short-term use in some patients with psychotic depression

• Developed as a conventional antipsychotic; i.e., reduces positive symptoms, but causes extrapyramidal symptoms and prolactin elevations

• Lower extrapyramidal symptoms than haloperidol in some studies, but not fixed dose studies and no low dose studies

✳ Causes less weight gain than other antipsychotics, both atypical and conventional, and may even be associated with weight loss

• No formal studies of negative symptoms, but some studies show superiority to conventional antipsychotics for emotional withdrawal and social competence

• Best use may be as low-cost augmentation agent to atypical antipsychotics

✳ Enhances efficacy in clozapine partial responders when given concomitantly with clozapine

• For previously stabilized patients with "breakthrough" agitation or incipient decompensation, "top-up" the atypical antipsychotic with as-needed intramuscular or oral single doses of loxapine

• Patients have very similar antipsychotic responses to any conventional antipsychotic, which is different from atypical antipsychotics where antipsychotic responses of individual patients can occasionally vary greatly from one atypical antipsychotic to another

• Patients with inadequate responses to atypical antipsychotics may benefit from a trial of augmentation with a conventional antipsychotic such as loxapine or from switching to a conventional antipsychotic such as loxapine

• However, long-term polypharmacy with a combination of a conventional antipsychotic such as loxapine with an atypical antipsychotic may combine their side effects without clearly augmenting the efficacy of either

• Although a frequent practice by some prescribers, adding 2 conventional antipsychotics together has little rationale and may reduce tolerability without clearly enhancing efficacy

Suggested Reading

Fenton M, Murphy B, Wood J, Bagnall A, Chue P, Leitner M. Loxapine for schizophrenia. Cochrane Database Syst Rev 2000; (2): CD001943.

Heel RC, Brogden RN, Speight TM, Avery GS. Loxapine: a review of its pharmacological properties and therapeutic efficacy as an antipsychotic agent. Drugs 1978; 15 (3): 198–217.

Zisook S, Click MA Jr. Evaluations of loxapine succinate in the ambulatory treatment of acute schizophrenic episodes. Int Pharmacopsychiatry 1980; 15 (6): 365–78.

MAPROTILINE

THERAPEUTICS

Brands • Ludiomil
see index for additional brand names

Generic? Yes

Class

- Tricyclic antidepressant (TCA), sometimes classified as a tetracyclic antidepressant (tetra)
- Predominantly a norepinephrine/noradrenaline reuptake inhibitor

Commonly Prescribed For
(bold for FDA approved)
- **Depression**
- Anxiety
- Insomnia
- Neuropathic pain/chronic pain
- Treatment-resistant depression

How The Drug Works

- Boosts neurotransmitter norepinephrine/noradrenaline
- Blocks norepinephrine reuptake pump (norepinephrine transporter), presumably increasing noradrenergic neurotransmission
- Since dopamine is inactivated by norepinephrine reuptake in frontal cortex, which largely lacks dopamine transporters, maprotiline can thus increase dopamine neurotransmission in this part of the brain
- A more potent inhibitor of norepinephrine reuptake pump than serotonin reuptake pump (serotonin transporter)
- At high doses may also boost neurotransmitter serotonin and presumably increase serotonergic neurotransmission

How Long Until It Works

- Onset of therapeutic actions usually not immediate, but often delayed 2 to 4 weeks
- If it is not working within 6 to 8 weeks for depression, it may require a dosage increase or it may not work at all
- May continue to work for many years to prevent relapse of symptoms

If It Works

- The goal of treatment of depression is complete remission of current symptoms as well as prevention of future relapses
- The goal of treatment of chronic neuropathic pain is to reduce symptoms as much as possible, especially in combination with other treatments
- Treatment of depression most often reduces or even eliminates symptoms, but not a cure since symptoms can recur after medicine stopped
- Treatment of chronic neuropathic pain may reduce symptoms, but rarely eliminates them completely, and is not a cure since symptoms can recur after medicine is stopped
- Continue treatment of depression until all symptoms are gone (remission)
- Once symptoms of depression are gone, continue treating for 1 year for the first episode of depression
- For second and subsequent episodes of depression, treatment may need to be indefinite
- Use in anxiety disorders and chronic pain may also need to be indefinite, but long-term treatment is not well-studied in these conditions

If It Doesn't Work

- Many depressed patients only have a partial response where some symptoms are improved but others persist (especially insomnia, fatigue, and problems concentrating)
- Other depressed patients may be nonresponders, sometimes called treatment-resistant or treatment-refractory
- Consider increasing dose, switching to another agent or adding an appropriate augmenting agent
- Consider psychotherapy
- Consider evaluation for another diagnosis or for a comorbid condition (e.g., medical illness, substance abuse, etc.)
- Some patients may experience apparent lack of consistent efficacy due to activation of latent or underlying bipolar disorder, and require antidepressant discontinuation and a switch to a mood stabilizer

Best Augmenting Combos for Partial Response or Treatment-Resistance

- Lithium, buspirone, thyroid hormone (for depression)
- Gabapentin, tiagabine, other anticonvulsants, even opiates if done by experts while monitoring carefully in difficult cases (for chronic pain)

Tests

- None for healthy individuals
- ✳ Since tricyclic and tetracyclic antidepressants are frequently associated with weight gain, before starting treatment, weigh all patients and determine if the patient is already overweight (BMI 25.0–29.9) or obese (BMI ≥30)
- Before giving a drug that can cause weight gain to an overweight or obese patient, consider determining whether the patient already has pre-diabetes (fasting plasma glucose 100–125 mg/dl), diabetes (fasting plasma glucose >126 mg/dl), or dyslipidemia (increased total cholesterol, LDL cholesterol and triglycerides; decreased HDL cholesterol), and treat or refer such patients for treatment, including nutrition and weight management, physical activity counseling, smoking cessation, and medical management
- ✳ Monitor weight and BMI during treatment
- ✳ While giving a drug to a patient who has gained >5% of initial weight, consider evaluating for the presence of pre-diabetes, diabetes, or dyslipidemia, or consider switching to a different antidepressant
- EKGs may be useful for selected patients (e.g., those with personal or family history of QTc prolongation; cardiac arrhythmia; recent myocardial infarction; uncompensated heart failure; or taking agents that prolong QTc interval such as pimozide, thioridazine, selected antiarrhythmics, moxifloxacin, sparfloxacin, etc.)
- Patients at risk for electrolyte disturbances (e.g., patients on diuretic therapy) should have baseline and periodic serum potassium and magnesium measurements

SIDE EFFECTS

How Drug Causes Side Effects

- Anticholinergic activity may explain sedative effects, dry mouth, constipation, and blurred vision
- Sedative effects and weight gain may be due to antihistamine properties
- Blockade of alpha adrenergic 1 receptors may explain dizziness, sedation, and hypotension
- Cardiac arrhythmias and seizures, especially in overdose, may be caused by blockade of ion channels

Notable Side Effects

- Blurred vision, constipation, urinary retention, increased appetite, dry mouth, nausea, diarrhea, heartburn, unusual taste in mouth, weight gain
- Fatigue, weakness, dizziness, sedation, headache, anxiety, nervousness, restlessness
- Sexual dysfunction (impotence, change in libido)
- Sweating, rash, itching

Life Threatening or Dangerous Side Effects

- Paralytic ileus, hyperthermia (TCAs/ tetracyclics + anticholinergic agents)
- Lowered seizure threshold and rare seizures
- Orthostatic hypotension, sudden death, arrhythmias, tachycardia
- QTc prolongation
- Hepatic failure, extrapyramidal symptoms
- Increased intraocular pressure
- Rare induction of mania and activation of suicidal ideation

Weight Gain

unusual   not unusual   common   problematic

- Many experience and/or can be significant in amount
- Can increase appetite and carbohydrate craving

Sedation

unusual   not unusual   common   problematic

- Many experience and/or can be significant in amount

- Tolerance to sedative effect may develop with long-term use

What To Do About Side Effects
- Wait
- Wait
- Wait
- Lower the dose
- Switch to an SSRI or newer antidepressant

Best Augmenting Agents for Side Effects
- Many side effects cannot be improved with an augmenting agent

DOSING AND USE

Usual Dosage Range
- 75–150 mg/day (for depression)
- 50–150 mg/day (for chronic pain)

Dosage Forms
- Tablet 25 mg, 50 mg, 75 mg

How to Dose
- Initial 25 mg/day at bedtime; increase by 25 mg every 3–7 days
- 75 mg/day; after 2 weeks increase dose gradually by 25 mg/day; maximum dose generally 225 mg/day

 Dosing Tips
- If given in a single dose, should generally be administered at bedtime because of its sedative properties
- If given in split doses, largest dose should generally be given at bedtime because of its sedative properties
- If patients experience nightmares, split dose and do not give large dose at bedtime
- Patients treated for chronic pain may only require lower doses
- ✳ Risk of seizures increases with dose, especially with maprotiline above 200 mg/day
- If intolerable anxiety, insomnia, agitation, akathisia, or activation occur either upon dosing initiation or discontinuation, consider the possibility of activated bipolar disorder, and switch to a mood stabilizer or an atypical antipsychotic

Overdose
- Death may occur; convulsions, cardiac dysrhythmias, severe hypotension, CNS depression, coma, changes in ECG

Long-Term Use
- Safe

Habit Forming
- No

How to Stop
- Taper to avoid withdrawal effects
- Even with gradual dose reduction some withdrawal symptoms may appear within the first 2 weeks
- Many patients tolerate 50% dose reduction for 3 days, then another 50% reduction for 3 days, then discontinuation
- If withdrawal symptoms emerge during discontinuation, raise dose to stop symptoms and then restart withdrawal much more slowly

Pharmacokinetics
- Substrate for CYP450 2D6
- Mean half-life approximately 51 hours
- Peak plasma concentration 8–24 hours

 Drug Interactions
- Tramadol increases the risk of seizures in patients taking TCAs
- Use of TCAs/tetracyclics with anticholinergic drugs may result in paralytic ileus or hyperthermia
- Fluoxetine, paroxetine, bupropion, duloxetine, and other CYP450 2D6 inhibitors may increase TCA/tetracyclic concentrations
- Cimetidine may increase plasma concentrations of TCAs/tetracyclics and cause anticholinergic symptoms
- Phenothiazines or haloperidol may raise TCA/tetracyclic blood concentrations
- May alter effects of antihypertensive drugs; may inhibit hypotensive effects of clonidine
- Use with sympathomimetic agents may increase sympathetic activity
- Methylphenidate may inhibit metabolism of TCAs/tetracyclics
- Activation and agitation, especially following switching or adding antidepressants, may represent the induction of a bipolar state, especially a

mixed dysphoric bipolar II condition sometimes associated with suicidal ideation, and require the addition of lithium, a mood stabilizer or an atypical antipsychotic, and/or discontinuation of maprotiline

 Other Warnings/ Precautions

- Add or initiate other antidepressants with caution for up to 2 weeks after discontinuing maprotiline
- Generally, do not use with MAO inhibitors, including 14 days after MAOIs are stopped; do not start an MAOI until 2 weeks after discontinuing maprotiline, but see Pearls
- Use with caution in patients with history of seizures, urinary retention, narrow angle-closure glaucoma, hyperthyroidism
- TCAs/tetracyclics can increase QTc interval, especially at toxic doses, which can be attained not only by overdose but also by combining with drugs that inhibit TCA/ tetracyclic metabolism via CYP450 2D6, potentially causing torsade de pointes-type arrhythmia or sudden death
- Because TCAs/tetracyclics can prolong QTc interval, use with caution in patients who have bradycardia or who are taking drugs that can induce bradycardia (e.g., beta blockers, calcium channel blockers, clonidine, digitalis)
- Because TCAs/tetracyclics can prolong QTc interval, use with caution in patients who have hypokalemia and/or hypomagnesemia or who are taking drugs that can induce hypokalemia and/or magnesemia (e.g., diuretics, stimulant laxatives, intravenous amphotericin B, glucocorticoids, tetracosactide)

Do Not Use

- If patient is recovering from myocardial infarction
- If patient is taking agents capable of significantly prolonging QTc interval (e.g., pimozide, thioridazine, selected antiarrhythmics, moxifloxacin, sparfloxacin)
- If there is a history of QTc prolongation or cardiac arrhythmia, recent acute myocardial infarction, uncompensated heart failure

- If patient is taking drugs that inhibit TCA/tetracyclic metabolism, including CYP450 2D6 inhibitors, except by an expert
- If there is reduced CYP450 2D6 function, such as patients who are poor 2D6 metabolizers, except by an expert and at low doses
- If there is a proven allergy to maprotiline

SPECIAL POPULATIONS

Renal Impairment
- Use with caution

Hepatic Impairment
- Use with caution

Cardiac Impairment

- TCAs/tetracyclics have been reported to cause arrhythmias, prolongation of conduction time, orthostatic hypotension, sinus tachycardia, and heart failure, especially in the diseased heart
- Myocardial infarction and stroke have been reported with TCAs/tetracyclics
- TCAs/tetracyclics produce QTc prolongation, which may be enhanced by the existence of bradycardia, hypokalemia, congenital or acquired long QTc interval, which should be evaluated prior to administering maprotiline
- Use with caution if treating concomitantly with a medication likely to produce prolonged bradycardia, hypokalemia, slowing of intracardiac conduction, or prolongation of the QTc interval
- Avoid TCAs/tetracyclics in patients with a known history of QTc prolongation, recent acute myocardial infarction, and uncompensated heart failure
- TCAs/tetracyclics may cause a sustained increase in heart rate in patients with ischemic heart disease and may worsen (decrease) heart rate variability, an independent risk of mortality in cardiac populations
- Since SSRIs may improve (increase) heart rate variability in patients following a myocardial infarct and may improve survival as well as mood in patients with acute angina or following a myocardial infarction, these are more appropriate agents for cardiac population than tricyclic/tetracyclic antidepressants

✻ Risk/benefit ratio may not justify use of TCAs/tetracyclics in cardiac impairment

Elderly
- May be more sensitive to anticholinergic, cardiovascular, hypotensive, and sedative effects
- Usual dose generally 50–75 mg/day

Children and Adolescents
- Use with caution, observing for activation of known or unknown bipolar disorder and/or suicidal ideation, and strongly consider informing parents or guardian of this risk so they can help observe child or adolescent patients
- Not recommended for use under age 18
- Several studies show lack of efficacy of TCAs/tetracyclics for depression
- May be used to treat enuresis or hyperactive/impulsive behaviors
- Some cases of sudden death have occurred in children taking TCAs/tetracyclics
- Maximum dose for children and adolescents is 75 mg/day

Pregnancy
- Risk Category B [animal studies do not show adverse effects, no controlled studies in humans]
- Adverse effects have been reported in infants whose mothers took a TCA/tetracyclic (lethargy, withdrawal symptoms, fetal malformations)
- Must weigh the risk of treatment (first trimester fetal development, third trimester newborn delivery) to the child against the risk of no treatment (recurrence of depression, maternal health, infant bonding) to the mother and child
- For many patients this may mean continuing treatment during pregnancy

Breast Feeding
- Some drug is found in mother's breast milk
- ✻ Recommended either to discontinue drug or bottle feed
- Immediate postpartum period is a high-risk time for depression, especially in women who have had prior depressive episodes, so drug may need to be reinstituted late in the third trimester or shortly after childbirth to prevent a recurrence during the postpartum period
- Must weigh benefits of breast feeding with risks and benefits of antidepressant treatment versus non-treatment to both the infant and the mother
- For many patients this may mean continuing treatment during breast feeding

---

THE ART OF PSYCHOPHARMACOLOGY

Potential Advantages
- Patients with insomnia
- Severe or treatment-resistant depression

Potential Disadvantages
- Pediatric and geriatric patients
- Patients concerned with weight gain
- Cardiac patients
- Patients with seizure disorders

Primary Target Symptoms
- Depressed mood
- Chronic pain

Pearls
- Tricyclic/tetracyclic antidepressants are often a first-line treatment option for chronic pain
- Tricyclic/tetracyclic antidepressants are no longer generally considered a first-line treatment option for depression because of their side effect profile
- Tricyclic/tetracyclic antidepressants continue to be useful for severe or treatment-resistant depression
- ✻ May have somewhat increased risk of seizures compared to some other TCAs, especially at higher doses
- TCAs/tetracyclics may aggravate psychotic symptoms
- Alcohol should be avoided because of additive CNS effects
- Underweight patients may be more susceptible to adverse cardiovascular effects
- Children, patients with inadequate hydration, and patients with cardiac disease may be more susceptible to TCA/tetracyclic-induced cardiotoxicity than healthy adults

- For the expert only: a heroic treatment (but potentially dangerous) for severely treatment-resistant patients is to give simultaneously with monoamine oxidase inhibitors for patients who fail to respond to numerous other antidepressants
- If this option is elected, start the MAOI with the tricyclic/tetracyclic antidepressant simultaneously at low doses after appropriate drug washout, then alternately increase doses of these agents every few days to a week as tolerated
- Although very strict dietary and concomitant drug restrictions must be observed to prevent hypertensive crises and serotonin syndrome, the most common side effects of MAOI/ tricyclic or tetracyclic combinations may be weight gain and orthostatic hypotension
- Patients on tricyclics/tetracyclics should be aware that they may experience symptoms such as photosensitivity or blue-green urine
- SSRIs may be more effective than TCAs/tetracyclics in women, and TCAs/tetracyclics may be more effective than SSRIs in men
* May have a more rapid onset of action than some other TCAs/tetracyclics
- Since tricyclic/tetracyclic antidepressants are substrates for CYP450 2D6, and 7% of the population (especially Caucasians) may have a genetic variant leading to reduced activity of 2D6, such patients may not safely tolerate normal doses of tricyclic/tetracyclic antidepressants and may require dose reduction
- Phenotypic testing may be necessary to detect this genetic variant prior to dosing with a tricyclic/tetracyclic antidepressant, especially in vulnerable populations such as children, elderly, cardiac populations, and those on concomitant medications
- Patients who seem to have extraordinarily severe side effects at normal or low doses may have this phenotypic CYP450 2D6 variant and require low doses or switching to another antidepressant not metabolized by 2D6

Suggested Reading

Anderson IM. Meta-analytical studies on new antidepressants. Br Med Bull. 2001; 57:161–178.

Anderson IM. Selective serotonin reuptake inhibitors versus tricyclic antidepressants: a meta-analysis of efficacy and tolerability. J Aff Disorders. 2000;58:19–36.

Kane JM, Lieberman J. The efficacy of amoxapine, maprotiline, and trazodone in comparison to imipramine and amitriptyline: a review of the literature. Psychopharmacol Bull. 1984;20:240–9.

MEMANTINE

Brands • Namenda
see index for additional brand names

Generic? No

Class
• NMDA receptor antagonist; N-methyl-d-aspartate (NMDA) subtype of glutamate receptor antagonist; cognitive enhancer

Commonly Prescribed For
(bold for FDA approved)
• **Moderate to severe dementia of the Alzheimer type**
• Mild to moderate Alzheimer dementia
• Memory disorders in other conditions
• Mild cognitive impairment
• Chronic pain

How The Drug Works
✳ Is a low to moderate affinity noncompetitive (open-channel) NMDA receptor antagonist, which binds preferentially to the NMDA receptor-operated cation channels
• Presumably interferes with the postulated persistent activation of NMDA receptors by excessive glutamate release in Alzheimer disease

How Long Until It Works
• Memory improvement is not expected and it may take months before any stabilization in degenerative course is evident

If It Works
• May slow progression of disease, but does not reverse the degenerative process

If It Doesn't Work
• Consider adjusting dose, switching to a cholinesterase inhibitor or adding a cholinesterase inhibitor
• Reconsider diagnosis and rule out other conditions such as depression or a dementia other than Alzheimer disease

Best Augmenting Combos for Partial Response or Treatment-Resistance
✳ Atypical antipsychotics to reduce behavioral disturbances
✳ Antidepressants if concomitant depression, apathy, or lack of interest
✳ May be combined with cholinesterase inhibitors
• Divalproex, carbamazepine, or oxcarbazepine for behavioral disturbances

Tests
• None for healthy individuals

How Drug Causes Side Effects
• Presumably due to excessive actions at NMDA receptors

Notable Side Effects
• Dizziness, headache
• Constipation

 Life Threatening or Dangerous Side Effects
• Seizures (rare)

Weight Gain

unusual   not unusual   common   problematic
• Reported but not expected

Sedation

unusual   not unusual   common   problematic
• Reported but not expected
• Fatigue may occur

What To Do About Side Effects
• Wait
• Wait
• Wait
• Consider lowering dose or switching to a different agent

Best Augmenting Agents for Side Effects
• Many side effects cannot be improved with an augmenting agent

MEMANTINE (continued)

NaN## DOSING AND USE

Usual Dosage Range
• 20 mg twice daily

Dosage Forms
• Tablet 5 mg, 10 mg

How to Dose
• Initial 5 mg/day; can increase by 5 mg each week; doses over 5 mg should be divided; maximum dose 20 mg twice daily

Dosing Tips
❋ Despite very long half-life, is generally dosed twice daily
• Both the patient and the patient's caregiver should be instructed on how to dose memantine since patients themselves have moderate to severe dementia and may require assistance
❋ Memantine is unlikely to affect pharmacokinetics of acetylcholinesterase inhibitors
• Absorption not affected by food

Overdose
• No fatalities have been reported; restlessness, psychosis, visual hallucinations, sedation, stupor, loss of consciousness

Long-Term Use
• Drug may lose effectiveness in slowing degenerative course of Alzheimer disease after 6 months

Habit Forming
• No

How to Stop
• No known withdrawal symptoms
• Theoretically, discontinuation could lead to notable deterioration in memory and behavior which may not be restored when drug is restarted or a cholinesterase inhibitor is initiated

Pharmacokinetics
• Little metabolism; mostly excreted unchanged in the urine
• Terminal elimination half-life approximately 60–80 hours
• Minimal inhibition of CYP450 enzymes

Drug Interactions
• No interactions with drugs metabolized by CYP450 enzymes
• Drugs that raise the urine pH (e.g., carbonic anhydrase inhibitors, sodium bicarbonate) may reduce elimination of memantine and raise plasma levels of memantine
❋ No interactions with cholinesterase inhibitors

Other Warnings/ Precautions
❋ Use cautiously if co-administering with other NMDA antagonists such as amantadine, ketamine, and dextromethorphan

Do Not Use
• If there is a proven allergy to memantine

SPECIAL POPULATIONS

Renal Impairment
• Use with caution; dose may need to be reduced
• Not recommended for use in severe renal impairment

Hepatic Impairment
• Not likely to require dosage adjustment

Cardiac Impairment
• Not likely to require dosage adjustment

Elderly
• Pharmacokinetics similar to younger adults

Children and Adolescents
• Memantine use has not been studied in children or adolescents

Pregnancy
• Risk Category B [animal studies do not show adverse effects; no controlled studies in humans]
❋ Not recommended for use in pregnant women or women of childbearing potential

Breast Feeding
- Unknown if memantine is secreted in human breast milk, but all psychotropics assumed to be secreted in breast milk
- ✳ Recommended either to discontinue drug or bottle feed
- Memantine is not recommended for use in nursing women

THE ART OF PSYCHOPHARMACOLOGY

Potential Advantages
- In patients with more advanced Alzheimer disease

Potential Disadvantages
- Unproven to be effective in mild to moderate Alzheimer disease
- Patients who have difficulty taking a medication twice daily

Primary Target Symptoms
- Memory loss in Alzheimer disease
- Behavioral symptoms in Alzheimer disease
- Memory loss in other dementias

Pearls
- ✳ In contrast to cholinesterase inhibitors, which are indicated for mild to moderate Alzheimer disease, memantine is indicated for moderate to severe Alzheimer disease
- Recently approved in the U.S. but available for many years in other countries (e.g., Germany)
- ✳ Memantine's actions are somewhat like the natural inhibition of NMDA receptors by magnesium, and thus memantine is a sort of "artificial magnesium"
- Theoretically, NMDA antagonism of memantine is strong enough to block chronic low level over-excitation of glutamate receptors associated with Alzheimer disease, but not strong enough to interfere with periodic high level utilization of glutamate for plasticity, learning, and memory
- Structurally related to the antiparkinsonian and anti-influenza agent amantadine, which is also a weak NMDA antagonist
- ✳ Memantine is well-tolerated with a low incidence of adverse effects
- Antagonist actions at 5HT3 receptors have unknown clinical consequences but may contribute to low incidence of gastrointestinal side effects
- Treat the patient but ask the caregiver about efficacy
- Delay in progression of Alzheimer disease is not evidence of disease-modifying actions of NMDA antagonism
- May or may not be effective in vascular dementia
- Under investigation for dementia associated with HIV/AIDS
- May or may not be effective in chronic neuropathic pain
- ✳ Theoretically, could be useful for any condition characterized by moderate over-activation of NMDA glutamate receptors (possibly neurodegenerative conditions or even bipolar disorder, anxiety disorders, or chronic neuropathic pain), but this is not proven

Suggested Reading

Areosa SA, Sherriff F. Memantine for dementia. Cochrane Database Syst Rev 2003;(3):CD003154.

Doggrell S. Is memantine a breakthrough in the treatment of moderate-to-severe Alzheimer's disease? Expert Opin Pharmacother 2003;4:1857–60.

Mobius HJ. Memantine: update on the current evidence. Int J Geriatr Psychiatry 2003;18(Suppl 1):S47–54.

Tariot PN, Federoff HJ. Current treatment for Alzheimer disease and future prospects. Alzheimer Dis Assoc Disord 2003;17 Suppl 4: S105–13.

MESORIDAZINE

THERAPEUTICS

Brands • Serentil
• Lidanil
see index for additional brand names

Generic? Yes

 Class

• Conventional antipsychotic (neuroleptic, phenothiazine, dopamine 2 antagonist)

Commonly Prescribed For
(bold for FDA approved)
• **Management of schizophrenic patients who fail to respond adequately to treatment with other antipsychotic drugs**

 How The Drug Works

• Blocks dopamine 2 receptors, reducing positive symptoms of psychosis

How Long Until It Works
• Psychotic symptoms can improve within 1 week, but it may take several weeks for full effect on behavior

If It Works
• Is a second-line treatment option
✳ Should evaluate for switching to an antipsychotic with a better risk/benefit ratio

If It Doesn't Work
• Consider trying one of the first-line atypical antipsychotics (risperidone, olanzapine, quetiapine, ziprasidone, aripiprazole, amisulpride)
• Consider trying another conventional antipsychotic
• If 2 or more antipsychotic monotherapies do not work, consider clozapine

 Best Augmenting Combos for Partial Response or Treatment-Resistance

• Augmentation of mesoridazine has not been systematically studied and can be dangerous, especially with drugs that can prolong QTc interval

Tests
✳ Baseline ECG and serum potassium levels should be determined
✳ Periodic evaluation of ECG and serum potassium levels
• Serum magnesium levels may also need to be monitored
✳ Since conventional antipsychotics are frequently associated with weight gain, before starting treatment, weigh all patients and determine if the patient is already overweight (BMI 25.0–29.9) or obese (BMI ≥30)
• Before giving a drug that can cause weight gain to an overweight or obese patient, consider determining whether the patient already has pre-diabetes (fasting plasma glucose 100–125 mg/dl), diabetes (fasting plasma glucose >126 mg/dl), or dyslipidemia (increased total cholesterol, LDL cholesterol and triglycerides; decreased HDL cholesterol), and treat or refer such patients for treatment, including nutrition and weight management, physical activity counseling, smoking cessation, and medical management
✳ Monitor weight and BMI during treatment
✳ While giving a drug to a patient who has gained >5% of initial weight, consider evaluating for the presence of pre-diabetes, diabetes, or dyslipidemia, or consider switching to a different antipsychotic
• Should check blood pressure in the elderly before starting and for the first few weeks of treatment
• Monitoring elevated prolactin levels of dubious clinical benefit
• Phenothiazines may cause false-positive phenylketonuria results

SIDE EFFECTS

How Drug Causes Side Effects
• By blocking dopamine 2 receptors in the striatum, it can cause motor side effects
• By blocking dopamine 2 receptors in the pituitary, it can cause elevations in prolactin
• By blocking dopamine 2 receptors excessively in the mesocortical and mesolimbic dopamine pathways, especially at high doses, it can cause worsening of

negative and cognitive symptoms (neuroleptic-induced deficit syndrome)
- Anticholinergic actions may cause sedation, blurred vision, constipation, dry mouth
- Antihistaminic actions may cause sedation, weight gain
- By blocking alpha 1 adrenergic receptors, it can cause dizziness, sedation, and hypotension
- Mechanism of weight gain and any possible increased incidence of diabetes or dyslipidemia with conventional antipsychotics is unknown
- ✳ Mechanism of potentially dangerous QTc prolongation may be related to actions at ion channels

Notable Side Effects
- ✳ Neuroleptic-induced deficit syndrome
- ✳ Akathisia
- ✳ Priapism
- ✳ Extrapyramidal symptoms, Parkinsonism, tardive dyskinesia
- ✳ Galactorrhea, amenorrhea
- ✳ Pigmentary retinopathy at high doses
- Dizziness, sedation
- Dry mouth, constipation, blurred vision
- Decreased sweating
- Sexual dysfunction
- Hypotension
- Weight gain

 Life Threatening or Dangerous Side Effects
- Rare neuroleptic malignant syndrome
- Rare jaundice, agranulocytosis
- Rare seizures
- ✳ Dose-dependent QTc prolongation
- Ventricular arrhythmias and sudden death

Weight Gain

unusual / **not unusual** / common / problematic
- Occurs in significant minority

Sedation

unusual / not unusual / **common** / problematic
- Many experience and/or can be significant in amount
- Sedation is usually transient

What To Do About Side Effects
- Wait
- Wait
- Wait
- For motor symptoms, add an anticholinergic agent
- Reduce the dose
- For sedation, give at night
- Switch to an atypical antipsychotic
- Weight loss, exercise programs, and medical management for high BMIs, diabetes, dyslipidemia

Best Augmenting Agents for Side Effects
- Augmentation of mesoridazine has not been systematically studied and can be dangerous

DOSING AND USE

Usual Dosage Range
- Oral: 100–400 mg/day
- Injection: 25–200 mg/day

Dosage Forms
- Tablet 10 mg, 25 mg, 50 mg, 100 mg
- Ampul 25 mg/mL, 1 mL
- Concentrate 25 mg/mL

How to Dose
- Oral: initial 50 mg 3 times a day; increase dose cautiously as needed
- Injection: initial 25 mg; repeat after 30–60 minutes if needed
- Take liquid formulation in water, orange juice, or grapefruit juice

 Dosing Tips
- ✳ The effects of mesoridazine on the QTc interval are dose-dependent, so start low and go slow while carefully monitoring QTc interval

Overdose
- Deaths have occurred; sedation, confusion, agitation, respiratory depression, cardiac disturbances, coma

Long-Term Use
- Some side effects may be irreversible (e.g., tardive dyskinesia)

Habit Forming
• No

How to Stop
• Slow down-titration of oral formulation (over 6 to 8 weeks), especially when simultaneously beginning a new antipsychotic while switching (i.e., cross-titration)
• Rapid oral discontinuation may lead to rebound psychosis and worsening of symptoms
• If antiparkinson agents are being used, they should be continued for a few weeks after mesoridazine is discontinued

Pharmacokinetics
• Half-life approximately 2–9 hours

 Drug Interactions
• May decrease the effects of levodopa, dopamine agonists
• May increase the effects of antihypertensive drugs
• May enhance QTc prolongation of other drugs capable of prolonging QTc interval
• Additive effects may occur if used with CNS depressants
• Respiratory depression or respiratory arrest may occur if mesoridazine is used with a barbiturate
• Some patients taking a neuroleptic and lithium have developed an encephalopathic syndrome similar to neuroleptic malignant syndrome
• Combined use with epinephrine may lower blood pressure

 Other Warnings/ Precautions
• If signs of neuroleptic malignant syndrome develop, treatment should be immediately discontinued
• Use with caution in patients with respiratory disorders, glaucoma, or urinary retention
• Use cautiously in patients with alcohol withdrawal or convulsive disorders because of possible lowering of seizure threshold
• Use with caution if at all in Parkinson's disease or Lewy Body dementia
• Avoid extreme heat exposure

• Antiemetic effect can mask signs of other disorders or overdose
• Do not use epinephrine in event of overdose as interaction with some pressor agents may lower blood pressure
• Because mesoridazine may dose-dependently prolong QTc interval, use with caution in patients who have bradycardia or who are taking drugs that can induce bradycardia (e.g., beta blockers, calcium channel blockers, clonidine, digitalis)
• Because mesoridazine may dose-dependently prolong QTc interval, use with caution in patients who have hypokalemia and/or hypomagnesemia or who are taking drugs that can induce hypokalemia and/or magnesemia (e.g., diuretics, stimulant laxatives, intravenous amphotericin B, glucocorticoids, tetracosactide)
• Mesoridazine can increase the QTc interval, potentially causing torsades de pointes-type arrhythmia or sudden death

Do Not Use
• If there is a history of QTc prolongation or cardiac arrhythmia, recent acute myocardial infarction, uncompensated heart failure
✱ If QTc interval greater than 450 msec or if taking an agent capable of prolonging the QTc interval
• If patient is in a comatose state or has CNS depression
• If there is a proven allergy to mesoridazine
• If there is a known sensitivity to any phenothiazine

SPECIAL POPULATIONS

Renal Impairment
• Use with caution

Hepatic Impairment
• Use with caution

Cardiac Impairment
• Mesoridazine produces a dose-dependent prolongation of QTc interval, which may be enhanced by the existence of bradycardia, hypokalemia, congenital or acquired long QTc interval, which should be evaluated prior to administering mesoridazine
• Use with caution if treating concomitantly with a medication likely to produce

prolonged bradycardia, hypokalemia, slowing of intracardiac conduction, or prolongation of the QTc interval
- Avoid mesoridazine in patients with a known history of QTc prolongation, recent acute myocardial infarction, and uncompensated heart failure
* Risk/benefit ratio may not justify use in cardiac impairment

Elderly
- Lower doses should be used and patient should be monitored closely

Children and Adolescents
- Safety and efficacy not established

Pregnancy
- Risk Category C [some animal studies show adverse effects, no controlled studies in humans]
- Reports of extrapyramidal symptoms, jaundice, hyperreflexia, hyporeflexia in infants whose mothers took a phenothiazine during pregnancy
- Psychotic symptoms may worsen during pregnancy and some form of treatment may be necessary
- Atypical antipsychotics may be preferable to conventional antipsychotics or anticonvulsant mood stabilizers if treatment is required during pregnancy
- Mesoridazine should generally not be used during the first trimester
- Should evaluate for an antipsychotic with a better risk/benefit ratio if treatment is required during pregnancy

Breast Feeding
- Some drug is found in mother's breast milk

- Effects on infant have been observed (dystonia, tardive dyskinesia, sedation)
* Recommended either to discontinue drug or bottle feed

THE ART OF PSYCHOPHARMACOLOGY

Potential Advantages
- Only for patients who respond to this agent and not other antipsychotics

Potential Disadvantages
- Vulnerable populations such as children or elderly
- Patients on other drugs

Primary Target Symptoms
- Positive symptoms of psychosis in patients who fail to respond to treatment with other antipsychotics
- Motor and autonomic hyperactivity in patients who fail to respond to treatment with other antipsychotics
- Violent or aggressive behavior in patients who fail to respond to treatment with other antipsychotics

Pearls
* Generally, the benefits of mesoridazine do not outweigh its risks for most patients
* Because of its effects on the QTc interval, mesoridazine is not intended for use unless other options (at least 2 antipsychotics) have failed
- Mesoridazine has not been systematically studied in treatment-refractory schizophrenia
- Conventional antipsychotics are much less expensive than atypical antipsychotics

Suggested Reading

Frankenburg FR. Choices in antipsychotic therapy in schizophrenia. Harv Rev Psychiatry 1999; 6: 241–9.

Gardos G, Tecce JJ, Hartmann E, Bowers P, Cole JO. Treatment with mesoridazine and thioridazine in chronic schizophrenia: II.

Potential predictors of drug response. Compr Psychiatry 1978; 19: 527–32.

Gershon S, Sakalis G, Bowers PA. Mesoridazine — a pharmacodynamic and pharmacokinetic profile. J Clin Psychiatry 1981; 42: 463–9.

MIDAZOLAM

THERAPEUTICS

Brands • Versed
see index for additional brand names

Generic? No

 Class
• Benzodiazepine (hypnotic)

Commonly Prescribed For
(bold for FDA approved)
• **Sedation in pediatric patients**
• **Sedation (adjunct to anesthesia)**
• **Pre-operative anxiolytic**
• **Drug-induced amnesia**

 How The Drug Works
• Binds to benzodiazepine receptors at the GABA-A ligand-gated chloride channel complex
• Enhances the inhibitory effects of GABA
• Boosts chloride conductance through GABA-regulated channels
• Inhibitory actions in sleep centers may provide sedative hypnotic effects

How Long Until It Works
• Intravenous injection: onset 3–5 minutes
• Intramuscular injection: onset 15 minutes, peak 30–60 minutes

If It Works
• Patients generally recover 2–6 hours after awakening

If It Doesn't Work
• Increase the dose
• Switch to another agent

 Best Augmenting Combos for Partial Response or Treatment-Resistance
• Augmenting agents have not been adequately studied

Tests
• None for healthy individuals

SIDE EFFECTS

How Drug Causes Side Effects
• Actions at benzodiazepine receptors that carry over to next day can cause daytime sedation, amnesia, and ataxia

Notable Side Effects
• Over-sedation, impaired recall, agitation, involuntary movements, headache
• Nausea, vomiting
• Hiccups, fluctuation in vital signs, irritation/pain at site of injection
• Hypotension

 Life Threatening or Dangerous Side Effects
• Respiratory depression, apnea, respiratory arrest
• Cardiac arrest

Weight Gain

unusual / not unusual / common / problematic
• Reported but not expected

Sedation

unusual / not unusual / **common** / problematic
• Many experience and/or can be significant in amount

What To Do About Side Effects
• Wait
• Switch to another agent
• Administer flumazenil if side effects are severe or life-threatening

Best Augmenting Agents for Side Effects
• Many side effects cannot be improved with an augmenting agent

DOSING AND USE

Usual Dosage Range
• Intravenous (adults): 1–2.5 mg
• Liquid (age 16 and under): 0.25–1.0 mg/kg

Dosage Forms
• Intravenous: 5 mg/mL – 1 mL vial, 2 mL vial, 5 mL vial, 10 mL vial
• Liquid: 2 mg/mL – 118 mL bottle

How to Dose
- Liquid single dose: 0.25–1.0 mg/kg; maximum dose generally 20 mg
- Intravenous (adults): administer over 2 minutes; monitor patient over the next 2 or more minutes to determine effects; allow 3–5 minutes between administrations; maximum 2.5 mg within 2 minutes

 Dosing Tips
- Better to underdose, observe for effects, and then prudently raise dose while monitoring carefully

Overdose
- Sedation, confusion, poor coordination, respiratory depression, coma

Long-Term Use
- Not generally intended for long-term use

Habit Forming
- Some patients may develop dependence and/or tolerance; risk may be greater with higher doses
- History of drug addiction may increase risk of dependence

How to Stop
- If administration was prolonged, do not stop abruptly

Pharmacokinetics
- Elimination half-life 1.8–6.4 hours
- Active metabolite

 Drug Interactions
- If CNS depressants are used concomitantly, midazolam dose should be reduced by half or more
- Increased depressive effects when taken with other CNS depressants
- Drugs that inhibit CYP450 3A4, such as nefazodone and fluvoxamine, may reduce midazolam clearance and thus raise midazolam levels
- Midazolam decreases the minimum alveolar concentration of halothane needed for general anesthesia

 Other Warnings/ Precautions
- Midazolam should only be used in an environment in which the patient can be closely monitored (e.g., hospital) because of the risk of respiratory depression and respiratory arrest
- Sedated pediatric patients should be monitored throughout the procedure
- Patients with chronic obstructive pulmonary disease should receive lower doses
- Use with caution in patients with impaired respiratory function

Do Not Use
- If patient has narrow angle-closure glaucoma
- If there is a proven allergy to midazolam or any benzodiazepine

Renal Impairment
- May have longer elimination half-life, prolonging time to recovery

Hepatic Impairment
- Longer elimination half-life; clearance is reduced

Cardiac Impairment
- Longer elimination half-life; clearance is reduced

Elderly
- Longer elimination half-life; clearance is reduced
- Intravenous: 1–3.5 mg; maximum 1.5 mg within 2 minutes

 Children and Adolescents
- In most pediatric populations, pharmacokinetic properties are similar to those in adults
- Seriously ill neonates have reduced clearance and longer elimination half-life
- Hypotension has occurred in neonates given midazolam and fentanyl
- Intravenous dose: dependent on age, weight, route, procedure

Pregnancy

- Risk Category D [positive evidence of risk to human fetus; potential benefits may still justify its use during pregnancy]
- Midazolam crosses the placenta
- Neonatal flaccidity has been reported in infants whose mother took a benzodiazepine during pregnancy

Breast Feeding

- Some drug is found in mother's breast milk
- Effects on infant have been observed and include feeding difficulties, sedation, and weight loss
- Midazolam can be used to relieve postoperative pain after cesarean section

THE ART OF PSYCHOPHARMACOLOGY

Potential Advantages

- Fast onset
- Parenteral dosage forms

Potential Disadvantages

- Can be oversedating

Primary Target Symptoms

- Anxiety

 Pearls

- Recovery (e.g., ability to stand/walk) generally takes from 2–6 hours after wakening
- Half-life may be longer in obese patients
- Patients with premenstrual syndrome may be less sensitive to midazolam than healthy women throughout the cycle
- Midazolam clearance may be reduced in postmenopausal women compared to premenopausal women

 Suggested Reading

Blumer JL. Clinical pharmacology of midazolam in infants and children. Clin Pharmacokinet 1998;35:37–47.

Fountain NB, Adams RE. Midazolam treatment of acute and refractory status epilepticus. Clin Neuropharmacol 1999;22:261–7.

Shafer A. Complications of sedation with midazolam in the intensive care unit and a comparison with other sedative regimens. Crit Care Med 1998;26:947–56.

Yuan R, Flockhart DA, Balian JD. Pharmacokinetic and pharmacodynamic consequences of metabolism-based drug interactions with alprazolam, midazolam, and triazolam. J Clin Pharmacol 1999;39:1109–25.

MILNACIPRAN

THERAPEUTICS

Brands • Toledomin
• Ixel
see index for additional brand names

Generic? No

Class
• SNRI (dual serotonin and norepinephrine reuptake inhibitor); antidepressant; chronic pain treatment

Commonly Prescribed For
(bold for FDA approved)
• Major depressive disorder
• Fibromyalgia
• Neuropathic pain/chronic pain

How The Drug Works
• Boosts neurotransmitters serotonin, norepinephrine/noradrenaline, and dopamine
• Blocks serotonin reuptake pump (serotonin transporter), presumably increasing serotonergic neurotransmission
• Blocks norepinephrine reuptake pump (norepinephrine transporter), presumably increasing noradrenergic neurotransmission
• Presumably desensitizes both serotonin 1A receptors and beta adrenergic receptors
✳ Weak noncompetitive NMDA-receptor antagonist (high doses), which may contribute to actions in chronic pain
• Since dopamine is inactivated by norepinephrine reuptake in frontal cortex, which largely lacks dopamine transporters, milnacipran can increase dopamine neurotransmission in this part of the brain

How Long Until It Works
• Onset of therapeutic actions usually not immediate, but often delayed 2 to 4 weeks
• If it is not working within 6 to 8 weeks, it may require a dosage increase or it may not work at all
• May continue to work for many years to prevent relapse of symptoms in depression

If It Works
• The goal of treatment of depression is complete remission of current symptoms as well as prevention of future relapses
• The goal of treatment of fibromyalgia and chronic neuropathic pain is to reduce symptoms as much as possible, especially in combination with other treatments
• Treatment of depression most often reduces or even eliminates symptoms, but is not a cure since symptoms can recur after medicine stopped
• Treatment of fibromyalgia and chronic neuropathic pain may reduce symptoms, but rarely eliminates them completely, and is not a cure since symptoms can recur after medicine is stopped
• Continue treatment of depression until all symptoms are gone (remission)
• Once symptoms of depression are gone, continue treating for 1 year for the first episode of depression
• For second and subsequent episodes of depression, treatment may need to be indefinite
• Use in fibromyalgia and chronic neuropathic pain may also need to be indefinite, but long-term treatment is not well-studied in these conditions

If It Doesn't Work
• Many depressed patients only have a partial response where some symptoms are improved but others persist (especially insomnia, fatigue, and problems concentrating)
• Other depressed patients may be nonresponders, sometimes called treatment-resistant or treatment-refractory
• Some depressed patients who have an initial response may relapse even though they continue treatment, sometimes called "poop-out"
• Consider increasing dose, switching to another agent or adding an appropriate augmenting agent
• Consider psychotherapy
• Consider evaluation for another diagnosis or for a comorbid condition (e.g., medical illness, substance abuse, etc.)
• Some patients may experience apparent lack of consistent efficacy due to activation of latent or underlying bipolar disorder, and require antidepressant discontinuation and switch to a mood stabilizer

Best Augmenting Combos for Partial Response or Treatment-Resistance

- Augmentation experience is limited compared to other antidepressants
- Benzodiazepines can reduce insomnia and anxiety
- Adding other agents to milnacipran for treating depression could follow the same practice for augmenting SSRIs or other SNRIs if done by experts while monitoring carefully in difficult cases
- Although no controlled studies and little clinical experience, adding other agents for treating fibromyalgia and chronic neuropathic pain could theoretically include gabapentin, tiagabine, other anticonvulsants, or even opiates if done by experts while monitoring carefully in difficult cases
- Mirtazapine, bupropion, reboxetine, atomoxetine (use combinations of antidepressants with caution as this may activate bipolar disorder and suicidal ideation)
- Modafinil, especially for fatigue, sleepiness, and lack of concentration
- Mood stabilizers or atypical antipsychotics for bipolar depression, psychotic depression or treatment-resistant depression
- Hypnotics or trazodone for insomnia
- Classically, lithium, buspirone, or thyroid hormone

Tests
- Check blood pressure before initiating treatment and regularly during treatment

SIDE EFFECTS

How Drug Causes Side Effects
- Theoretically due to increases in serotonin and norepinephrine concentrations at receptors in parts of the brain and body other than those that cause therapeutic actions (e.g., unwanted actions of serotonin in sleep centers causing insomnia, unwanted actions of norepinephrine on acetylcholine release causing urinary retention or constipation)
- Most side effects are immediate but often go away with time

Notable Side Effects
- Most side effects increase with higher doses, at least transiently
- Headache, nervousness, insomnia, sedation
- Nausea, diarrhea, decreased appetite
- Sexual dysfunction (abnormal ejaculation/orgasm, impotence)
- Asthenia, sweating
- SIADH (syndrome of inappropriate antidiuretic hormone secretion)
- Dose-dependent increased blood pressure
- Dry mouth, constipation
- Dysuria, urological complaints, urinary hesitancy, urinary retention
- Increase in heart rate
- Palpitations

 Life Threatening or Dangerous Side Effects

- Rare induction of mania and activation of suicidal ideation
- Rare seizures

Weight Gain

unusual not unusual common problematic

- Reported but not expected

Sedation

unusual not unusual **common** problematic

- Many experience and/or can be significant in amount

What To Do About Side Effects
- Wait
- Wait
- Wait
- Lower the dose
- In a few weeks, switch or add other drugs

Best Augmenting Agents for Side Effects
- ✳ For urinary hesitancy, give an alpha 1 blocker such as tamsulosin or naftopidil
- Often best to try another antidepressant monotherapy prior to resorting to augmentation strategies to treat side effects
- Trazodone or a hypnotic for insomnia
- Bupropion, sildenafil, vardenafil, or tadalafil for sexual dysfunction

- Benzodiazepines for anxiety, agitation
- Mirtazapine for insomnia, agitation, and gastrointestinal side effects
- Many side effects are dose-dependent (i.e., they increase as dose increases, or they reemerge until tolerance re-develops)
- Many side effects are time-dependent (i.e., they start immediately upon dosing and upon each dose increase, but go away with time)
- Activation and agitation may represent the induction of a bipolar state, especially a mixed dysphoric bipolar II condition sometimes associated with suicidal ideation, and require the addition of lithium, a mood stabilizer or an atypical antipsychotic, and/or discontinuation of milnacipran

DOSING AND USE

Usual Dosage Range
- 30–200 mg/day in 2 doses

Dosage Forms
- Capsule 25 mg, 50 mg (France, other European countries, and worldwide markets)
- Capsule 15 mg, 25 mg, 50 mg (Japan)

How to Dose
- Should be administered in 2 divided doses
- Begin at 25 mg twice daily and increase as necessary and as tolerated up to 100 mg twice daily; maximum dose 300 mg/day

 Dosing Tips

* Once daily dosing has far less consistent efficacy, so only give as twice daily
- Higher doses (>200 mg/day) not consistently effective in all studies of depression
- Nevertheless, some patients respond better to higher doses (200–300 mg/day) than to lower doses
- Different doses in different countries
- Different doses in different indications and different populations
- Preferred dose for depression may be 50 mg twice daily to 100 mg twice daily in France

- Preferred dose for depression in the elderly may be 15 mg twice daily to 25 mg twice daily in Japan
- Preferred dosing for depression in other adults may be 25 mg twice daily to 50 mg twice daily in Japan
- Preferred dose for fibromyalgia may be 100 mg twice daily
* Thus, clinicians must be aware that titration of twice daily dosing across a 10-fold range (30 mg – 300 mg total daily dose) can optimize milnacipran's efficacy in broad clinical use
- Patients with agitation or anxiety may require slower titration to optimize tolerability
- Higher doses usually well tolerated in fibromyalgia patients
- No pharmacokinetic drug interactions (not an inhibitor of CYP450 2D6 or 3A4)
- As milnacipran is a more potent norepinephrine reuptake inhibitor than a serotonin reuptake inhibitor, some patients may require dosing at the higher end of the dosing range to obtain robust dual SNRI actions
- At high doses, NMDA glutamate antagonist actions may be a factor

Overdose
- Vomiting, hypertension, sedation, tachycardia
- The emetic effect of high doses of milnacipran may reduce the risk of serious adverse effects

Long-Term Use
- Safe

Habit Forming
- No

How to Stop
- Taper is prudent, but usually not necessary

Pharmacokinetics
- Half-life 8 hours
- No active metabolite

 Drug Interactions
- Tramadol increases the risk of seizures in patients taking an antidepressant
- Can cause a fatal "serotonin syndrome" when combined with MAO inhibitors, so do

not use with MAO inhibitors or for at least 14 days after MAOIs are stopped
- Do not start an MAO inhibitor for at least 2 weeks after discontinuing milnacipran
- Switching from or addition of other norepinephrine reuptake inhibitors should be done with caution, as the additive pro-noradrenergic effects may enhance therapeutic actions in depression, but also enhance noradrenergically-mediated side effects
- Few known adverse pharmacokinetic drug interactions

 Other Warnings/ Precautions

- Use with caution in patients with history of seizures
- Use with caution in patients with bipolar disorder unless treated with concomitant mood stabilizing agent
- Monitor patients for activation of suicidal ideation, especially children and adolescents

Do Not Use
- If patient has uncontrolled narrow angle-closure glaucoma
- If patient is taking an MAO inhibitor
- If there is a proven allergy to milnacipran

SPECIAL POPULATIONS

Renal Impairment
- Should receive lower doses; amount of dose adjustment related to degree of impairment

Hepatic Impairment
- No dose adjustment necessary

Cardiac Impairment
- Drug should be used with caution

Elderly
- Some patients may tolerate lower doses better

 Children and Adolescents
- Use with caution, observing for activation of known or unknown bipolar disorder and/or suicidal ideation, and strongly

consider informing parents or guardian of this risk so they can help observe child or adolescent patients
- Not well-studied

 Pregnancy
- Not generally recommended for use during pregnancy, especially during first trimester
- Nonetheless, continuous treatment during pregnancy may be necessary and has not been proven to be harmful to the fetus
- Must weigh the risk of treatment (first trimester fetal development, third trimester newborn delivery) to the child against the risk of no treatment (recurrence of depression, maternal health, infant bonding) to the mother and child
- For many patients this may mean continuing treatment during pregnancy
- Neonates exposed to SSRIs or SNRIs late in the third trimester have developed complications requiring prolonged hospitalization, respiratory support, and tube feeding; reported symptoms are consistent with either a direct toxic effect of SSRIs and SNRIs or, possibly, a drug discontinuation syndrome, and include respiratory distress, cyanosis, apnea, seizures, temperature instability, feeding difficulty, vomiting, hypoglycemia, hypotonia, hypertonia, hyperreflexia, tremor, jitteriness, irritability, and constant crying

Breast Feeding
- Unknown if milnacipran is secreted in human breast milk, but all psychotropics assumed to be secreted in breast milk
- Immediate postpartum period is a high-risk time for depression, especially in women who have had prior depressive episodes, so drug may need to be reinstituted late in the third trimester or shortly after childbirth to prevent a recurrence during the postpartum period
- Must weigh benefits of breast feeding with risks and benefits of antidepressant treatment versus non-treatment to both the infant and the mother
- For many patients, this may mean continuing treatment during breast feeding

THE ART OF PSYCHOPHARMACOLOGY

Potential Advantages

- Patients with retarded depression
- Patients with hypersomnia
- Patients with atypical depression
- Patients with depression may have higher remission rates on SNRIs than on SSRIs
- Depressed patients with somatic symptoms, fatigue, and pain
- Fibromyalgia, chronic pain syndrome

Potential Disadvantages

- Patients with urologic disorders, prostate disorders
- Patients with borderline or uncontrolled hypertension
- Patients with agitation and anxiety (short-term)

Primary Target Symptoms

- Depressed mood
- Energy, motivation, and interest
- Sleep disturbance
- Physical symptoms
- Pain

 Pearls

- Not studied in stress urinary incontinence
- Not well studied in ADHD or anxiety disorders, but may be effective
- ✳ Has greater potency for norepinephrine reuptake blockade than for serotonin reuptake blockade, but this is of unclear clinical significance as a differentiating feature from other SNRIs, although it might contribute to its therapeutic activity in fibromyalgia and chronic pain
- ✳ Onset of action in fibromyalgia may be somewhat faster than depression (i.e., 2 weeks rather than 2–8 weeks)
- Therapeutic actions in fibromyalgia are partial, with symptom reduction but not necessarily remission of painful symptoms in many patients
- ✳ Potent noradrenergic actions may account for possibly higher incidence of sweating and urinary hesitancy than other SNRIs
- Urinary hesitancy more common in men than women and in older men than in younger men
- Alpha 1 antagonists such as tamsulosin or naftopidil can reverse urinary hesitancy or retention
- Alpha 1 antagonists given prophylactically may prevent urinary hesitancy or retention in patients at higher risk, such as elderly men with borderline urine flow
- May be better tolerated than tricyclic or tetracyclic antidepressants in the treatment of fibromyalgia or other chronic pain syndromes
- No pharmacokinetic interactions or elevations in plasma drug levels of tricyclic or tetracyclic antidepressants when adding or switching to or from milnacipran

 Suggested Reading

Bisserbe JC. Clinical utility of milnacipran in comparison with other antidepressants. Int Clin Psychopharmacol 2002;17 Suppl 1:S43–50.

Montgomery SA, Prost JF, Solles A, Briley M. Efficacy and tolerability of milnacipran: an overview. Int Clin Psychopharmacol 1996;11 Suppl 4:47–51.

Puozzo C, Panconi E, Deprez D. Pharmacology and pharmacokinetics of milnacipran. Int Clin Psychopharmacol 2002;17 Suppl 1:S25–35.

Spencer CM, Wilde MI. Milnacipran. A review of its use in depression. Drugs 1998; 56:405–27.

MIRTAZAPINE

THERAPEUTICS

Brands • Remeron
see index for additional brand names

Generic? Yes

Class
- Alpha 2 antagonist; NaSSA (noradrenaline and specific serotonergic agent); dual serotonin and norepinephrine agent; antidepressant

Commonly Prescribed For
(bold for FDA approved)
- **Major depressive disorder**
- Panic disorder
- Generalized anxiety disorder
- Posttraumatic stress disorder

How The Drug Works
- Boost neurotransmitters serotonin and norepinephrine/noradrenaline
- Blocks alpha 2 adrenergic presynaptic receptor, thereby increasing norepinephrine neurotransmission
- Blocks alpha 2 adrenergic presynaptic receptor on serotonin neurons (heteroreceptors), thereby increasing serotonin neurotransmission
- This is a novel mechanism independent of norepinephrine and serotonin reuptake blockade
- Blocks 5HT2A, 5HT2C, and 5HT3 serotonin receptors
- Blocks H1 histamine receptors

How Long Until It Works
- ✳ Actions on insomnia and anxiety can start shortly after initiation of dosing
- Onset of therapeutic actions in depression, however, is usually not immediate, but often delayed 2 to 4 weeks
- If it is not working within 6 to 8 weeks for depression, it may require a dosage increase or it may not work at all
- May continue to work for many years to prevent relapse of symptoms

If It Works
- The goal of treatment is complete remission of current symptoms as well as prevention of future relapses
- Treatment most often reduces or even eliminates symptoms, but not a cure since symptoms can recur after medicine stopped
- Continue treatment until all symptoms are gone (remission)
- Once symptoms gone, continue treating for 1 year for the first episode of depression
- For second and subsequent episodes of depression, treatment may need to be indefinite
- Use in anxiety disorders may also need to be indefinite

If It Doesn't Work
- Many patients only have a partial response where some symptoms are improved but others persist (especially insomnia, fatigue, and problems concentrating)
- Other patients may be nonresponders, sometimes called treatment-resistant or treatment-refractory
- Consider increasing dose, switching to another agent or adding an appropriate augmenting agent
- Consider psychotherapy
- Consider evaluation for another diagnosis or for a comorbid condition (e.g., medical illness, substance abuse, etc.)
- Some patients may experience apparent lack of consistent efficacy due to activation of latent or underlying bipolar disorder, and require antidepressant discontinuation and a switch to a mood stabilizer

Best Augmenting Combos for Partial Response or Treatment-Resistance
- SSRIs, bupropion, reboxetine, atomoxetine (use combinations of antidepressants with caution as this may activate bipolar disorder and suicidal ideation)
- ✳ Venlafaxine ("California rocket fuel"; a potentially powerful dual serotonin and norepinephrine combination, but observe for activation of bipolar disorder and suicidal ideation)
- Modafinil, especially for fatigue, sleepiness, and lack of concentration

- Mood stabilizers or atypical antipsychotics for bipolar depression, psychotic depression or treatment-resistant depression
- Benzodiazepines
- Hypnotics or trazodone for insomnia

Tests

- None for healthy individuals
- May need liver function tests for those with hepatic abnormalities before initiating treatment
- May need to monitor blood count during treatment for those with blood dyscrasias, leucopenia, or granulocytopenia
- Since some antidepressants such as mirtazapine can be associated with significant weight gain, before starting treatment, weigh all patients and determine if the patient is already overweight (BMI>25.0–29.9) or obese (BMI>30)
- Before giving a drug that can cause weight gain to an overweight or obese patient, consider determining whether the patient already has pre-diabetes (fasting plasma glucose 100–125 mg/dl), diabetes (fasting plasma glucose >126 mg/dl), or dyslipidemia (increased total cholesterol, LDL cholesterol and triglycerides; decreased HDL cholesterol), and treat or refer such patients for treatment, including nutrition and weight management, physical activity counseling, smoking cessation, and medical management
- ✳ Monitor weight and BMI during treatment
- ✳ While giving a drug to a patient who has gained >5% of initial weight, consider evaluating for the presence of pre-diabetes, diabetes, or dyslipidemia, or consider switching to a different antipsychotic

SIDE EFFECTS

How Drug Causes Side Effects

- Most side effects are immediate but often go away with time
- ✳ Histamine 1 receptor antagonism may explain sedative effects
- ✳ Histamine 1 receptor antagonism plus 5HT2C antagonism may explain some aspects of weight gain

Notable Side Effects

- Dry mouth, constipation, increased appetite, weight gain
- Sedation, dizziness, abnormal dreams, confusion
- Flu-like symptoms (may indicate low white blood cell or granulocyte count)
- Change in urinary function
- Hypotension

 ### Life Threatening or Dangerous Side Effects

- Rare seizures
- Rare induction of mania and activation of suicidal ideation

Weight Gain

unusual not unusual **common** problematic

- Many experience and/or can be significant in amount

Sedation

unusual not unusual **common** problematic

- Many experience and/or can be significant in amount

What To Do About Side Effects

- Wait
- Wait
- Wait
- Switch to another drug

Best Augmenting Agents for Side Effects

- Often best to try another antidepressant monotherapy prior to resorting to augmentation strategies to treat side effects
- Many side effects are dose-dependent (i.e., they increase as dose increases, or they reemerge until tolerance re-develops)
- Many side effects are time-dependent (i.e., they start immediately upon dosing and upon each dose increase, but go away with time)
- Trazodone or a hypnotic for insomnia
- Many side effects cannot be improved with an augmenting agent
- Activation and agitation may represent the induction of a bipolar state, especially a mixed dysphoric bipolar II condition

sometimes associated with suicidal ideation, and require the addition of lithium, a mood stabilizer or an atypical antipsychotic, and/or discontinuation of mirtazapine

DOSING AND USE

Usual Dosage Range
• 15–45 mg at night

Dosage Forms
• Tablet 15 mg scored, 30 mg scored, 45 mg
• SolTab disintegrating tablet 15 mg, 30 mg, 45 mg

How to Dose
• Initial 15 mg/day in the evening; increase every 1–2 weeks until desired efficacy is reached; maximum generally 45 mg/day

 Dosing Tips
• Sedation may not worsen as dose increases
* Breaking a 15 mg tablet in half and administering 7.5 mg dose may actually increase sedation
• Some patients require more than 45 mg daily, including up to 90 mg in difficult patients who tolerate these doses
• If intolerable anxiety, insomnia, agitation, akathisia, or activation occur either upon dosing initiation or discontinuation, consider the possibility of activated bipolar disorder and switch to a mood stabilizer or an atypical antipsychotic

Overdose
• Rarely lethal; all fatalities have involved other medications; symptoms include sedation, disorientation, memory impairment, rapid heartbeat

Long-Term Use
• Safe

Habit Forming
• Not expected

How to Stop
• Taper is prudent to avoid withdrawal effects, but tolerance, dependence, and withdrawal effects not reliably reported

Pharmacokinetics
• Half-life 20–40 hours

 Drug Interactions
• Tramadol increases the risk of seizures in patients taking an antidepressant
• No significant pharmacokinetic drug interactions
• Can cause a fatal "serotonin syndrome" when combined with MAO inhibitors, so do not use with MAO inhibitors or for at least 14 days after MAOIs are stopped
• Do not start an MAO inhibitor for at least 2 weeks after discontinuing mirtazapine

 Other Warnings/ Precautions
• Drug may lower white blood cell count (rare; may not be increased compared to other antidepressants but controlled studies lacking; not a common problem reported in post marketing surveillance)
• Drug may increase cholesterol
• May cause photosensitivity
• Avoid alcohol, which may increase sedation and cognitive and motor effects
• Use with caution in patients with history of seizures
• Use with caution in patients with bipolar disorder unless treated with concomitant mood stabilizing agent
• Monitor patients for activation of suicidal ideation, especially children and adolescents

Do Not Use
• If patient is taking an MAO inhibitor
• If there is a proven allergy to mirtazapine

SPECIAL POPULATIONS

Renal Impairment
• Drug should be used with caution

Hepatic Impairment
• Drug should be used with caution
• May require lower dose

Cardiac Impairment
• Drug should be used with caution
• The potential risk of hypotension should be considered

Elderly
• Some patients may tolerate lower doses better

Children and Adolescents
• Use with caution, observing for activation of known or unknown bipolar disorder and/or suicidal ideation, and strongly consider informing parents or guardian of this risk so they can help observe child or adolescent patients
• Safety and efficacy have not been established

Pregnancy
• Risk Category C [some animal studies show adverse effects; no controlled studies in humans]
• Not generally recommended for use during pregnancy, especially during first trimester
• Must weigh the risk of treatment (first trimester fetal development, third trimester newborn delivery) to the child against the risk of no treatment (recurrence of depression, maternal health, infant bonding) to the mother and child
• For many patients this may mean continuing treatment during pregnancy

Breast Feeding
• Unknown if mirtazapine is secreted in human breast milk, but all psychotropics assumed to be secreted in breast milk
• If child becomes irritable or sedated, breast feeding or drug may need to be discontinued
• Immediate postpartum period is a high-risk time for depression, especially in women who have had prior depressive episodes, so drug may need to be reinstituted late in the third trimester or shortly after childbirth to prevent a recurrence during the postpartum period
• Must weigh benefits of breast feeding with risks and benefits of antidepressant treatment versus non-treatment to both the infant and the mother
• For many patients, this may mean continuing treatment during breast feeding

THE ART OF PSYCHOPHARMACOLOGY

Potential Advantages
• Patients particularly concerned about sexual side effects
• Patients with symptoms of anxiety
• Patients on concomitant medications
• As an augmenting agent to boost the efficacy of other antidepressants

Potential Disadvantages
• Patients particularly concerned about gaining weight
• Patients with low energy

Primary Target Symptoms
• Depressed mood
• Sleep disturbance
• Anxiety

Pearls
✱ Adding alpha 2 antagonism to agents that block serotonin and/or norepinephrine reuptake may be synergistic for severe depression
• Adding mirtazapine to venlafaxine or SSRIs may reverse drug-induced anxiety and insomnia
• Adding mirtazapine's 5HT3 antagonism to venlafaxine or SSRIs may reverse drug-induced nausea, diarrhea, stomach cramps, and gastrointestinal side effects
• SSRIs, venlafaxine, bupropion, phentermine, or stimulants may mitigate mirtazapine-induced weight gain
• If weight gain has not occurred by week 6 of treatment, it is less likely for there to be significant weight gain
• Has been demonstrated to have an earlier onset of action than SSRIs
✱ Does not affect the CYP450 system, and so may be preferable in patients requiring concomitant medications
• Preliminary evidence suggests efficacy as an augmenting agent to haloperidol in treating negative symptoms of schizophrenia
• Anecdotal reports of efficacy in recurrent brief depression
• Weight gain as a result of mirtazapine treatment is more likely in women than in men, and before menopause rather than after

✳ May cause sexual dysfunction only
  infrequently
• Patients can have carryover sedation and
  intoxicated-like feeling if particularly
  sensitive to sedative side effects when
  initiating dosing
• Rarely, patients may complain of visual
  "trails" or after-images on mirtazapine

Suggested Reading

Anttila SA, Leinonen EV. A review of the
pharmacological and clinical profile of
mirtazapine. CNS Drug Rev 2001;7(3):249–64.

Benkert O, Muller M, Szegedi A. An overview
of the clinical efficacy of mirtazapine. Hum
Psychopharmacol. 2002;17 Suppl 1:S23–6.

Falkai P. Mirtazapine: other indications. J Clin
Psychiatry 1999;60(suppl 17):36–40.

Fawcett J, Barkin RL. A meta-analysis of eight
randomized, double-blind, controlled clinical
trials of mirtazapine for the treatment of
patients with major depression and symptoms
of anxiety. J Clin Psychiatry. 1998;
59:123–127.

Masand PS, Gupta S. Long-term side effects
of newer-generation antidepressants: SSRIS,
venlafaxine, nefazodone, bupropion, and
mirtazapine. Ann Clin Psychiatry 2002;
14:175–82.

MOCLOBEMIDE

THERAPEUTICS

Brands
- Aurorix
- Arima
- Manerix

see index for additional brand names

Generic? No

Class
- Reversible inhibitor of monoamine oxidase A (MAO-A) (RIMA)

Commonly Prescribed For
(bold for FDA approved)
- Depression
- Social anxiety disorder

How The Drug Works
- Reversibly blocks MAO-A from breaking down norepinephrine, dopamine, and serotonin
- This presumably boosts noradrenergic, serotonergic, and dopaminergic neurotransmission
- MAO-A inhibition predominates unless significant concentrations of monoamines build up (e.g., due to dietary tyramine), in which case MAO-A inhibition is theoretically reversed

How Long Until It Works
- Onset of therapeutic actions usually not immediate, but often delayed 2 to 4 weeks
- If it is not working within 6 to 8 weeks, it may require a dosage increase or it may not work at all
- May continue to work for many years to prevent relapse of symptoms

If It Works
- The goal of treatment is complete remission of current symptoms as well as prevention of future relapses
- Treatment most often reduces or even eliminates symptoms, but not a cure since symptoms can recur after medicine stopped
- Continue treatment until all symptoms are gone (remission)
- Once symptoms gone, continue treating for 1 year for the first episode of depression
- For second and subsequent episodes of depression, treatment may need to be indefinite
- Use in anxiety disorders may also need to be indefinite

If It Doesn't Work
- Many patients only have a partial response where some symptoms are improved but others persist (especially insomnia, fatigue, and problems concentrating)
- Other patients may be nonresponders, sometimes called treatment-resistant or treatment-refractory
- Consider increasing dose, switching to another agent or adding an appropriate augmenting agent
- Consider psychotherapy
- Consider evaluation for another diagnosis or for a comorbid condition (e.g., medical illness, substance abuse, etc.)
- Some patients may experience apparent lack of consistent efficacy due to activation of latent or underlying bipolar disorder, and require antidepressant discontinuation and a switch to a mood stabilizer

 Best Augmenting Combos for Partial Response or Treatment-Resistance
* Augmentation of MAOIs has not been systematically studied, and this is something for the expert, to be done with caution and with careful monitoring, but may be somewhat less risky with moclobemide than with other MAO inhibitors
* A stimulant such as d-amphetamine or methylphenidate (with caution; may activate bipolar disorder and suicidal ideation)
- Lithium
- Mood stabilizing anticonvulsants
- Atypical antipsychotics (with special caution for those agents with monoamine reuptake blocking properties, such as ziprasidone and zotepine)

Tests
- Patients should be monitored for changes in blood pressure

SIDE EFFECTS

How Drug Causes Side Effects
- Theoretically due to increases in monoamines in parts of the brain and body and at receptors other than those that cause therapeutic actions (e.g., unwanted actions of serotonin in sleep centers causing insomnia, unwanted actions of norepinephrine on vascular smooth muscle causing changes in blood pressure)
- Side effects are generally immediate, but immediate side effects often disappear in time

Notable Side Effects
- Insomnia, dizziness, agitation, anxiety, restlessness
- Dry mouth, diarrhea, constipation, nausea, vomiting
- Galactorrhea
- Rare hypertension

 Life Threatening or Dangerous Side Effects
- Hypertensive crisis (especially when MAOIs are used with certain tyramine containing foods – reduced risk compared to irreversible MAOIs)
- Induction of mania and activation of suicidal ideation
- Seizures

Weight Gain

unusual   not unusual   common   problematic
- Reported but not expected

Sedation

unusual   not unusual   common   problematic
- Occurs in significant minority

What To Do About Side Effects
- Wait
- Wait
- Wait
- Lower the dose
- Switch to an SSRI or newer antidepressant

Best Augmenting Agents for Side Effects
- Trazodone (with caution) for insomnia
- Benzodiazepines for insomnia

- ✱ Single oral or sublingual dose of a calcium channel blocker (e.g., nifedipine) for urgent treatment of hypertension due to drug interaction or dietary tyramine
- Many side effects cannot be improved with an augmenting agent

DOSING AND USE

Usual Dosage Range
- 300–600 mg/day

Dosage Forms
- Tablet 100 mg scored, 150 mg scored

How to Dose
- Initial 300 mg/day in 3 divided doses after a meal; increase dose gradually; maximum dose generally 600 mg/day; minimum dose generally 150 mg/day

 Dosing Tips
- ✱ At higher doses, moclobemide also inhibits MAO-B and thereby loses its selectivity for MAO-A, with uncertain clinical consequences
- ✱ Taking moclobemide after meals as opposed to before may minimize the chances of interactions with tyramine
- May be less toxic in overdose than tricyclic antidepressants and older MAOIs
- Clinical duration of action may be longer than biological half-life and allow twice daily dosing in some patients, or even once daily dosing, especially at lower doses

Overdose
- Agitation, aggression, behavioral disturbances, gastrointestinal irritation

Long-Term Use
- MAOIs may lose efficacy long-term

Habit Forming
- Some patients have developed dependence to MAOIs

How to Stop
- Taper not generally necessary

Pharmacokinetics
- Partially metabolized by CYP450 2C19 and 2D6

- Inactive metabolites
- Elimination half-life approximately 1–4 hours
- Clinical duration of action at least 24 hours

 Drug Interactions

- Tramadol may increase the risk of seizures in patients taking an MAO inhibitor
- Can cause a fatal "serotonin syndrome" when combined with drugs that block serotonin reuptake (e.g., SSRIs, SNRIs, sibutramine, tramadol, etc.), so do not use with a serotonin reuptake inhibitor or for up to 5 weeks after stopping the serotonin reuptake inhibitor
- Hypertensive crisis with headache, intracranial bleeding, and death may result from combining MAO inhibitors with sympathomimetic drugs (e.g., amphetamines, methylphenidate, cocaine, dopamine, epinephrine, norepinephrine, and related compounds methyldopa, levodopa, L-tryptophan, L-tyrosine, and phenylalanine)
- Excitation, seizures, delirium, hyperpyrexia, circulatory collapse, coma, and death may result from combining MAO inhibitors with mepiridine or dextromethorphan
- Do not combine with another MAO inhibitor, alcohol, buspirone, bupropion, or guanethidine
- Adverse drug reactions can result from combining MAO inhibitors with tricyclic/tetracyclic antidepressants and related compounds, including carbamazepine, cyclobenzaprine, and mirtazapine, and should be avoided except by experts to treat difficult cases
- MAO inhibitors in combination with spinal anesthesia may cause combined hypotensive effects
- Combination of MAOIs and CNS depressants may enhance sedation and hypotension
- Cimetidine may increase plasma concentrations of moclobemide
- Moclobemide may enhance the effects of non-steroidal anti-inflammatory drugs such as ibuprofen
- Risk of hypertensive crisis may be increased if moclobemide is used concurrently with levodopa or other dopaminergic agents

 Other Warnings/ Precautions

- Use still requires low tyramine diet, although more tyramine may be tolerated with moclobemide than with other MAO inhibitors before eliciting a hypertensive reaction
- Patients taking MAO inhibitors should avoid high protein food that has undergone protein breakdown by aging, fermentation, pickling, smoking, or bacterial contamination
- Patients taking MAO inhibitors should avoid cheeses (especially aged varieties), pickled herring, beer, wine, liver, yeast extract, dry sausage, hard salami, pepperoni, Lebanon bologna, pods of broad beans (fava beans), yogurt, and excessive use of caffeine and chocolate
- Patient and prescriber must be vigilant to potential interactions with any drug, including antihypertensives and over-the-counter cough/cold preparations
- Over-the-counter medications to avoid include cough and cold preparations, including those containing dextromethorphan, nasal decongestants (tablets, drops, or spray), hay-fever medications, sinus medications, asthma inhalant medications, anti-appetite medications, weight reducing preparations, "pep" pills
- Use cautiously in hypertensive patients
- Moclobemide is not recommended for use in patients who cannot be monitored closely
- Monitor patients for activation of suicidal ideation, especially children and adolescents

Do Not Use

- If patient is taking meperidine (pethidine)
- If patient is taking a sympathomimetic agent or taking guanethidine
- If patient is taking another MAOI
- If patient is taking any agent that can inhibit serotonin reuptake (e.g., SSRIs, sibutramine, tramadol, milnacipran, duloxetine, venlafaxine, clomipramine, etc.)
- If patient is in an acute confusional state
- If patient has pheochromocytoma or thyrotoxicosis
- If patient has frequent or severe headaches

- If patient is undergoing elective surgery and requires general anesthesia
- If there is a proven allergy to moclobemide

- Should evaluate patient for treatment with an antidepressant with a better risk/benefit ratio

SPECIAL POPULATIONS

Renal Impairment
- Use with caution

Hepatic Impairment
- Plasma concentrations are increased
- May require one-half to one-third of usual adult dose

Cardiac Impairment
- Cardiac impairment may require lower than usual adult dose
- Patients with angina pectoris or coronary artery disease should limit their exertion

Elderly
- Elderly patients may have greater sensitivity to adverse effects

Children and Adolescents
- Not recommended for use under age 18
- Use with caution, observing for activation of known or unknown bipolar disorder and/or suicidal ideation, and strongly consider informing parents or guardian of this risk so they can help observe child or adolescent patients

Pregnancy
- Not generally recommended for use during pregnancy, especially during first trimester
- Should evaluate patient for treatment with an antidepressant with a better risk/benefit ratio

Breast Feeding
- Some drug is found in mother's breast milk
- Effects on infant are unknown
- Immediate postpartum period is a high-risk time for depression, especially in women who have had prior depressive episodes, so drug may need to be reinstituted late in the third trimester or shortly after childbirth to prevent a recurrence during the postpartum period

THE ART OF PSYCHOPHARMACOLOGY

Potential Advantages
- Atypical depression
- Severe depression
- Treatment-resistant depression or anxiety disorders

Potential Disadvantages
- Patients noncompliant with dietary restrictions, concomitant drug restrictions, and twice daily dosing after meals

Primary Target Symptoms
- Depressed mood

 Pearls

- MAOIs are generally reserved for second-line use after SSRIs, SNRIs, and combinations of newer antidepressants have failed
- Patient should be advised not to take any prescription or over-the-counter drugs without consulting their doctor because of possible drug interactions with the MAOI
- Headache is often the first symptom of hypertensive crisis
- Moclobemide has a much reduced risk of interactions with tyramine than nonselective MAOIs
- Especially at higher doses of moclobemide, foods with high tyramine need to be avoided: dry sausage, pickled herring, liver, broad bean pods, sauerkraut, cheese, yogurt, alcoholic beverages, nonalcoholic beer and wine, chocolate, caffeine, meat and fish
- The rigid dietary restrictions may reduce compliance
- ✳ May be a safer alternative to classical irreversible nonselective MAO-A and MAO-B inhibitors with less propensity for tyramine and drug interactions and hepatotoxicity (although not entirely free of interactions)
- May not be as effective at low doses, and may have more side effects at higher doses

- Moclobemide's profile at higher doses may be more similar to classical MAOIs
- MAOIs are a viable second-line treatment option in depression, but are not frequently used
- ✻ Myths about the danger of dietary tyramine can be exaggerated, but prohibitions against concomitant drugs often not followed closely enough
- Orthostatic hypotension, insomnia, and sexual dysfunction are often the most troublesome common side effects
- ✻ MAOIs should be for the expert, especially if combining with agents of potential risk (e.g., stimulants, trazodone, TCAs)
- ✻ MAOIs should not be neglected as therapeutic agents for the treatment-resistant
- Although generally prohibited, a heroic but potentially dangerous treatment for severely treatment-resistant patients is for an expert to give a tricyclic/tetracyclic antidepressant other than clomipramine simultaneously with an MAO inhibitor for patients who fail to respond to numerous other antidepressants
- Use of MAOIs with clomipramine is always prohibited because of the risk of serotonin syndrome and death
- Amoxapine may be the preferred trycyclic/tetracyclic antidepressant to combine with an MAOI in heroic cases due to its theoretically protective 5HT2A antagonist properties
- If this option is elected, start the MAOI with the tricyclic/tetracyclic antidepressant simultaneously at low doses after appropriate drug washout, then alternately increase doses of these agents every few days to a week as tolerated
- Although very strict dietary and concomitant drug restrictions must be observed to prevent hypertensive crises and serotonin syndrome, the most common side effects of MAOI and tricyclic/tetracyclic combinations may be weight gain and orthostatic hypotension

 Suggested Reading

Amrein R, Martin JR, Cameron AM. Moclobemide in patients with dementia and depression. Adv Neurol 1999;80:509–19.

Fulton B, Benfield P. Moclobemide. An update of its pharmacological properties and therapeutic use. Drugs 1996;52:450–74.

Kennedy SH. Continuation and maintenance treatments in major depression: the neglected role of monoamine oxidase inhibitors. J Psychiatry Neurosci 1997;22:127–31.

Lippman SB, Nash K. Monoamine oxidase inhibitor update. Potential adverse food and drug interactions. Drug Saf 1990;5:195–204

Nutt D, Montgomery SA. Moclobemide in the treatment of social phobia. Int Clin Psychopharmacol 1996;11 (Suppl 3):77–82.

MODAFINIL

MODAFINIL

THERAPEUTICS

Brands
- Provigil
- Alertec
- Modiodal

see index for additional brand names

Generic? No

Class
- Wake-promoting

Commonly Prescribed For
(bold for FDA approved)
- **Reducing excessive sleepiness in patients with narcolepsy and shift work sleep disorder**
- **Reducing excessive sleepiness in patients with obstructive sleep apnea/hypopnea syndrome (OSAHS) (adjunct to standard treatment for underlying airway obstruction)**
- Fatigue and sleepiness in depression
- Fatigue in multiple sclerosis
- Attention deficit hyperactivity disorder

How The Drug Works
- Unknown, but clearly different from classical stimulants such as methylphenidate and amphetamine
- Increases neuronal activity selectively in the hypothalamus
- ✳ Presumably enhances activity in hypothalamic wakefulness center (TMN, tuberomammillary nucleus) within the hypothalamic sleep wake switch by an unknown mechanism
- ✳ Activates tuberomammillary nucleus neurons that release histamine
- ✳ Activates other hypothalamic neurons that release orexin/hypocretin

How Long Until It Works
- Can immediately reduce daytime sleepiness and improve cognitive task performance within 2 hours of first dosing
- Can take several days to optimize dosing and clinical improvement

If It Works
- ✳ Improves daytime sleepiness and may improve attention as well as fatigue

- ✳ Does not prevent one from falling asleep when needed
- May not completely normalize wakefulness
- Treat until improvement stabilizes and then continue treatment indefinitely as long as improvement persists

If It Doesn't Work
- ✳ Change dose; some patients do better with an increased dose but some actually do better with a decreased dose
- Augment or consider an alternative treatment for daytime sleepiness, fatigue, or ADHD

 ### Best Augmenting Combos for Partial Response or Treatment-Resistance
- ✳ Modafinil is itself an adjunct to standard treatments for obstructive sleep apnea/hypopnea syndrome (OSAHS); if continuous positive airway pressure (CPAP) is the treatment of choice, a maximal effort to treat first with CPAP should be made prior to initiating modafinil and CPAP should be continued after initiation of modafinil
- ✳ Modafinil is itself an augmenting therapy to antidepressants for residual sleepiness and fatigue in major depressive disorder
- Best to attempt another monotherapy prior to augmenting with other drugs in the treatment of sleepiness associated with sleep disorders or problems concentrating in ADHD
- Combination of modafinil with stimulants such as methylphenidate or amphetamine or with atomoxetine for ADHD has not been systematically studied
- However, such combinations may be useful options for experts, with close monitoring, when numerous monotherapies for sleepiness or ADHD have failed

Tests
- None for healthy individuals

SIDE EFFECTS

How Drug Causes Side Effects
- Unknown
- CNS side effects presumably due to excessive CNS actions on various neurotransmitter systems

Notable Side Effects

* ❋ Headache
* Anxiety, nervousness, insomnia
* Dry mouth, diarrhea, nausea, anorexia
* Pharyngitis, rhinitis, infection
* Hypertension
* Palpitations

 Life Threatening or Dangerous Side Effects

* Transient EKG ischemic changes in patients with mitral valve prolapse or left ventricular hypertrophy have been reported (rare)
* Theoretically, could activate hypomania or mania

Weight Gain

unusual   not unusual   common   problematic

* Reported but not expected

Sedation

unusual   not unusual   common   problematic

* Reported but not expected
* Patients are usually awakened and some may be activated

What To Do About Side Effects

* Wait
* Lower the dose
* Give only once daily
* Give smaller split doses 2 or more times daily
* For activation or insomnia, do not give in the evening
* If unacceptable side effects persist, discontinue use

Best Augmenting Agents for Side Effects

* Many side effects cannot be improved with an augmenting agent

---

DOSING AND USE

Usual Dosage Range

* 200 mg/day in the morning

Dosage Forms

* Tablet 100 mg, 200 mg (scored)

How to Dose

* Titration up or down only necessary if not optimally efficacious at the standard starting dose of 200 mg once a day in the morning

 Dosing Tips

* ❋ For sleepiness, more may be more: higher doses (200–800 mg/day) may be better than lower doses (50–200 mg/day) in patients with daytime sleepiness in sleep disorders
* ❋ For problems concentrating and fatigue, less may be more: lower doses (50–200 mg/day) may be paradoxically better than higher doses (200–800 mg/day) in some patients
* At high doses, may slightly induce its own metabolism, possibly by actions of inducing CYP450 3A4
* Dose may creep upward in some patients with long-term treatment due to autoinduction; drug holiday may restore efficacy at original dose

Overdose

* No fatalities; agitation, insomnia, increase in hemodynamic parameters

Long-Term Use

* Efficacy in reducing excessive sleepiness in sleep disorders has been demonstrated in 9 to 12 week trials
* Unpublished data show safety for up to 136 weeks
* The need for continued treatment should be reevaluated periodically

Habit Forming

* Schedule IV; may have some potential for abuse but unusual in clinical practice

How to Stop

* Taper not necessary; patients may have sleepiness on discontinuation

Pharmacokinetics

* Metabolized by the liver
* Excreted renally
* Elimination half-life 10–12 hours
* Inhibits CYP450 2C19 (and perhaps 2C9)
* Induces CYP450 3A4 (and slightly 1A2 and 2B6)

Drug Interactions

- May increase plasma levels of drugs metabolized by CYP450 2C19 (e.g., diazepam, phenytoin, propranolol)
- Modafinil may increase plasma levels of CYP450 2D6 substrates such as tricyclic antidepressants and SSRIs, perhaps requiring downward dose adjustments of these agents
- Modafinil may decrease plasma levels of CYP450 3A4 substrates such as ethinyl estradiol and triazolam
- Due to induction of CYP450 3A4, effectiveness of steroidal contraceptives may be reduced by modafinil, including 1 month after discontinuation
- Inducers or inhibitors of CYP450 3A4 may affect levels of modafinil (e.g., carbamazepine may lower modafinil plasma levels; fluvoxamine and fluoxetine may raise modafinil plasma levels)
- Modafinil may slightly reduce its own levels by autoinduction of CYP450 3A4
- Modafinil may increase clearance of drugs dependent on CYP450 1A2 and reduce their plasma levels
- Patients on modafinil and warfarin should have prothrombin times monitored
- Methylphenidate may delay absorption of modafinil by an hour
- ✱ However, co-administration with methylphenidate does not significantly change the pharmacokinetics of either modafinil or methylphenidate
- ✱ Co-administration with dextroamphetamine also does not significantly change the pharmacokinetics of either modafinil or dextroamphetamine
- Interaction studies with MAO inhibitors have not been performed, but MAOIs can be given with modafinil by experts with cautious monitoring

⚠️ **Other Warnings/ Precautions**

- Patients with history of drug abuse should be monitored closely
- Modafinil may cause CNS effects similar to those caused by other CNS agents (e.g., changes in mood and, theoretically, activation of psychosis, mania, or suicidal ideation)

- Modafinil should be used in patients with sleep disorders that have been completely evaluated for narcolepsy, obstructive sleep apnea/hypopnea syndrome (OSAHS), and shift work sleep disorder
- In OSAHS patients for whom continuous positive airway pressure (CPAP) is the treatment of choice, a maximal effort to treat first with CPAP should be made prior to initiating modafinil, and then CPAP should be continued after initiating modafinil
- The effectiveness of steroidal contraceptives may be reduced when used with modafinil and for 1 month after discontinuation of modafinil
- Modafinil is not a replacement for sleep

Do Not Use

- If patient has severe hypertension
- If patient has cardiac arrhythmias
- If there is a proven allergy to modafinil

SPECIAL POPULATIONS

Renal Impairment

- Use with caution; dose reduction is recommended

Hepatic Impairment

- Reduce dose by half in severely impaired patients

Cardiac Impairment

- Use with caution
- Not recommended for use in patients with a history of left ventricular hypertrophy, ischemic ECG changes, chest pain, arrhythmias, or recent myocardial infarction

Elderly

- Limited experience in patients over 65
- Clearance of modafinil may be reduced in elderly patients

 Children and Adolescents

- Safety and efficacy not established under age 16
- Can be used cautiously by experts for children and adolescents

Pregnancy

- Risk Category C [some animal studies show adverse effects, no controlled studies in humans]
- Animal studies were conducted at doses lower than necessary to elucidate the effects of modafinil on the developing fetus
- Use in women of childbearing potential requires weighing potential benefits to the mother against potential risks to the fetus
- ✳ Generally, modafinil should be discontinued prior to anticipated pregnancies

Breast Feeding

- Unknown if modafinil is secreted in human breast milk, but all psychotropics assumed to be secreted in breast milk
- ✳ Recommended either to discontinue drug or bottle feed

THE ART OF PSYCHOPHARMACOLOGY

Potential Advantages

- Selective for areas of brain involved in sleep/wake promotion
- Less activating and less abuse potential than stimulants

Potential Disadvantages

- May not work as well as stimulants in some patients

Primary Target Symptoms

- Sleepiness
- Concentration
- Physical and mental fatigue

Pearls

- ✳ Only agent approved for treating sleepiness associated with obstructive sleep apnea/hypopnea syndrome (OSAHS)
- ✳ Only agent approved for treating sleepiness associated with shift work sleep disorder

- ✳ Anecdotal usefulness for jet lag short-term (off-label)
- ✳ Modafinil is not a replacement for sleep
- ✳ The treatment for sleep deprivation is sleep, not modafinil
- Controlled studies suggest modafinil improves attention in OSAHS, shift work sleep disorder, and ADHD (both children and adults), but controlled studies of attention have not been performed in major depressive disorder
- ✳ May be useful to treat fatigue in patients with depression as well as other disorders, such as multiple sclerosis, myotonic dystrophy, HIV/AIDS
- In depression, modafinil's actions on fatigue appear to be independent of actions (if any) on mood
- In depression, modafinil's actions on sleepiness also appear to be independent of actions (if any) on mood but may be linked to actions on fatigue or on global functioning
- Several controlled studies in depression show improvement in sleepiness or global functioning, especially for depressed patients with sleepiness and fatigue
- May be useful in treating sleepiness associated with opioid analgesia, particularly in end-of-life management
- Subjective sensation associated with modafinil is usually one of normal wakefulness, not of stimulation, although jitteriness can rarely occur
- Anecdotally, some patients may experience wearing off of efficacy over time, especially for off-label uses, with restoration of efficacy after a drug holiday; such wearing off is less likely with intermittent dosing
- ✳ Compared to stimulants, modafinil has a novel mechanism of action, novel therapeutic uses, and less abuse potential, but is often inaccurately classified as a stimulant
- Alpha 1 antagonists such as prazosin may block the therapeutic actions of modafinil
- The active R-enantiomer of modafinil, also called armodafinil, is in development

Suggested Reading

Batejat DM, Lagarde DP. Naps and modafinil as countermeasures for the effects of sleep deprivation on cognitive performance. Aviat Space Environ Med 1999;70:493–8.

Bourdon L, Jacobs I, Bateman WA, Vallerand AL. Effect of modafinil on heat production and regulation of body temperatures in cold-exposed humans. Aviat Space Environ Med 1994;65:999–1004.

Cox JM, Pappagallo M. Modafinil: a gift to portmanteau. Am J Hosp Palliat Care 2001;18:408–10.

Jasinski DR, Koyacevic-Ristanovic. Evaluation of the abuse liability of modafinil and other drugs for excessive daytime sleepiness associated with narcolepsy. Clin Neuropharmacol 2000;23:149–56.

Wesensten NJ, Belenky G, Kautz MA, Thorne DR, Reichardt RM, Balkin TJ. Maintaining alertness and performance during sleep deprivation: modafinil versus caffeine. Psychopharmacology (Berl) 2002;159:238–47.

MOLINDONE

THERAPEUTICS

Brands • Moban
see index for additional brand names

Generic? Yes

 Class
• Conventional antipsychotic (neuroleptic, dopamine 2 antagonist)

Commonly Prescribed For
(bold for FDA approved)
• **Schizophrenia**
• Other psychotic disorders
• Bipolar disorder

 How The Drug Works
• Blocks dopamine 2 receptors, reducing positive symptoms of psychosis

How Long Until It Works
• Psychotic symptoms can improve within 1 week, but it may take several weeks for full effect on behavior

If It Works
• Most often reduces positive symptoms in schizophrenia but does not eliminate them
• Most schizophrenic patients do not have a total remission of symptoms but rather a reduction of symptoms by about a third
• Continue treatment in schizophrenia until reaching a plateau of improvement
• After reaching a satisfactory plateau, continue treatment for at least a year after first episode of psychosis in schizophrenia
• For second and subsequent episodes of psychosis in schizophrenia, treatment may need to be indefinite
• Reduces symptoms of acute psychotic mania but not proven as a mood stabilizer or as an effective maintenance treatment in bipolar disorder
• After reducing acute psychotic symptoms in mania, switch to a mood stabilizer and/or an atypical antipsychotic for mood stabilization and maintenance

If It Doesn't Work
• Consider trying one of the first-line atypical antipsychotics (risperidone, olanzapine, quetiapine, ziprasidone, aripiprazole, amisulpride)
• Consider trying another conventional antipsychotic
• If 2 or more antipsychotic monotherapies do not work, consider clozapine

 Best Augmenting Combos for Partial Response or Treatment-Resistance
• Augmentation of conventional antipsychotics has not been systematically studied
• Addition of a mood stabilizing anticonvulsant such as valproate, carbamazepine, or lamotrigine may be helpful in both schizophrenia and bipolar mania
• Augmentation with lithium in bipolar mania may be helpful
• Addition of a benzodiazepine, especially short-term for agitation

Tests
✱ Since conventional antipsychotics are frequently associated with weight gain, before starting treatment, weigh all patients and determine if the patient is already overweight (BMI 25.0–29.9) or obese (BMI ≥30)
• Before giving a drug that can cause weight gain to an overweight or obese patient, consider determining whether the patient already has pre-diabetes (fasting plasma glucose 100–125 mg/dl), diabetes (fasting plasma glucose >126 mg/dl), or dyslipidemia (increased total cholesterol, LDL cholesterol and triglycerides; decreased HDL cholesterol), and treat or refer such patients for treatment, including nutrition and weight management, physical activity counseling, smoking cessation, and medical management
✱ Monitor weight and BMI during treatment
✱ While giving a drug to a patient who has gained >5% of initial weight, consider evaluating for the presence of pre-diabetes, diabetes, or dyslipidemia, or consider switching to a different antipsychotic
• Should check blood pressure in the elderly before starting and for the first few weeks of treatment
• Monitoring elevated prolactin levels of dubious clinical benefit

SIDE EFFECTS

How Drug Causes Side Effects

- By blocking dopamine 2 receptors in the striatum, it can cause motor side effects
- By blocking dopamine 2 receptors in the pituitary, it can cause elevations in prolactin
- By blocking dopamine 2 receptors excessively in the mesocortical and mesolimbic dopamine pathways, especially at high doses, it can cause worsening of negative and cognitive symptoms (neuroleptic-induced deficit syndrome)
- Anticholinergic actions may cause sedation, blurred vision, constipation, dry mouth
- Antihistaminic actions may cause sedation, weight gain
- By blocking alpha 1 adrenergic receptors, it can cause dizziness, sedation, and hypotension
- Mechanism of weight gain and any possible increased incidence of diabetes or dyslipidemia with conventional antipsychotics is unknown

Notable Side Effects

- ✳ Neuroleptic-induced deficit syndrome
- ✳ Akathisia
- ✳ Extrapyramidal symptoms, Parkinsonism, tardive dyskinesia
- ✳ Galactorrhea, amenorrhea
- Sedation
- Dry mouth, constipation, vision disturbance, urinary retention
- Hypotension, tachycardia

Life Threatening or Dangerous Side Effects

- Rare neuroleptic malignant syndrome
- Rare leukopenia
- Rare seizures

Weight Gain

unusual — not unusual — common — problematic

✳ Reported but not expected

Sedation

unusual — not unusual — **common** — problematic

- Many experience and/or can be significant in amount

- Sedation is usually transient

What To Do About Side Effects

- Wait
- Wait
- Wait
- For motor symptoms, add an anticholinergic agent
- Reduce the dose
- For sedation, give at night
- Switch to an atypical antipsychotic
- Weight loss, exercise programs, and medical management for high BMIs, diabetes, dyslipidemia

Best Augmenting Agents for Side Effects

- Benztropine or trihexyphenidyl for motor side effects
- Sometimes amantadine can be helpful for motor side effects
- Benzodiazepines may be helpful for akathisia
- Many side effects cannot be improved with an augmenting agent

DOSING AND USE

Usual Dosage Range

- 40–100 mg/day in divided doses

Dosage Forms

- Tablet 5 mg, 10 mg, 25 mg scored, 50 mg scored, 100 mg scored
- Liquid 20 mg/mL

How to Dose

- Initial 50–75 mg/day; increase to 100 mg/day after 3–4 days; maximum 225 mg/day

Dosing Tips

- Very short half-life, but some patients may only require once daily dosing
- Other patients may do better with 3 or 4 divided doses daily
- Patients receiving atypical antipsychotics may occasionally require a "top up" of a conventional antipsychotic to control aggression or violent behavior

Overdose
- Deaths have occurred; extrapyramidal symptoms, sedation, hypotension, respiratory depression, coma

Long-Term Use
- Some side effects may be irreversible (e.g., tardive dyskinesia)

Habit Forming
- No

How to Stop
- Slow down-titration (over 6 to 8 weeks), especially when simultaneously beginning a new antipsychotic while switching (i.e., cross-titration)
- Rapid discontinuation may lead to rebound psychosis and worsening of symptoms
- If antiparkinson agents are being used, they should be continued for a few weeks after molindone is discontinued

Pharmacokinetics
- Half-life approximately 1.5 hours

 Drug Interactions
- Additive effects may occur if used with CNS depressants
- Some patients taking a neuroleptic and lithium have developed an encephalopathic syndrome similar to neuroleptic malignant syndrome
- Molindone tablets contain calcium sulfate, which may interfere with absorption of phenytoin sodium or tetracyclines
- Combined use with epinephrine may lower blood pressure
- May increase the effects of antihypertensive drugs

 Other Warnings/ Precautions
- If signs of neuroleptic malignant syndrome develop, treatment should be immediately discontinued
- Liquid molindone contains sodium metabisulfite, which may cause allergic reactions in some people, especially in asthmatic people
- Use cautiously in patients with alcohol withdrawal or convulsive disorders

because of possible lowering of seizure threshold
- Antiemetic effect can mask signs of other disorders or overdose
- Do not use epinephrine in event of overdose as interaction with some pressor agents may lower blood pressure
- Use cautiously in patients with glaucoma, urinary retention
- Observe for signs of ocular toxicity (pigmentary retinopathy, lenticular pigmentation)
- Use only with caution if at all in Parkinson's disease or Lewy Body dementia

Do Not Use
- If patient is in a comatose state or has CNS depression
- If there is a proven allergy to molindone

SPECIAL POPULATIONS

Renal Impairment
- Should receive initial lower dose

Hepatic Impairment
- Should receive initial lower dose

Cardiac Impairment
- Use with caution

Elderly
- Should receive initial lower dose

 Children and Adolescents
- Safety and efficacy not well established
- Generally consider second-line after atypical antipsychotics

 Pregnancy
- Animal studies have not shown adverse effects
- No studies in pregnant women
- Psychotic symptoms may worsen during pregnancy and some form of treatment may be necessary
- Atypical antipsychotics may be preferable to conventional antipsychotics or anticonvulsant mood stabilizers if treatment is required during pregnancy

Breast Feeding

- Unknown if molindone is secreted in human breast milk, but all psychotropics assumed to be secreted in breast milk
- ✱ Recommended either to discontinue drug or bottle feed

Potential Advantages

- Some patients benefit from molindone's sedative properties

Potential Disadvantages

- Patients with tardive dyskinesia

Primary Target Symptoms

- Positive symptoms of psychosis
- Motor and autonomic hyperactivity
- Violent or aggressive behavior

 Pearls

- ✱ May have less weight gain than some other antipsychotics
- Conventional antipsychotics are much less expensive than atypical antipsychotics

- Not shown to be effective for behavioral problems in mental retardation
- Patients have very similar antipsychotic responses to any conventional antipsychotic, which is different from atypical antipsychotics where antipsychotic responses of individual patients can occasionally vary greatly from one atypical antipsychotic to another
- Patients with inadequate responses to atypical antipsychotics may benefit from a trial of augmentation with a conventional antipsychotic such as molindone or from switching to a conventional antipsychotic such as molindone
- However, long-term polypharmacy with a combination of a conventional antipsychotic such as molindone with an atypical antipsychotic may combine their side effects without clearly augmenting the efficacy of either
- Although a frequent practice by some prescribers, adding two conventional antipsychotics together has little rationale and may reduce tolerability without clearly enhancing efficacy

 Suggested Reading

Bagnall A, Fenton M, Lewis R, Leitner ML, Kleijnen J. Molindone for schizophrenia and severe mental illness. Cochrane Database Syst Rev 2000; (2): CD002083.

Owen RR Jr, Cole JO. Molindone hydrochloride: a review of laboratory and clinical findings. J Clin Psychopharmacol 1989; 9 (4): 268–76.

NEFAZODONE

THERAPEUTICS

Brands • Serzone
see index for additional brand names

Generic? Yes

 Class

• SARI (serotonin 2 antagonist/reuptake inhibitor); antidepressant

Commonly Prescribed For
(bold for FDA approved)
• **Depression**
• **Relapse prevention in MDD**
• Panic disorder
• Posttraumatic stress disorder

 How The Drug Works

• Blocks serotonin 2A receptors potently
• Blocks serotonin reuptake pump (serotonin transporter) and norepinephrine reuptake pump (norepinephrine transporter) less potently

How Long Until It Works
• Can improve insomnia and anxiety early after initiating dosing
• Onset of therapeutic actions usually not immediate, but often delayed 2 to 4 weeks
• If it is not working within 6 to 8 weeks for depression, it may require a dosage increase or it may not work at all
• May continue to work for many years to prevent relapse of symptoms

If It Works
• The goal of treatment is complete remission of current symptoms as well as prevention of future relapses
• Treatment most often reduces or even eliminates symptoms, but not a cure since symptoms can recur after medicine stopped
• Continue treatment until all symptoms are gone (remission)
• Once symptoms gone, continue treating for 1 year for the first episode of depression
• For second and subsequent episodes of depression, treatment may need to be indefinite
• Use in anxiety disorders may also need to be indefinite

If It Doesn't Work
• Many patients only have a partial response where some symptoms are improved but others persist (especially insomnia, fatigue, and problems concentrating)
• Other patients may be nonresponders, sometimes called treatment-resistant or treatment-refractory
• Some patients who have an initial response may relapse even though they continue treatment, sometimes called "poop-out"
• Consider increasing dose, switching to another agent or adding an appropriate augmenting agent
• Consider psychotherapy, especially cognitive-behavioral psychotherapies, which have been specifically shown to enhance nefazodone's antidepressant actions
• Consider evaluation for another diagnosis or for a comorbid condition (e.g., medical illness, substance abuse, etc.)
• Some patients may experience apparent lack of consistent efficacy due to activation of latent or underlying bipolar disorder, and require antidepressant discontinuation and a switch to a mood stabilizer

 Best Augmenting Combos for Partial Response or Treatment-Resistance

✳ Venlafaxine and escitalopram may be the best tolerated when switching or augmenting with a serotonin reuptake inhibitor, as neither is a potent CYP450 2D6 inhibitor (use combinations of antidepressants with caution as this may activate bipolar disorder and suicidal ideation)
• Modafinil, especially for fatigue, sleepiness, and lack of concentration
• Mood stabilizers or atypical antipsychotics for bipolar depression, psychotic depression or treatment-resistant depression
• Benzodiazepines for anxiety, but give alprazolam cautiously with nefazodone as alprazolam levels can be much higher in the presence of nefazodone
• Classically, lithium, buspirone, or thyroid hormone

Tests

* Liver function testing is not required but is often prudent given the small but finite risk of serious hepatoxicity
* However, to date no clinical strategy, including routine liver function tests, has been identified to reduce the risk of irreversible liver failure

SIDE EFFECTS

How Drug Causes Side Effects

* Blockade of alpha adrenergic 1 receptors may explain dizziness, sedation, and hypotension
* A metabolite of nefazodone, mCPP (meta-chloro-phenyl-piperazine), can cause side effects if its levels rise significantly
* If CYP450 2D6 is absent (7% of Caucasians lack CYP450 2D6) or inhibited (concomitant treatment with CYP450 2D6 inhibitors such as fluoxetine or paroxetine), increased levels of mCPP can form, leading to stimulation of 5HT2C receptors and causing dizziness, insomnia, and agitation
* Most side effects are immediate but often go away with time

Notable Side Effects

* Nausea, dry mouth, constipation, dyspepsia, increased appetite
* Headache, dizziness, vision changes, sedation, insomnia, agitation, confusion, memory impairment
* Ataxia, paresthesia, asthenia
* Cough increased
* Rare postural hypotension

 Life Threatening or Dangerous Side Effects

* Rare seizures
* Rare induction of mania and activation of suicidal ideation
* Rare priapism (no causal relationship established)
* Hepatic failure requiring liver transplant and/or fatal

Weight Gain

unusual   not unusual   common   problematic

* Reported but not expected

Sedation

unusual   not unusual   common   problematic

* Many experience and/or can be significant in amount

What To Do About Side Effects

* Wait
* Wait
* Wait
* Take once-daily at night to reduce daytime sedation
* Lower the dose and try titrating again more slowly as tolerated
* Switch to another agent

Best Augmenting Agents for Side Effects

* Often best to try another antidepressant monotherapy prior to resorting to augmentation strategies to treat side effects
* Many side effects cannot be improved with an augmenting agent
* Many side effects are dose-dependent (i.e., they increase as dose increases, or they reemerge until tolerance re-develops)
* Many side effects are time-dependent (i.e., they start immediately upon dosing and upon each dose increase, but go away with time)
* Activation and agitation may represent the induction of a bipolar state, especially a mixed dysphoric bipolar II condition sometimes associated with suicidal ideation, and require the addition of lithium, a mood stabilizer or an atypical antipsychotic, and/or discontinuation of nefazodone

DOSING AND USE

Usual Dosage Range

* 300–600 mg/day

Dosage Forms

* Tablet 50 mg, 100 mg scored, 150 mg scored, 200 mg, 250 mg

How to Dose

* Initial dose 100 mg twice a day; increase by 100–200 mg/day each week until

desired efficacy is reached; maximum dose 600 mg twice a day

Dosing Tips

- Take care switching from or adding to SSRIs (especially fluoxetine or paroxetine) because of side effects due to the drug interaction
- Do not underdose the elderly
- Normally twice daily dosing, especially when initiating treatment
- Patients may tolerate all dosing once daily at night once titrated
- Often much more effective at 400–600 mg/day than at lower doses if tolerated
- Slow titration can enhance tolerability when initiating dosing

Overdose
- Rarely lethal; sedation, nausea, vomiting, low blood pressure

Long-Term Use
- Safe

Habit Forming
- No

How to Stop
- Taper is prudent to avoid withdrawal effects, but problems in withdrawal not common

Pharmacokinetics
- Half-life of parent compound is 2–4 hours
- Half-life of active mebatolites up to 12 hours
- Inhibits CYP450 3A4

Drug Interactions
- Tramadol increases the risk of seizures in patients taking an antidepressant
- May interact with SSRIs such as paroxetine, fluoxetine, and others that inhibit CYP450 2D6
- * Since a metabolite of nefazodone, mCPP, is a substrate of CYP450 2D6, combination of 2D6 inhibitors with nefazodone will raise mCPP levels, leading to stimulation of 5HT2C receptors and causing dizziness and agitation

- Can cause a fatal "serotonin syndrome" when combined with MAO inhibitors, so do not use with MAO inhibitors or for at least 14 days after MAOIs are stopped
- Do not start an MAO inhibitor for at least 2 weeks after discontinuing nefazodone
- Via CYP450 3A4 inhibition, nefazodone may increase the half-life of alprazolam and triazolam, so their dosing may need to be reduced by half or more
- Via CYP450 3A4, nefazodone may increase plasma concentrations of buspirone, so buspirone dose may need to be reduced
- Via CYP450 3A4 inhibition, nefazodone could theoretically increase concentrations of certain cholesterol lowering HMG CoA reductase inhibitors, especially simvastatin, atorvastatin, and lovastatin, but not pravastatin or fluvastatin, which would increase the risk of rhabdomyolysis; thus, coadministration of nefazodone with certain HMG CoA reductase inhibitors should proceed with caution
- Via CYP450 3A4 inhibition, nefazodone could theoretically increase the concentrations of pimozide, and cause QTc prolongation and dangerous cardiac arrhythmias
- Nefazodone may reduce clearance of haloperidol, so haloperidol dose may need to be reduced
- It is recommended to discontinue nefazodone prior to elective surgery because of the potential for interaction with general anesthetics

Other Warnings/ Precautions

- * Hepatotoxicity, sometimes requiring liver transplant and/or fatal, has occurred with nefazodone use. Risk may be one in every 250,000 to 300,000 patient years. Patients should be advised to report symptoms such as jaundice, dark urine, loss of appetite, nausea, and abdominal pain to prescriber immediately. If patient develops signs of hepatocellular injury, such as increased serum AST or serum ALPT levels >3 times the upper limit of normal, nefazodone treatment should be discontinued.
- * No risk factor yet predicts who will develop irreversible liver failure with nefazodone and no clinical strategy,

including routine monitoring of liver function tests, is known to reduce the risk of liver failure
- Use with caution in patients with history of seizures
- Use with caution in patients with bipolar disorder unless treated with concomitant mood stabilizing agent
- Monitor patients for activation of suicidal ideation, especially children and adolescents

Do Not Use
- If patient is taking an MAO inhibitor
- If patient has acute hepatic impairment or elevated baseline serum transaminases
- If patient was previously withdrawn from nefazodone treatment due to hepatic injury
- If patient is taking pimozide, as nefazodone could raise pimozide levels and increase QTc interval, perhaps causing dangerous arrhythmia
- If patient is taking carbamazepine, as this agent can dramatically reduce nefazodone levels and thus interfere with its antidepressant actions
- If there is a proven allergy to nefazodone

SPECIAL POPULATIONS

Renal Impairment
- No dose adjustment necessary

Hepatic Impairment
- Contraindicated in patients with known hepatic impairment

Cardiac Impairment
- Use in patients with cardiac impairment has not been studied, so use with caution because of risk of orthostatic hypotension

Elderly
- Recommended to initiate treatment at half the usual adult dose, but to follow the same titration schedule as with younger patients, including same ultimate dose

 Children and Adolescents
- Use with caution, observing for activation of known or unknown bipolar disorder and/or suicidal ideation, and strongly

consider informing parents or guardian of this risk so they can help observe child or adolescent patients
- Safety and efficacy have not been established
- Preliminary research indicates efficacy and tolerability of nefazodone in children and adolescents with depression

 Pregnancy
- Risk Category C [some animal studies show adverse effects; no controlled studies in humans]
- Not generally recommended for use during pregnancy, especially during first trimester
- Must weigh the risk of treatment (first trimester fetal development, third trimester newborn delivery) to the child against the risk of no treatment (recurrence of depression, maternal health, infant bonding) to the mother and child
- For many patients this may mean continuing treatment during pregnancy

Breast Feeding
- Unknown if nefazodone is secreted in human breast milk, but all psychotropics assumed to be secreted in breast milk
- Trace amounts may be present in nursing children whose mothers are on nefazodone
- If child becomes irritable or sedated, breast feeding or drug may need to be discontinued
- Immediate postpartum period is a high-risk time for depression, especially in women who have had prior depressive episodes, so drug may need to be reinstituted late in the third trimester or shortly after childbirth to prevent a recurrence during the postpartum period
- Must weigh benefits of breast feeding with risks and benefits of antidepressant treatment versus non-treatment to both the infant and the mother
- For many patients, this may mean continuing treatment during breast feeding

THE ART OF PSYCHOPHARMACOLOGY

Potential Advantages
- Depressed patients with anxiety or insomnia who do not respond to other antidepressants
- Patients with SSRI-induced sexual dysfunction

Potential Disadvantages
- Patients who have difficulty with a long titration period or twice-daily dosing
- Patients with hepatic impairment

Primary Target Symptoms
- Depressed mood
- Sleep disturbance
- Anxiety

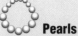 **Pearls**
- Preliminary data for efficacy in panic disorder and PTSD
- Fluoxetine and paroxetine may not be tolerated when switching or augmenting
- For elderly patients with early dementia and agitated depression, consider nefazodone in the morning and additional trazodone at night
- Anecdotal reports suggest that nefazodone may be effective in treating PMDD
- ✴ Studies suggest that cognitive-behavioral psychotherapy enhances the efficacy of nefazodone in chronic depression
- ✴ Risk of hepatotoxicity makes this agent a second-line choice and has led to its withdrawal from some markets
- Rarely, patients may complain of visual "trails" or after-images on nefazodone

 Suggested Reading

DeVane CL, Grothe DR, Smith SL. Pharmacology of antidepressants: focus on nefazodone. J Clin Psychiatry 2002; 63(1):10–7.

Dunner DL, Laird LK, Zajecka J, Bailey L, Sussman N, Seabolt JL. Six-year perspectives on the safety and tolerability of nefazodone. J Clin Psychiatry 2002;63(1):32–41.

Khouzam HR. The antidepressant nefazodone. A review of its pharmacology, clinical efficacy, adverse effects, dosage, and administration. Journal of Psychosocial Nursing and Mental Health Services 2000;38:20–25.

Masand PS, Gupta S. Long-term side effects of newer-generation antidepressants: SSRIS, venlafaxine, nefazodone, bupropion, and mirtazapine. Ann Clin Psychiatry 2002; 14:175–82.

Schatzberg AF, Prather MR, Keller MB, Rush AJ, Laird LK, Wright CW. Clinical use of nefazodone in major depression: a 6-year perspective. J Clin Psychiatry 2002; 63(1):18–31.

NORTRIPTYLINE

THERAPEUTICS

Brands • Pamelor
see index for additional brand names

Generic? Yes

Class
- Tricyclic antidepressant (TCA)
- Predominantly a norepinephrine/ noradrenaline reuptake inhibitor

Commonly Prescribed For
(bold for FDA approved)
- **Major depressive disorder**
- Anxiety
- Insomnia
- Neuropathic pain/chronic pain
- Treatment-resistant depression

How The Drug Works
- Boosts neurotransmitter norepinephrine/ noradrenaline
- Blocks norepinephrine reuptake pump (norepinephrine transporter), presumably increasing noradrenergic neurotransmission
- Since dopamine is inactivated by norepinephrine reuptake in frontal cortex, which largely lacks dopamine transporters, nortriptyline can increase dopamine neurotransmission in this part of the brain
- A more potent inhibitor of norepinephrine reuptake pump than serotonin reuptake pump (serotonin transporter)
- At high doses may also boost neurotransmitter serotonin and presumably increase serotonergic neurotransmission

How Long Until It Works
- May have immediate effects in treating insomnia or anxiety
- Onset of therapeutic actions usually not immediate, but often delayed 2 to 4 weeks
- If it is not working within 6 to 8 weeks for depression, it may require a dosage increase or it may not work at all
- May continue to work for many years to prevent relapse of symptoms

If It Works
- The goal of treatment of depression is complete remission of current symptoms as well as prevention of future relapses

- The goal of treatment of chronic neuropathic pain is to reduce symptoms as much as possible, especially in combination with other treatments
- Treatment of depression most often reduces or even eliminates symptoms, but not a cure since symptoms can recur after medicine stopped
- Treatment of chronic neuropathic pain may reduce symptoms, but rarely eliminates them completely, and is not a cure since symptoms can recur after medicine is stopped
- Continue treatment of depression until all symptoms are gone (remission)
- Once symptoms of depression are gone, continue treating for 1 year for the first episode of depression
- For second and subsequent episodes of depression, treatment may need to be indefinite
- Use in anxiety disorders and chronic pain may also need to be indefinite, but long-term treatment is not well studied in these conditions

If It Doesn't Work
- Many depressed patients only have a partial response where some symptoms are improved but others persist (especially insomnia, fatigue, and problems concentrating)
- Other depressed patients may be nonresponders, sometimes called treatment-resistant or treatment-refractory
- Consider increasing dose, switching to another agent or adding an appropriate augmenting agent
- Consider psychotherapy
- Consider evaluation for another diagnosis or for a comorbid condition (e.g., medical illness, substance abuse, etc.)
- Some patients may experience apparent lack of consistent efficacy due to activation of latent or underlying bipolar disorder, and require antidepressant discontinuation and a switch to a mood stabilizer

Best Augmenting Combos for Partial Response or Treatment-Resistance
- Lithium, buspirone, thyroid hormone (for depression)
- Gabapentin, tiagabine, other anticonvulsants, even opiates if done by

experts while monitoring carefully in difficult cases (for chronic pain)

Tests

✳ None for healthy individuals, although monitoring of plasma drug levels is available

✳ Since tricyclic and tetracyclic antidepressants are frequently associated with weight gain, before starting treatment, weigh all patients and determine if the patient is already overweight (BMI 25.0–29.9) or obese (BMI ≥30)

• Before giving a drug that can cause weight gain to an overweight or obese patient, consider determining whether the patient already has pre-diabetes (fasting plasma glucose 100–125 mg/dl), diabetes (fasting plasma glucose >126 mg/dl), or dyslipidemia (increased total cholesterol, LDL cholesterol and triglycerides; decreased HDL cholesterol), and treat or refer such patients for treatment, including nutrition and weight management, physical activity counseling, smoking cessation, and medical management

✳ Monitor weight and BMI during treatment

✳ While giving a drug to a patient who has gained >5% of initial weight, consider evaluating for the presence of pre-diabetes, diabetes, or dyslipidemia, or consider switching to a different antidepressant

• EKGs may be useful for selected patients (e.g., those with personal or family history of QTc prolongation; cardiac arrhythmia; recent myocardial infarction; uncompensated heart failure; or taking agents that prolong QTc interval such as pimozide, thioridazine, selected antiarrhythmics, moxifloxacin, sparfloxacin, etc.)

• Patients at risk for electrolyte disturbances (e.g., patients on diuretic therapy) should have baseline and periodic serum potassium and magnesium measurements

SIDE EFFECTS

How Drug Causes Side Effects

• Anticholinergic activity may explain sedative effects, dry mouth, constipation, and blurred vision

• Sedative effects and weight gain may be due to antihistamine properties

• Blockade of alpha adrenergic 1 receptors may explain dizziness, sedation, and hypotension

• Cardiac arrhythmias and seizures, especially in overdose, may be caused by blockade of ion channels

Notable Side Effects

• Blurred vision, constipation, urinary retention, increased appetite, dry mouth, nausea, diarrhea, heartburn, unusual taste in mouth, weight gain

• Fatigue, weakness, dizziness, sedation, headache, anxiety, nervousness, restlessness

• Sexual dysfunction (impotence, change in libido)

• Sweating, rash, itching

 Life Threatening or Dangerous Side Effects

• Paralytic ileus, hyperthermia (TCAs + anticholinergic agents)

• Lowered seizure threshold and rare seizures

• Orthostatic hypotension, sudden death, arrhythmias, tachycardia

• QTc prolongation

• Hepatic failure, extrapyramidal symptoms

• Increased intraocular pressure

• Rare induction of mania and activation of suicidal ideation

Weight Gain

unusual   not unusual   **common**   problematic

• Many experience and/or can be significant in amount

• Can increase appetite and carbohydrate craving

Sedation

unusual   not unusual   **common**   problematic

• Many experience and/or can be significant in amount

• Tolerance to sedative effect may develop with long-term use

What To Do About Side Effects

• Wait

• Wait

• Wait

- Lower the dose
- Switch to an SSRI or newer antidepressant

Best Augmenting Agents for Side Effects
- Many side effects cannot be improved with an augmenting agent

---

DOSING AND USE

Usual Dosage Range
- 75–150 mg/day once daily or in up to 4 divided doses (for depression)
- 50–150 mg/day (for chronic pain)

Dosage Forms
- Capsule 10 mg, 25 mg, 50 mg, 75 mg
- Liquid 10 mg/5mL

How to Dose
- Initial 10–25 mg/day at bedtime; increase by 25 mg every 3–7 days; can be dosed once daily or in divided doses; maximum dose 300 mg/day
- When treating nicotine dependence, nortriptyline should be initiated 10–28 days before cessation of smoking to achieve steady drug states

 Dosing Tips
- If given in a single dose, should generally be administered at bedtime because of its sedative properties
- If given in split doses, largest dose should generally be given at bedtime because of its sedative properties
- If patients experience nightmares, split dose and do not give large dose at bedtime
- Patients treated for chronic pain may only require lower doses
- Risk of seizure increases with dose
- ✳ Monitoring plasma levels of nortriptyline is recommended in patients who do not respond to the usual dose or whose treatment is regarded as urgent
- Some formulations of nortriptyline contain sodium bisulphate, which may cause allergic reactions in some patients, perhaps more frequently in asthmatics
- If intolerable anxiety, insomnia, agitation, akathisia, or activation occur either upon dosing initiation or discontinuation,

consider the possibility of activated bipolar disorder, and switch to a mood stabilizer or an atypical antipsychotic

Overdose
- Death may occur; CNS depression, convulsions, cardiac dysrhythmias, severe hypotension, ECG changes, coma

Long-Term Use
- Safe

Habit Forming
- No

How to Stop
- Taper to avoid withdrawal effects
- Even with gradual dose reduction some withdrawal symptoms may appear within the first two weeks
- Many patients tolerate 50% dose reduction for 3 days, then another 50% reduction for 3 days, then discontinuation
- If withdrawal symptoms emerge during discontinuation, raise dose to stop symptoms and then restart withdrawal much more slowly

Pharmacokinetics
- Substrate for CYP450 2D6
- Nortriptyline is the active metabolite of amitriptyline, formed by demethylation via CYP450 1A2
- Half-life approximately 36 hours

 Drug Interactions
- Tramadol increases the risk of seizures in patients taking TCAs
- Use of TCAs with anticholinergic drugs may result in paralytic ileus or hyperthermia
- Fluoxetine, paroxetine, bupropion, duloxetine and other CYP450 2D6 inhibitors may increase TCA concentrations and cause side effects including dangerous arrhythmias
- Cimetidine may increase plasma concentrations of TCAs and cause anticholinergic symptoms
- Phenothiazines or haloperidol may raise TCA blood concentrations
- May alter effects of antihypertensive drugs; may inhibit hypotensive effects of clonidine

NORTRIPTYLINE (continued)

- Use of TCAs with sympathomimetic agents may increase sympathetic activity
- Methylphenidate may inhibit metabolism of TCAs
- Nortriptyline may raise plasma levels of dicumarol
- Activation and agitation, especially following switching or adding antidepressants, may represent the induction of a bipolar state, especially a mixed dysphoric bipolar II condition sometimes associated with suicidal ideation, and require the addition of lithium, a mood stabilizer or an atypical antipsychotic, and/or discontinuation of nortriptyline

 Other Warnings/ Precautions

- Add or initiate other antidepressants with caution for up to 2 weeks after discontinuing nortriptyline
- Generally, do not use with MAO inhibitors, including 14 days after MAOIs are stopped; do not start an MAOI until 2 weeks after discontinuing nortriptyline, but see Pearls
- Use with caution in patients with history of seizures, urinary retention, narrow angle-closure glaucoma, hyperthyroidism
- TCAs can increase QTc interval, especially at toxic doses, which can be attained not only by overdose but also by combining with drugs that inhibit TCA metabolism via CYP450 2D6, potentially causing torsade de pointes-type arrhythmia or sudden death
- Because TCAs can prolong QTc interval, use with caution in patients who have bradycardia or who are taking drugs that can induce bradycardia (e.g., beta blockers, calcium channel blockers, clonidine, digitalis)
- Because TCAs can prolong QTc interval, use with caution in patients who have hypokalemia and/or hypomagnesemia or who are taking drugs that can induce hypokalemia and/or magnesemia (e.g., diuretics, stimulant laxatives, intravenous amphotericin B, glucocorticoids, tetracosactide)

Do Not Use

- If patient is recovering from myocardial infarction

- If patient is taking agents capable of significantly prolonging QTc interval (e.g., pimozide, thioridazine, selected antiarrhythmics, moxifloxacin, sparfloxacin)
- If there is a history of QTc prolongation or cardiac arrhythmia, recent acute myocardial infarction, uncompensated heart failure
- If patient is taking drugs that inhibit TCA metabolism, including CYP450 2D6 inhibitors, except by an expert
- If there is reduced CYP450 2D6 function, such as patients who are poor 2D6 metabolizers, except by an expert and at low doses
- If there is a proven allergy to nortriptyline or amitriptyline

SPECIAL POPULATIONS

Renal Impairment

- Use with caution; may need to lower dose
- May need to monitor plasma levels

Hepatic Impairment

- Use with caution
- May need to monitor plasma levels
- May require a lower dose with slower titration

Cardiac Impairment

- TCAs have been reported to cause arrhythmias, prolongation of conduction time, orthostatic hypotension, sinus tachycardia, and heart failure, especially in the diseased heart
- Myocardial infarction and stroke have been reported with TCAs
- TCAs produce QTc prolongation, which may be enhanced by the existence of bradycardia, hypokalemia, congenital or acquired long QTc interval, which should be evaluated prior to administering nortriptyline
- Use with caution if treating concomitantly with a medication likely to produce prolonged bradycardia, hypokalemia, slowing of intracardiac conduction, or prolongation of the QTc interval
- Avoid TCAs in patients with a known history of QTc prolongation, recent acute myocardial infarction, and uncompensated heart failure

- TCAs may cause a sustained increase in heart rate in patients with ischemic heart disease and may worsen (decrease) heart rate variability, an independent risk of mortality in cardiac populations
- Since SSRIs may improve (increase) heart rate variability in patients following a myocardial infarct and may improve survival as well as mood in patients with acute angina or following a myocardial infarction, these are more appropriate agents for cardiac population than tricyclic/tetracyclic antidepressants
- ✱ Risk/benefit ratio may not justify use of TCAs in cardiac impairment

Elderly

- May be more sensitive to anticholinergic, cardiovascular, hypotensive, and sedative effects
- May require lower dose; it may be useful to monitor plasma levels in elderly patients

 Children and Adolescents

- Use with caution, observing for activation of known or unknown bipolar disorder and/or suicidal ideation, and strongly consider informing parents or guardian of this risk so they can help observe child or adolescent patients
- Not recommended for use under age 12
- Not intended for use under age 6
- Several studies show lack of efficacy of TCAs for depression
- May be used to treat enuresis or hyperactive/impulsive behaviors
- Some cases of sudden death have occurred in children taking TCAs
- Plasma levels may need to be monitored
- Dose in children generally less than 50 mg/day
- May be useful to monitor plasma levels in children and adolescents

Pregnancy

- Risk Category D [positive evidence of risk to human fetus; potential benefits may still justify its use during pregnancy]
- Crosses the placenta
- Should be used only if potential benefits outweigh potential risks

- Adverse effects have been reported in infants whose mothers took a TCA (lethargy, withdrawal symptoms, fetal malformations)
- Evaluate for treatment with an antidepressant with a better risk/benefit ratio

Breast Feeding

- Some drug is found in mother's breast milk
- ✱ Recommended either to discontinue drug or bottle feed
- Immediate postpartum period is a high-risk time for depression, especially in women who have had prior depressive episodes, so drug may need to be reinstituted late in the third trimester or shortly after childbirth to prevent a recurrence during the postpartum period
- Must weigh benefits of breast feeding with risks and benefits of antidepressant treatment versus non-treatment to both the infant and the mother
- For many patients this may mean continuing treatment during breast feeding

THE ART OF PSYCHOPHARMACOLOGY

Potential Advantages

- Patients with insomnia
- Severe or treatment-resistant depression
- Patients for whom therapeutic drug monitoring is desirable

Potential Disadvantages

- Pediatric and geriatric patients
- Patients concerned with weight gain
- Cardiac patients

Primary Target Symptoms

- Depressed mood
- Chronic pain

 Pearls

- Tricyclic antidepressants are often a first-line treatment option for chronic pain
- Tricyclic antidepressants are no longer generally considered a first-line option for depression because of their side effect profile
- Tricyclic antidepressants continue to be useful for severe or treatment-resistant depression

- Noradrenergic reuptake inhibitors such as nortriptyline can be used as a second-line treatment for smoking cessation, cocaine dependence, and attention deficit disorder
- TCAs may aggravate psychotic symptoms
- Alcohol should be avoided because of additive CNS effects
- Underweight patients may be more susceptible to adverse cardiovascular effects
- Children, patients with inadequate hydration, and patients with cardiac disease may be more susceptible to TCA-induced cardiotoxicity than healthy adults
- For the expert only: although generally prohibited, a heroic but potentially dangerous treatment for severely treatment-resistant patients is for an expert to give a tricyclic/tetracyclic antidepressant other than clomipramine simultaneously with an MAO inhibitor for patients who fail to respond to numerous other antidepressants
- If this option is elected, start the MAOI with the tricyclic/tetracyclic antidepressant simultaneously at low doses after appropriate drug washout, then alternately increase doses of these agents every few days to a week as tolerated
- Although very strict dietary and concomitant drug restrictions must be observed to prevent hypertensive crises and serotonin syndrome, the most common side effects of MAOI and tricyclic/tetracyclic antidepressant combinations may be weight gain and orthostatic hypotension

- Patients on TCAs should be aware that they may experience symptoms such as photosensitivity or blue-green urine
- SSRIs may be more effective than TCAs in women, and TCAs may be more effective than SSRIs in men
- Not recommended for first-line use in children with ADHD because of the availability of safer treatments with better documented efficacy and because of nortriptyline's potential for sudden death in children
* Nortriptyline is one of the few TCAs where monitoring of plasma drug levels has been well studied
- Since tricyclic/tetracyclic antidepressants are substrates for CYP450 2D6, and 7% of the population (especially Caucasians) may have a genetic variant leading to reduced activity of 2D6, such patients may not safely tolerate normal doses of tricyclic/tetracyclic antidepressants and may require dose reduction
- Phenotypic testing may be necessary to detect this genetic variant prior to dosing with a tricyclic/tetracyclic antidepressant, especially in vulnerable populations such as children, elderly, cardiac populations, and those on concomitant medications
- Patients who seem to have extraordinarily severe side effects at normal or low doses may have this phenotypic CYP450 2D6 variant and require low doses or switching to another antidepressant not metabolized by 2D6

Suggested Reading

Anderson IM. Meta-analytical studies on new antidepressants. Br Med Bull 2001; 57:161–178.

Anderson IM. Selective serotonin reuptake inhibitors versus tricyclic antidepressants: a meta-analysis of efficacy and tolerability. J Aff Disorders 2000;58:19–36.

Hughes JR, Stead LF, Lancaster T. Antidepressants for smoking cessation. Cochrane Database Syst Rev 2000;4:CD000031.

Wilens TE, Biederman J, Baldessarini RJ, Geller B, Schleifer D, Spencer TJ, Birmajer B, Goldblatt A. Cardiovascular effects of therapeutic doses of tricyclic antidepressants in children and adolescents. J Am Acad Child Adolesc Psychiatry 1996;35(11):1491–501.

OLANZAPINE

THERAPEUTICS

Brands
- Zyprexa
- Olasek
- Ziprexa
- Symbyax (olanzapine-fluoxetine combination)

see index for additional brand names

Generic? Not in U.S., Europe, or Japan

Class
- Atypical antipsychotic (serotonin-dopamine antagonist; second generation antipsychotic; also a mood stabilizer)

Commonly Prescribed For
(bold for FDA approved)
- **Schizophrenia**
- **Maintaining response in schizophrenia**
- **Acute agitation associated with schizophrenia (intramuscular)**
- **Acute mania (monotherapy and adjunct to lithium or valproate)**
- **Bipolar maintenance**
- **Acute agitation associated with bipolar I mania (intramuscular)**
- **Bipolar depression [in combination with fluoxetine (Symbyax)]**
- Other psychotic disorders
- Unipolar depression unresponsive to antidepressants
- Behavioral disturbances in dementias
- Behavioral disturbances in children and adolescents
- Disorders associated with problems with impulse control

How The Drug Works
- Blocks dopamine 2 receptors, reducing positive symptoms of psychosis and stabilizing affective symptoms
- Blocks serotonin 2A receptors, causing enhancement of dopamine release in certain brain regions and thus reducing motor side effects and possibly improving cognitive and affective symptoms
- Interactions at a myriad of other neurotransmitter receptors may contribute to olanzapine's efficacy
- ✳ Specifically, antagonist actions at 5HT2C receptors may contribute to efficacy for cognitive and affective symptoms in some patients
- ✳ 5HT2C antagonist actions plus serotonin reuptake blockade of fluoxetine add to the actions of olanzapine when given as Symbyax (olanzapine-fluoxetine combination)

How Long Until It Works
- Psychotic symptoms can improve within 1 week, but it may take several weeks for full effect on behavior as well as on cognition and affective stabilization
- Classically recommended to wait at least 4–6 weeks to determine efficacy of drug, but in practice some patients require up to 16–20 weeks to show a good response, especially on cognitive symptoms

If It Works
- Most often reduces positive symptoms in schizophrenia but does not eliminate them
- Can improve negative symptoms, as well as aggressive, cognitive, and affective symptoms in schizophrenia
- Most schizophrenic patients do not have a total remission of symptoms but rather a reduction of symptoms by about a third
- Perhaps 5–15% of schizophrenic patients can experience an overall improvement of greater than 50–60%, especially when receiving stable treatment for more than a year
- Such patients are considered super-responders or "awakeners" since they may be well enough to be employed, live independently, and sustain long-term relationships
- Many bipolar patients may experience a reduction of symptoms by half or more
- Continue treatment until reaching a plateau of improvement
- After reaching a satisfactory plateau, continue treatment for at least a year after first episode of psychosis
- For second and subsequent episodes of psychosis, treatment may need to be indefinite
- Even for first episodes of psychosis, it may be preferable to continue treatment indefinitely to avoid subsequent episodes
- Treatment may not only reduce mania but also prevent recurrences of mania in bipolar disorder

If It Doesn't Work

- Try one of the other atypical antipsychotics (risperidone, quetiapine, ziprasidone, aripiprazole, amisulpride)
- If 2 or more antipsychotic monotherapies do not work, consider clozapine
- If no first-line atypical antipsychotic is effective, consider higher doses or augmentation with valproate or lamotrigine
- Some patients may require treatment with a conventional antipsychotic
- Consider noncompliance and switch to another antipsychotic with fewer side effects or to an antipsychotic that can be given by depot injection
- Consider initiating rehabilitation and psychotherapy
- Consider presence of concomitant drug abuse

 ### Best Augmenting Combos for Partial Response or Treatment-Resistance

- Valproic acid (valproate, divalproex, divalproex ER)
- Other mood stabilizing anticonvulsants (carbamazepine, oxcarbazepine, lamotrigine)
- Lithium
- Benzodiazepines
- Fluoxetine and other antidepressants may be effective augmenting agents to olanzapine for bipolar depression, psychotic depression, and for unipolar depression not responsive to antidepressants alone (e.g., olanzapine-fluoxetine combination)

Tests

Before starting an atypical antipsychotic

✳ Weigh all patients and track BMI during treatment
- Get baseline personal and family history of obesity, dyslipidemia, hypertension, and cardiovascular disease
✳ Get waist circumference (at umbilicus), blood pressure, fasting plasma glucose, and fasting lipid profile
- Determine if the patient is
  - overweight (BMI 25.0–29.9)
  - obese (BMI ≥30)
  - has pre-diabetes (fasting plasma glucose 100–125 mg/dl)
  - has diabetes (fasting plasma glucose >126 mg/dl)
  - has hypertension (BP >140/90 mm Hg)
  - has dyslipidemia (increased total cholesterol, LDL cholesterol, and triglycerides; decreased HDL cholesterol)
- Treat or refer such patients for treatment, including nutrition and weight management, physical activity counseling, smoking cessation, and medical management

Monitoring after starting an atypical antipsychotic

✳ BMI monthly for 3 months, then quarterly
✳ Blood pressure, fasting plasma glucose, fasting lipids within 3 months and then annually, but earlier and more frequently for patients with diabetes or who have gained >5% of initial weight
- Treat or refer for treatment and consider switching to another atypical antipsychotic for patients who become overweight, obese, pre-diabetic, diabetic, hypertensive, or dyslipidemic while receiving an atypical antipsychotic
✳ Even in patients without known diabetes, be vigilant for the rare but life threatening onset of diabetic ketoacidosis, which always requires immediate treatment, by monitoring for the rapid onset of polyuria, polydipsia, weight loss, nausea, vomiting, dehydration, rapid respiration, weakness and clouding of sensorium, even coma
- Patients with liver disease should have blood tests a few times a year

SIDE EFFECTS

How Drug Causes Side Effects

- By blocking histamine 1 receptors in the brain, it can cause sedation and possibly weight gain
- By blocking alpha 1 adrenergic receptors, it can cause dizziness, sedation, and hypotension
- By blocking muscarinic 1 receptors, it can cause dry mouth, constipation, and sedation
- By blocking dopamine 2 receptors in the striatum, it can cause motor side effects (unusual)

- Mechanism of weight gain and increased incidence of diabetes and dyslipidemia with atypical antipsychotics is unknown

Notable Side Effects

✳ Probably increases risk for diabetes mellitus and dyslipidemia
- Dizziness, sedation
- Dry mouth, constipation, dyspepsia, weight gain
- Joint pain, back pain, chest pain, extremity pain, abnormal gait, ecchymosis, peripheral edema
- Tachycardia
- Rare orthostatic hypotension, usually during initial dose titration
- Rare tardive dyskinesia (much reduced risk compared to conventional antipsychotics)
- Rare rash on exposure to sunlight

 Life Threatening or Dangerous Side Effects

- Hyperglycemia, in some cases extreme and associated with ketoacidosis or hyperosmolar coma or death, has been reported in patients taking atypical antipsychotics
- Increased incidence of cerebrovascular events, including stoke, transient ischemic attacks, and fatalities, in elderly patients with dementia
- Increased incidence of mortality in elderly patients with dementia-related psychosis
- Rare neuroleptic malignant syndrome (much reduced risk compared to conventional antipsychotics)
- Rare seizures

Weight Gain

unusual   not unusual   common   problematic

- Frequent and can be significant in amount
- Can become a health problem in some
- More than for some other antipsychotics, but never say always as not a problem in everyone

Sedation

unusual   not unusual   common   problematic

- Many patients experience and/or can be significant in amount
- Usually transient

- May be less than for some antipsychotics, more than for others

What To Do About Side Effects

- Wait
- Wait
- Wait
- Take at bedtime to help reduce daytime sedation
- Anticholinergics may reduce motor side effects such as akathisia when present, but rarely necessary
- Weight loss, exercise programs, and medical management for high BMIs, diabetes, dyslipidemia
- Switch to another atypical antipsychotic

Best Augmenting Agents for Side Effects

- Benztropine or trihexyphenidyl for motor side effects
- Many side effects cannot be improved with an augmenting agent

DOSING AND USE

Usual Dosage Range

- 10–20 mg/day (oral or intramuscular)
- 6–12 mg olanzapine / 25–50 mg fluoxetine (olanzapine-fluoxetine combination)

Dosage Forms

- Tablets 2.5 mg, 5 mg, 7.5 mg, 10 mg, 15 mg, 20 mg
- Orally disintegrating tablets 5 mg, 10 mg, 15 mg, 20 mg
- Intramuscular formulation 5 mg/mL, each vial contains 10 mg (available in some countries)
- Olanzapine-fluoxetine combination capsule (mg equivalent olanzapine/mg equivalent fluoxetine) 6 mg/25 mg, 6 mg/50 mg, 12 mg/25 mg, 12 mg/50 mg

How to Dose

- Initial 5–10 mg once daily orally; increase by 5 mg/day once a week until desired efficacy is reached; maximum approved dose is 20 mg/day
- For intramuscular formulation, recommended initial dose 10 mg; second injection of 5–10 mg may be administered 2 hours after first injection; maximum daily

dose of olanzapine is 20 mg, with no more than 3 injections per 24 hours
- For olanzapine-fluoxetine combination, recommended initial dose 6 mg/25 mg once daily in evening; increase dose based on efficacy and tolerability; maximum generally 18 mg/75 mg

 Dosing Tips

✳ **More may be more:** raising usual dose above 15 mg/day can be useful for acutely ill and agitated patients and some treatment-resistant patients, gaining efficacy without many more side effects

✳ Some heroic uses for patients who do not respond to other antipsychotics can occasionally justify dosing over 30 mg/day
- Usual doses (>15 mg/day range) can be among the most costly among atypical antipsychotics, and dosing >30 mg/day can be very expensive
- Rather than raise the dose above these levels in acutely agitated patients requiring acute antipsychotic actions, consider augmentation with a benzodiazepine or conventional antipsychotic, either orally or intramuscularly
- Rather than raise the dose above these levels in partial responders, consider augmentation with a mood stabilizing anticonvulsant, such as valproate or lamotrigine
- Clearance of olanzapine is reduced in women compared to men, so women may need lower doses than men
- Children and elderly should generally be dosed at the lower end of the dosage spectrum

✳ Olanzapine intramuscularly can be given short-term, both to initiate dosing with oral olanzapine or another oral antipsychotic and to treat breakthrough agitation in patients maintained on oral antipsychotics

Overdose
- Rarely lethal in monotherapy overdose; sedation, slurred speech

Long-Term Use
- Approved to maintain response in long-term treatment of schizophrenia
- Approved for long-term maintenance in bipolar disorder
- Often used for long-term maintenance in various behavioral disorders

Habit Forming
- No

How to Stop
- Slow down-titration of oral formulation (over 6 to 8 weeks), especially when simultaneously beginning a new antipsychotic while switching (i.e., cross-titration)
- Rapid oral discontinuation may lead to rebound psychosis and worsening of symptoms

Pharmacokinetics
- Metabolites are inactive
- Parent drug has 21–54 hour half-life

 Drug Interactions
- May increase effect of anti-hypertensive agents
- May antagonize levodopa, dopamine agonists
- Dose may need to be lowered if given with CYP450 1A2 inhibitors (e.g., fluvoxamine); raised if given in conjunction with CYP450 1A2 inducers (e.g., cigarette smoke, carbamazepine)

 Other Warnings/ Precautions
- Use with caution in patients with conditions that predispose to hypotension (dehydration, overheating)
- Use with caution in patients with prostatic hypertrophy, narrow angle-closure glaucoma, paralytic ileus
- Patients receiving the intramuscular formulation of olanzapine should be observed closely for hypotension
- Intramuscular formulation is not generally recommended to be administered with parenteral benzodiazepines; if patient requires a parenteral benzodiazepine it should be given at least 1 hour after intramuscular olanzapine
- Olanzapine should be used cautiously in patients at risk for aspiration pneumonia, as dysphagia has been reported

Do Not Use

- If there is a known risk of narrow angle-closure glaucoma (intramuscular formulation)
- If patient has unstable medical condition (e.g., acute myocardial infarction, unstable angina pectoris, severe hypotension and/or bradycardia, sick sinus syndrome, recent heart surgery) (intramuscular formulation)
- If there is a proven allergy to olanzapine

SPECIAL POPULATIONS

Renal Impairment

- No dose adjustment required for oral formulation
- Not removed by hemodialysis
- For intramuscular formulation, consider lower starting dose (5 mg)

Hepatic Impairment

- May need to lower dose
- Patients with liver disease should have liver function tests a few times a year
- For moderate to severe hepatic impairment, starting oral dose 5 mg; increase with caution
- For intramuscuar formulation, consider lower starting dose (5 mg)

Cardiac Impairment

- Drug should be used with caution because of risk of orthostatic hypotension

Elderly

- Some patients may tolerate lower doses better
- Increased incidence of stroke
- For intramuscular formulation, recommended starting dose is 2.5–5 mg; a second injection of 2.5–5 mg may be administered 2 hours after first injection; no more than 3 injections should be administered within 24 hours

Children and Adolescents

- Not officially recommended under age 18; however, olanzapine is often used for patients under 18
- Clinical experience and early data suggest olanzapine is probably safe and effective

for behavioral disturbances in children and adolescents
- Children and adolescents using olanzapine may need to be monitored more often than adults
- Intramuscular formulation has not been studied in patients under 18 and is not recommended for use in this population

Pregnancy

- Risk Category C [some animal studies show adverse effects, no controlled studies in humans]
- Psychotic symptoms may worsen during pregnancy, and some form of treatment may be necessary
- Early findings of infants exposed to olanzapine in utero currently do not show adverse consequences
- Olanzapine may be preferable to anticonvulsant mood stabilizers if treatment is required during pregnancy

Breast Feeding

- Unknown if olanzapine is secreted in human breast milk, but all psychotropics assumed to be secreted in breast milk
- ✳ Recommended either to discontinue drug or bottle feed
- Infants of women who choose to breast feed while on olanzapine should be monitored for possible adverse effects

THE ART OF PSYCHOPHARMACOLOGY

Potential Advantages

- ✳ Some cases of psychosis and bipolar disorder refractory to treatment with other antipsychotics
- ✳ Often a preferred augmenting agent in bipolar depression or treatment-resistant unipolar depression
- ✳ Patients needing rapid onset of antipsychotic action without drug titration
- Patients switching from intramuscular olanzapine to an oral preparation

Potential Disadvantages

- Patients concerned about gaining weight
- ✳ Patients with diabetes mellitus

OLANZAPINE (continued)

Primary Target Symptoms
- Positive symptoms of psychosis
- Negative symptoms of psychosis
- Cognitive symptoms
- Unstable mood (both depressed mood and mania)
- Aggressive symptoms

Pearls
- Well accepted for use in schizophrenia and bipolar disorder, including difficult cases
- ✱ Documented utility in treatment-refractory cases, especially at higher doses
- ✱ Documented efficacy as augmenting agent to SSRIs (especially fluoxetine) in nonpsychotic treatment-resistant major depressive disorder
- ✱ Documented efficacy in bipolar depression, especially in combination with fluoxetine

- More weight gain than other antipsychotics —does not mean every patient gains weight
- Motor side effects unusual at low- to mid-doses
- Less sedation than for some other antipsychotics, more than for others
- ✱ Controversial as to whether olanzapine has more risk of diabetes and dyslipidemia than other antipsychotics
- One of the most expensive atypical antipsychotics within the usual therapeutic dosing range
- Cigarette smoke can decrease olanzapine levels and patients may require a dose increase if they begin or increase smoking
- ✱ One of only two atypical antipsychotics with a short-acting intramuscular dosage formulation

Suggested Reading

Duggan L, Fenton M, Dardennes RM, El-Dosoky A, Indran S. Olanzapine for schizophrenia. Cochrane Database Syst Rev 2003;(1):CD001359.

Kapur S, Remington G. Atypical antipsychotics: new directions and new challenges in the treatment of schizophrenia. Annu Rev Med 2001;52:503–17.

Tandon R. Safety and tolerability: how do new generation "atypical" antipsychotics compare? Psychiatric Quarterly 2002;73:297–311.

Tandon R, Jibson MD. Efficacy of newer generation antipsychotics in the treatment of schizophrenia. Psychoneuroendocrinology 2003;28:9–26.

Yatham LN. Efficacy of atypical antipsychotics in mood disorders. J Clin Psychopharmacol 2003;23(3 Suppl 1):S9–14.

OXAZEPAM

THERAPEUTICS

Brands • Serax
see index for additional brand names

Generic? Yes

Class
• Benzodiazepine (anxiolytic)

Commonly Prescribed For
(bold for FDA approved)
• **Anxiety**
• **Anxiety associated with depression**
• **Alcohol withdrawal**

 How The Drug Works
• Binds to benzodiazepine receptors at the GABA-A ligand-gated chloride channel complex
• Enhances the inhibitory effects of GABA
• Boosts chloride conductance through GABA-regulated channels
• Inhibits neuronal activity presumably in amygdala-centered fear circuits to provide therapeutic benefits in anxiety disorders

How Long Until It Works
• Some immediate relief with first dosing is common; can take several weeks with daily dosing for maximal therapeutic benefit

If It Works
• For short-term symptoms of anxiety – after a few weeks, discontinue use or use on an "as-needed" basis
• For chronic anxiety disorders, the goal of treatment is complete remission of symptoms as well as prevention of future relapses
• For chronic anxiety disorders, treatment most often reduces or even eliminates symptoms, but not a cure since symptoms can recur after medicine stopped
• For long-term symptoms of anxiety, consider switching to an SSRI or SNRI for long-term maintenance
• If long-term maintenance with a benzodiazepine is necessary, continue treatment for 6 months after symptoms resolve, and then taper dose slowly
• If symptoms reemerge, consider treatment with an SSRI or SNRI, or consider

restarting the benzodiazepine; sometimes benzodiazepines have to be used in combination with SSRIs or SNRIs for best results

If It Doesn't Work
• Consider switching to another agent or adding an appropriate augmenting agent
• Consider psychotherapy, especially cognitive behavioral psychotherapy
• Consider presence of concomitant substance abuse
• Consider presence of oxazepam abuse
• Consider another diagnosis, such as a comorbid medical condition

 Best Augmenting Combos for Partial Response or Treatment-Resistance
• Benzodiazepines are frequently used as augmenting agents for antipsychotics and mood stabilizers in the treatment of psychotic and bipolar disorders
• Benzodiazepines are frequently used as augmenting agents for SSRIs and SNRIs in the treatment of anxiety disorders
• Not generally rational to combine with other benzodiazepines
• Caution if using as an anxiolytic concomitantly with other sedative hypnotics for sleep

Tests
• In patients with seizure disorders, concomitant medical illness, and/or those with multiple concomitant long-term medications, periodic liver tests and blood counts may be prudent

SIDE EFFECTS

How Drug Causes Side Effects
• Same mechanism for side effects as for therapeutic effects – namely due to excessive actions at benzodiazepine receptors
• Long-term adaptations in benzodiazepine receptors may explain the development of dependence, tolerance, and withdrawal
• Side effects are generally immediate, but immediate side effects often disappear in time

Notable Side Effects

* ✱ Sedation, fatigue, depression
* ✱ Dizziness, ataxia, slurred speech, weakness
* ✱ Forgetfulness, confusion
* ✱ Hyper-excitability, nervousness
* Rare hallucinations, mania
* Rare hypotension
* Hypersalivation, dry mouth

Life Threatening or Dangerous Side Effects

* Respiratory depression, especially when taken with CNS depressants in overdose
* Rare hepatic dysfunction, renal dysfunction, blood dyscrasias

Weight Gain

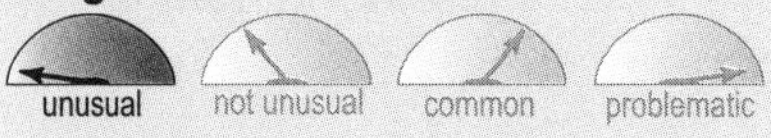
unusual
not unusual
common
problematic

* Reported but not expected

Sedation

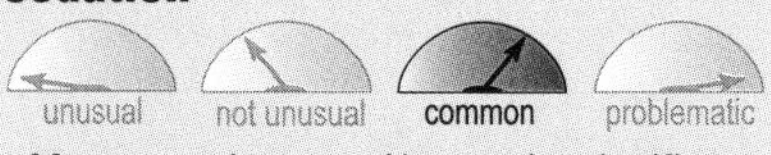
unusual
not unusual
common
problematic

* Many experience and/or can be significant in amount
* Especially at initiation of treatment or when dose increases
* Tolerance often develops over time

What To Do About Side Effects

* Wait
* Wait
* Wait
* Lower the dose
* Take largest dose at bedtime to avoid sedative effects during the day
* Switch to another agent
* Administer flumazenil if side effects are severe or life-threatening

Best Augmenting Agents for Side Effects

* Many side effects cannot be improved with an augmenting agent

DOSING AND USE

Usual Dosage Range

* Mild to moderate anxiety: 30–60 mg/day in 3–4 divided doses
* Severe anxiety, anxiety associated with alcohol withdrawal: 45–120 mg/day in 3–4 divided doses

Dosage Forms

* Capsule 10 mg, 15 mg, 30 mg
* Tablet 15 mg

How to Dose

* Titration generally not necessary

Dosing Tips

* Use lowest possible effective dose for the shortest possible period of time (a benzodiazepine-sparing strategy)
* 15 mg tablet contains tartrazine, which may cause allergic reactions in certain patients, particularly those who are sensitive to aspirin
* For inter-dose symptoms of anxiety, can either increase dose or maintain same total daily dose but divide into more frequent doses
* Can also use an as-needed occasional "top up" dose for inter-dose anxiety
* Because anxiety disorders can require higher doses, the risk of dependence may be greater in these patients
* Some severely ill patients may require doses higher than the generally recommended maximum dose
* Frequency of dosing in practice is often greater than predicted from half-life, as duration of biological activity is often shorter than pharmacokinetic terminal half-life

Overdose

* Fatalities can occur; hypotension, tiredness, ataxia, confusion, coma

Long-Term Use

* Risk of dependence, particularly for treatment periods longer than 12 weeks and especially in patients with past or current polysubstance abuse

Habit Forming

* Oxazepam is a Schedule IV drug
* Patients may develop dependence and/or tolerance with long-term use

How to Stop

- Patients with history of seizure may seize upon withdrawal, especially if withdrawal is abrupt
- Taper by 15 mg every 3 days to reduce chances of withdrawal effects
- For difficult to taper cases, consider reducing dose much more slowly once reaching 45 mg/day, perhaps by as little as 10 mg per week or less
- For other patients with severe problems discontinuing a benzodiazepine, dosing may need to be tapered over many months (i.e., reduce dose by 1% every 3 days by crushing tablet and suspending or dissolving in 100 ml of fruit juice and then disposing of 1 ml while drinking the rest; 3–7 days later, dispose of 2 ml, and so on). This is both a form of very slow biological tapering and a form of behavioral desensitization
- Be sure to differentiate reemergence of symptoms requiring reinstitution of treatment from withdrawal symptoms
- Benzodiazepine-dependent anxiety patients and insulin-dependent diabetics are not addicted to their medications. When benzodiazepine-dependent patients stop their medication, disease symptoms can reemerge, disease symptoms can worsen (rebound), and/or withdrawal symptoms can emerge

Pharmacokinetics

- Elimination half-life 3–21 hours
- No active metabolites

 Drug Interactions

- Increased depressive effects when taken with other CNS depressants

 Other Warnings/ Precautions

- Dosage changes should be made in collaboration with prescriber
- Use with caution in patients with pulmonary disease; rare reports of death after initiation of benzodiazepines in patients with severe pulmonary impairment
- History of drug or alcohol abuse often creates greater risk for dependency

- Some depressed patients may experience a worsening of suicidal ideation
- Some patients may exhibit abnormal thinking or behavioral changes similar to those caused by other CNS depressants (i.e., either depressant actions or disinhibiting actions)

Do Not Use

- If patient has narrow angle-closure glaucoma
- If there is a proven allergy to oxazepam or any benzodiazepine

SPECIAL POPULATIONS

Renal Impairment

- Use with caution; oxazepam levels may be increased

Hepatic Impairment

- Use with caution; oxazepam levels may be increased
- Because of its short half-life and inactive metabolites, oxazepam may be a preferred benzodiazepine in some patients with liver disease

Cardiac Impairment

- Benzodiazepines have been used to treat anxiety associated with acute myocardial infarction

Elderly

- Initial 30 mg in 3 divided doses; can be increased to 30–60 mg/day in 3–4 divided doses

 Children and Adolescents

- Safety and efficacy not established under age 6
- No clear dosing guidelines for children ages 6–12
- Long-term effects of oxazepam in children/adolescents are unknown
- Should generally receive lower doses and be more closely monitored

Pregnancy

- Risk Category D [positive evidence of risk to human fetus; potential benefits may still justify its use during pregnancy]
- Possible increased risk of birth defects when benzodiazepines taken during pregnancy
- Because of the potential risks, oxazepam is not generally recommended as treatment for anxiety during pregnancy, especially during the first trimester
- Drug should be tapered if discontinued
- Infants whose mothers received a benzodiazepine late in pregnancy may experience withdrawal effects
- Neonatal flaccidity has been reported in infants whose mothers took a benzodiazepine during pregnancy
- Seizures, even mild seizures, may cause harm to the embryo/fetus

Breast Feeding

- Some drug is found in mother's breast milk
- ✳ Recommended either to discontinue drug or bottle feed
- Effects on infant have been observed and include feeding difficulties, sedation, and weight loss

THE ART OF PSYCHOPHARMACOLOGY

Potential Advantages
- Rapid onset of action

Potential Disadvantages
- Euphoria may lead to abuse
- Abuse especially risky in past or present substance abusers

Primary Target Symptoms
- Panic attacks
- Anxiety
- Agitation

 Pearls

- Can be a very useful adjunct to SSRIs and SNRIs in the treatment of numerous anxiety disorders
- Not effective for treating psychosis as a monotherapy, but can be used as an adjunct to antipsychotics
- Not effective for treating bipolar disorder as a monotherapy, but can be used as an adjunct to mood stabilizers and antipsychotics
- ✳ Because of its short half-life and inactive metabolites, oxazepam may be preferred over some benzodiazepines for patients with liver disease
- Oxazepam may be preferred over some other benzodiazepines for the treatment of delirium
- Can both cause and treat depression in different patients
- When using to treat insomnia, remember that insomnia may be a symptom of some other primary disorder itself, and thus warrant evaluation for comorbid psychiatric and/or medical conditions

 Suggested Reading

Ayd FJ Jr. Oxazepam: update 1989. Int Clin Psychopharmacol 1990;5:1–15.

Garattini S. Biochemical and pharmacological properties of oxazepam. Acta Psychiatr Scand Suppl 1978;274:9–18.

Greenblatt DJ. Clinical pharmacokinetics of oxazepam and lorazepam. Clin Pharmacokinet 1981;6:89–105.

OXCARBAZEPINE

THERAPEUTICS

Brands • Trileptal
see index for additional brand names

Generic? No

 Class

• Anticonvulsant, voltage-sensitive sodium channel antagonist

Commonly Prescribed For
(bold for FDA approved)
• **Partial seizures in adults with epilepsy (monotherapy or adjunctive)**
• **Partial seizures in children ages 4–16 with epilepsy (monotherapy or adjunctive)**
• Bipolar disorder

 How The Drug Works

✻ Acts as a use-dependent blocker of voltage-sensitive sodium channels
✻ Interacts with the open channel conformation of voltage-sensitive sodium channels
✻ Interacts at a specific site of the alpha pore-forming subunit of voltage-sensitive sodium channels
• Inhibits release of glutamate

How Long Until It Works
• For acute mania, effects should occur within a few weeks
• May take several weeks to months to optimize an effect on mood stabilization
• Should reduce seizures by 2 weeks

If It Works
• The goal of treatment is complete remission of symptoms (e.g., seizures, mania)
• Continue treatment until all symptoms are gone or until improvement is stable and then continue treating indefinitely as long as improvement persists
• Continue treatment indefinitely to avoid recurrence of mania and seizures

If It Doesn't Work (for bipolar disorder)
✻ Many patients only have a partial response where some symptoms are improved but others persist or continue to wax and wane without stabilization of mood
• Other patients may be nonresponders, sometimes called treatment-resistant or treatment-refractory
• Consider increasing dose, switching to another agent or adding an appropriate augmenting agent
• Consider adding psychotherapy
• For bipolar disorder, consider the presence of noncompliance and counsel patient
• Switch to another mood stabilizer with fewer side effects
• Consider evaluation for another diagnosis or for a comorbid condition (e.g., medical illness, substance abuse, etc.)

 Best Augmenting Combos for Partial Response or Treatment-Resistance

• Oxcarbazepine is itself a second-line augmenting agent for numerous other anticonvulsants, lithium, and atypical antipsychotics in treating bipolar disorder, although its use in bipolar disorder is not yet well-studied
• Oxcarbazepine may be a second or third-line augmenting agent for antipsychotics in treating schizophrenia, although its use in schizophrenia is also not yet well-studied

Tests
• Consider monitoring sodium levels because of possibility of hyponatremia, especially during the first 3 months

SIDE EFFECTS

How Drug Causes Side Effects
• CNS side effects theoretically due to excessive actions at voltage-sensitive sodium channels

Notable Side Effects
✻ Sedation, dizziness, headache, ataxia, nystagmus, abnormal gait, confusion, nervousness, fatigue
✻ Nausea, vomiting, abdominal pain, dyspepsia
• Diplopia, vertigo, abnormal vision
✻ Rash

Life Threatening or Dangerous Side Effects
- Hyponatremia

Weight Gain

unusual not unusual common problematic

- Occurs in significant minority
- Some patients experience increased appetite

Sedation

unusual not unusual common problematic

- Occurs in significant minority
- Dose-related
- Less than carbamazepine
- More when combined with other anticonvulsants
- Can wear off with time, but may not wear off at high doses

What To Do About Side Effects
- Wait
- Wait
- Wait
- Switch to another agent

Best Augmenting Agents for Side Effects
- Many side effects cannot be improved with an augmenting agent

DOSING AND USE

Usual Dosage Range
- 1200–2400 mg/day

Dosage Forms
- Tablet 150 mg, 300 mg, 600 mg
- Liquid 300 mg/5 mL

How to Dose
- Monotherapy for seizures or bipolar disorder: initial 600 mg/day in 2 doses; increase every 3 days by 300 mg/day; maximum dose generally 2400 mg/day
- Adjunctive: initial 600 mg/day in 2 doses; each week can increase by 600 mg/day; recommended dose 1200 mg/day; maximum dose generally 2400 mg/day

- When converting from adjunctive to monotherapy in the treatment of epilepsy, titrate concomitant drug down over 3–6 weeks while titrating oxcarbazepine up over 2–4 weeks, with an initial daily oxcarbazepine dose of 600 mg divided in 2 doses

 Dosing Tips
- ✳ Doses of oxcarbazepine need to be about one-third higher than those of carbamazepine for similar results
- Usually administered as adjunctive medication to other anticonvulsants, lithium, or atypical antipsychotics for bipolar disorder
- Side effects may increase with dose
- Although increased efficacy for seizures is seen at 2400 mg/day compared to 1200 mg/day, CNS side effects may be intolerable at the higher dose
- Liquid formulation can be administered mixed in a glass of water or directly from the oral dosing syringe supplied
- Slow dose titration may delay onset of therapeutic action but enhance tolerability to sedating side effects
- Should titrate slowly in the presence of other sedating agents, such as other anticonvulsants, in order to best tolerate additive sedative side effects

Overdose
- No fatalities reported

Long-Term Use
- Safe
- Monitoring of sodium may be required, especially during the first 3 months

Habit Forming
- No

How to Stop
- Taper
- Epilepsy patients may seize upon withdrawal, especially if withdrawal is abrupt
- ✳ Rapid discontinuation may increase the risk of relapse in bipolar disorder
- Discontinuation symptoms uncommon

Pharmacokinetics
- Metabolized in the liver

- Renally excreted
- Inhibits CYP450 2C19
* Oxcarbazepine is a prodrug for 10-hydroxy carbazepine
* This main active metabolite is sometimes called the monohydroxy derivative or MHD, and is also known as licarbazepine
* Half-life of parent drug is approximately 2 hours; half-life of MHD is approximately 9 hours; thus oxcarbazepine is essentially a prodrug rapidly converted to its MHD, licarbazepine
- A mild inducer of CYP450 3A4

 Drug Interactions

- Depressive effects may be increased by other CNS depressants (alcohol, MAOIs, other anticonvulsants, etc.)
- Strong inducers of CYP450 cytochromes (e.g., carbamazepine, phenobarbital, phenytoin, and primidone) can decrease plasma levels of the active metabolite MHD
- Verapamil may decrease plasma levels of the active metabolite MHD
- Oxcarbazepine can decrease plasma levels of hormonal contraceptives and dihydropyridine calcium antagonists
- Oxcarbazepine at doses greater than 1200 mg/day may increase plasma levels of phenytoin, possibly requiring dose reduction of phenytoin

 Other Warnings/ Precautions

- Because oxcarbazepine has a tricyclic chemical structure, it is not recommended to be taken with MAOIs, including 14 days after MAOIs are stopped; do not start an MAOI until 2 weeks after discontinuing oxcarbazepine
- Because oxcarbazepine can lower plasma levels of hormonal contraceptives, it may also reduce their effectiveness
- May exacerbate narrow angle-closure glaucoma
- May need to restrict fluids and/or monitor sodium because of risk of hyponatremia
- Use cautiously in patients who have demonstrated hypersensitivity to carbamazepine

Do Not Use

- If patient is taking an MAOI

- If there is a proven allergy to any tricyclic compound
- If there is a proven allergy to oxcarbazepine

SPECIAL POPULATIONS

Renal Impairment

- Oxcarbazepine is renally excreted
- Elimination half-life of active metabolite MHD is increased
- Reduce initial dose by half; may need to use slower titration

Hepatic Impairment

- No dose adjustment recommended for mild to moderate hepatic impairment

Cardiac Impairment

- No dose adjustment recommended

Elderly

- Older patients may have reduced creatinine clearance and require reduced dosing
- Elderly patients may be more susceptible to adverse effects
- Some patients may tolerate lower doses better

 Children and Adolescents

- Approved as adjunctive therapy or monotherapy for partial seizures in children 4 and older
- Ages 4–16 (adjunctive): initial 8–10 mg/kg/day or less than 600 mg/day in 2 doses; increase over 2 weeks to 900 mg/day (20–29 kg), 1200 mg/day (29.1–39 kg), or 1800 mg/day (>39 kg)
- When converting from adjunctive to monotherapy, titrate concomitant drug down over 3–6 weeks while titrating oxcarbazepine up by no more than 10 mg/kg/day each week, with an initial daily oxcarbazepine dose of 8–10 mg/kg/day divided in 2 doses
- Monotherapy: Initial 8–10 mg/kg/day in 2 doses; increase every 3 days by 5 mg/kg/day; recommended maintenance dose dependent on weight
- 0–20 kg (600–900 mg/day); 21–30 kg (900–1200 mg/day); 31–40 kg (900–1500 mg/day);

41–45 kg (1200–1500 mg/day);
46–55 kg (1200–1800 mg/day);
56–65 kg (1200–2100 mg/day);
over 65 kg (1500–2100 mg)

- Children below age 8 may have increased clearance compared to adults

Pregnancy

- Risk category C [some animal studies show adverse effects, no controlled studies in humans]
- ❋ Oxcarbazepine is structurally similar to carbamazepine, which is thought to be teratogenic in humans
- ❋ Use during first trimester may raise risk of neural tube defects (e.g., spina bifida) or other congenital anomalies
- Use in women of childbearing potential requires weighing potential benefits to the mother against the risks to the fetus
- ❋ If drug is continued, perform tests to detect birth defects
- ❋ If drug is continued, start on folate 1 mg/day to reduce risk of neural tube defects
- Taper drug if discontinuing
- ❋ For bipolar patients, oxcarbazepine should generally be discontinued before anticipated pregnancies
- Seizures, even mild seizures, may cause harm to the embryo/fetus
- Recurrent bipolar illness during pregnancy can be quite disruptive
- ❋ For bipolar patients, given the risk of relapse in the postpartum period, some form of mood stabilizer treatment may need to be restarted immediately after delivery if patient is unmedicated during pregnancy
- ❋ Atypical antipsychotics may be preferable to lithium or anticonvulsants such as oxcarbazepine if treatment of bipolar disorder is required during pregnancy
- Bipolar symptoms may recur or worsen during pregnancy and some form of treatment may be necessary

Breast Feeding

- Some drug is found in mother's breast milk
- ❋ Recommended either to discontinue drug or bottle feed

- If drug is continued while breast feeding, infant should be monitored for possible adverse effects
- If infant shows signs of irritability or sedation, drug may need to be discontinued
- Bipolar disorder may recur during the postpartum period, particularly if there is a history of prior postpartum episodes of either depression or psychosis
- ❋ Relapse rates may be lower in women who receive prophylactic treatment for postpartum episodes of bipolar disorder
- Atypical antipsychotics and anticonvulsants such as valproate may be safer than oxcarbazepine during the postpartum period when breast feeding

THE ART OF PSYCHOPHARMACOLOGY

Potential Advantages

- Treatment-resistant bipolar and psychotic disorders
- Those unable to tolerate carbamazepine but who respond to carbamazepine

Potential Disadvantages

- Patients at risk for hyponatremia

Primary Target Symptoms

- Incidence of seizures
- Severity of seizures
- Unstable mood, especially mania

Pearls

- ❋ Some evidence of effectiveness in treating acute mania; included in American Psychiatric Association's bipolar treatment guidelines as an option for acute treatment and maintenance treatment of bipolar disorder
- Some evidence of effectiveness as adjunctive treatment in schizophrenia and schizoaffective disorders
- Oxcarbazepine is the 10-keto analog of carbamazepine, but not a metabolite of carbamazepine
- ❋ Oxcarbazepine seems to have the same mechanism of therapeutic action as carbamazepine but with fewer side effects
- ❋ Specifically, risk of leukopenia, aplastic anemia, agranulocytosis, elevated liver

enzymes, or Stevens Johnson syndrome and serious rash associated with carbamazepine does <u>not</u> seem to be associated with oxcarbazepine

- Skin rash reactions to carbamazepine may resolve in 75% of patients with epilepsy when switched to oxcarbazepine; thus, 25% of patients who experience rash with carbamazepine may also experience it with oxcarbazepine
- Oxcarbazepine has much less prominent actions on CYP 450 enzyme systems than carbamazepine, and thus fewer drug-drug interactions
- Specifically, oxcarbazepine and its active metabolite, the monohydroxy derivative (MHD), cause less enzyme induction of CYP450 3A4 than the structurally-related carbamazepine
- The active metabolite MHD, also called licarbazepine, is a racemic mixture of 80% S-MHD (active) and 20% R-MHD (inactive)
- R, S-licarbazepine is also in clinical development as a novel mood stabilizer

- The active S enantiomer of licarbazepine is another related compound in development as yet another novel mood stabilizer
- ✱ Most significant risk of oxcarbazepine may be clinically significant hyponatremia (sodium level <125 m mol/L), most likely occurring within the first 3 months of treatment, and occurring in 2–3% of patients
- Unknown if this risk is higher than for carbamazepine
- ✱ Since SSRIs can sometimes also reduce sodium due to SIADH (syndrome of inappropriate antidiuretic hormone production), patients treated with combinations of oxcarbazepine and SSRIs should be carefully monitored, especially in the early stages of treatment
- By analogy with carbamazepine, could theoretically be useful in chronic neuropathic pain

Suggested Reading

Beydoun A. Safety and efficacy of oxcarbazepine: results of randomized, double-blind trials. Pharmacotherapy. 2000; 20(8 Pt 2):152S–158S.

Centorrino F, Albert MJ, Berry JM, Kelleher JP, Fellman V, Line G, Koukopoulos AE, Kidwell JE, Fogarty KV, Baldessarini RJ. Oxcarbazepine: clinical experience with hospitalized psychiatric patients. Bipolar Disord. 2003;5:370–4.

Dietrich DE, Kropp S, Emrich HM. Oxcarbazepine in affective and schizoaffective disorders. Pharmacopsychiatry. 2001;34:242–50.

Glauser TA. Oxcarbazepine in the treatment of epilepsy. Pharmacotherapy. 2001;21:904–19.

Hellewell JS. Oxcarbazepine (Trileptal) in the treatment of bipolar disorders: a review of efficacy and tolerability. J Affect Disord. 2002;72(Suppl 1):S23–34.

PAROXETINE

Brands • Paxil
• Paxil CR
see index for additional brand names

Generic? Yes (not for paroxetine CR)

 Class

- SSRI (selective serotonin reuptake inhibitor); often classified as an antidepressant, but it is not just an antidepressant

Commonly Prescribed For
(bold for FDA approved)

- **Major depressive disorder (paroxetine and paroxetine CR)**
- **Obsessive-compulsive disorder (OCD)**
- **Panic disorder (paroxetine and paroxetine CR)**
- **Social anxiety disorder (social phobia) (paroxetine and paroxetine CR)**
- **Posttraumatic stress disorder (PTSD)**
- **Generalized anxiety disorder (GAD)**
- **Premenstrual dysphoric disorder (PMDD) (paroxetine CR)**

 How The Drug Works

- Boosts neurotransmitter serotonin
- Blocks serotonin reuptake pump (serotonin transporter)
- Desensitizes serotonin receptors, especially serotonin 1A autoreceptors
- Presumably increases serotonergic neurotransmission
- Paroxetine also has mild anticholinergic actions
- Paroxetine may have mild norepinephrine reuptake blocking actions

How Long Until It Works

❋ Some patients may experience relief of insomnia or anxiety early after initiation of treatment
- Onset of therapeutic actions usually not immediate, but often delayed 2 to 4 weeks
- If it is not working within 6 to 8 weeks for depression, it may require a dosage increase or it may not work at all
- By contrast, for generalized anxiety, onset of response and increases in remission rates may still occur after 8 weeks of treatment and for up to 6 months after initiating dosing
- May continue to work for many years to prevent relapse of symptoms

If It Works

- The goal of treatment is complete remission of current symptoms as well as prevention of future relapses
- Treatment most often reduces or even eliminates symptoms, but not a cure since symptoms can recur after medicine stopped
- Continue treatment until all symptoms are gone (remission) or significantly reduced (e.g., OCD, PTSD)
- Once symptoms are gone, continue treating for 1 year for the first episode of depression
- For second and subsequent episodes of depression, treatment may need to be indefinite
- Use in anxiety disorders may also need to be indefinite

If It Doesn't Work

- Many patients only have a partial response where some symptoms are improved but others persist (especially insomnia, fatigue, and problems concentrating in depression)
- Other patients may be nonresponders, sometimes called treatment-resistant or treatment-refractory
- Some patients who have an initial response may relapse even though they continue treatment, sometimes called "poop-out"
- Consider increasing dose, switching to another agent or adding an appropriate augmenting agent
- Consider psychotherapy
- Consider evaluation for another diagnosis or for a comorbid condition (e.g., medical illness, substance abuse, etc.)
- Some patients may experience apparent lack of consistent efficacy due to activation of latent or underlying bipolar disorder, and require antidepressant discontinuation and a switch to a mood stabilizer

 Best Augmenting Combos for Partial Response or Treatment-Resistance

- Trazodone, especially for insomnia
- Bupropion, mirtazapine, reboxetine, or atomoxetine (add with caution and at lower

351

doses since paroxetine could theoretically raise atomoxetine levels); use combinations of antidepressants with caution as this may activate bipolar disorder and suicidal ideation
- Modafinil, especially for fatigue, sleepiness, and lack of concentration
- Mood stabilizers or atypical antipsychotics for bipolar depression, psychotic depression, treatment-resistant depression, or treatment-resistant anxiety disorders
- Benzodiazepines
- If all else fails for anxiety disorders, consider gabapentin or tiagabine
- Hypnotics for insomnia
- Classically, lithium, buspirone, or thyroid hormone

Tests
- None for healthy individuals

SIDE EFFECTS

How Drug Causes Side Effects
- Theoretically due to increases in serotonin concentrations at serotonin receptors in parts of the brain and body other than those that cause therapeutic actions (e.g., unwanted actions of serotonin in sleep centers causing insomnia, unwanted actions of serotonin in the gut causing diarrhea, etc.)
- Increasing serotonin can cause diminished dopamine release and might contribute to emotional flattening, cognitive slowing, and apathy in some patients
- Most side effects are immediate but often go away with time, in contrast to most therapeutic effects which are delayed and are enhanced over time
- ✳ Paroxetine's weak antimuscarinic properties can cause constipation, dry mouth, sedation

Notable Side Effects
- Sexual dysfunction (men: delayed ejaculation, erectile dysfunction; men and women: decreased sexual desire, anorgasmia)
- Gastrointestinal (decreased appetite, nausea, diarrhea, constipation, dry mouth)
- Mostly central nervous system (insomnia but also sedation, agitation, tremors, headache, dizziness)

- Note: patients with diagnosed or undiagnosed bipolar or psychotic disorders may be more vulnerable to CNS-activating actions of SSRIs
- Autonomic (sweating)
- Bruising and rare bleeding
- Rare hyponatremia (mostly in elderly patients and generally reversible on discontinuation of paroxetine)

 ### Life Threatening or Dangerous Side Effects
- Rare seizures
- Rare induction of mania and activation of suicidal ideation

Weight Gain

unusual · not unusual · common · problematic

- Occurs in significant minority

Sedation

unusual · not unusual · common · problematic

- Many experience and/or can be significant in amount
- Generally transient

What To Do About Side Effects
- Wait
- Wait
- Wait
- If paroxetine is sedating, take at night to reduce daytime drowsiness
- Reduce dose to 5–10 mg (12.5 mg for CR) until side effects abate, then increase as tolerated, usually to at least 20 mg (25 mg CR)
- In a few weeks, switch or add other drugs

Best Augmenting Agents for Side Effects
- Often best to try another SSRI or another antidepressant monotherapy prior to resorting to augmentation strategies to treat side effects
- Trazodone or a hypnotic for insomnia
- Bupropion, sildenafil, vardenafil, or tadalafil for sexual dysfunction
- Bupropion for emotional flattening, cognitive slowing, or apathy
- Mirtazapine for insomnia, agitation, and gastrointestinal side effects

- Benzodiazepines for jitteriness and anxiety, especially at initiation of treatment and especially for anxious patients
- Many side effects are dose-dependent (i.e., they increase as dose increases, or they reemerge until tolerance re-develops)
- Many side effects are time-dependent (i.e., they start immediately upon dosing and upon each dose increase, but go away with time)
- Activation and agitation may represent the induction of a bipolar state, especially a mixed dysphoric bipolar II condition sometimes associated with suicidal ideation, and require the addition of lithium, a mood stabilizer or an atypical antipsychotic, and/or discontinuation of paroxetine

DOSING AND USE

Usual Dosage Range
- Depression: 20–50 mg (25–62.5 mg CR)

Dosage Forms
- Tablets 10 mg scored, 20 mg scored, 30 mg, 40 mg
- Controlled release tablets 12.5 mg, 25 mg
- Liquid 10 mg/5mL – 250 mL bottle

How to Dose
- Depression: initial 20 mg (25 mg CR); usually wait a few weeks to assess drug effects before increasing dose, but can increase by 10 mg/day (12.5 mg/day CR) once a week; maximum generally 50 mg/day (62.5 mg/day CR); single dose
- Panic disorder: initial 10 mg/day (12.5 mg/day CR); usually wait a few weeks to assess drug effects before increasing dose, but can increase by 10 mg/day (12.5 mg/day CR) once a week; maximum generally 60 mg/day (75 mg/day CR); single dose
- Social anxiety disorder: initial 20 mg/day (25 mg/day CR); usually wait a few weeks to assess drug effects before increasing dose, but can increase by 10 mg/day (12.5 mg/day CR) once a week; maximum 60 mg/day (75 mg/day CR); single dose
- Other anxiety disorders: initial 20 mg/day (25 mg/day CR); usually wait a few weeks to assess drug effects before increasing dose, but can increase by 10 mg/day

(12.5 mg/day CR) once a week; maximum 60 mg/day (75 mg/day CR); single dose

 Dosing Tips

- 20 mg tablet is scored, so to save costs, give 10 mg as half of 20 mg tablet, since 10 mg and 20 mg tablets cost about the same in many markets
- Given once daily, often at bedtime, but any time of day tolerated
- 20 mg/day (25 mg/day CR) is often sufficient for patients with social anxiety disorder and depression
- Other anxiety disorders, as well as difficult cases in general, may require higher dosing
- Occasional patients are dosed above 60 mg/day (75 mg/day CR), but this is for experts and requires caution
- If intolerable anxiety, insomnia, agitation, akathisia, or activation occur either upon dosing initiation or discontinuation, consider the possibility of activated bipolar disorder and switch to a mood stabilizer or an atypical antipsychotic
- Liquid formulation easiest for doses below 10 mg when used for cases that are very intolerant to paroxetine or especially for very slow down-titration during discontinuation for patients with withdrawal symptoms
- Paroxetine CR tablets not scored, so chewing or cutting in half can destroy controlled release properties
- Unlike other SSRIs and antidepressants where dosage increments can be double and triple the starting dose, paroxetine's dosing increments are in 50% increments (i.e., 20, 30, 40; or 25, 37.5, 50 CR)
- Paroxetine inhibits its own metabolism and thus plasma concentrations can double when oral doses increase by 50%; plasma concentrations can increase 2–7 fold when oral doses are doubled
* Main advantage of CR is reduced side effects, especially nausea and perhaps sedation, sexual dysfunction, and withdrawal
* For patients with severe problems discontinuing paroxetine, dosing may need to be tapered over many months (i.e., reduce dose by 1% every 3 days by crushing tablet and suspending or

dissolving in 100 mL of fruit juice and then disposing of 1 mL while drinking the rest; 3–7 days later, dispose of 2 mL, and so on). This is both a form of very slow biological tapering and a form of behavioral desensitization
- For some patients with severe problems discontinuing paroxetine, it may be useful to add an SSRI with a long half-life, especially fluoxetine, prior to taper of paroxetine; while maintaining fluoxetine dosing, first slowly taper paroxetine and then taper fluoxetine
- Be sure to differentiate between re-emergence of symptoms requiring re-institution of treatment and withdrawal symptoms

Overdose
- Rarely lethal in monotherapy overdose; vomiting, sedation, heart rhythm disturbances, dilated pupils, dry mouth

Long-Term Use
- Safe

Habit Forming
- No

How to Stop
- Taper to avoid withdrawal effects (dizziness, nausea, stomach cramps, sweating, tingling, dysesthesias)
- Many patients tolerate 50% dose reduction for 3 days, then another 50% reduction for 3 days, then discontinuation
- If withdrawal symptoms emerge during discontinuation, raise dose to stop symptoms and then restart withdrawal much more slowly
- ✱ Withdrawal effects can be more common or more severe with paroxetine than with some other SSRIs
- Paroxetine's withdrawal effects may be related in part to the fact that it inhibits its own metabolism
- Thus, when paroxetine is withdrawn, the rate of its decline can be faster as it stops inhibiting its metabolism
- Controlled release paroxetine may slow the rate of decline and thus reduce withdrawal reactions in some patients
- Re-adaptation of cholinergic receptors after prolonged blockade may contribute to withdrawal effects of paroxetine

Pharmacokinetics
- Inactive metabolites
- Half-life approximately 24 hours
- Inhibits CYP450 2D6

 Drug Interactions
- Tramadol increases the risk of seizures in patients taking an antidepressant
- Can increase tricyclic antidepressant levels; use with caution with tricyclic antidepressants or when switching from a TCA to paroxetine
- Can cause a fatal "serotonin syndrome" when combined with MAO inhibitors, so do not use with MAO inhibitors or for at least 14 days after MAOIs are stopped
- Do not start an MAO inhibitor for at least 2 weeks after discontinuing paroxetine
- May displace highly protein bound drugs (e.g., warfarin)
- There are reports of elevated theophylline levels associated with paroxetine treatment, so it is recommended that theophylline levels be monitored when these drugs are administered together
- May increase anticholinergic effects of procyclidine and other drugs with anticholinergic properties
- Can rarely cause weakness, hyperreflexia, and incoordination when combined with sumatriptan or possibly with other triptans, requiring careful monitoring of patient
- Via CYP450 2D6 inhibition, paroxetine could theoretically interfere with the analgesic actions of codeine, and increase the plasma levels of some beta blockers and of atomoxetine
- Via CYP450 2D6 inhibition, paroxetine could theoretically increase concentrations of thioridazine and cause dangerous cardiac arrhythmias

 Other Warnings/ Precautions
- Add or initiate other antidepressants with caution for up to 2 weeks after discontinuing paroxetine
- Use with caution in patients with history of seizures
- Use with caution in patients with bipolar disorder unless treated with concomitant mood stabilizing agent

- Monitor patients for activation of suicidal ideation, especially children and adolescents

Do Not Use
- If patient is taking an MAO inhibitor
- If patient is taking thioridazine
- If there is a proven allergy to paroxetine

Renal Impairment
- Lower dose [initial 10 mg/day (12.5 mg CR), maximum 40 mg/day (50 mg/day CR)]

Hepatic Impairment
- Lower dose [initial 10 mg/day (12.5 mg CR), maximum 40 mg/day (50 mg/day CR)]

Cardiac Impairment
- Preliminary research suggests that paroxetine is safe in these patients
- Treating depression with SSRIs in patients with acute angina or following myocardial infarction may reduce cardiac events and improve survival as well as mood

Elderly
- Lower dose [initial 10 mg/day (12.5 mg CR), maximum 40 mg/day (50 mg/day CR)]

Children and Adolescents
- Use with caution, observing for activation of known or unknown bipolar disorder and/or suicidal ideation, and strongly consider informing parents or guardian of this risk so they can help observe child or adolescent patients
- Not specifically approved, but preliminary evidence suggests efficacy in children and adolescents with OCD, social phobia, or depression

Pregnancy
- Risk Category C [some animal studies show adverse effects, no controlled studies in humans]

- Not generally recommended for use during pregnancy, especially during first trimester
- Nonetheless, continuous treatment during pregnancy may be necessary and has not been proven to be harmful to the fetus
- Preliminary research has not shown birth defects in children whose mothers took paroxetine during pregnancy
- Paroxetine use late in pregnancy may be associated with higher risk of neonatal complications, including respiratory distress
- At delivery there may be more bleeding in the mother and transient irritability or sedation in the newborn
- Must weigh the risk of treatment (first trimester fetal development, third trimester newborn delivery) to the child against the risk of no treatment (recurrence of depression, maternal health, infant bonding) to the mother and child
- For many patients this may mean continuing treatment during pregnancy
- Neonates exposed to SSRIs or SNRIs late in the third trimester have developed complications requiring prolonged hospitalization, respiratory support, and tube feeding; reported symptoms are consistent with either a direct toxic effect of SSRIs and SNRIs or, possibly, a drug discontinuation syndrome, and include respiratory distress, cyanosis, apnea, seizures, temperature instability, feeding difficulty, vomiting, hypoglycemia, hypotonia, hypertonia, hyperreflexia, tremor, jitteriness, irritability, and constant crying

Breast Feeding
- Some drug is found in mother's breast milk
- Trace amounts may be present in nursing children whose mothers are on paroxetine
- If child becomes irritable or sedated, breast feeding or drug may need to be discontinued
- Immediate postpartum period is a high-risk time for depression, especially in women who have had prior depressive episodes, so drug may need to be reinstituted late in the third trimester or shortly after childbirth to prevent a recurrence during the postpartum period
- Must weigh benefits of breast feeding with risks and benefits of antidepressant

treatment versus non-treatment to both the infant and the mother
- For many patients, this may mean continuing treatment during breast feeding

THE ART OF PSYCHOPHARMACOLOGY

Potential Advantages
- Patients with anxiety disorders and insomnia
- Patients with mixed anxiety/depression

Potential Disadvantages
- Patients with hypersomnia
- Alzheimer/cognitive disorders
- Patients with psychomotor retardation, fatigue, and low energy

Primary Target Symptoms
- Depressed mood
- Anxiety
- Sleep disturbance, especially insomnia
- Panic attacks, avoidant behavior, re-experiencing, hyperarousal

 Pearls

✳ Often a preferred treatment of anxious depression as well as major depressive disorder comorbid with anxiety disorders
✳ Withdrawal effects may be more likely than for some other SSRIs when discontinued (especially akathisia, restlessness, gastrointestinal symptoms, dizziness, tingling, dysesthesias, nausea, stomach cramps, restlessness)

- Inhibits own metabolism, so dosing is not linear
✳ Paroxetine has mild anticholinergic actions that can enhance the rapid onset of anxiolytic and hypnotic efficacy but also cause mild anticholinergic side effects
- Can cause cognitive and affective "flattening"
- May be less activating than other SSRIs
- Paroxetine is a potent CYP450 2D6 inhibitor
- SSRIs may be less effective in women over 50, especially if they are not taking estrogen
- SSRIs may be useful for hot flushes in perimenopausal women
- Some anecdotal reports suggest greater weight gain and sexual dysfunction than some other SSRIs, but the clinical significance of this is unknown
- For sexual dysfunction, can augment with bupropion, sildenafil, tadalafil, or switch to a non-SSRI such as bupropion or mirtazapine
- Some postmenopausal women's depression will respond better to paroxetine plus estrogen augmentation than to paroxetine alone
- Nonresponse to paroxetine in elderly may require consideration of mild cognitive impairment or Alzheimer disease
- CR formulation may enhance tolerability, especially for nausea
- Can be better tolerated than some SSRIs for patients with anxiety and insomnia and can reduce these symptoms early in dosing

 Suggested Reading

Bourin M, Chue P, Guillon Y. Paroxetine: a review. CNS Drug Rev. 2001;7:25–47.

Edwards JG, Anderson I. Systematic review and guide to selection of selective serotonin reuptake inhibitors. Drugs. 1999;57:507–533.

Green B. Focus on paroxetine. Curr Med Res Opin. 2003;19:13–21.

Wagstaff AJ, Cheer SM, Matheson AJ, Ormrod D, Goa KL. Paroxetine: an update of its use in psychiatric disorders in adults. Drugs. 2002;62:655–703.

PEMOLINE

THERAPEUTICS

Brands • Cylert
see index for additional brand names

Generic? Yes

 Class
• Stimulant

Commonly Prescribed For
(bold for FDA approved)
• **Attention deficit hyperactivity disorder (ADHD) for patients who fail to respond to other treatments**

 How The Drug Works
• Unknown
• Theoretically enhances dopaminergic neurotransmission by an unknown mechanism
• Structurally unrelated to amphetamine or methylphenidate

How Long Until It Works
• First dose effects may not occur, as is common with other stimulants
• Substantial clinical benefits should occur within 3 weeks of dosage titration or the patient should be withdrawn from treatment

If It Works
✳ Monitor need for continued treatment
✳ Monitor liver function
• The goal of treatment of ADHD is reduction of symptoms of inattentiveness, motor hyperactivity, and/or impulsiveness that disrupt social, school, and/or occupational functioning
• Continue treatment until all symptoms are under control or improvement is stable and then continue treatment indefinitely as long as improvement persists
• Treatment begun in childhood may need to be continued into adolescence and adulthood if continued benefit is documented

If It Doesn't Work
✳ If no response is seen 3 weeks after dose titration, discontinue use and try another agent

 Best Augmenting Combos for Partial Response or Treatment-Resistance
• Best to attempt another monotherapy prior to augmenting
✳ Drug combinations with pemoline have not been systematically studied and this is best left to the expert if used at all

Tests
✳ At present, there is no way to predict who is likely to develop liver failure; however, only patients without liver disease and with normal baseline liver function tests should initiate pemoline therapy
✳ Liver function tests: Serum ALT (SGPT) levels taken at baseline and every 2 weeks
• If liver function tests increase to > twice baseline, discontinue treatment
• In children, monitor height and weight

SIDE EFFECTS

How Drug Causes Side Effects
• Unknown
• CNS side effects presumably due to excessive dopamine actions
• Mechanism of hepatic toxicity unknown

Notable Side Effects
✳ Insomnia
• Headache, exacerbation of tics, irritability, drowsiness, dizziness
• Anorexia, weight loss
• Rash
• Can temporarily slow normal growth in children (controversial)

 Life Threatening or Dangerous Side Effects
✳ Liver failure, hepatitis, jaundice
• Psychotic episodes
• Seizures
• Isolated reports of aplastic anemia
• Theoretically, could activate mania or suicidal ideation

Weight Gain

unusual · not unusual · common · problematic

• Reported but not expected

• Some patients may experience weight loss, which is generally regained in 3–6 months

Sedation

unusual   not unusual   common   problematic

• Occurs in significant minority
• Activation may also occur

What To Do About Side Effects

• Wait
• Adjust dose
• If side effects persist, discontinue use
• If signs of hepatic failure develop, discontinue use

Best Augmenting Agents for Side Effects

• Short-term use of hypnotics for insomnia
• Dose reduction or switching to another agent may be more effective since most side effects cannot be improved with an augmenting agent

DOSING AND USE

Usual Dosage Range

• 56.25–75 mg/day

Dosage Forms

• Tablet 18.75 mg scored, 37.5 mg scored, 37.5 mg scored chewable, 75 mg

How to Dose

• Initial 37.5 mg/day in morning; increase by 18.75 mg each week; maximum 112.5 mg/day

 Dosing Tips

✻ Has a relatively long half-life and sustained duration of clinical activity, so it only needs to be administered once daily in the morning and there are no sustained release formulations
• Chlorpromazine or atypical antipsychotics may treat the stimulant effects of pemoline overdose
• May wish to stop treatment intermittently to determine if behavioral symptoms return or if treatment is no longer necessary
• Administer in the morning to avoid insomnia

• Most side effects appear to be dose-dependent

Overdose

• Vomiting, agitation, tremor, hyperreflexia, twitching, convulsion, coma, euphoria, confusion, hallucination, sweating, headache, hyperpyrexia, tachycardia, hypertension, mydriasis

Long-Term Use

• Dependence and abuse less likely than with amphetamine or methylphenidate
• Long-term stimulant use may be associated with growth suppression in children (controversial)
✻ Must monitor serum ALT (SGPT) levels every 2 weeks for the duration of treatment
✻ Pemoline should be discontinued if serum ALT (SGPT) is increased to a clinically significant level, if any increase >2 times the upper limit of normal occurs, or if clinical signs and symptoms suggest liver failure
✻ If pemoline therapy is discontinued and then restarted, the liver testing should be done prior to reinitiating treatment and then every 2 weeks
• Periodic monitoring of weight and height may be prudent

Habit Forming

• Low abuse potential, Schedule IV
• Some patients may develop tolerance, but abuse and psychological dependence are rare

How to Stop

• Taper generally unnecessary and not recommended when discontinuing for hepatic toxicity
• Discontinuation symptoms uncommon

Pharmacokinetics

• Serum half-life approximately 12 hours
• Metabolized by the liver
• Excreted primarily by the kidneys

 Drug Interactions

✻ Drug interactions involving pemoline have not been evaluated in humans
• Due to risk of hepatic toxicity, concomitant therapy should generally be avoided whenever possible

**Other Warnings/
Precautions**

✴ May cause liver failure; patients should
be advised to be alert for signs of liver
dysfunction (jaundice, anorexia,
gastrointestinal distress, malaise, etc.) and
to report them immediately to their
physician

✴ Pemoline should be discontinued if
serum ALT (SGPT) increases to twice the
normal upper limit

• Children who are not growing or gaining
weight should stop treatment, at least
temporarily

• May worsen motor and phonic tics

• May worsen symptoms of thought disorder
and behavioral disturbance in psychotic
patients

• Use with caution in patients with history of
drug abuse

• Pemoline may be associated with growth
suppression

• May lower seizure threshold

• Emergence or worsening of activation and
agitation could theoretically represent the
induction of a bipolar state, especially a
mixed dysphoric bipolar II condition
sometimes associated with suicidal
ideation, and require the addition of a
mood stabilizer and/or discontinuation of
pemoline

Do Not Use

• If patient has hepatic impairment
• If patient has extreme anxiety or agitation
• If patient has Tourette's syndrome
• If there is a proven allergy to pemoline

SPECIAL POPULATIONS

Renal Impairment
• Use with caution

Hepatic Impairment
• Contraindicated

Cardiac Impairment
• Use with caution; less likely than other
stimulants to raise blood pressure

Elderly
• Use with caution; elderly patients are more
likely to have hepatic impairment

• Not extensively studied in elderly patients

 Children and Adolescents

• Safety and efficacy not established under
age 6

• Use in children should be reserved for the
expert

• Pemoline may worsen symptoms of
behavioral disturbance and thought
disorder in psychotic children

• Pemoline may affect growth (predicted
height, weight) in children with long-term
use (controversial); weight and height
should be monitored during long-term
treatment

 Pregnancy

• Risk Category B [animal studies do not
show adverse effects, no controlled studies
in humans]

• Use in women of childbearing potential
requires weighing potential benefits to the
mother against potential risks to the fetus

✴ For ADHD patients, pemoline should
generally be discontinued before
anticipated pregnancies

Breast Feeding

• Unknown if pemoline is secreted in human
breast milk, but all psychotropics assumed
to be secreted in breast milk

✴ Recommended either to discontinue drug
or bottle feed

THE ART OF PSYCHOPHARMACOLOGY

Potential Advantages
• Only for ADHD patients who respond to
this agent and not to other treatments of
ADHD

Potential Disadvantages
• Hepatic toxicity may not justify its use

Primary Target Symptoms
• Concentration, attention span
• Motor hyperactivity
• Impulsiveness

Pearls

* Rarely if ever appropriate for off-label uses
* Not used first-line because of the risk of hepatotoxicity
* Written informed consent from the patient is required before initiating treatment with pemoline
- Consent form available in manufacturer's package insert and published in the Physician's Desk Reference, Thompson PDR, Montvale, NJ. 58th edition, 2004 pp 419–420
- Although pharmacologic activity similar to other CNS stimulants, pemoline has minimal sympathomimetic effects
- Has a more gradual onset of action than some other stimulants
- Insomnia often occurs prior to the onset of therapeutic actions
- It is not clear if baseline and periodic liver function testing is predictive of active liver failure
- However, it is generally believed that early detection of drug-induced hepatic injury along with immediate withdrawal of the suspect drug enhances the likelihood for recovery
- Thus, liver function monitoring is a necessary component of pemoline therapy

Suggested Reading

Cyr M, Brown CS. Current drug therapy recommendations for the treatment of attention deficit hyperactivity disorder. Drugs. 1998; 56: 215–23.

Greenhill LL, Pliszka S, Dulcan MK, Bernet W, Arnold V, Beitchman J, Benson RS, Bukstein O, Kinlan J, McClellan J, Rue D, Shaw JA, Stock S. Practice parameter for the use of stimulant medications in the treatment of children, adolescents, and adults. J Am Acad Child Adolesc Psychiatry. 2002;41 (2 Suppl): 26S–49S.

Shevell M, Schreiber R. Pemoline-associated hepatic failure: a critical analysis of the literature. Pediatr Neurol. 1997; 16: 14–6.

Wender PH, Wolf LE, Wasserstein J. Adults with ADHD. An overview. Ann N Y Acad Sci. 2001; 931: 1–16.

PEROSPIRONE

Brands • Lullan
see index for additional brand names

Generic? No

Class
• Atypical antipsychotic (serotonin-dopamine antagonist, second generation antipsychotic)

Commonly Prescribed For
(bold for FDA approved)
• Schizophrenia (Japan)

How The Drug Works
• Blocks dopamine 2 receptors, reducing positive symptoms of psychosis
• Blocks serotonin 2A receptors, causing enhancement of dopamine release in certain brain regions and thus reducing motor side effects and possibly improving cognitive and affective symptoms
✱ Interactions at 5HT1A receptors may contribute to efficacy for cognitive and affective symptoms in some patients

How Long Until It Works
• Psychotic symptoms can improve within 1 week, but it may take several weeks for full effect on behavior as well as on cognition and affective stabilization
• Classically recommended to wait at least 4–6 weeks to determine efficacy of drug, but in practice some patients require up to 16–20 weeks to show a good response, especially on cognitive symptoms

If It Works
• Most often reduces positive symptoms in schizophrenia but does not eliminate them
• Can improve negative symptoms, as well as aggressive, cognitive, and affective symptoms in schizophrenia
• Most schizophrenic patients do not have a total remission of symptoms but rather a reduction of symptoms by about a third
• Perhaps 5–15% of schizophrenic patients can experience an overall improvement of greater than 50–60%, especially when receiving stable treatment for more than a year

• Such patients are considered super-responders or "awakeners" since they may be well enough to be employed, live independently, and sustain long-term relationships
• Continue treatment until reaching a plateau of improvement
• After reaching a satisfactory plateau, continue treatment for at least a year after first episode of psychosis
• For second and subsequent episodes of psychosis, treatment may need to be indefinite
• Even for first episodes of psychosis, it may be preferable to continue treatment

If It Doesn't Work
• Consider trying one of the first-line atypical antipsychotics (e.g. risperidone, olanzapine, quetiapine, aripiprazole)
• If 2 or more antipsychotic monotherapies do not work, consider clozapine
• If no first-line atypical antipsychotic is effective, consider higher doses or augmentation with valproate or lamotrigine
• Some patients may require treatment with a conventional antipsychotic
• Consider noncompliance and switch to another antipsychotic with fewer side effects or to an antipsychotic that can be given by depot injection
• Consider initiating rehabilitation and psychotherapy
• Consider presence of concomitant drug abuse

Best Augmenting Combos for Partial Response or Treatment-Resistance
• Augmentation of perospirone has not been systematically studied
• Addition of a benzodiazepine, especially short-term for agitation
• Addition of a mood stabilizing anticonvulsant such as valproate, carbamazepine, or lamotrigine may theoretically be helpful in both schizophrenia and bipolar mania
• Augmentation with lithium in bipolar mania may be helpful

Tests
✱ Potential of weight gain, diabetes, and dyslipidemia associated with perospirone has not been systematically studied, but

patients should be monitored the same as for other atypical antipsychotics

Before starting an atypical antipsychotic

✱ Weigh all patients and track BMI during treatment
- Get baseline personal and family history of obesity, dyslipidemia, hypertension, and cardiovascular disease
✱ Get waist circumference (at umbilicus), blood pressure, fasting plasma glucose, and fasting lipid profile
- Determine if patient is
  - overweight (BMI 25.0–29.9)
  - obese (BMI ≥30)
  - has pre-diabetes (fasting plasma glucose 100–125 mg/dl)
  - has diabetes (fasting plasma glucose >126 mg/dl)
  - has hypertension (BP >140/90 mm Hg)
  - has dyslipidemia (increased total cholesterol, LDL cholesterol, and triglycerides; decreased HDL cholesterol)
- Treat or refer such patients for treatment, including nutrition and weight management, physical activity counseling, smoking cessation, and medical management

Monitoring after starting an atypical antipsychotic

✱ BMI monthly for 3 months, then quarterly
✱ Blood pressure, fasting plasma glucose, fasting lipids within 3 months and then annually, but earlier and more frequently for patients with diabetes or who have gained >5% of initial weight
- Treat or refer for treatment and consider switching to another atypical antipsychotic for patients who become overweight, obese, pre-diabetic, diabetic, hypertensive, or dyslipidemic while receiving an atypical antipsychotic
✱ Even in patients without known diabetes, be vigilant for the rare but life threatening onset of diabetic ketoacidosis, which always requires immediate treatment, by monitoring for the rapid onset of polyuria, polydipsia, weight loss, nausea, vomiting, dehydration, rapid respiration, weakness and clouding of sensorium, even coma
- Should check blood pressure in the elderly before starting and for the first few weeks of treatment

SIDE EFFECTS

How Drug Causes Side Effects

- By blocking dopamine 2 receptors in the striatum, it can cause motor side effects
- By blocking dopamine 2 receptors in the pituitary, it can cause increased prolactin (unusual)
- Mechanism of weight gain and increased incidence of diabetes and dyslipidemia with some atypical antipsychotics is unknown
- Receptor binding portfolio of perospirone is not well-characterized

Notable Side Effects

✱ Extrapyramidal symptoms, akathisia
✱ Insomnia
- Sedation, anxiety, weakness, headache, anorexia, constipation
- Theoretically, tardive dyskinesia (should be reduced risk compared to conventional antipsychotics)
- Elevated creatine phosphokinase levels

 Life Threatening or Dangerous Side Effects
- Rare neuroleptic malignant syndrome
- Theoretically, seizures are rarely associated with atypical antipsychotics

Weight Gain

✱ Not well characterized

Sedation

unusual — not unusual — common — problematic

- Occurs in significant minority

What To Do About Side Effects

- Wait
- Wait
- Wait
- For motor symptoms, add an anticholinergic agent
- Reduce the dose
- Switch to another atypical antipsychotic

Best Augmenting Agents for Side Effects

- Benztropine or trihexyphenidyl for motor side effects
- Sometimes amantadine can be helpful for motor side effects

- Benzodiazepines may be helpful for akathisia
- Many side effects cannot be improved with an augmenting agent

DOSING AND USE

Usual Dosage Range
- 8–48 mg/day in 3 divided doses

Dosage Forms
- Tablet 4 mg, 8 mg

How to Dose
- Begin at 4 mg 3 times a day, increasing as tolerated up to 16 mg 3 times a day

 Dosing Tips
- Some patients have been treated with up to 96 mg/day in 3 divided doses
- Unknown whether dosing frequency can be reduced to once or twice daily, but by analogy with other agents in this class with half-lives shorter than 24 hours, this may be possible

Overdose
- Not reported

Long-Term Use
- Long-term studies not reported, but as for other atypical antipsychotics, long-term use for treatment of schizophrenia is common

Habit Forming
- No

How to Stop
- Slow down-titration (over 6 to 8 weeks), especially when simultaneously beginning a new antipsychotic while switching (i.e., cross-titration)
- Rapid discontinuation may lead to rebound psychosis and worsening of symptoms
- If antiparkinson agents are being used, they should be continued for a few weeks after perospirone is discontinued

Pharmacokinetics
- Metabolized primarily by CYP450 3A4
- No active metabolites

 Drug Interactions
- Ketaconazole and possibly other CYP450 3A4 inhibitors such as nefazodone, fluvoxamine, and fluoxetine may increase plasma levels of perospirone
- Carbamazepine and possibly other inducers of CYP450 3A4 may decrease plasma levels of perospirone

 Other Warnings/ Precautions
- Not reported

Do Not Use
- If there is a proven allergy to perospirone

SPECIAL POPULATIONS

Renal Impairment
- Use with caution

Hepatic Impairment
- Use with caution

Cardiac Impairment
- Use with caution

Elderly
- Some patients may tolerate lower doses better

 Children and Adolescents
- Use with caution

 Pregnancy
- Psychotic symptoms may worsen during pregnancy and some form of treatment may be necessary

Breast Feeding
- Unknown if perospirone is secreted in human breast milk, but all psychotropics assumed to be secreted in breast milk
- ✳ Recommended either to discontinue drug or bottle feed
- Infants of women who choose to breast feed should be monitored for possible adverse effects

THE ART OF PSYCHOPHARMACOLOGY

Potential Advantages
- In Japan, studies suggest efficacy for negative symptoms of schizophrenia

Potential Disadvantages
- Patients who have difficulty complying with three times daily administration

Primary Target Symptoms
- Positive symptoms of psychosis
- Negative symptoms of psychosis
- Affective symptoms (depression, anxiety)
- Cognitive symptoms

 Pearls
- Extrapyramidal symptoms may be more frequent than with some other atypical antipsychotics
- Potent 5HT1A binding properties may be helpful for improving cognitive symptoms of schizophrenia in long-term treatment
- Theoretically, should be effective in acute bipolar mania

 Suggested Reading

Ohno Y. Pharmacological characteristics of perospirone hydrochloride, a novel antipsychotic agent. Nippon Yakurigaku Zasshi 2000; 116 (4): 225–31.

PERPHENAZINE

THERAPEUTICS

Brands • Trilafon
see index for additional brand names

Generic? Yes

Class

- Conventional antipsychotic (neuroleptic, phenothiazine, dopamine 2 antagonist, antiemetic)

Commonly Prescribed For
(bold for FDA approved)

- **Schizophrenia**
- **Nausea, vomiting**
- Other psychotic disorders
- Bipolar disorder

How The Drug Works

- Blocks dopamine 2 receptors, reducing positive symptoms of psychosis
- Combination of dopamine D2, histamine H1, and cholinergic M1 blockade in the vomiting center may reduce nausea and vomiting

How Long Until It Works

- Psychotic symptoms can improve within 1 week, but may take several weeks for full effect on behavior
- Injection: initial effect after 10 minutes, peak after 1–2 hours
- Actions on nausea and vomiting are immediate

If It Works

- Most often reduces positive symptoms in schizophrenia but does not eliminate them
- Most schizophrenic patients do not have a total remission of symptoms but rather a reduction of symptoms by about a third
- Continue treatment in schizophrenia until reaching a plateau of improvement
- After reaching a satisfactory plateau, continue treatment for at least a year after first episode of psychosis in schizophrenia
- For second and subsequent episodes of psychosis in schizophrenia, treatment may need to be indefinite
- Reduces symptoms of acute psychotic mania but not proven as a mood stabilizer

or as an effective maintenance treatment in bipolar disorder
- After reducing acute psychotic symptoms in mania, switch to a mood stabilizer and/or an atypical antipsychotic for mood stabilization and maintenance

If It Doesn't Work

- Consider trying one of the first-line atypical antipsychotics (risperidone, olanzapine, quetiapine, ziprasidone, aripiprazole, amisulpride)
- Consider trying another conventional antipsychotic
- If 2 or more antipsychotic monotherapies do not work, consider clozapine

 ### Best Augmenting Combos for Partial Response or Treatment-Resistance

- Augmentation of conventional antipsychotics has not been systematically studied
- Addition of a mood stabilizing anticonvulsant such as valproate, carbamazepine, or lamotrigine may be helpful in both schizophrenia and bipolar mania
- Augmentation with lithium in bipolar mania may be helpful
- Addition of a benzodiazepine, especially short-term for agitation

Tests

- ✻ Since conventional antipsychotics are frequently associated with weight gain, before starting treatment, weigh all patients and determine if the patient is already overweight (BMI 25.0–29.9) or obese (BMI ≥30)
- Before giving a drug that can cause weight gain to an overweight or obese patient, consider determining whether the patient already has pre-diabetes (fasting plasma glucose 100–125 mg/dl), diabetes (fasting plasma glucose >126 mg/dl), or dyslipidemia (increased total cholesterol, LDL cholesterol and triglycerides; decreased HDL cholesterol), and treat or refer such patients for treatment, including nutrition and weight management, physical activity counseling, smoking cessation, and medical management
- ✻ Monitor weight and BMI during treatment

* While giving a drug to a patient who has gained >5% of initial weight, consider evaluating for the presence of pre-diabetes, diabetes, or dyslipidemia, or consider switching to a different antipsychotic
• Should check blood pressure in the elderly before starting and for the first few weeks of treatment
• Monitoring elevated prolactin levels of dubious clinical benefit
• Phenothiazines may cause false-positive phenylketonuria results

SIDE EFFECTS

How Drug Causes Side Effects
• By blocking dopamine 2 receptors in the striatum, it can cause motor side effects
• By blocking dopamine 2 receptors in the pituitary, it can cause elevations in prolactin
• By blocking dopamine 2 receptors excessively in the mesocortical and mesolimbic dopamine pathways, especially at high doses, it can cause worsening of negative and cognitive symptoms (neuroleptic-induced deficit syndrome)
• Anticholinergic actions may cause sedation, blurred vision, constipation, dry mouth
• Antihistaminic actions may cause sedation, weight gain
• By blocking alpha 1 adrenergic receptors, it can cause dizziness, sedation, and hypotension
• Mechanism of weight gain and any possible increased incidence of diabetes or dyslipidemia with conventional antipsychotics is unknown

Notable Side Effects
* Neuroleptic-induced deficit syndrome
* Akathisia
* Extrapyramidal symptoms, Parkinsonism, tardive dyskinesia
* Galactorrhea, amenorrhea
• Dizziness, sedation
• Dry mouth, constipation, urinary retention, blurred vision
• Decreased sweating
• Sexual dysfunction
• Hypotension, tachycardia, syncope
• Weight gain

 ### Life Threatening or Dangerous Side Effects
• Rare neuroleptic malignant syndrome
• Rare jaundice, agranulocytosis
• Rare seizures

Weight Gain

unusual   not unusual   common   problematic

• Many experience and/or can be significant in amount

Sedation

unusual   not unusual   common   problematic

• Many experience and/or can be significant in amount
• Sedation is usually transient

What To Do About Side Effects
• Wait
• Wait
• Wait
• For motor symptoms, add an anticholinergic agent
• Reduce the dose
• For sedation, give at night
• Switch to an atypical antipsychotic
• Weight loss, exercise programs, and medical management for high BMIs, diabetes, dyslipidemia

Best Augmenting Agents for Side Effects
• Benztropine or trihexyphenidyl for motor side effects
• Sometimes amantadine can be helpful for motor side effects
• Benzodiazepines may be helpful for akathisia
• Many side effects cannot be improved with an augmenting agent

DOSING AND USE

Usual Dosage Range
• Psychosis: oral: 12–24 mg/day; 16–64 mg/day in hospitalized patients
• Nausea/vomiting: 8–16 mg/day oral, 5 mg intramuscularly

Dosage Forms
- Tablet 2 mg, 4 mg, 8 mg, 16 mg
- Injection 5 mg/mL

How to Dose
- Oral: Psychosis: 4–8 mg 3 times a day; 8–16 mg 2 times a day to 4 times a day in hospitalized patients; maximum 64 mg/day
- Oral: Nausea/vomiting: 8–16 mg/day in divided doses; maximum 24 mg/day
- Intramuscular: Psychosis: initial 5 mg; can repeat every 6 hours, maximum 15 mg/day (30 mg/day in hospitalized patients)

 Dosing Tips
- Injection contains sulfites that may cause allergic reactions, particularly in patients with asthma
- Oral perphenazine is less potent than the injection, so patients should receive equal or higher dosage when switched from injection to tablet

Overdose
- Extrapyramidal symptoms, coma, hypotension, sedation, seizures, respiratory depression

Long-Term Use
- Some side effects may be irreversible (e.g., tardive dyskinesia)

Habit Forming
- No

How to Stop
- Slow down-titration of oral formulation (over 6 to 8 weeks), especially when simultaneously beginning a new antipsychotic while switching (i.e., cross-titration)
- Rapid oral discontinuation may lead to rebound psychosis and worsening of symptoms
- If antiparkinson agents are being used, they should be continued for a few weeks after perphenazine is discontinued

Pharmacokinetics
- Half-life approximately 9.5 hours

 Drug Interactions
- May decrease the effects of levodopa, dopamine agonists
- May increase the effects of antihypertensive drugs except for guanethidine, whose antihypertensive actions perphenazine may antagonize
- Additive effects may occur if used with CNS depressants
- Anticholinergic effects may occur if used with atropine or related compounds
- Some patients taking a neuroleptic and lithium have developed an encephalopathic syndrome similar to neuroleptic malignant syndrome
- Epinephrine may lower blood pressure; diuretics and alcohol may increase risk of hypotension

 Other Warnings/ Precautions
- If signs of neruoleptic malignant syndrome develop, treatment should be immediately discontinued
- Use cautiously in patients with respiratory disorders
- Use cautiously in patients with alcohol withdrawal or convulsive disorders because of possible lowering of seizure threshold
- Do not use epinephrine in event of overdose as interaction with some pressor agents may lower blood pressure
- Avoid undue exposure to sunlight
- Avoid extreme heat exposure
- Use with caution in patients with respiratory disorders, glaucoma or urinary retention
- Antiemetic effect of perphenazine may mask signs of other disorders or overdose; suppression of cough reflex may cause asphyxia
- Observe for signs of ocular toxicity (corneal and lenticular deposits)
- Use only with caution if at all in Parkinson's disease or Lewy Body dementia

Do Not Use
- If patient is in a comatose state or has CNS depression

- If there is the presence of blood dyscrasias, subcortical brain damage, bone marrow depression, or liver disease
- If there is a proven allergy to perphenazine
- If there is a known sensitivity to any phenothiazine

Breast Feeding

- Unknown if perphenazine is secreted in human breast milk, but all psychotropics assumed to be secreted in breast milk
- ✱ Recommended either to discontinue drug or bottle feed

SPECIAL POPULATIONS

Renal Impairment

- Use with caution

Hepatic Impairment

- Use with caution; may not be recommended as long-term treatment because perphenazine may increase risk of further liver damage

Cardiac Impairment

- Cardiovascular toxicity can occur, especially orthostatic hypotension

Elderly

- Lower doses should be used and patient should be monitored closely

Children and Adolescents

- Not recommended for use under age 12
- Over age 12: if given intramuscularly, should receive lowest adult dose
- Generally consider second-line after atypical antipsychotics

Pregnancy

- Risk Category C [some animal studies show adverse effects, no controlled studies in humans]
- Reports of extrapyramidal symptoms, jaundice, hyperreflexia, hyporeflexia in infants whose mothers took a phenothiazine during pregnancy
- Perphenazine should only be used during pregnancy if clearly needed
- Psychotic symptoms may worsen during pregnancy and some form of treatment may be necessary
- Atypical antipsychotics may be preferable to conventional antipsychotics or anticonvulsant mood stabilizers if treatment is required during pregnancy

THE ART OF PSYCHOPHARMACOLOGY

Potential Advantages

- Intramuscular formulation for emergency use

Potential Disadvantages

- Patients with tardive dyskinesia
- Children
- Elderly

Primary Target Symptoms

- Positive symptoms of psychosis
- Motor and autonomic hyperactivity
- Violent or aggressive behavior

Pearls

- Perphenazine is a higher potency phenothiazine
- Less risk of sedation and orthostatic hypotension but greater risk of extrapyramidal symptoms than with low potency phenothiazines
- Conventional antipsychotics are much less expensive than atypical antipsychotics
- Patients have very similar antipsychotic responses to any conventional antipsychotic, which is different from atypical antipsychotics where antipsychotic responses of individual patients can occasionally vary greatly from one atypical antipsychotic to another
- Patients with inadequate responses to atypical antipsychotics may benefit from a trial of augmentation with a conventional antipsychotic such as perphenazine or from switching to a conventional antipsychotic such as perphenazine
- However, long-term polypharmacy with a combination of a conventional antipsychotic such as perphenazine with an atypical antipsychotic may combine their side effects without clearly augmenting the efficacy of either

- Although a frequent practice by some prescribers, adding 2 conventional antipsychotics together has little rationale and may reduce tolerability without clearly enhancing efficacy
- Availability of alternative treatments and risk of tardive dyskinesia make utilization of perphenazine for nausea and vomiting a short-term and second-line treatment option

Suggested Reading

Dencker SJ, Gios I, Martensson E, Norden T, Nyberg G, Persson R, Roman G, Stockman O, Syard KO. A long-term cross-over pharmacokinetic study comparing perphenazine decanoate and haloperidol decanoate in schizophrenic patients. Psychopharmacology (Berl) 1994; 114: 24–30.

Frankenburg FR. Choices in antipsychotic therapy in schizophrenia. Harv Rev Psychiatry 1999; 6: 241–9.

Quraishi S, David A. Depot perphenazine decanoate and enanthate for schizophrenia. Cochrane Database Syst Rev 2000; (2): CD001717.

PHENELZINE

THERAPEUTICS

Brands • Nardil
• Nardelzine
see index for additional brand names

Generic? Yes

Class
• Monoamine oxidase inhibitor (MAOI)

Commonly Prescribed For
(bold for FDA approved)
• **Depressed patients characterized as "atypical", "nonendogenous", or "neurotic"**
• Treatment-resistant depression
• Treatment-resistant panic disorder
• Treatment-resistant social anxiety disorder

How The Drug Works
• Irreversibly blocks monoamine oxidase (MAO) from breaking down norepinephrine, serotonin, and dopamine
• This presumably boosts noradrenergic, serotonergic, and dopaminergic neurotransmission

How Long Until It Works
• Onset of therapeutic actions usually not immediate, but often delayed 2 to 4 weeks
• If it is not working within 6 to 8 weeks, it may require a dosage increase or it may not work at all
• May continue to work for many years to prevent relapse of symptoms

If It Works
• The goal of treatment is complete remission of current symptoms as well as prevention of future relapses
• Treatment most often reduces or even eliminates symptoms, but not a cure since symptoms can recur after medicine stopped
• Continue treatment until all symptoms are gone (remission)
• Once symptoms gone, continue treating for 1 year for the first episode of depression
• For second and subsequent episodes of depression, treatment may need to be indefinite

• Use in anxiety disorders may also need to be indefinite

If It Doesn't Work
• Many patients only have a partial response where some symptoms are improved but others persist (especially insomnia, fatigue, and problems concentrating)
• Other patients may be nonresponders, sometimes called treatment-resistant or treatment-refractory
• Some patients who have an initial response may relapse even though they continue treatment, sometimes called "poop-out"
• Consider increasing dose, switching to another agent, or adding an appropriate augmenting agent
• Consider psychotherapy
• Consider evaluation for another diagnosis or for a comorbid condition (e.g., medical illness, substance abuse, etc.)
• Some patients may experience apparent lack of consistent efficacy due to activation of latent or underlying bipolar disorder, and require antidepressant discontinuation and a switch to a mood stabilizer

Best Augmenting Combos for Partial Response or Treatment-Resistance
✳ Augmentation of MAOIs has not been systematically studied, and this is something for the expert, to be done with caution and with careful monitoring
✳ A stimulant such as d-amphetamine or methylphenidate (with caution; may activate bipolar disorder and suicidal ideation; may elevate blood pressure)
• Lithium
• Mood stabilizing anticonvulsants
• Atypical antipsychotics (with special caution for those agents with monoamine reuptake blocking properties, such as ziprasidone and zotepine)

Tests
• Patients should be monitored for changes in blood pressure
• Patients receiving high doses or long-term treatment should have hepatic function evaluated periodically
✳ Since MAO inhibitors are frequently associated with weight gain, before starting treatment, weigh all patients and determine

if the patient is already overweight (BMI 25.0–29.9) or obese (BMI ≥30)
• Before giving a drug that can cause weight gain to an overweight or obese patient, consider determining whether the patient already has pre-diabetes (fasting plasma glucose 100–125 mg/dl), diabetes (fasting plasma glucose >126 mg/dl), or dyslipidemia (increased total cholesterol, LDL cholesterol and triglycerides; decreased HDL cholesterol), and treat or refer such patients for treatment, including nutrition and weight management, physical activity counseling, smoking cessation, and medical management
✳ Monitor weight and BMI during treatment
✳ While giving a drug to a patient who has gained >5% of initial weight, consider evaluating for the presence of pre-diabetes, diabetes, or dyslipidemia, or consider switching to a different antidepressant

SIDE EFFECTS

How Drug Causes Side Effects
• Theoretically due to increases in monoamines in parts of the brain and body and at receptors other than those that cause therapeutic actions (e.g., unwanted actions of serotonin in sleep centers causing insomnia, unwanted actions of norepinephrine on vascular smooth muscle causing changes in blood pressure, etc.)
• Side effects are generally immediate, but immediate side effects often disappear in time

Notable Side Effects
• Dizziness, sedation, headache, sleep disturbances, fatigue, weakness, tremor, movement problems, blurred vision, increased sweating
• Constipation, dry mouth, nausea, change in appetite, weight gain
• Sexual dysfunction
• Orthostatic hypotension (dose-related); syncope may develop at high doses

 Life Threatening or Dangerous Side Effects
• Hypertensive crisis (especially when MAOIs are used with certain tyramine-containing foods or prohibited drugs)

• Induction of mania and activation of suicidal ideation
• Seizures
• Hepatotoxicity

Weight Gain

• Many experience and/or can be significant in amount

Sedation

• Many experience and/or can be significant in amount
• Can also cause activation

What To Do About Side Effects
• Wait
• Wait
• Wait
• Lower the dose
• Take at night if daytime sedation
• Switch after appropriate washout to an SSRI or newer antidepressant

Best Augmenting Agents for Side Effects
• Trazodone (with caution) for insomnia
• Benzodiazepines for insomnia
✳ Single oral or sublingual dose of a calcium channel blocker (e.g., nifedipine) for urgent treatment of hypertension due to drug interaction or dietary tyramine
• Many side effects cannot be improved with an augmenting agent

DOSING AND USE

Usual Dosage Range
• 45–75 mg/day

Dosage Forms
• Tablet 15 mg

How to Dose
• Initial 45 mg/day in 3 divided doses; increase to 60–90 mg/day; after desired therapeutic effect is achieved lower dose as far as possible

Dosing Tips

- Once dosing is stabilized, some patients may tolerate once or twice daily dosing rather than 3-times-a-day dosing
- Orthostatic hypotension, especially at high doses, may require splitting into 4 daily doses
- Patients receiving high doses may need to be evaluated periodically for effects on the liver
- Little evidence to support efficacy of phenelzine below doses of 45 mg/day

Overdose

- Death may occur; dizziness, ataxia, sedation, headache, insomnia, restlessness, anxiety, irritability, cardiovascular effects, confusion, respiratory depression, coma

Long-Term Use

- May require periodic evaluation of hepatic function
- MAOIs may lose efficacy long-term

Habit Forming

- Some patients have developed dependence to MAOIs

How to Stop

- Generally no need to taper, as the drug wears off slowly over 2–3 weeks

Pharmacokinetics

- Clinical duration of action may be up to 21 days due to irreversible enzyme inhibition

Drug Interactions

- Tramadol may increase the risk of seizures in patients taking an MAO inhibitor
- Can cause a fatal "serotonin syndrome" when combined with drugs that block serotonin reuptake (e.g., SSRIs, SNRIs, sibutramine, tramadol, etc.), so do not use with a serotonin reuptake inhibitor or for up to 5 weeks after stopping the serotonin reuptake inhibitor
- Hypertensive crisis with headache, intracranial bleeding, and death may result from combining MAO inhibitors with sympathomimetic drugs (e.g., amphetamines, methylphenidate, cocaine, dopamine, epinephrine, norepinephrine, and related compounds methyldopa, levodopa, L-tryptophan, L-tyrosine, and phenylalanine)
- Excitation, seizures, delirium, hyperpyrexia, circulatory collapse, coma, and death may result from combining MAO inhibitors with mepiridine or dextromethorphan
- Do not combine with another MAO inhibitor, alcohol, buspirone, bupropion, or guanethidine
- Adverse drug reactions can result from combining MAO inhibitors with tricyclic/tetracyclic antidepressants and related compounds, including carbamazepine, cyclobenzaprine, and mirtazapine, and should be avoided except by experts to treat difficult cases
- MAO inhibitors in combination with spinal anesthesia may cause combined hypotensive effects
- Combination of MAOIs and CNS depressants may enhance sedation and hypotension

Other Warnings/ Precautions

- Use requires low tyramine diet
- Patients taking MAO inhibitors should avoid high protein food that has undergone protein breakdown by aging, fermentation, pickling, smoking, or bacterial contamination
- Patients taking MAO inhibitors should avoid cheeses (especially aged varieties), pickled herring, beer, wine, liver, yeast extract, dry sausage, hard salami, pepperoni, Lebanon bologna, pods of broad beans (fava beans), yogurt, and excessive use of caffeine and chocolate
- Patient and prescriber must be vigilant to potential interactions with any drug, including antihypertensives and over-the-counter cough/cold preparations
- Over-the-counter medications to avoid include cough and cold preparations, including those containing dextromethorphan, nasal decongestants (tablets, drops, or spray), hay-fever medications, sinus medications, asthma inhalant medications, anti-appetite medications, weight reducing preparations, "pep" pills

- Hypoglycemia may occur in diabetic patients receiving insulin or oral antidiabetic agents
- Use cautiously in patients receiving reserpine, anesthetics, disulfiram, metrizamide, anticholinergic agents
- Phenelzine is not recommended for use in patients who cannot be monitored closely
- Monitor patients for activation of suicidal ideation, especially children and adolescents

Do Not Use

- If patient is taking meperidine (pethidine)
- If patient is taking a sympathomimetic agent or taking guanethidine
- If patient is taking another MAOI
- If patient is taking any agent that can inhibit serotonin reuptake (e.g., SSRIs, sibutramine, tramadol, milnacipran, duloxetine, venlafaxine, clomipramine, etc.)
- If patient is taking diuretics, dextromethorphan, buspirone, bupropion
- If patient has pheochromocytoma
- If patient has cardiovascular or cerebrovascular disease
- If patient has frequent or severe headaches
- If patient is undergoing elective surgery and requires general anesthesia
- If patient has a history of liver disease or abnormal liver function tests
- If patient is taking a prohibited drug
- If patient is not compliant with a low-tyramine diet
- If there is a proven allergy to phenelzine

SPECIAL POPULATIONS

Renal Impairment

- Use with caution – drug may accumulate in plasma
- May require lower than usual adult dose

Hepatic Impairment

- Phenelzine should not be used

Cardiac Impairment

- Contraindicated in patients with congestive heart failure or hypertension
- Any other cardiac impairment may require lower than usual adult dose
- Patients with angina pectoris or coronary artery disease should limit their exertion

Elderly

- Initial dose 7.5 mg/day; increase every few days by 7.5–15 mg/day
- Elderly patients may have greater sensitivity to adverse effects

 Children and Adolescents

- Not recommended for use under age 16
- Use with caution, observing for activation of known or unknown bipolar disorder and/or suicidal ideation, and strongly consider informing parents or guardian of this risk so they can help observe child or adolescent patients

Pregnancy

- Risk Category C [some animal studies show adverse effects, no controlled studies in humans]
- Not generally recommended for use during pregnancy, especially during first trimester
- Possible increased incidence of fetal malformations if phenelzine is taken during the first trimester
- Should evaluate patient for treatment with an antidepressant with a better risk/benefit ratio

Breast Feeding

- Some drug is found in mother's breast milk
- If child becomes irritable or sedated, breast feeding or drug may need to be discontinued
- Immediate postpartum period is a high-risk time for depression, especially in women who have had prior depressive episodes, so drug may need to be reinstituted late in the third trimester or shortly after childbirth to prevent a recurrence during the postpartum period
- Should evaluate patient for treatment with an antidepressant with a better risk/benefit ratio

THE ART OF PSYCHOPHARMACOLOGY

Potential Advantages

- Atypical depression
- Severe depression
- Treatment-resistant depression or anxiety disorders

Potential Disadvantages

- Requires compliance to dietary restrictions, concomitant drug restrictions
- Patients with cardiac problems or hypertension
- Multiple daily doses

Primary Target Symptoms

- Depressed mood
- Somatic symptoms
- Sleep and eating disturbances
- Psychomotor retardation
- Morbid preoccupation

 Pearls

- MAOIs are generally reserved for second-line use after SSRIs, SNRIs, and combinations of newer antidepressants have failed
- Patient should be advised not to take any prescription or over-the-counter drugs without consulting their doctor because of possible drug interactions with the MAOI
- Headache is often the first symptom of hypertensive crisis
- Foods generally to avoid as they are usually high in tyramine content: dry sausage, pickled herring, liver, broad bean pods, sauerkraut, cheese, yogurt, alcoholic beverages, nonalcoholic beer and wine, chocolate, caffeine, meat and fish
- The rigid dietary restrictions may reduce compliance
- Mood disorders can be associated with eating disorders (especially in adolescent females), and phenelzine can be used to treat both depression and bulimia
- MAOIs are a viable second-line treatment option in depression, but are not frequently used
- ✳ Myths about the danger of dietary tyramine can be exaggerated, but prohibitions against concomitant drugs often not followed closely enough
- Orthostatic hypotension, insomnia, and sexual dysfunction are often the most troublesome common side effects
- ✳ MAOIs should be for the expert, especially if combining with agents of potential risk (e.g., stimulants, trazodone, TCAs)
- ✳ MAOIs should not be neglected as therapeutic agents for the treatment-resistant
- Although generally prohibited, a heroic but potentially dangerous treatment for severely treatment-resistant patients is for an expert to give a tricyclic/tetracyclic antidepressant other than clomipramine simultaneously with an MAO inhibitor for patients who fail to respond to numerous other antidepressants
- Use of MAOIs with clomipramine is always prohibited because of the risk of serotonin syndrome and death
- Amoxapine may be the preferred trycyclic/tetracyclic antidepressant to combine with an MAOI in heroic cases due to its theoretically protective 5HT2A antagonist properties
- If this option is elected, start the MAOI with the tricyclic/tetracyclic antidepressant simultaneously at low doses after appropriate drug washout, then alternately increase doses of these agents every few days to a week as tolerated
- Although very strict dietary and concomitant drug restrictions must be observed to prevent hypertensive crises and serotonin syndrome, the most common side effects of MAOI and tricyclic/tetracyclic combinations may be weight gain and orthostatic hypotension

 Suggested Reading

Kennedy SH. Continuation and maintenance treatments in major depression: the neglected role of monoamine oxidase inhibitors. J Psychiatry Neurosci 1997;22:127–31.

Lippman SB, Nash K. Monoamine oxidase inhibitor update. Potential adverse food and drug interactions. Drug Saf 1990;5:195–204.

Parsons B, Quitkin FM, McGrath PJ, Stewart JW, Tricamo E, Ocepek-Welikson K, Harrison W, Rabkin JG, Wager SG, Nunes E. Phenelzine, imipramine, and placebo in borderline patients meeting criteria for atypical depression. Psychopharmacol Bull 1989; 25:524–34.

PIMOZIDE

THERAPEUTICS

Brands • Orap
see index for additional brand names

Generic? Not in U.S.

Class
• Tourette's syndrome/tic suppressant; conventional antipsychotic (neuroleptic, dopamine 2 antagonist)

Commonly Prescribed For
(bold for FDA approved)
• **Suppression of motor and phonic tics in patients with Tourette Disorder who have failed to respond satisfactorily to standard treatment**
• Psychotic disorders in patients who have failed to respond satisfactorily to standard treatment

How The Drug Works
• Blocks dopamine 2 receptors in the nigrostriatal dopamine pathway, reducing tics in Tourette's syndrome
• When used for psychosis, can block dopamine 2 receptors in the mesolimbic dopamine pathway, reducing positive symptoms of psychosis

How Long Until It Works
• Relief from tics may occur more rapidly than antipsychotic actions
• Psychotic symptoms can improve within 1 week, but it may take several weeks for full effect on behavior

If It Works
✻ Is a second-line treatment option for Tourette's syndrome
✻ Is a secondary or tertiary treatment option for psychosis or other behavioral disorders
• Should evaluate for switching to an antipsychotic with a better/risk benefit ratio

If It Doesn't Work
• Consider trying one of the first-line atypical antipsychotics (risperidone, olanzapine, quetiapine, ziprasidone, aripiprazole, amisulpride)

• Consider trying another conventional antipsychotic
• If 2 or more antipsychotic monotherapies do not work, consider clozapine

Best Augmenting Combos for Partial Response or Treatment-Resistance
✻ Augmentation of pimozide has not been systematically studied and can be dangerous, especially with drugs that can either prolong QTc interval or raise pimozide plasma levels

Tests
✻ Baseline ECG and serum potassium levels should be determined
✻ Periodic evaluation of ECG and serum potassium levels, especially during dose titration
• Serum magnesium levels may also need to be monitored
✻ Since conventional antipsychotics are frequently associated with weight gain, before starting treatment, weigh all patients and determine if the patient is already overweight (BMI 25.0–29.9) or obese (BMI ≥30)
• Before giving a drug that can cause weight gain to an overweight or obese patient, consider determining whether the patient already has pre-diabetes (fasting plasma glucose 100–125 mg/dl), diabetes (fasting plasma glucose >126 mg/dl), or dyslipidemia (increased total cholesterol, LDL cholesterol and triglycerides; decreased HDL cholesterol), and treat or refer such patients for treatment, including nutrition and weight management, physical activity counseling, smoking cessation, and medical management
✻ Monitor weight and BMI during treatment
✻ While giving a drug to a patient who has gained >5% of initial weight, consider evaluating for the presence of pre-diabetes, diabetes, or dyslipidemia, or consider switching to a different antipsychotic
• Should check blood pressure in the elderly before starting and for the first few weeks of treatment
• Monitoring elevated prolactin levels of dubious clinical benefit

SIDE EFFECTS

How Drug Causes Side Effects
- By blocking dopamine 2 receptors in the striatum, it can cause motor side effects
- By blocking dopamine 2 receptors in the pituitary, it can cause elevations in prolactin
- By blocking dopamine 2 receptors excessively in the mesocortical and mesolimbic dopamine pathways, especially at high doses, it can cause worsening of negative and cognitive symptoms (neuroleptic-induced deficit syndrome)
- Anticholinergic actions may cause sedation, blurred vision, constipation, dry mouth
- Antihistaminic actions may cause sedation, weight gain
- By blocking alpha 1 adrenergic receptors, it can cause dizziness, sedation, and hypotension
- Mechanism of weight gain and any possible increased incidence of diabetes or dyslipidemia with conventional antipsychotics is unknown
- ✳ Mechanism of potentially dangerous QTc prolongation may be related to actions at ion channels

Notable Side Effects
- ✳ Neuroleptic-induced deficit syndrome
- ✳ Akathisia
- ✳ Extrapyramidal symptoms, Parkinsonism, tardive dyskinesia
- ✳ Hypotension
- Sedation, akinesia
- Galactorrhea, amenorrhea
- Dry mouth, constipation, blurred vision
- Sexual dysfunction
- ✳ Weight gain

 Life Threatening or Dangerous Side Effects
- Rare neuroleptic malignant syndrome
- Rare seizures
- ✳ Dose-dependent QTc prolongation
- Ventricular arrhythmias and sudden death

Weight Gain

unusual / not unusual / common / problematic
- Occurs in significant minority

Sedation

unusual / not unusual / common / problematic
- Occurs in significant minority

What To Do About Side Effects
- Wait
- Wait
- Wait
- For motor symptoms, add an anticholinergic agent
- Reduce the dose
- For sedation, give at night
- Switch to an atypical antipsychotic
- Weight loss, exercise programs, and medical management for high BMIs, diabetes, dyslipidemia

Best Augmenting Agents for Side Effects
- ✳ Augmentation of pimozide has not been systematically studied and can be dangerous, especially with drugs that can either prolong QTc interval or raise pimozide plasma levels

DOSING AND USE

Usual Dosage Range
- Less than 10 mg/day

Dosage Forms
- Tablet 1 mg scored, 2 mg scored

How to Dose
- Initial 1–2 mg/day in divided doses; can increase dose every other day; maximum 10 mg/day or 0.2 mg/kg/day
- Children: initial 0.05 mg/kg/day at night; can increase every 3 days; maximum 10 mg/day or 0.2 mg/kg/day

 Dosing Tips
- ✳ The effects of pimozide on the QTc interval are dose-dependent, so start low and go slow while carefully monitoring QTc interval

Overdose
- Deaths have occurred; extrapyramidal symptoms, ECG changes, hypotension, respiratory depression, coma

Long-Term Use
- Some side effects may be irreversible (e.g., tardive dyskinesia)

Habit Forming
- No

How to Stop
- Slow down-titration (over 6 to 8 weeks), especially when simultaneously beginning a new antipsychotic while switching (i.e., cross-titration)
- Rapid discontinuation may lead to rebound psychosis and worsening of symptoms
- If antiparkinson agents are being used, they should be continued for a few weeks after pimozide is discontinued

Pharmacokinetics
- Metabolized by CYP450 3A and to a lesser extent by CYP450 1A2
- Mean elimination half-life approximately 55 hours

 Drug Interactions
- May decrease the effects of levodopa, dopamine agonists
- May enhance QTc prolongation of other drugs capable of prolonging QTc interval
- May increase the effects of antihypertensive drugs
- ❋ Use with CYP450 3A4 inhibitors (e.g., drugs such as fluoxetine, sertraline, fluvoxamine, and nefazodone; foods such as grapefruit juice) can raise pimozide levels and increase the risks of dangerous arrhythmias
- Use of pimozide and fluoxetine may lead to bradycardia
- Additive effects may occur if used with CNS depressants
- Some patients taking a neuroleptic and lithium have developed an encephalopathic syndrome similar to neuroleptic malignant syndrome
- Combined use with epinephrine may lower blood pressure

 Other Warnings/ Precautions
- If signs of neuroleptic malignant syndrome develop, treatment should be immediately discontinued

- Use cautiously in patients with alcohol withdrawal or convulsive disorders because of possible lowering of seizure threshold
- Antiemetic effect can mask signs of other disorders or overdose
- Do not use epinephrine in event of overdose as interaction with some pressor agents may lower blood pressure
- Use only with caution if at all in Parkinson's disease or Lewy Body dementia
- Because pimozide may dose-dependently prolong QTc interval, use with caution in patients who have bradycardia or who are taking drugs that can induce bradycardia (e.g., beta blockers, calcium channel blockers, clonidine, digitalis)
- Because pimozide may dose-dependently prolong QTc interval, use with caution in patients who have hypokalemia and/or hypomagnesemia or who are taking drugs that can induce hypokalemia and/or magnesemia (e.g., diuretics, stimulant laxatives, intravenous amphotericin B, glucocorticoids, tetracosactide)
- Pimozide can increase tumors in mice (dose-related effect)
- ❋ Pimozide can increase the QTc interval and potentially cause arrhythmia or sudden death, especially in combination with drugs that raise its levels

Do Not Use
- If patient is in a comatose state or has CNS depression
- ❋ If patient is taking an agent capable of significanty prolonging QTc interval (e.g., thioridazine, selected antiarrhythmics, moxifoxacin, and sparfloxacin)
- ❋ If there is a history of QTc prolongation or cardiac arrhythmia, recent acute myocardial infarction, uncompensated heart failure
- If patient is taking drugs that can cause tics
- ❋ If patient is taking drugs that inhibit pimozide metabolism, such as macrolide antibiotics, azole antifungal agents (ketoconazole, itraconazole), protease inhibitors, nefazodone, fluvoxamine, fluoxetine, sertaline, etc.
- If there is a proven allergy to pimozide
- If there is a known sensitivity to other antipsychotics

PIMOZIDE (continued)

Renal Impairment
• Use with caution

Hepatic Impairment
• Use with caution

Cardiac Impairment
• Pimozide produces a dose-dependent prolongation of QTc interval, which may be enhanced by the existence of bradycardia, hypokalemia, congenital or acquired long QTc interval, which should be evaluated prior to administering pimozide
• Use with caution if treating concomitantly with a medication likely to produce prolonged bradycardia, hypokalemia, slowing of intracardiac conduction, or prolongation of the QTc interval
• Avoid pimozide in patients with a known history of QTc prolongation, recent acute myocardial infarction, and uncompensated heart failure

Elderly
• Some patients may tolerate lower doses better

Children and Adolescents
• Safety and efficacy established for patients over age 12
• Preliminary data show similar safety for patients age 2–12 as for patients over 12
• Generally use second-line after atypical antipsychotics and other conventional antipsychotics

Pregnancy
• Risk Category C [some animal studies show adverse effects, no controlled studies in humans]
• Renal papillary abnormalities have been seen in rats during pregnancy
• No studies in pregnant women
• Psychotic symptoms may worsen during pregnancy and some form of treatment may be necessary
• Atypical antipsychotics may be preferable to conventional antipsychotics or anticonvulsant mood stabilizers if treatment is required during pregnancy

• Should evaluate for an antipsychotic with a better risk/benefit ratio if treatment required during pregnancy

Breast Feeding
• Unknown if pimozide is secreted in human breast milk, but all psychotropics assumed to be secreted in breast milk
• Not recommended for use because of potential for tumorigenicity or cardiovascular effects on infant
✳ Recommended either to discontinue drug or bottle feed

Potential Advantages
• Only for patients who respond to this agent and not to other antipsychotics

Potential Disadvantages
• Vulnerable populations such as children and elderly
• Patients on other drugs

Primary Target Symptoms
• Vocal and motor tics in patients who fail to respond to treatment with other antipsychotics
• Psychotic symptoms in patients who fail to respond to treatment with other antipsychotics

Pearls
✳ In the past, was a first-line choice for Tourette's syndrome and for certain behavioral disorders, including monosymptomatic hypochondriasis; however, it is now recognized that the benefits of pimozide generally do not outweigh its risks in most patients
✳ Because of its effects on the QTc interval, pimozide is not intended for use unless other options for tic disorders (or psychotic disorders) have failed

Suggested Reading

Shapiro AK, Shapiro E, Fulop G. Pimozide treatment of tic and Tourette disorders. Pediatrics 1987; 79 (6): 1032–9.

Sultana A, McMonagle T. Pimozide for schizophrenia or related psychoses. Cochrane Database Syst Rev 2000; (3): CD001949.

Tueth MJ, Cheong JA. Clinical uses of pimozide. South Med J 1993; 86 (3): 344–9.

PIPOTHIAZINE

THERAPEUTICS

Brands • Piportil
see index for additional brand names

Generic? No

Class
• Conventional antipsychotic (neuroleptic, phenothiazine, dopamine 2 antagonist)

Commonly Prescribed For
(bold for FDA approved)
• Maintenance treatment of schizophrenia
• Other psychotic disorders
• Bipolar disorder

How The Drug Works
• Blocks dopamine 2 receptors, reducing positive symptoms of psychosis

How Long Until It Works
• Psychotic symptoms can improve within 1 week, but it may take several weeks for full effect on behavior

If It Works
• Most often reduces positive symptoms in schizophrenia but does not eliminate them
• Most schizophrenic patients do not have a total remission of symptoms but rather a reduction of symptoms by about a third
• Continue treatment in schizophrenia until reaching a plateau of improvement
• After reaching a satisfactory plateau, continue treatment for at least a year after first episode of psychosis in schizophrenia
• For second and subsequent episodes of psychosis in schizophrenia, treatment may need to be indefinite
• Reduces symptoms of acute psychotic mania but not proven as a mood stabilizer or as an effective maintenance treatment in bipolar disorder
• After reducing acute psychotic symptoms in mania, switch to a mood stabilizer and/or an atypical antipsychotic for mood stabilization and maintenance

If It Doesn't Work
• Consider trying one of the first-line atypical antipsychotics (risperidone, olanzapine,

quetiapine, ziprasidone, aripiprazole, amisulpride)
• Consider trying another conventional antipsychotic
• If 2 or more antipsychotic monotherapies do not work, consider clozapine

Best Augmenting Combos for Partial Response or Treatment-Resistance
• Augmentation of conventional antipsychotics has not been systematically studied
• Addition of a mood stabilizing anticonvulsant such as valproate, carbamazepine, or lamotrigine may be helpful in both schizophrenia and bipolar mania
• Augmentation with lithium in bipolar mania may be helpful
• Addition of a benzodiazepine, especially short-term for agitation

Tests
✱ Since conventional antipsychotics are frequently associated with weight gain, before starting treatment, weigh all patients and determine if the patient is already overweight (BMI 25.0–29.9) or obese (BMI ≥30)
• Before giving a drug that can cause weight gain to an overweight or obese patient, consider determining whether the patient already has pre-diabetes (fasting plasma glucose 100–125 mg/dl), diabetes (fasting plasma glucose >126 mg/dl), or dyslipidemia (increased total cholesterol, LDL cholesterol and triglycerides; decreased HDL cholesterol), and treat or refer such patients for treatment, including nutrition and weight management, physical activity counseling, smoking cessation, and medical management
✱ Monitor weight and BMI during treatment
✱ While giving a drug to a patient who has gained >5% of initial weight, consider evaluating for the presence of pre-diabetes, diabetes, or dyslipidemia, or consider switching to a different antipsychotic
• Should check blood pressure in the elderly before starting and for the first few weeks
• Monitoring elevated prolactin levels of dubious clinical benefit
• Phenothiazines may cause false-positive phenylketonuria results

SIDE EFFECTS

How Drug Causes Side Effects
- By blocking dopamine 2 receptors in the striatum, it can cause motor side effects
- By blocking dopamine 2 receptors in the pituitary, it can cause elevations in prolactin
- By blocking dopamine 2 receptors excessively in the mesocortical and mesolimbic dopamine pathways, especially at high doses, it can cause worsening of negative and cognitive symptoms (neuroleptic-induced deficit syndrome)
- Anticholinergic actions may cause sedation, blurred vision, constipation, dry mouth
- Antihistaminic actions may cause sedation, weight gain
- By blocking alpha 1 adrenergic receptors, it can cause dizziness, sedation, and hypotension
- Mechanism of weight gain and any possible increased incidence of diabetes or dyslipidemia with conventional antipsychotics is unknown

Notable Side Effects
- ✳ Excitement, insomnia, restlessness
- ✳ Rare tardive dyskinesia (risk increases with duration of treatment and with dose)
- ✳ Galactorrhea, amenorrhea
- Dry mouth, nausea, blurred vision, sweating, appetite change
- Sexual dysfunction (impotence)
- Hypotension, arrhythmia, tachycardia
- Weight gain
- Rare rash

 Life Threatening or Dangerous Side Effects
- Rare neuroleptic malignant syndrome
- Jaundice, leucopenia
- Rare seizures

Weight Gain

unusual / not unusual / **common** / problematic

- Many experience and/or can be significant in amount

Sedation

unusual / not unusual / common / problematic

- Reported but not expected

What To Do About Side Effects
- Wait
- Wait
- Wait
- For motor symptoms, add an anticholinergic agent
- Reduce the dose
- For sedation, take at night
- Switch to an atypical antipsychotic
- Weight loss, exercise programs, and medical management for high BMIs, diabetes, dyslipidemia

Best Augmenting Agents for Side Effects
- Benztropine or trihexyphenidyl for motor side effects
- Sometimes amantadine can be helpful for motor side effects
- Benzodiazepines may be helpful for akathisia
- Many side effects cannot be improved with an augmenting agent

DOSING AND USE

Usual Dosage Range
- 50–100 mg once a month

Dosage Forms
- Injection 50 mg/mL

How to Dose
- Initial 25 mg; can be increased by 25–50 mg; maximum 200 mg once a month
- Drug should be administerd intramuscularly in the gluteal region

 Dosing Tips
- ✳ Only available as long acting intramuscular formulation and not as oral formulation
- The peak of action generally occurs after 9–10 days
- May need to treat with an oral antipsychotic for 1–2 weeks when initiating treatment
- One of the few conventional antipsychotics available in a depot formulation lasting for up to a month

Overdose
- Sedation, tachycardia, extrapyramidal symptoms, arrhythmia, hypothermia, ECG changes, hypotension

Long-Term Use
- Some side effects may be irreversible (e.g., tardive dyskinesia)

Habit Forming
- No

How to Stop
- If antiparkinson agents are being used, they should be continued for a few weeks after pipothiazine is discontinued

Pharmacokinetics
- Onset of action of palmitic ester formulation within 2–3 days
- Duration of action of palmitic ester formulation 3–6 weeks

 Drug Interactions
- Use with tricyclic antidepressants may increase risk of cardiac symptoms
- CNS effects may be increased if used with other CNS depressants
- May increase the effects of antihypertensive agents
- May decrease the effects of amphetamines, levodopa, dopamine agonists, clonidine, guanethidine, adrenaline
- Effects may be reduced by anticholinergic agents
- Antacids, antiparkinson drugs, and lithium may reduce pipothiazine absorption
- Combined use with epinephrine may lower blood pressure
- Some patients taking a neuroleptic and lithium have developed an encephalopathic syndrome similar to neuroleptic malignant syndrome

 Other Warnings/ Precautions
- Patients may be more sensitive to extreme temperatures
- Use with caution in patients with Parkinson's disease, Lewy Body dementia, or extrapyramidal symptoms with previous treatments
- Avoid undue exposure to sunlight

- Use with caution in patients with respiratory disease, Lewy Body dementia, narrow angle-closure glaucoma (including family history), alcohol withdrawal syndrome, brain damage, epilepsy, hypothyroidism, myaesthenia gravis, prostatic hypertrophy, thyrotoxicosis
- Contact with skin can cause rash
- Antiemetic effect can mask signs of other disorders or overdose
- Do not use epinephrine in event of overdose as interaction with some pressor agents may lower blood pressure

Do Not Use
- If patient is comatose
- If there is cerebral atherosclerosis
- If patient has phaeochromocytoma
- If patient has renal or liver failure, blood dyscrasias
- If patient has severe cardiac impairment
- If patient has subcortical brain damage
- If there is a proven allergy to pipothiazine
- If there is a known sensitivity to any phenothiazine

SPECIAL POPULATIONS

Renal Impairment
- Use with caution

Hepatic Impairment
- Use with caution

Cardiac Impairment
- Use with caution

Elderly
- Elderly patients do not metabolize the drug as quickly
- Dose should be reduced
- Recommended starting dose 5–10 mg

 Children and Adolescents
- Not recommended for use in children

 Pregnancy
- Risk Category C [some animal studies show adverse effects, no controlled studies in humans]

- Reports of extrapyramidal symptoms, jaundice, hyperreflexia, hyporeflexia in infants whose mothers took a phenothiazine during pregnancy
- Not recommended unless absolutely necessary
- Psychotic symptoms may worsen during pregnancy and some form of treatment may be necessary
- Atypical antipsychotics may be preferable to conventional antipsychotics or anticonvulsant mood stabilizers if treatment is required during pregnancy

Breast Feeding

- Unknown if pipothiazine is secreted in human breast milk, but all psychotropics assumed to be secreted in breast milk
- ✳ Recommended either to discontinue drug or bottle feed

THE ART OF PSYCHOPHARMACOLOGY

Potential Advantages

- Non-compliant patients

Potential Disadvantages

- Patients who need immediate onset of antipsychotic actions

Primary Target Symptoms

- Positive symptoms of psychosis
- Negative symptoms of psychosis
- Aggressive symptoms

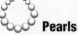 **Pearls**

- Pipothiazine is a higher potency phenothiazine
- Less risk of sedation and orthostatic hypotension but greater risk of extrapyramidal symptoms than with low potency phenothiazines
- ✳ Only available in long-acting parenteral formulation
- Generally, patients must be stabilized on an oral antipsychotic prior to switching to parenteral long-acting pipothiazine
- Patients have very similar antipsychotic responses to any conventional antipsychotic, which is different from atypical antipsychotics where antipsychotic responses of individual patients can occasionally vary greatly from one atypical antipsychotic to another
- Patients with inadequate responses to atypical antipsychotics may benefit from a trial of augmentation with a conventional antipsychotic such as pipothiazine or from switching to a conventional antipsychotic such as pipothiazine
- However, long-term polypharmacy with a combination of a conventional antipsychotic with an atypical antipsychotic such as pipothiazine may combine their side effects without clearly augmenting the efficacy of either
- Although a frequent practice by some prescribers, adding 2 conventional antipsychotics together has little rationale and may reduce tolerability without clearly enhancing efficacy

---

 Suggested Reading

Leong OK, Wong KE, Tay WK, Gill RC. A comparative study of pipothiazine palmitate and fluphenazine decanoate in the maintenance of remission of schizophrenia. Singapore Med J 1989; 30 (5): 436–40.

Quraishi S, David A. Depot pipothiazine palmitate and undecylenate for schizophrenia. Cochrane Database Syst Rev 2001; (3): CD001720.

Schmidt K. Pipothiazine palmitate: a versatile, sustained-action neuroleptic in psychiatric practice. Curr Med Res Opin 1986; 10 (5): 326–9.

PREGABALIN

THERAPEUTICS

Brands • Lyrica
see index for additional brand names

Generic? No

Class
• Anticonvulsant, antineuralgic for chronic pain, alpha 2 delta ligand at voltage-sensitive calcium channels

Commonly Prescribed For
(bold for FDA approved)
• Peripheral neuropathic pain
• Partial seizures with or without secondary generalization (adjunctive)
• Generalized anxiety disorder
• Panic disorder
• Social anxiety disorder
• Fibromyalgia

How The Drug Works
• Is a leucine analogue and is transported both into the blood from the gut and also across the blood-brain barrier into the brain from the blood by the system L transport system (a sodium independent transporter) as well as by additional sodium-dependent amino acid transporter systems
* Binds to the alpha 2 delta subunit of voltage-sensitive calcium channels
• This closes N and P/Q presynaptic calcium channels, diminishing excessive neuronal activity and neurotransmitter release
• Although structurally related to gamma-aminobutyric acid (GABA), no known direct actions on GABA or its receptors

How Long Until It Works
• Can reduce neuropathic pain and anxiety within a week
• Should reduce seizures by 2 weeks
• If it is not producing clinical benefits within 6–8 weeks, it may require a dosage increase or it may not work at all

If It Works
• The goal of treatment of neuropathic pain, seizures, and anxiety disorders is to reduce symptoms as much as possible, and if necessary in combination with other treatments
• Treatment of neuropathic pain most often reduces but does not eliminate all symptoms and is not a cure since symptoms usually recur after medicine stopped
• Continue treatment until all symptoms are gone or until improvement is stable and then continue treating indefinitely as long as improvement persists

If It Doesn't Work (for neuropathic pain)
• Many patients only have a partial response where some symptoms are improved but others persist
• Other patients may be nonresponders, sometimes called treatment-resistant or treatment-refractory
• Consider increasing dose, switching to another agent or adding an appropriate augmenting agent
• Consider biofeedback or hypnosis for pain
• Consider psychotherapy for anxiety
• Consider the presence of noncompliance and counsel patient
• Consider evaluation for another diagnosis or for a comorbid condition (e.g., medical illness, substance abuse, etc.)

Best Augmenting Combos for Partial Response or Treatment-Resistance
* In addition to being a first-line treatment for neuropathic pain and anxiety disorders, pregabalin is itself an augmenting agent to numerous other anticonvulsants in treating epilepsy
• For postherpetic neuralgia, pregabalin can decrease concomitant opiate use
* For neuropathic pain, tricyclic antidepressants and SNRIs as well as tiagabine, other anticonvulsants, and even opiates can augment pregabalin if done by experts while carefully monitoring in difficult cases
• For anxiety, SSRIs, SNRIs, or benzodiazepines can augment pregabalin

Tests
• None for healthy individuals

SIDE EFFECTS

How Drug Causes Side Effects
• CNS side effects may be due to excessive blockade of voltage-sensitive calcium channels

Notable Side Effects
❋ Sedation, dizziness
• Ataxia, fatigue, tremor, dysarthria, paraesthesia, memory impairment, coordination abnormal, impaired attention, confusion, euphoric mood, irritability
• Vomiting, dry mouth, constipation, weight gain, increased appetite, flatulence
• Blurred vision, diplopia
• Peripheral edema
• Libido decreased, erectile dysfunction

Life Threatening or Dangerous Side Effects
• None

Weight Gain

 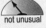
unusual • not unusual • common • problematic

• Occurs in significant minority

Sedation

unusual • not unusual • common • problematic

• Many experience and/or can be significant in amount
• Dose-related
• Can wear off with time

What To Do About Side Effects
• Wait
• Wait
• Wait
• Take more of the dose at night to reduce daytime sedation
• Lower the dose
• Switch to another agent

Best Augmenting Agents for Side Effects
• Many side effects cannot be improved with an augmenting agent

DOSING AND USE

Usual Dosage Range
• 150–600 mg/day in 2–3 doses

Dosage Forms
• Capsule 25 mg, 50 mg, 75 mg, 100 mg, 150 mg, 200 mg, 300 mg

How to Dose
• Neuropathic pain: initial 150 mg/day in 2–3 doses; can increase to 300 mg/day in 2–3 doses after 3–7 days; can increase to 600 mg/day in 2–3 doses after 7 more days; maximum dose generally 600 mg/day
• Seizures: initial 150 mg/day in 2–3 doses; can increase to 300 mg/day in 2–3 doses after 7 days; can increase to 600 mg/day in 2–3 doses after 7 more days; maximum dose generally 600 mg/day

Dosing Tips
❋ Generally given in one-third to one-sixth the dose of gabapentin
• If pregabalin is added to a second sedating agent, such as another anticonvulsant, a benzodiazepine, or an opiate, the titration period should be at least a week to improve tolerance to sedation
• Most patients only need to take pregabalin twice daily
• At the high end of the dosing range, tolerability may be enhanced by splitting dose into 3 or more divided doses
• For intolerable sedation, can give most of the dose at night and less during the day
• To improve slow-wave sleep, may only need to take pregabalin at bedtime
• May be taken with or without food

Overdose
• No fatalities

Long-Term Use
• Safe

Habit Forming
• No

How to Stop
• Taper over a minimum of 1 week
• Epilepsy patients may seize upon withdrawal, especially if withdrawal is abrupt

- Discontinuation symptoms uncommon

Pharmacokinetics
- Pregabalin is not metabolized but excreted intact renally
- Elimination half-life approximately 5–7 hours

 Drug Interactions
- Pregabalin has not been shown to have significant pharmacokinetic drug interactions
- Because pregabalin is excreted unchanged, it is unlikely to have significant pharmacokinetic drug interactions
- May add to or potentiate the sedative effects of oxycodone, lorazepam, and alcohol

Other Warnings/ Precautions
- Dizziness and sedation could increase the chances of accidental injury (falls) in the elderly
- Increased incidence of hemangiosarcoma at high doses in mice involves platelet changes and associated endothelial cell proliferation not present in rats or humans; no evidence to suggest an associated risk for humans

Do Not Use
- If there is a proven allergy to pregabalin or gabapentin
- If patient has a problem of galactose intolerance, the Lapp lactase deficiency, or glucose-galactose malabsorption

SPECIAL POPULATIONS

Renal Impairment
- Pregabalin is renally excreted, so the dose may need to be lowered
- Dosing can be adjusted according to creatinine clearance, such that patients with clearance below 15 mL/min should receive 25–75 mg/day in 1 dose, patients with clearance between 15–29 mL/min should receive 25–150 mg/day in 1–2 doses, and patients with clearance between 30–59 mL/min should receive 75–300 mg/day in 2–3 doses

- Starting dose should be at the bottom of the range; titrate as usual up to maximum dose
- Can be removed by hemodialysis; patients receiving hemodialysis may require a supplemental dose of pregabalin following hemodialysis (25–100 mg)

Hepatic Impairment
- Dose adjustment not necessary

Cardiac Impairment
- No specific recommendations

Elderly
- Some patients may tolerate lower doses better
- Elderly patients may be more susceptible to adverse effects

 Children and Adolescents
- Safety and efficacy have not been established
- Use should be reserved for the expert

 Pregnancy
- Some animal studies have shown adverse effects, no controlled studies in humans
- Use in women of childbearing potential requires weighing potential benefits to the mother against the risks to the fetus
- Taper drug if discontinuing
- Seizures, even mild seizures, may cause harm to the embryo/fetus

Breast Feeding
- Unknown if pregabalin is secreted in human breast milk, but all psychotropics assumed to be secreted in breast milk
- ✳ Recommended either to discontinue drug or bottle feed
- If drug is continued while breast feeding, infant should be monitored for possible adverse effects
- If infant becomes irritable or sedated, breast feeding or drug may need to be discontinued

THE ART OF PSYCHOPHARMACOLOGY

Potential Advantages
- First-line for diabetic peripheral neuropathy
- Fibromyalgia
- Anxiety disorders
- Sleep
- Has relatively mild side effect profile
- Has few pharmacokinetic drug interactions
- More potent and probably better tolerated than gabapentin

Potential Disadvantages
- Requires 2–3 times a day dosing
- Not yet approved for anxiety disorders
- Not yet available in the United States

Primary Target Symptoms
- Seizures
- Pain
- Anxiety

 Pearls

* First and only treatment currently approved for neuropathic pain associated with diabetic peripheral neuropathy
- Also effective in postherpetic neuralgia
- Improves sleep interference as well as pain in patients with painful diabetic peripheral neuropathy or postherpetic neuralgia
- Improves pain and sleep interference associated with fibromyalgia

- Well-studied in epilepsy, peripheral neuropathic pain, and generalized anxiety disorder
* Off-label use for generalized anxiety disorder, panic disorder, and social anxiety disorder may be justified
- May have uniquely robust therapeutic actions for both the somatic and the psychic symptoms of generalized anxiety disorder
* Off-label use as an adjunct for bipolar disorder may not be justified
* One of the few agents that enhances slow-wave delta sleep, which may be helpful in chronic neuropathic pain syndromes
- Pregabalin is generally well-tolerated, with only mild adverse effects
* Although no head-to-head studies, appears to be better tolerated and more consistently efficacious at high doses than gabapentin
* Drug absorption and clinical efficacy may be more consistent at high doses for pregabalin compared to gabapentin because of the higher potency of pregabalin and the fact that, unlike gabapentin, it is transported by more than one transport system

 Suggested Reading

Hovinga CA. Novel anticonvulsant medications in development. Expert Opin Investig Drugs 2002;11:1387–406.

Lauria-Horner BA, Pohl RB. Pregabalin: a new anxiolytic. Expert Opin Investig Drugs 2003; 12:663–72.

Stahl SM. Anticonvulsants and the relief of chronic pain: pregabalin and gabapentin as alpha(2)delta ligands at voltage-gated calcium channels. J Clin Psychiatry 2004;65:596–7.

Stahl SM. Anticonvulsants as anxiolytics, part 2: Pregabalin and gabapentin as alpha(2)delta ligands at voltage-gated calcium channels. J Clin Psychiatry 2004;65:460–1.

PROTRIPTYLINE

THERAPEUTICS

Brands • Triptil
• Vivactil
see index for additional brand names

Generic? Yes

Class
• Tricyclic antidepressant (TCA)
• Predominantly a norepinephrine/
noradrenaline reuptake inhibitor

Commonly Prescribed For
(bold for FDA approved)
• **Mental depression**
• Treatment-resistant depression

How The Drug Works
• Boosts neurotransmitter
norepinephrine/noradrenaline
• Blocks norepinephrine reuptake pump
(norepinephrine transporter), presumably
increasing noradrenergic
neurotransmission
• Since dopamine is inactivated by
norepinephrine reuptake in frontal cortex,
which largely lacks dopamine transporters,
protriptyline can increase dopamine
neurotransmission in this part of the brain
• A more potent inhibitor of norepinephrine
reuptake pump than serotonin reuptake
pump (serotonin transporter)
• At high doses may also boost
neurotransmitter serotonin and presumably
increase serotonergic neurotransmission

How Long Until It Works
❋ Some evidence it may have an early onset
of action with improvement in activity and
energy as early as 1 week
• Onset of therapeutic actions usually not
immediate, but often delayed 2 to 4 weeks
• If it is not working within 6 to 8 weeks for
depression, it may require a dosage
increase or it may not work at all
• May continue to work for many years to
prevent relapse of symptoms

If It Works
• The goal of treatment is complete
remission of current symptoms as well as
prevention of future relapses
• Treatment most often reduces or even
eliminates symptoms, but not a cure since
symptoms can recur after medicine
stopped
• Continue treatment until all symptoms are
gone (remission)
• Once symptoms gone, continue treating for
1 year for the first episode of depression
• For second and subsequent episodes of
depression, treatment may need to be
indefinite
• Use in anxiety disorders may also need to
be indefinite

If It Doesn't Work
• Many patients only have a partial response
where some symptoms are improved but
others persist (especially insomnia, fatigue,
and problems concentrating)
• Other patients may be nonresponders,
sometimes called treatment-resistant or
treatment-refractory
• Consider increasing dose, switching to
another agent or adding an appropriate
augmenting agent
• Consider psychotherapy
• Consider evaluation for another diagnosis
or for a comorbid condition (e.g., medical
illness, substance abuse, etc.)
• Some patients may experience apparent
lack of consistent efficacy due to activation
of latent or underlying bipolar disorder, and
require antidepressant discontinuation and
a switch to a mood stabilizer

Best Augmenting Combos for Partial Response or Treatment-Resistance

• Lithium, buspirone, thyroid hormone

Tests
• None for healthy individuals
❋ Since tricyclic and tetracyclic
antidepressants are frequently associated
with weight gain, before starting treatment,
weigh all patients and determine if the
patient is already overweight
(BMI 25.0–29.9) or obese (BMI ≥30)
• Before giving a drug that can cause weight
gain to an overweight or obese patient,
consider determining whether the patient

already has pre-diabetes (fasting plasma glucose 100–125 mg/dl), diabetes (fasting plasma glucose >126 mg/dl), or dyslipidemia (increased total cholesterol, LDL cholesterol and triglycerides; decreased HDL cholesterol), and treat or refer such patients for treatment, including nutrition and weight management, physical activity counseling, smoking cessation, and medical management

✳ Monitor weight and BMI during treatment

✳ While giving a drug to a patient who has gained >5% of initial weight, consider evaluating for the presence of pre-diabetes, diabetes, or dyslipidemia, or consider switching to a different antidepressant

• EKGs may be useful for selected patients (e.g., those with personal or family history of QTc prolongation; cardiac arrhythmia; recent myocardial infarction; uncompensated heart failure; or taking agents that prolong QTc interval such as pimozide, thioridazine, selected antiarrhythmics, moxifloxacin, sparfloxacin, etc.)

• Patients at risk for electrolyte disturbances (e.g., patients on diuretic therapy) should have baseline and periodic serum potassium and magnesium measurements

SIDE EFFECTS

How Drug Causes Side Effects

✳ Anticholinergic activity for protriptyline may be more potent than for some other TCAs and may explain sedative effects, dry mouth, constipation, blurred vision, tachycardia, and hypotension

• Sedative effects and weight gain may be due to antihistamine properties

• Blockade of alpha adrenergic 1 receptors may explain dizziness, sedation, and hypotension

• Cardiac arrhythmias, especially in overdose, may be caused by blockade of ion channels

Notable Side Effects

• Blurred vision, constipation, urinary retention, increased appetite, dry mouth, nausea, diarrhea, heartburn, unusual taste in mouth, weight gain

• Fatigue, weakness, dizziness, sedation, headache, anxiety, nervousness, restlessness

• Sexual dysfunction (impotence, change in libido)

• Sweating, rash, itching

 Life Threatening or Dangerous Side Effects

• Paralytic ileus, hyperthermia (TCAs + anticholinergic agents)

• Lowered seizure threshold and rare seizures

• Orthostatic hypotension, sudden death, arrhythmias, tachycardia

• QTc prolongation

• Hepatic failure, extrapyramidal symptoms

• Increased intraocular pressure

• Rare induction of mania and activation of suicidal ideation

Weight Gain

unusual   not unusual   common   problematic

• Many experience and/or can be significant in amount

• Can increase appetite and carbohydrate craving

Sedation

unusual   not unusual   common   problematic

• Many experience and/or can be significant in amount

✳ Not as sedating as other TCAs; more likely to be activating than other TCAs

What To Do About Side Effects

• Wait

• Wait

• Wait

• Lower the dose

• Switch to an SSRI or newer antidepressant

Best Augmenting Agents for Side Effects

• Trazodone or a hypnotic for insomnia

• Benzodiazepines for agitation and anxiety

• Many side effects cannot be improved with an augmenting agent

DOSING AND USE

Usual Dosage Range
• 15–40 mg/day in 3–4 divided doses

Dosage Forms
• Tablets 5 mg, 10 mg

How to Dose
• Initial 15 mg/day in divided doses; increase morning dose as needed; maximum dose 60 mg/day

 Dosing Tips

✳ Be aware that among this class of agents (tricyclic/tetracyclic antidepressants), protriptyline has uniquely low dosing (15–40 mg/day for protriptyline compared to 75–300 mg/day for most other tricyclic/tetracyclic antidepressants)
✳ Be aware that among this class of agents (tricyclic/tetracyclic antidepressants), protriptyline has uniquely frequent dosing (3–4 times a day compared to once daily for most other tricyclic/tetracyclic antidepressants)
• If intolerable anxiety, insomnia, agitation, akathisia, or activation occur either upon dosing initiation or discontinuation, consider the possibility of activated bipolar disorder, and switch to a mood stabilizer or an atypical antipsychotic

Overdose
• Death may occur; CNS depression, convulsions, cardiac dysrhythmias, severe hypotension, ECG changes, coma

Long-Term Use
• Safe

Habit Forming
• No

How to Stop
• Taper to avoid withdrawal effects
• Even with gradual dose reduction some withdrawal symptoms may appear within the first 2 weeks
• Many patients tolerate 50% dose reduction for 3 days, then another 50% reduction for 3 days, then discontinuation
• If withdrawal symptoms emerge during discontinuation, raise dose to stop

symptoms and then restart withdrawal much more slowly

Pharmacokinetics
• Substrate for CYP450 2D6
• Half-life approximately 74 hours

 Drug Interactions

• Tramadol increases the risk of seizures in patients taking TCAs
• Use of TCAs with anticholinergic drugs may result in paralytic ileus or hyperthermia
• Fluoxetine, paroxetine, bupropion, duloxetine, and other 2D6 inhibitors may increase TCA concentrations
• Cimetidine may increase plasma concentrations of TCAs and cause anti-cholinergic symptoms
• Phenothiazines or haloperidol may raise TCA blood concentrations
• May alter effects of antihypertensive drugs; may inhibit hypotensive effects of clonidine
• Use with sympathomimetic agents may increase sympathetic activity
• Methylphenidate may inhibit metabolism of TCAs
• Activation and agitation, especially following switching or adding antidepressants, may represent the induction of a bipolar state, especially a mixed dysphoric bipolar II condition sometimes associated with suicidal ideation, and require the addition of lithium, a mood stabilizer or an atypical antipsychotic, and/or discontinuation of protriptyline

 Other Warnings/ Precautions

• Add or initiate other antidepressants with caution for up to 2 weeks after discontinuing protriptyline
• Generally, do not use with MAO inhibitors, including 14 days after MAOIs are stopped; do not start an MAOI until 2 weeks after discontinuing protriptyline
• Use with caution in patients with history of seizures, urinary retention, narrow angle-closure glaucoma, hyperthyroidism
• TCAs can increase QTc interval, especially at toxic doses, which can be attained not only by overdose but also by combining

with drugs that inhibit TCA metabolism via CYP450 2D6, potentially causing torsade de pointes-type arrhythmia or sudden death
- Because TCAs can prolong QTc interval, use with caution in patients who have bradycardia or who are taking drugs that can induce bradycardia (e.g., beta blockers, calcium channel blockers, clonidine, digitalis)
- Because TCAs can prolong QTc interval, use with caution in patients who have hypokalemia and/or hypomagnesemia or who are taking drugs that can induce hypokalemia and/or magnesemia (e.g., diuretics, stimulant laxatives, intravenous amphotericin B, glucocorticoids, tetracosactide)

Do Not Use
- If patient is recovering from myocardial infarction
- If patient is taking agents capable of significantly prolonging QTc interval (e.g., pimozide, thioridazine, selected antiarrhythmics, moxifloxacin, sparfloxacin)
- If there is a history of QTc prolongation or cardiac arrhythmia, recent acute myocardial infarction, uncompensated heart failure
- If patient is taking drugs that inhibit TCA metabolism, including CYP450 2D6 inhibitors, except by an expert
- If there is reduced CYP450 2D6 function, such as patients who are poor 2D6 metabolizers, except by an expert and at low doses
- If there is a proven allergy to protriptyline

SPECIAL POPULATIONS

Renal Impairment
- Use with caution; may need to lower dose
- Patient may need to be monitored closely

Hepatic Impairment
- Use with caution; may need to lower dose
- Patient may need to be monitored closely

Cardiac Impairment
- TCAs have been reported to cause arrhythmias, prolongation of conduction time, orthostatic hypotension, sinus tachycardia, and heart failure, especially in the diseased heart
- Myocardial infarction and stroke have been reported with TCAs
- TCAs produce QTc prolongation, which may be enhanced by the existence of bradycardia, hypokalemia, congenital or acquired long QTc interval, which should be evaluated prior to administering protriptyline
- Use with caution if treating concomitantly with a medication likely to produce prolonged bradycardia, hypokalemia, slowing of intracardiac conduction, or prolongation of the QTc interval
- Avoid TCAs in patients with a known history of QTc prolongation, recent acute myocardial infarction, and uncompensated heart failure
- TCAs may cause a sustained increase in heart rate in patients with ischemic heart disease and may worsen (decrease) heart rate variability, an independent risk of mortality in cardiac populations
- Since SSRIs may improve (increase) heart rate variability in patients following a myocardial infarct and may improve survival as well as mood in patients with acute angina or following a myocardial infarction, these are more appropriate agents for cardiac population than tricyclic/tetracyclic antidepressants
- ✳ Risk/benefit ratio may not justify use of TCAs in cardiac impairment

Elderly
- May be more sensitive to anticholinergic, cardiovascular, hypotensive, and sedative effects
- Recommended dose is between 15–20 mg/day; doses >20 mg/day require close monitoring of patient

Children and Adolescents
- Use with caution, observing for activation of known or unknown bipolar disorder and/or suicidal ideation, and strongly consider informing parents or guardian of this risk so they can help observe child or adolescent patients
- Not recommended for use under age 12
- Not intended for use under age 6

- Several studies show lack of efficacy of TCAs for depression
- Some cases of sudden death have occurred in children taking TCAs
- Recommended dose: 15–20 mg/day

 Pregnancy

- Risk Category C [some animal studies show adverse effects, no controlled studies in humans]
- Crosses the placenta
- Adverse effects have been reported in infants whose mothers took a TCA (lethargy, withdrawal symptoms, fetal malformations)
- Must weigh the risk of treatment (first trimester fetal development, third trimester newborn delivery) to the child against the risk of no treatment (recurrence of depression, maternal health, infant bonding) to the mother and child
- For many patients this may mean continuing treatment during pregnancy

Breast Feeding

- Some drug is found in mother's breast milk
- ✳ Recommended either to discontinue drug or bottle feed
- Immediate postpartum period is a high-risk time for depression, especially in women who have had prior depressive episodes, so drug may need to be reinstituted late in the third trimester or shortly after childbirth to prevent a recurrence during the postpartum period
- Must weigh benefits of breast feeding with risks and benefits of antidepressant treatment versus non-treatment to both the infant and the mother
- For many patients this may mean continuing treatment during breast feeding

THE ART OF PSYCHOPHARMACOLOGY

Potential Advantages

- Severe or treatment-resistant depression
- Withdrawn, anergic patients

Potential Disadvantages

- Pediatric, geriatric, and cardiac patients
- Patients concerned with weight gain

- Patients noncompliant with 3–4 times daily dosing

Primary Target Symptoms

- Depressed mood

 Pearls

- Tricyclic antidepressants are no longer generally considered a first-line treatment option for depression because of their side effect profile
- Tricyclic antidepressants continue to be useful for severe or treatment-resistant depression
- ✳ Has some potential advantages for withdrawn, anergic patients
- ✳ May have a more rapid onset of action than some other TCAs
- ✳ May aggravate agitation and anxiety more than some other TCAs
- ✳ May have more anticholinergic side effects, hypotension, and tachycardia than some other TCAs
- Noradrenergic reuptake inhibitors such as protriptyline can be used as a second-line treatment for smoking cessation, cocaine dependence, and attention deficit disorder
- TCAs may aggravate psychotic symptoms
- Alcohol should be avoided because of additive CNS effects
- Underweight patients may be more susceptible to adverse cardiovascular effects
- Children, patients with inadequate hydration, and patients with cardiac disease may be more susceptible to TCA-induced cardiotoxicity than healthy adults
- For the expert only: a heroic treatment (but potentially dangerous) for severely treatment-resistant patients is to give simultaneously with monoamine oxidase inhibitors for patients who fail to respond to numerous other antidepressants, but generally recommend a different TCA than protriptyline for this use
- If this option is elected, start the MAOI with the tricyclic/tetracyclic antidepressant simultaneously at low doses after appropriate drug washout, then alternately increase doses of these agents every few days to a week as tolerated
- Although very strict dietary and concomitant drug restrictions must be

observed to prevent hypertensive crises and serotonin syndrome, the most common side effects of MAOI and tricyclic/tetracyclic antidepressant combinations may be weight gain and orthostatic hypotension
• Patients on TCAs should be aware that they may experience symptoms such as photosensitivity or blue-green urine
• SSRIs may be more effective than TCAs in women, and TCAs may be more effective than SSRIs in men
• Since tricyclic/tetracyclic antidepressants are substrates for CYP450 2D6, and 7% of the population (especially Caucasians) may have a genetic variant leading to reduced

activity of 2D6, such patients may not safely tolerate normal doses of tricyclic/tetracyclic antidepressants and may require dose reduction
• Phenotypic testing may be necessary to detect this genetic variant prior to dosing with a tricyclic/tetracyclic antidepressant, especially in vulnerable populations such as children, elderly, cardiac populations, and those on concomitant medications
• Patients who seem to have extraordinarily severe side effects at normal or low doses may have this phenotypic CYP450 2D6 variant and require low doses or switching to another antidepressant not metabolized by 2D6

 Suggested Reading

Anderson IM. Meta-analytical studies on new antidepressants. Br Med Bull. 2001; 57: 161–178.

Anderson IM. Selective serotonin reuptake inhibitors versus tricyclic antidepressants: a meta-analysis of efficacy and tolerability. J Aff Disorders. 2000; 58: 19–36.

Rudorfer MV, Potter WZ. Metabolism of tricyclic antidepressants. Cell Mol Neurobiol. 1999; 19 (3): 373–409.

QUAZEPAM

THERAPEUTICS

Brands • Doral
see index for additional brand names

Generic? No

 Class
• Benzodiazepine (hypnotic)

Commonly Prescribed For
(bold for FDA approved)
• **Short-term treatment of insomnia**

 How The Drug Works
• Binds to benzodiazepine receptors at the GABA-A ligand-gated chloride channel complex
• Enhances the inhibitory effects of GABA
• Boosts chloride conductance through GABA-regulated channels
• Inhibitory actions in sleep centers may provide sedative hypnotic effects

How Long Until It Works
• Generally takes effect in less than an hour

If It Works
• Improves quality of sleep
• Effects on total wake-time and number of nighttime awakenings may be decreased over time

If It Doesn't Work
• If insomnia does not improve after 7–10 days, it may be a manifestation of a primary psychiatric or physical illness such as obstructive sleep apnea or restless leg syndrome, which requires independent evaluation
• Increase the dose
• Improve sleep hygiene
• Switch to another agent

 Best Augmenting Combos for Partial Response or Treatment-Resistance
• Generally, best to switch to another agent
• Trazodone
• Agents with antihistamine actions (e.g., diphenhydramine, tricyclic antidepressants)

Tests
• In patients with seizure disorders, concomitant medical illness, and/or those with multiple concomitant long-term medications, periodic liver tests and blood counts may be prudent

SIDE EFFECTS

How Drug Causes Side Effects
• Same mechanism for side effects as for therapeutic effects – namely due to excessive actions at benzodiazepine receptors
• Actions at benzodiazepine receptors that carry over to the next day can cause daytime sedation, amnesia, and ataxia
• Long-term adaptations in benzodiazepine receptors may explain the development of dependence, tolerance, and withdrawal

Notable Side Effects
✳ Sedation, fatigue, depression
✳ Dizziness, ataxia, slurred speech, weakness
✳ Forgetfulness, confusion
✳ Hyper-excitability, nervousness
• Rare hallucinations, mania
• Rare hypotension
• Hypersalivation, dry mouth
• Rebound insomnia when withdrawing from long-term treatment

 Life Threatening or Dangerous Side Effects
• Respiratory depression, especially when taken with CNS depressants in overdose
• Rare hepatic dysfunction, renal dysfunction, blood dyscrasias

Weight Gain

unusual · not unusual · common · problematic
• Reported but not expected

Sedation

unusual · not unusual · common · problematic
• Many experience and/or can be significant in amount

What To Do About Side Effects
- Wait
- To avoid problems with memory, only take quazepam if planning to have a full night's sleep
- Lower the dose
- Switch to a shorter-acting sedative hypnotic
- Switch to a non-benzodiazepine hypnotic
- Administer flumazenil if side effects are severe or life-threatening

Best Augmenting Agents for Side Effects
- Many side effects cannot be improved with an augmenting agent

DOSING AND USE

Usual Dosage Range
- 15 mg/day at bedtime

Dosage Forms
- Tablet 7.5 mg, 15 mg

How to Dose
- 15 mg/day at bedtime; increase to 30 mg/day if ineffective; maximum dose 30 mg/day

 Dosing Tips
- Use lowest possible effective dose and assess need for continued treatment regularly
- Quazepam should generally not be prescribed in quantities greater than a 1-month supply
- Patients with lower body weights may require lower doses
- Risk of dependence may increase with dose and duration of treatment

Overdose
- No death reported in monotherapy; sedation, respiratory depression, poor coordination, confusion, coma

Long-Term Use
- Not generally intended for use beyond 4 weeks
- ✳ Because of its relatively longer half-life, quazepam may cause some daytime sedation and/or impaired motor/cognitive function, and may do so progressively over time

Habit Forming
- Quazepam is a Schedule IV drug
- Some patients may develop dependence and/or tolerance; risk may be greater with higher doses
- History of drug addiction may increase risk of dependence

How to Stop
- If taken for more than a few weeks, taper to reduce chances of withdrawal effects
- Patients with seizure history may seize upon sudden withdrawal
- Rebound insomnia may occur the first 1–2 nights after stopping
- For patients with severe problems discontinuing a benzodiazepine, dosing may need to be tapered over many months (i.e., reduce dose by 1% every 3 days by crushing tablet and suspending or dissolving in 100 ml of fruit juice and then disposing of 1 ml while drinking the rest; 3–7 days later, dispose of 2 ml, and so on). This is both a form of very slow biological tapering and a form of behavioral desensitization

Pharmacokinetics
- Half life 25–41 hours
- Active metabolite
- Metabolized in part by CYP450 3A4

 Drug Interactions
- Increased depressive effects when taken with other CNS depressants
- Effects of quazepam may be increased by CYP450 3A4 inhibitors such as nefazodone or fluvoxamine

 Other Warnings/ Precautions
- Insomnia may be a symptom of a primary disorder, rather than a primary disorder itself
- Some patients may exhibit abnormal thinking or behavioral changes similar to those caused by other CNS depressants (i.e., either depressant actions or disinhibiting actions)

- Some depressed patients may experience a worsening of suicidal ideation
- Use only with extreme caution in patients with impaired respiratory function or obstructive sleep apnea
- Quazepam should only be administered at bedtime

Do Not Use
- If patient is pregnant
- If patient has narrow angle-closure glaucoma
- If there is a proven allergy to quazepam or any benzodiazepine

SPECIAL POPULATIONS

Renal Impairment
- Recommended dose: 7.5 mg/day

Hepatic Impairment
- Recommended dose: 7.5 mg/day

Cardiac Impairment
- Benzodiazepines have been used to treat insomnia associated with acute myocardial infarction

Elderly
- Recommended dose: 7.5 mg/day
- If 15 mg/day is given initially, try to reduce the dose to 7.5 mg/day after the first 1–2 nights

 Children and Adolescents
- Safety and efficacy have not been established
- Long-term effects of quazepam in children/adolescents are unknown
- Should generally receive lower doses and be more closely monitored

 Pregnancy
- Risk Category X [positive evidence of risk to human fetus; contraindicated for use in pregnancy]
- Infants whose mothers received a benzodiazepine late in pregnancy may experience withdrawal effects

- Neonatal flaccidity has been reported in infants whose mothers took a benzodiazepine during pregnancy

Breast Feeding
- Some drug is found in mother's breast milk
* Recommended either to discontinue drug or bottle feed
- Effects on infant have been observed and include feeding difficulties, sedation, and weight loss

THE ART OF PSYCHOPHARMACOLOGY

Potential Advantages
- Transient insomnia

Potential Disadvantages
- Chronic nightly insomnia

Primary Target Symptoms
- Time to sleep onset
- Total night sleep
- Nighttime awakening

 Pearls
* Because quazepam tends to accumulate over time, perhaps not the best hypnotic for chronic nightly use
- If tolerance develops, it may result in increased anxiety during the day and/or increased wakefulness during the latter part of the night
- Quazepam has a longer half-life than some other sedative hypnotics, so it may be less likely to cause rebound insomnia on discontinuation
* Long-term accumulation of quazepam and its active metabolites may cause insidious onset of confusion or falls, especially in the elderly

Suggested Reading

Ankier SI, Goa KL. Quazepam. A preliminary review of its pharmacodynamic and pharmacokinetic properties, and therapeutic efficacy in insomnia. Drugs 1988;35:42–62.

Hilbert JM, Battista D. Quazepam and flurazepam: differential pharmacokinetic and pharmacodynamic characteristics. J Clin Psychiatry 1991;52(Suppl):21–6.

Kales A. Quazepam: hypnotic efficacy and side effects. Pharmacotherapy 1990;10:1–10.

Kirkwood CK. Management of insomnia. J Am Pharm Assoc (Wash) 1999;39:688–96.

Roth T, Roehrs TA. A review of the safety profiles of benzodiazepine hypnotics. J Clin Psychiatry 1991;52 (Suppl):38–41.

QUETIAPINE

THERAPEUTICS

Brands • Seroquel
see index for additional brand names

Generic? Not in U.S., Europe, or Japan

Class
• Atypical antipsychotic (serotonin-dopamine antagonist; second generation antipsychotic; also a mood stabilizer)

Commonly Prescribed For
(bold for FDA approved)
• **Schizophrenia**
• **Acute mania (monotherapy and adjunct to lithium or valproate)**
• Other psychotic disorders
• Bipolar maintenance
• Bipolar depression
• Behavioral disturbances in dementias
• Behavioral disturbances in Parkinson's disease and Lewy Body dementia
• Psychosis associated with levodopa treatment in Parkinson's disease
• Behavioral disturbances in children and adolescents
• Disorders associated with problems with impulse control

How The Drug Works
• Blocks dopamine 2 receptors, reducing positive symptoms of psychosis and stabilizing affective symptoms
• Blocks serotonin 2A receptors, causing enhancement of dopamine release in certain brain regions and thus reducing motor side effects and possibly improving cognitive and affective symptoms
• Interactions at a myriad of other neurotransmitter receptors may contribute to quetiapine's efficacy
✱ Specifically, actions at 5HT1A receptors may contribute to efficacy for cognitive and affective symptoms in some patients, especially at moderate to high doses

How Long Until It Works
• Psychotic symptoms can improve within 1 week, but it may take several weeks for full effect on behavior as well as on cognition and affective stabilization

• Classically recommended to wait at least 4–6 weeks to determine efficacy of drug, but in practice some patients require up to 16–20 weeks to show a good response, especially on cognitive symptoms

If It Works
• Most often reduces positive symptoms in schizophrenia but does not eliminate them
• Can improve negative symptoms, as well as aggressive, cognitive, and affective symptoms in schizophrenia
• Most schizophrenic patients do not have a total remission of symptoms but rather a reduction of symptoms by about a third
• Perhaps 5–15% of schizophrenic patients can experience an overall improvement of greater than 50–60%, especially when receiving stable treatment for more than a year
• Such patients are considered super-responders or "awakeners" since they may be well enough to be employed, live independently, and sustain long-term relationships
• Many bipolar patients may experience a reduction of symptoms by half or more
• Continue treatment until reaching a plateau of improvement
• After reaching a satisfactory plateau, continue treatment for at least a year after first episode of psychosis
• For second and subsequent episodes of psychosis, treatment may need to be indefinite
• Even for first episodes of psychosis, it may be preferable to continue treatment indefinitely to avoid subsequent episodes
• Treatment may not only reduce mania but also prevent recurrences of mania in bipolar disorder

If It Doesn't Work
• Try one of the other atypical antipsychotics (risperidone, olanzapine, ziprasidone, aripiprazole, amisulpride)
• If 2 or more antipsychotic monotherapies do not work, consider clozapine
• If no first-line atypical antipsychotic is effective, consider higher doses or augmentation with valproate or lamotrigine
• Some patients may require treatment with a conventional antipsychotic
• Consider noncompliance and switch to another antipsychotic with fewer side

QUETIAPINE (continued)

effects or to an antipsychotic that can be given by depot injection
- Consider initiating rehabilitation and psychotherapy
- Consider presence of concomitant drug abuse

Best Augmenting Combos for Partial Response or Treatment-Resistance

- Valproic acid (valproate, divalproex, divalproex ER)
- Other mood stabilizing anticonvulsants (carbamazepine, oxcarbazepine, lamotrigine)
- Lithium
- Benzodiazepines

Tests

Before starting an atypical antipsychotic
✶ Weigh all patients and track BMI during treatment
- Get baseline personal and family history of obesity, dyslipidemia, hypertension, and cardiovascular disease
✶ Get waist circumference (at umbilicus), blood pressure, fasting plasma glucose, and fasting lipid profile
- Determine if the patient is
  - overweight (BMI 25.0–29.9)
  - obese (BMI ≥30)
  - has pre-diabetes (fasting plasma glucose 100–125 mg/dl)
  - has diabetes (fasting plasma glucose >126 mg/dl)
  - has hypertension (BP >140/90 mm Hg)
  - has dyslipidemia (increased total cholesterol, LDL cholesterol, and triglycerides; decreased HDL cholesterol)
- Treat or refer such patients for treatment, including nutrition and weight management, physical activity counseling, smoking cessation, and medical management

Monitoring after starting an atypical antipsychotic
✶ BMI monthly for 3 months, then quarterly
✶ Blood pressure, fasting plasma glucose, fasting lipids within 3 months and then annually, but earlier and more frequently for patients with diabetes or who have gained >5% of initial weight
- Treat or refer for treatment and consider switching to another atypical antipsychotic

for patients who become overweight, obese, pre-diabetic, diabetic, hypertensive, or dyslipidemic while receiving an atypical antipsychotic
✶ Even in patients without known diabetes, be vigilant for the rare but life threatening onset of diabetic ketoacidosis, which always requires immediate treatment, by monitoring for the rapid onset of polyuria, polydipsia, weight loss, nausea, vomiting, dehydration, rapid respiration, weakness and clouding of sensorium, even coma
- Although U.S. manufacturer recommends 6-month eye checks for cataracts, clinical experience suggests this may be unnecessary

SIDE EFFECTS

How Drug Causes Side Effects
- By blocking histamine 1 receptors in the brain, it can cause sedation and possibly weight gain
- By blocking alpha 1 adrenergic receptors, it can cause dizziness, sedation, and hypotension
- By blocking muscarinic 1 receptors, it can cause dry mouth, constipation, and sedation
- By blocking dopamine 2 receptors in the striatum, it can cause motor side effects (rare)
- Mechanism of weight gain and increased incidence of diabetes and dyslipidemia with atypical antipsychotics is unknown

Notable Side Effects
✶ May increase risk for diabetes and dyslipidemia
✶ Dizziness, sedation
- Dry mouth, constipation, dyspepsia, abdominal pain, weight gain
- Tachycardia
- Orthostatic hypotension, usually during initial dose titration
- Theoretical risk of tardive dyskinesia

Life Threatening or Dangerous Side Effects
- Hyperglycemia, in some cases extreme and associated with ketoacidosis or hyperosmolar coma or death, has been

reported in patients taking atypical antipsychotics
- Rare neuroleptic malignant syndrome (much reduced risk compared to conventional antipsychotics)
- Rare seizures

Weight Gain

- Many patients experience and/or can be significant in amount at effective antipsychotic doses
- Can become a health problem in some
- May be less than for some antipsychotics, more than for others

Sedation

- Frequent and can be significant in amount
- Some patients may not tolerate it
- More than for some other antipsychotics, but never say always as not a problem in everyone
- Can wear off over time
- Can reemerge as dose increases and then wear off again over time

What To Do About Side Effects
- Wait
- Wait
- Wait
- Usually dosed twice daily, so take more of the total daily dose at bedtime to help reduce daytime sedation
- Start dosing low and increase slowly as side effects wear off at each dosing increment
- Weight loss, exercise programs, and medical management for high BMIs, diabetes, dyslipidemia
- Switch to another atypical antipsychotic

Best Augmenting Agents for Side Effects
- Many side effects cannot be improved with an augmenting agent

 DOSING AND USE

Usual Dosage Range
- 150–750 mg/day (in divided doses) for schizophrenia
- 400–800 mg/day (in divided doses) for acute bipolar mania

Dosage Forms
- Tablets 25 mg, 100 mg, 200 mg, 300 mg

How to Dose
- (according to manufacturer for schizophrenia): initial 25 mg/day twice a day; increase by 25–50 mg twice a day each day until desired efficacy is reached; maximum approved dose 800 mg/day
- In practice, can start adults with schizophrenia under age 65 with same doses as recommended for acute bipolar mania
- (according to manufacturing for acute bipolar mania): initiate in twice daily doses, totaling 100 mg/day on day 1, increasing to 400 mg/day on day 4 in increments of up to 100 mg/day; further dosage adjustments up to 800 mg/day by day 6 should be in increments of no greater than 200 mg/day

 Dosing Tips

✴ **More may be much more:** Clinical practice suggests quetiapine often underdosed, then switched prior to adequate trials
- Clinical practice suggests that at low doses it may be a sedative hypnotic, possibly due to potent H1 antihistamine actions, but this is an expensive use for which there are many other options
✴ Initial target dose of 400–800 mg/day should be reached in most cases to optimize the chances of success in treating acute psychosis and acute mania, but only a minority of patients are adequately dosed in clinical practice
- May be lower cost than some other atypical antipsychotics at 200 mg twice daily, but higher doses can be among the most costly for atypical antipsychotics
- Recommended titration to 400 mg/day by the fourth day can often be achieved when necessary to control acute symptoms
✴ Higher doses generally achieve greater response

✳ Occasional patients may require more than 800–1000 mg/day
- Rather than raise the dose above these levels in acutely agitated patients requiring acute antipsychotic actions, consider augmentation with a benzodiazepine or conventional antipsychotic, either orally or intramuscularly
- Rather than raise the dose above these levels in partial responders, consider augmentation with a mood stabilizing anticonvulsant such as valproate or lamotrigine
- Children and elderly should generally be dosed at the lower end of the dosage spectrum

Overdose
- Rarely lethal in monotherapy overdose; sedation, slurred speech, hypotension

Long-Term Use
- Often used for long-term maintenance in schizophrenia, bipolar disorder, and various behavioral disorders

Habit Forming
- No

How to Stop
- Slow down-titration (over 6 to 8 weeks), especially when simultaneously beginning a new antipsychotic while switching (i.e., cross-titration)
- Rapid discontinuation may lead to rebound psychosis and worsening of symptoms

Pharmacokinetics
- Metabolites are inactive
- Parent drug has 6–7 hour half-life

 Drug Interactions
- CYP450 3A inhibitors and CYP450 2D6 inhibitors may reduce clearance of quetiapine and thus raise quetiapine plasma levels, but dosage reduction of quetiapine usually not necessary
- May increase effect of anti-hypertensive agents

 Other Warnings/ Precautions
- In the U.S., manufacturer recommends examination for cataracts before and every 6 months after initiating quetiapine, but this does not seem to be necessary in clinical practice
- Quetiapine should be used cautiously in patients at risk for aspiration pneumonia, as dysphagia has been reported
- Priapism has been reported
- Use with caution in patients with known cardiovascular disease, cerebrovascular disease
- Use with caution in patients with conditions that predispose to hypotension (dehydration, overheating)

Do Not Use
- If there is a proven allergy to quetiapine

SPECIAL POPULATIONS

Renal Impairment
- No dose adjustment required

Hepatic Impairment
- Downward dose adjustment may be necessary

Cardiac Impairment
- Drug should be used with caution because of risk of orthostatic hypotension

Elderly
- Lower dose is generally used (e.g., 25–100 mg twice a day), although higher doses may be used if tolerated

 Children and Adolescents
- Not officially recommended for patients under age 18
- Clinical experience and early data suggest quetiapine may be safe and effective for behavioral disturbances in children and adolescents
- Children and adolescents using quetiapine may need to be monitored more often than adults
- May tolerate lower doses better

Pregnancy

- Risk Category C [some animal studies show adverse effects, no controlled studies in humans]
- Psychotic symptoms may worsen during pregnancy and some form of treatment may be necessary
- Quetiapine may be preferable to anticonvulsant mood stabilizers if treatment is required during pregnancy

Breast Feeding

- Unknown if quetiapine is secreted in human breast milk, but all psychotropics assumed to be secreted in breast milk
- Recommended either to discontinue drug or bottle feed
- Infants of women who choose to breast feed while on quetiapine should be monitored for possible adverse effects

THE ART OF PSYCHOPHARMACOLOGY

Potential Advantages

- Some cases of psychosis and bipolar disorder refractory to treatment with other antipsychotics
- ✳ Patients with Parkinson's disease who need an antipsychotic or mood stabilizer
- ✳ Patients with Lewy Body dementia who need an antipsychotic or mood stabilizer

Potential Disadvantages

- Patients requiring rapid onset of action
- Patients noncompliant with twice daily dosing

Primary Target Symptoms

- Positive symptoms of psychosis
- Negative symptoms of psychosis
- Cognitive symptoms
- Unstable mood (both depression and mania)
- Aggressive symptoms

 Pearls

- ✳ May be the preferred antipsychotic for psychosis in Parkinson's disease and Lewy Body dementia
- Anecdotal reports of efficacy in treatment-refractory cases and positive symptoms of psychoses other than schizophrenia
- ✳ Efficacy may be underestimated since quetiapine is mostly under-dosed in clinical practice
- More sedation than some other antipsychotics
- ✳ Essentially no motor side effects or prolactin elevation
- May have less weight gain than some antipsychotics, more than others
- ✳ Controversial as to whether quetiapine has more or less risk of diabetes and dyslipidemia than some other antipsychotics
- Can be a more expensive atypical antipsychotic than some others when dosed appropriately in schizophrenia or acute mania; some patients respond to moderate doses, which are less expensive
- Commonly used at low doses to augment other atypical antipsychotics, but such antipsychotic polypharmacy has not been systematically studied and can be quite expensive

 Suggested Reading

Kapur S, Remington G. Atypical antipsychotics: new directions and new challenges in the treatment of schizophrenia. Annu Rev Med 2001;52:503–17.

Srisurapanont M, Disayavanish C, Taimkaew K. Quetiapine for schizophrenia. Cochrane Database Syst Rev 2000;3:CD000967.

Tandon R. Safety and tolerability: how do new generation "atypical" antipsychotics compare? Psychiatric Quarterly 2002;73:297–311.

Tandon R, Jibson MD. Efficacy of newer generation antipsychotics in the treatment of schizophrenia. Psychoneuroendocrinology 2003;28:9–26.

Yatham LN. Efficacy of atypical antipsychotics in mood disorders. J Clin Psychopharmacol 2003;23(3 Suppl 1):S9–14.

REBOXETINE

THERAPEUTICS

Brands • Norebox
• Edronax
see index for additional brand names

Generic? No

 Class

• Selective norepinephrine reuptake inhibitor (NRI); antidepressant

Commonly Prescribed For
(bold for FDA approved)
• Major depressive disorder
• Dysthymia
• Panic disorder
• Attention deficit hyperactivity disorder

 How The Drug Works

• Boost neurotransmitters norepinephrine/ noradrenaline and dopamine
• Blocks norepinephrine reuptake pump (norepinephrine transporter)
• Presumably, this increases noradrenergic neurotransmission
• Since dopamine is inactivated by norepinephrine reuptake in frontal cortex which largely lacks dopamine transporters, reboxetine can increase dopamine neurotransmission in this part of the brain

How Long Until It Works
• Onset of therapeutic actions usually not immediate, but often delayed 2 to 4 weeks
• If it is not working within 6 to 8 weeks for depression, it may require a dosage increase or it may not work at all
• May continue to work for many years to prevent relapse of symptoms

If It Works
• The goal of treatment is complete remission of current symptoms as well as prevention of future relapses
• Treatment most often reduces or even eliminates symptoms, but not a cure since symptoms can recur after medicine stopped
• Continue treatment until all symptoms are gone (remission)
• Once symptoms gone, continue treating for 1 year for the first episode of depression

• For second and subsequent episodes of depression, treatment may need to be indefinite

If It Doesn't Work
• Many patients only have a partial response where some symptoms are improved but others persist (especially insomnia, fatigue, and problems concentrating)
• Other patients may be nonresponders, sometimes called treatment-resistant or treatment-refractory
• Consider increasing dose, switching to another agent or adding an appropriate augmenting agent
• Consider psychotherapy
• Consider evaluation for another diagnosis or for a comorbid condition (e.g., medical illness, substance abuse, etc.)
• Some patients may experience apparent lack of consistent efficacy due to activation of latent or underlying bipolar disorder, and require antidepressant discontinuation and a switch to a mood stabilizer

 Best Augmenting Combos for Partial Response or Treatment-Resistance

• Trazodone, especially for insomnia
• SSRIs, SNRIs, mirtazapine (use combinations of antidepressants with caution as this may activate bipolar disorder and suicidal ideation)
• Modafinil, especially for fatigue, sleepiness, and lack of concentration
• Mood stabilizers or atypical antipsychotics for bipolar depression, psychotic depression or treatment-resistant depression
• Benzodiazepines for anxiety
• Hypnotics for insomnia
• Classically, lithium, buspirone, or thyroid hormone

Tests
• None for healthy individuals

SIDE EFFECTS

How Drug Causes Side Effects
• Norepinephrine increases in parts of the brain and body and at receptors other than those that cause therapeutic actions (e.g., unwanted actions of norepinephrine on

acetylcholine release causing constipation and dry mouth, etc.)
- Most side effects are immediate but often go away with time

Notable Side Effects

- Insomnia, dizziness, anxiety, agitation
- Dry mouth, constipation
- Urinary hesitancy, urinary retention
- Sexual dysfunction (impotence)
- Dose-dependent hypotension

 ### Life Threatening or Dangerous Side Effects

- Rare seizures
- Rare induction of mania and activation of suicidal ideation

Weight Gain

unusual   not unusual   common   problematic

- Reported but not expected

Sedation

unusual   not unusual   common   problematic

- Reported but not expected

What To Do About Side Effects

- Wait
- Wait
- Wait
- Lower the dose
- In a few weeks, switch or add other drugs

Best Augmenting Agents for Side Effects

- For urinary hesitancy, give an alpha 1 blocker such as tamsulosin
- Often best to try another antidepressant monotherapy prior to resorting to augmentation strategies to treat side effects
- Trazodone or a hypnotic for drug-induced insomnia
- Benzodiazepines for drug-induced anxiety and activation
- Mirtazapine for drug-induced insomnia or anxiety
- Many side effects are dose-dependent (i.e., they increase as dose increases, or they reemerge until tolerance re-develops)
- Many side effects are time-dependent (i.e., they start immediately upon dosing and

upon each dose increase, but go away with time)
- Activation and agitation may represent the induction of a bipolar state, especially a mixed dysphoric bipolar II condition sometimes associated with suicidal ideation, and require the addition of lithium, a mood stabilizer or an atypical antipsychotic, and/or discontinuation of reboxetine

DOSING AND USE

Usual Dosage Range

- 8 mg/day in 2 doses (10 mg usual maximum daily dose)

Dosage Forms

- Tablet 2 mg, 4 mg scored

How to Dose

- Initial 2 mg/day twice a day for 1 week, 4 mg/day twice a day for second week

 ### Dosing Tips

- When switching from another antidepressant or adding to another antidepressant, dosing may need to be lower and titration slower to prevent activating side effects (e.g., 2 mg in the daytime for 2–3 days, then 2 mg bid for 1–2 weeks)
- Give second daily dose in late afternoon rather than at bedtime to avoid undesired activation or insomnia in the evening
- May not need full dose of 8 mg/day when given in conjunction with another antidepressant
- Some patients may need 10 mg/day or more if well-tolerated without orthostatic hypotension and if additional efficacy is seen at high doses in difficult cases
- Early dosing in patients with panic and anxiety may need to be lower and titration slower, perhaps with the use of concomitant short-term benzodiazepines to increase tolerability

Overdose

- Postural hypotension, anxiety, hypertension

Long-Term Use

- Safe

Habit Forming
- No

How to Stop
- Taper not necessary

Pharmacokinetics
- Metabolized by CYP450 3A4
- Inhibits CYP450 2D6 and 3A4 at high doses
- Elimination half-life approximately 13 hours

 Drug Interactions
- Tramadol increases the risk of seizures in patients taking an antidepressant
- May need to reduce reboxetine dose or avoid concomitant use with inhibitors of CYP450 3A4, such as azole and antifungals, macrolide antibiotics, fluvoxamine, nefazodone, fluoxetine, sertraline, etc.
- Via CYP450 2D6 inhibition, reboxetine could theoretically interfere with the analgesic actions of codeine, and increase the plasma levels of some beta blockers and of atomoxetine and TCAs
- Via CYP450 2D6 inhibition, reboxetine could theoretically increase concentrations of thioridazine and cause dangerous cardiac arrhythmias
- Via CYP450 3A4 inhibition, reboxetine may increase the levels of alprazolam, buspirone, and triazolam
- Via CYP450 3A4 inhibition, reboxetine could theoretically increase concentrations of certain cholesterol lowering HMG CoA reductase inhibitors, especially simvastatin, atorvastatin, and lovastatin, but not pravastatin or fluvastatin, which would increase the risk of rhabdomyolysis; thus, coadministration of reboxetine with certain HMG CoA reductase inhibitors should proceed with caution
- Via CYP450 3A4 inhibition, reboxetine could theoretically increase the concentrations of pimozide, and cause QTc prolongation and dangerous cardiac arrhythmias
- Use with ergotamine may increase blood pressure
- Hypokalemia may occur if reboxetine is used with diuretics
- Do not use with MAO inhibitors, including 14 days after MAOIs are stopped

 Other Warnings/ Precautions
- Use with caution in patients with bipolar disorder unless treated with concomitant mood stabilizing agent
- Use with caution in patients with urinary retention, benign prostatic hyperplasia, glaucoma, epilepsy
- Use with caution with drugs that lower blood pressure
- Monitor patients for activation of suicidal ideation, especially children and adolescents

Do Not Use
- If patient has narrow angle-closure glaucoma
- If patient is taking an MAO inhibitor
- If patient is taking pimozide or thioridazine
- If there is a proven allergy to reboxetine

SPECIAL POPULATIONS

Renal Impairment
- Plasma concentrations are increased
- May need to lower dose

Hepatic Impairment
- Plasma concentrations are increased
- May need to lower dose

Cardiac Impairment
- Use with caution

Elderly
- Lower dose is recommended (4–6 mg/day)

 Children and Adolescents
- Use with caution, observing for activation of known or unknown bipolar disorder and/or suicidal ideation, and strongly consider informing parents or guardian of this risk so they can help observe child or adolescent patients
- No guidelines for children; safety and efficacy have not been established

 Pregnancy
- No controlled studies in humans
- Not generally recommended for use during pregnancy, especially during first trimester

- Must weigh the risk of treatment (first trimester fetal development, third trimester newborn delivery) to the child against the risk of no treatment (recurrence of depression, maternal health, infant bonding) to the mother and child
- For many patients this may mean continuing treatment during pregnancy

Breast Feeding

- Some drug is found in mother's breast milk
- Immediate postpartum period is a high-risk time for depression, especially in women who have had prior depressive episodes, so drug may need to be reinstituted late in the third trimester or shortly after childbirth to prevent a recurrence during the postpartum period
- Must weigh benefits of breast feeding with risks and benefits of antidepressant treatment versus non-treatment to both the infant and the mother
- For many patients, this may mean continuing treatment during breast feeding

THE ART OF PSYCHOPHARMACOLOGY

Potential Advantages

- Tired, unmotivated patients
- Patients with cognitive disturbances
- Patients with psychomotor retardation

Potential Disadvantages

- Patients unable to comply with twice-daily dosing
- Patients unable to tolerate activation

Primary Target Symptoms

- Depressed mood
- Energy, motivation, and interest
- Suicidal ideation
- Cognitive disturbance
- Psychomotor retardation

 Pearls

- May be effective if SSRIs have failed or for SSRI "poop-out"
- ✳ May be more likely than SSRIs to improve social and work functioning
- Reboxetine is a mixture of an active and an inactive enantiomer, and the active enantiomer may be developed in future clinical testing
- ✳ Side effects may appear "anticholinergic", but reboxetine does not directly block muscarinic receptors
- Constipation, dry mouth, and urinary retention are noradrenergic, due in part to peripheral alpha 1 receptor stimulation causing decreased acetylcholine release
- ✳ Thus, antidotes for these side effects can be alpha 1 antagonists such as tamsulosin, especially for urinary retention in men over 50 with borderline urine flow
- Novel use of reboxetine may be for attention deficit disorder, analogous to the actions of another norepinephrine selective reuptake inhibitor, atomoxetine, but few controlled studies
- Another novel use may be for neuropathic pain, alone or in combination with other antidepressants, but few controlled studies
- Some studies suggest efficacy in panic disorder

 Suggested Reading

Fleishaker JC. Clinical pharmacokinetics of reboxetine, a selective norepinephrine reuptake inhibitor for the treatment of patients with depression. Clin Pharmacokinet 2000;39(6):413–27.

Kasper S, el Giamal N, Hilger E. Reboxetine: the first selective noradrenaline re-uptake inhibitor. Expert Opin Pharmacother 2000;1(4):771–82.

Keller M. Role of serotonin and noradrenaline in social dysfunction: a review of data on reboxetine and the Social Adaptation Self-evaluation Scale (SASS). Gen Hosp Psychiatry 2001;23(1):15–9.

Tanum L. Reboxetine: tolerability and safety profile in patients with major depression. Acta Psychiatr Scand Suppl 2000;402:37–40.

RISPERIDONE

THERAPEUTICS

Brands • Risperdal • CONSTA
see index for additional brand names

Generic? Not in U.S., Europe, or Japan

Class
- Atypical antipsychotic (serotonin-dopamine antagonist; second generation antipsychotic; also a mood stabilizer)

Commonly Prescribed For
(bold for FDA approved)
- **Schizophrenia (oral, long-acting microspheres intramuscularly)**
- **Delaying relapse in schizophrenia (oral)**
- **Other psychotic disorders (oral)**
- **Acute mania (oral, monotherapy and adjunct to lithium or valproate)**
- Bipolar maintenance
- Bipolar depression
- Behavioral disturbances in dementias
- Behavioral disturbances in children and adolescents
- Disorders associated with problems with impulse control

How The Drug Works
- Blocks dopamine 2 receptors, reducing positive symptoms of psychosis and stabilizing affective symptoms
- Blocks serotonin 2A receptors, causing enhancement of dopamine release in certain brain regions and thus reducing motor side effects and possibly improving cognitive and affective symptoms
- Interactions at a myriad of other neurotransmitter receptors may contribute to risperidone's efficacy
- * Specifically, alpha 2 antagonist properties may contribute to antidepressant actions

How Long Until It Works
- Psychotic symptoms can improve within 1 week, but it may take several weeks for full effect on behavior as well as on cognition and affective stabilization
- Classically recommended to wait at least 4–6 weeks to determine efficacy of drug, but in practice some patients require up to 16–20 weeks to show a good response, especially on cognitive symptoms

If It Works
- Most often reduces positive symptoms in schizophrenia but does not eliminate them
- Can improve negative symptoms, as well as aggressive, cognitive, and affective symptoms in schizophrenia
- Most schizophrenic patients do not have a total remission of symptoms but rather a reduction of symptoms by about a third
- Perhaps 5–15% of schizophrenic patients can experience an overall improvement of greater than 50–60%, especially when receiving stable treatment for more than a year
- Such patients are considered super-responders or "awakeners" since they may be well enough to be employed, live independently, and sustain long-term relationships
- Many bipolar patients may experience a reduction of symptoms by half or more
- Continue treatment until reaching a plateau of improvement
- After reaching a satisfactory plateau, continue treatment for at least a year after first episode of psychosis
- For second and subsequent episodes of psychosis, treatment may need to be indefinite
- Even for first episodes of psychosis, it may be preferable to continue treatment indefinitely to avoid subsequent episodes
- Treatment may not only reduce mania but also prevent recurrences of mania in bipolar disorder

If It Doesn't Work
- Try one of the other atypical antipsychotics (olanzapine, quetiapine, ziprasidone, aripiprazole, amisulpride)
- If 2 or more antipsychotic monotherapies do not work, consider clozapine
- If no first-line atypical antipsychotic is effective, consider higher doses or augmentation with valproate or lamotrigine
- Some patients may require treatment with a conventional antipsychotic
- Consider noncompliance and switch to another antipsychotic with fewer side effects or to an antipsychotic that can be given by depot injection
- Consider initiating rehabilitation and psychotherapy
- Consider presence of concomitant drug abuse

Best Augmenting Combos for Partial Response or Treatment-Resistance
- Valproic acid (valproate, divalproex, divalproex ER)
- Other mood stabilizing anticonvulsants (carbamazepine, oxcarbazepine, lamotrigine)
- Lithium
- Benzodiazepines

Tests

Before starting an atypical antipsychotic
✻ Weigh all patients and track BMI during treatment
- Get baseline personal and family history of obesity, dyslipidemia, hypertension, and cardiovascular disease
✻ Get waist circumference (at umbilicus), blood pressure, fasting plasma glucose, and fasting lipid profile
- Determine if the patient is
  - overweight (BMI 25.0–29.9)
  - obese (BMI ≥30)
  - has pre-diabetes (fasting plasma glucose 100–125 mg/dl)
  - has diabetes (fasting plasma glucose >126 mg/dl)
  - has hypertension (BP >140/90 mm Hg)
  - has dyslipidemia (increased total cholesterol, LDL cholesterol, and triglycerides; decreased HDL cholesterol)
- Treat or refer such patients for treatment, including nutrition and weight management, physical activity counseling, smoking cessation, and medical management

Monitoring after starting an atypical antipsychotic
✻ BMI monthly for 3 months, then quarterly
✻ Blood pressure, fasting plasma glucose, fasting lipids within 3 months and then annually, but earlier and more frequently for patients with diabetes or who have gained >5% of initial weight
- Treat or refer for treatment and consider switching to another atypical antipsychotic for patients who become overweight, obese, pre-diabetic, diabetic, hypertensive, or dyslipidemic while receiving an atypical antipsychotic
✻ Even in patients without known diabetes, be vigilant for the rare but life threatening onset of diabetic ketoacidosis, which always requires immediate treatment, by monitoring for the rapid onset of polyuria,

polydipsia, weight loss, nausea, vomiting, dehydration, rapid respiration, weakness and clouding of sensorium, even coma
- Should check blood pressure in the elderly before starting and for the first few weeks of treatment
- Monitoring elevated prolactin levels of dubious clinical benefit

SIDE EFFECTS

How Drug Causes Side Effects
- By blocking alpha 1 adrenergic receptors, it can cause dizziness, sedation, and hypotension
- By blocking dopamine 2 receptors in the striatum, it can cause motor side effects, especially at high doses
- By blocking dopamine 2 receptors in the pituitary, it can cause elevations in prolactin
- Mechanism of weight gain and increased incidence of diabetes and dyslipidemia with atypical antipsychotics is unknown

Notable Side Effects
✻ May increase risk for diabetes and dyslipidemia
✻ Dose-dependent extrapyramidal symptoms
✻ Dose-related hyperprolactinemia
- Rare tardive dyskinesia (much reduced risk compared to conventional antipsychotics)
- Dizziness, insomnia, headache, anxiety, sedation
- Nausea, constipation, abdominal pain, weight gain
- Rare orthostatic hypotension, usually during initial dose titration
- Tachycardia, sexual dysfunction

Life Threatening or Dangerous Side Effects
- Hyperglycemia, in some cases extreme and associated with ketoacidosis or hyperosmolar coma or death, has been reported in patients taking atypical antipsychotics
- Increased incidence of cerebrovascular events, including stroke, transient ischemic attacks, and fatalities in elderly patients with dementia
- Increased incidence of mortality in elderly patients with dementia-related psychosis

- Rare neuroleptic malignant syndrome (much reduced risk compared to conventional antipsychotics)
- Rare seizures

Weight Gain

unusual   not unusual   **common**   problematic

- Many patients experience and/or can be significant in amount
- Can become a health problem in some
- May be less than for some antipsychotics, more than for others

Sedation

unusual   not unusual   **common**   problematic

- Many patients experience and/or can be significant in amount
- Usually transient
- May be less than for some antipsychotics, more than for others

What To Do About Side Effects

- Wait
- Wait
- Wait
- Take at bedtime to help reduce daytime sedation
- Anticholinergics may reduce motor side effects when present
- Weight loss, exercise programs, and medical management for high BMIs, diabetes, dyslipidemia
- Switch to another atypical antipsychotic

Best Augmenting Agents for Side Effects

- Benztropine or trihexyphenidyl for motor side effects
- Many side effects cannot be improved with an augmenting agent

DOSING AND USE

Usual Dosage Range

- 2–8 mg/day orally for acute psychosis and bipolar disorder
- 0.5–2.0 mg/day orally for children and elderly
- 25–50 mg depot intramuscularly every 2 weeks

Dosage Forms

- Tablets 0.25 mg, 0.5 mg, 1 mg, 2 mg, 3 mg, 4 mg
- Orally disintegrating tablets 0.5 mg, 1 mg, 2 mg
- Liquid 1 mg/mL — 30 mL bottle
- Risperidone long-acting depot microspheres formulation for deep intramuscular administration 25 mg vial/kit, 37.5 mg vial/kit, 50 mg vial/kit

How to Dose

- In adults with psychosis in non-emergent settings, initial dosage recommendation is 1 mg/day orally in 2 divided doses
- Increase each day by 1 mg/day orally until desired efficacy is reached
- Maximum generally 16 mg/day orally
- Typically maximum effect is seen at 4–8 mg/day orally
- Can be administered on a once daily schedule as well as twice daily orally
- Long-acting risperidone is not recommended for patients who have not first demonstrated tolerability to oral risperidone
- Long-acting risperidone should be administered every 2 weeks by deep intramuscular gluteal injection
- Oral antipsychotic medication should be given with the first injection of long-acting risperidone and continued for 3 weeks, then discontinued
- Long-acting risperidone should only be administered by a health care professional
- Typically maximum effect with long-acting risperidone is seen at 25–50 mg every 2 weeks; maximum recommended dose is 50 mg every 2 weeks
- Titration of long-acting risperidone should occur at intervals of no less than 4 weeks
- Two different dosage strengths of long-acting risperidone should not be combined in a single administration

 Dosing Tips – Oral Formulation

* **Less may be more:** lowering the dose in some patients with stable efficacy but side effects may reduce side effects without loss of efficacy, especially for doses over 6 mg/day orally
* Target doses for best efficacy/best tolerability in many adults with psychosis

or bipolar disorder may be 2–6 mg/day (average 4.5 mg/day) orally
- Patients who respond to these doses may have one of the lowest drug costs among the atypical antipsychotics
- Low doses may not be adequate in difficult patients
- Rather than raise the dose above these levels in acutely agitated patients requiring acute antipsychotic actions, consider augmentation with a benzodiazepine or conventional antipsychotic, either orally or intramuscularly
- Rather than raise the dose above these levels in partial responders, consider augmentation with a mood stabilizing anticonvulsant, such as valproate or lamotrigine
- Approved for use up to 16 mg/day orally, but data suggest that risk of extrapyramidal symptoms is increased above 6 mg/day
- Risperidone oral solution is not compatible with cola or tea
- Children and elderly may need to have oral twice daily dosing during initiation and titration of drug dosing and then can switch to oral once daily when maintenance dose is reached
- Children and elderly should generally be dosed at the lower end of the dosage spectrum

 Dosing Tips – Long-Acting Microsphere Depot Formulation

* When initiating long-acting risperidone formulation by intramuscular injection, onset of action can be delayed for 2 weeks while microspheres are being absorbed
* For antipsychotic coverage during initiation of long-acting risperidone, continue ongoing treatment with an oral antipsychotic or initiate treatment with some oral antipsychotic for 3 weeks
- Steady-state plasma concentrations are reached after 4 injections of long-acting risperidone and maintained for 4–6 weeks after the last injection
- For missed long-acting risperidone injections 2 or more weeks late (i.e., 28 or more days following last injection), may need to provide antipsychotic coverage with oral administration for 3 weeks while reinitiating injections

- For missed long-acting risperidone injections up to 2 weeks late (i.e., within 28 days of last injection), may not need to provide oral coverage
- Long-acting risperidone must be kept refrigerated
- Must deliver each syringe in full since drug is not in a solution (i.e., half a syringe is not necessarily half the drug dose)

Overdose
- Rarely lethal in monotherapy overdose; sedation, rapid heartbeat, convulsions, low blood pressure, difficulty breathing

Long-Term Use
- Approved to delay relapse in long-term treatment of schizophrenia
- Often used for long-term maintenance in bipolar disorder and various behavioral disorders

Habit Forming
- No

How to Stop
- Slow down-titration of oral formulation (over 6 to 8 weeks), especially when simultaneously beginning a new antipsychotic while switching (i.e., cross-titration)
- Rapid oral discontinuation may lead to rebound psychosis and worsening of symptoms

Pharmacokinetics
- Metabolites are active
- Metabolized by CYP450 2D6
- Parent drug of oral formulation has 20–24 hour half-life
- Long-acting risperidone has 3–6 day half-life
- Long-acting risperidone has elimination phase of approximately 7–8 weeks after last injection

 Drug Interactions
- May increase effect of anti-hypertensive agents
- May antagonize levodopa, dopamine agonists
- Clearance of risperidone may be reduced and thus plasma levels increased by clozapine; dosing adjustment usually not necessary

- Co-administration with carbamazepine may decrease plasma levels of risperidone
- Co-administration with fluoxetine and paroxetine may increase plasma levels of risperidone
- Since risperidone is metabolized by CYP450 2D6, any agent that inhibits this enzyme could theoretically raise risperidone plasma levels; however, dose reduction of risperidone is usually not necessary when such combinations are used

⚠ Other Warnings/ Precautions

- Use with caution in patients with conditions that predispose to hypotension (dehydration, overheating)
- Risperidone should be used cautiously in patients at risk for aspiration pneumonia, as dysphagia has been reported
- Priapism has been reported

Do Not Use

- If there is a proven allergy to risperidone

SPECIAL POPULATIONS

Renal Impairment

- Initial 0.5 mg orally twice a day for first week; increase to 1 mg twice a day during second week
- Long-acting risperidone should not be administered unless patient has demonstrated tolerability of at least 2 mg/day orally
- Long-acting risperidone should be dosed at 25 mg every 2 weeks; oral administration should be continued for 3 weeks after the first injection

Hepatic Impairment

- Initial 0.5 mg orally twice a day for first week; increase to 1 mg twice a day during second week
- Long-acting risperidone should not be administered unless patient has demonstrated tolerability of at least 2 mg/day orally
- Long-acting risperidone should be dosed at 25 mg every two weeks; oral administration should be continued for 3 weeks after the first injection

Cardiac Impairment

- Drug should be used with caution because of risk of orthostatic hypotension
- ✳ When administered to elderly patients with atrial fibrillation, may increase the chances of stroke

Elderly

- Initial 0.5 mg orally twice a day; increase by 0.5 mg twice a day; titrate once a week for doses above 1.5 mg twice a day
- Recommended dose of long-acting risperidone is 25 mg every 2 weeks; oral administration should be continued for 3 weeks after the first injection

 Children and Adolescents

- Safety and effectiveness have not been established
- ✳ However, risperidone is the most frequently used atypical antipsychotic in children and adolescents
- Clinical experience and early data suggest risperidone is safe and effective for behavioral disturbances in children and adolescents
- Children and adolescents using risperidone may need to be monitored more often than adults

 Pregnancy

- Risk Category C [some animal studies show adverse effects, no controlled studies in humans]
- Psychotic symptoms may worsen during pregnancy and some form of treatment may be necessary
- Early findings of infants exposed to risperidone in utero do not show adverse consequences
- Risperidone may be preferable to anticonvulsant mood stabilizers if treatment is required during pregnancy
- Effects of hyperprolactinemia on the fetus are unknown

Breast Feeding

- Unknown if risperidone is secreted in human breast milk, but all psychotropics assumed to be secreted in breast milk
- ✳ Recommended either to discontinue drug or bottle feed

• Infants of women who choose to breast feed while on risperidone should be monitored for possible adverse effects

THE ART OF PSYCHOPHARMACOLOGY

Potential Advantages

• Some cases of psychosis and bipolar disorder refractory to treatment with other antipsychotics
✳ Often a preferred treatment for dementia with aggressive features
✳ Often a preferred atypical antipsychotic for children with behavioral disturbances of multiple causations
✳ Non-compliant patients (long-acting risperidone)
✳ Long-term outcomes may be enhanced when compliance is enhanced (long-acting risperidone)

Potential Disadvantages

• Patients for whom elevated prolactin may not be desired (e.g., possibly pregnant patients; pubescent girls with amenorrhea; postmenopausal women with low estrogen who do not take estrogen replacement therapy)

Primary Target Symptoms

• Positive symptoms of psychosis
• Negative symptoms of psychosis
• Cognitive functioning
• Unstable mood (both depression and mania)
• Aggressive symptoms

Pearls

✳ Well accepted for treatment of agitation and aggression in elderly demented patients
✳ Well accepted for treatment of behavioral symptoms in children and adolescents, but may have more sedation and weight gain in pediatric populations than in adult populations
• Many anecdotal reports of utility in treatment-refractory cases and for positive symptoms of psychosis in disorders other than schizophrenia
• Only atypical antipsychotic to consistently raise prolactin, but this is of unproven and uncertain clinical significance
• Hyperprolactinemia in women with low estrogen may accelerate osteoporosis
• Less weight gain than some antipsychotics, more than others
• Less sedation than some antipsychotics, more than others
• Risperidone is one of the least expensive atypical antipsychotics within the usual therapeutic dosing range
• Increased risk of stroke may be most relevant in the elderly with atrial fibrillation
✳ Controversial as to whether risperidone has more or less risk of diabetes and dyslipidemia than some other antipsychotics
• May cause more motor side effects than some other atypical antipsychotics, especially when administered to patients with Parkinson's disease or Lewy Body dementia
✳ Only atypical antipsychotic with a long-acting depot formulation

Suggested Reading

Kapur S, Remington G. Atypical antipsychotics: new directions and new challenges in the treatment of schizophrenia. Annu Rev Med 2001;52:503–17.

Schweitzer I. Does risperidone have a place in the treatment of nonschizophrenic patients? International Clinical Psychopharmacology 2001;16:1–19.

Tandon R. Safety and tolerability: how do new generation "atypical" antipsychotics compare? Psychiatric Quarterly 2002;73:297–311.

Tandon R, Jibson MD. Efficacy of newer generation antipsychotics in the treatment of schizophrenia. Psychoneuroendocrinology 2003;28:9–26.

Yatham LN. Efficacy of atypical antipsychotics in mood disorders. J Clin Psychopharmacol 2003;23(3 Suppl 1):S9–14.

RIVASTIGMINE

THERAPEUTICS

Brands • Exelon
see index for additional brand names

Generic? No

Class
• Cholinesterase inhibitor
(acetylcholinesterase inhibitor and
butyrylcholinesterase inhibitor); cognitive
enhancer

Commonly Prescribed For
(bold for FDA approved)
• **Alzheimer disease**
• Memory disorders in other conditions
• Mild cognitive impairment

How The Drug Works
✶ Pseudoirreversibly inhibits centrally-
active acetylcholinesterase (AChE), making
more acetylcholine available
• Increased availability of acetylcholine
compensates in part for degenerating
cholinergic neurons in neocortex that
regulate memory
✶ Inhibits butyrylcholinesterase (BuChE)
• May release growth factors or interfere
with amyloid deposition

How Long Until It Works
• May take up to 6 weeks before any
improvement in baseline memory or
behavior is evident
• May take months before any stabilization in
degenerative course is evident

If It Works
• May improve symptoms and slow
progression of disease, but does not
reverse the degenerative process

If It Doesn't Work
• Consider adjusting dose, switching to a
different cholinesterase inhibitor or adding
an appropriate augmenting agent
• Reconsider diagnosis and rule out other
conditions such as depression or a
dementia other than Alzheimer disease

Best Augmenting Combos for Partial Response or Treatment-Resistance
✶ Atypical antipsychotics to reduce
behavioral disturbances
✶ Antidepressants if concomitant
depression, apathy, or lack of interest
✶ Memantine for moderate to severe
Alzheimer disease
• Divalproex, carbamazepine, or
oxcarbazepine for behavioral disturbances

Tests
• None for healthy individuals

SIDE EFFECTS

How Drug Causes Side Effects
• Peripheral inhibition of acetylcholinesterase
can cause gastrointestinal side effects
• Peripheral inhibition of
butyrylcholinesterase can cause
gastrointestinal side effects
• Central inhibition of acetylcholinesterase
may contribute to nausea, vomiting, weight
loss, and sleep disturbances

Notable Side Effects
✶ Nausea, diarrhea, vomiting, appetite loss,
weight loss, dyspepsia, increased gastric
acid secretion
• Headache, dizziness
• Fatigue, asthenia, sweating

Life Threatening or Dangerous Side Effects
• Rare seizures
• Rare syncope

Weight Gain

unusual   not unusual   common   problematic

• Reported but not expected
• Some patients may experience weight loss

Sedation

unusual   not unusual   common   problematic

• Reported but not expected

What To Do About Side Effects
• Wait

- Wait
- Wait
- Use slower dose titration
- Consider lowering dose, switching to a different agent or adding an appropriate augmenting agent

Best Augmenting Agents for Side Effects

- Many side effects cannot be improved with an augmenting agent

DOSING AND USE

Usual Dosage Range

- 6–12 mg/day

Dosage Forms

- Capsule 1.5 mg, 3 mg, 4.5 mg, 6 mg
- Liquid 2 mg/mL – 120 mL bottle

How to Dose

- Initial 1.5 mg twice daily; increase by 3 mg every 2 weeks; titrate to tolerability; maximum dose generally 6 mg twice daily

 Dosing Tips

- Incidence of nausea is generally higher during the titration phase than during maintenance treatment
- ✳ If restarting treatment after a lapse of several days or more, dose titration should occur as when starting drug for the first time
- Doses between 6–12 mg/day have been shown to be more effective than doses between 1–4 mg/day
- Recommended to take rivastigmine with food
- Rapid dose titration increases the incidence of gastrointestinal side effects
- Probably best to utilize highest tolerated dose within the usual dosage range
- ✳ When switching to another cholinesterase inhibitor, probably best to cross-titrate from one to the other to prevent precipitous decline in function if the patient washes out of one drug entirely

Overdose

- Can be lethal; nausea, vomiting, excess salivation, sweating, hypotension, bradycardia, collapse, convulsions, muscle weakness (weakness of respiratory muscles can lead to death)

Long-Term Use

- Drug may lose effectiveness in slowing degenerative course of Alzheimer disease after 6 months
- Can be effective in many patients for several years

Habit Forming

- No

How to Stop

- Taper not necessary
- Discontinuation may lead to notable deterioration in memory and behavior which may not be restored when drug is restarted or another cholinesterase inhibitor is initiated

Pharmacokinetics

- Elimination half-life 1–2 hours
- Not hepatically metabolized; no CYP450-mediated pharmacokinetic drug interactions

 Drug Interactions

- Rivastigmine may increase the effects of anesthetics and should be discontinued prior to surgery
- Rivastigmine may interact with anticholinergic agents and the combination may decrease the efficacy of both
- Clearance of rivastigmine may be increased by nicotine
- May have synergistic effect if administered with cholinomimetics (e.g., bethanechol)
- Bradycardia may occur if combined with beta blockers
- Theoretically, could reduce the efficacy of levodopa in Parkinson's disease
- Not rational to combine with another cholinesterase inhibitor

 Other Warnings/ Precautions

- May exacerbate asthma or other pulmonary disease
- Increased gastric acid secretion may increase the risk of ulcers

• Bradycardia or heart block may occur in patients with or without cardiac impairment
❋ Severe vomiting with esophageal rupture may occur if rivastigmine therapy is resumed without re-titrating the drug to full dosing

Do Not Use

• If there is a proven allergy to rivastigmine or other carbamates

Renal Impairment

• Dose adjustment not necessary; titrate to point of tolerability

Hepatic Impairment

• Dose adjustment not necessary; titrate to point of tolerability

Cardiac Impairment

• Should be used with caution
• Syncopal episodes have been reported with the use of rivastigmine

Elderly

• Some patients may tolerate lower doses better

 Children and Adolescents

• Safety and efficacy have not been established

 Pregnancy

• Risk Category B [animal studies do not show adverse effects, no controlled studies in humans]
❋ Not recommended for use in pregnant women or women of childbearing potential

Breast Feeding

• Unknown if rivastigmine is secreted in human breast milk, but all psychotropics assumed to be secreted in breast milk
❋ Recommended either to discontinue drug or bottle feed
• Rivastigmine is not recommended for use in nursing women

Potential Advantages

• Theoretically, butyrylcholinesterase inhibition centrally could enhance therapeutic efficacy
• May be useful in some patients who do not respond to or do not tolerate other cholinesterase inhibitors
• Later stages or rapidly progressive Alzheimer disease

Potential Disadvantages

• Theoretically, butyrylcholinesterase inhibition peripherally could enhance side effects

Primary Target Symptoms

• Memory loss in Alzheimer disease
• Behavioral symptoms in Alzheimer disease
• Memory loss in other dementias

 Pearls

• Dramatic reversal of symptoms of Alzheimer disease is not generally seen with cholinesterase inhibitors
• Can lead to therapeutic nihilism among prescribers and lack of an appropriate trial of a cholinesterase inhibitor
❋ Perhaps only 50% of Alzheimer patients are diagnosed, and only 50% of those diagnosed are treated, and only 50% of those treated are given a cholinesterase inhibitor, and then only for 200 days in a disease that lasts 7–10 years
• Must evaluate lack of efficacy and loss of efficacy over months, not weeks
❋ Treats behavioral and psychological symptoms of Alzheimer dementia as well as cognitive symptoms (i.e., especially apathy, disinhibition, delusions, anxiety, cooperation, pacing)
• Patients who complain themselves of memory problems may have depression, whereas patients whose spouses or children complain of the patient's memory problems may have Alzheimer disease
• Treat the patient but ask the caregiver about efficacy
• What you see may depend upon how early you treat
• The first symptoms of Alzheimer disease are generally mood changes; thus,

Alzheimer disease may initially be diagnosed as depression

- Women may experience cognitive symptoms in perimenopause as a result of hormonal changes that are not a sign of dementia or Alzheimer disease
- Aggressively treat concomitant symptoms with augmentation (e.g., atypical antipsychotics for agitation, antidepressants for depression)
- If treatment with antidepressants fails to improve apathy and depressed mood in the elderly, it is possible that this represents early Alzheimer disease and a cholinesterase inhibitor like rivastigmine may be helpful
- What to expect from a cholinesterase inhibitor:
  - Patients do not generally improve dramatically although this can be observed in a significant minority of patients
  - Onset of behavioral problems and nursing home placement can be delayed
  - Functional outcomes, including activities of daily living, can be preserved
  - Caregiver burden and stress can be reduced
- Delay in progression in Alzheimer disease is not evidence of disease-modifying actions of cholinesterase inhibition
- Cholinesterase inhibitors like rivastigmine depend upon the presence of intact targets for acetylcholine for maximum effectiveness and thus may be most effective in the early stages of Alzheimer disease
- The most prominent side effects of rivastigmine are gastrointestinal effects, which are usually mild and transient
- ✳ May cause more gastrointestinal side effects than some other cholinesterase inhibitors, especially if not slowly titrated
- Use with caution in underweight or frail patients
- Weight loss can be a problem in Alzheimer patients with debilitation and muscle wasting
- Women over 85, particularly with low body weights, may experience more adverse effects
- For patients with intolerable side effects, generally allow a washout period with

resolution of side effects prior to switching to another cholinesterase inhibitor

- Cognitive improvement may be linked to substantial (>65%) inhibition of acetylcholinesterase
- Rivastigmine may be more selective for the form of acetylcholinesterase in hippocampus (G1)
- ✳ More potent inhibitor of the G1 form of acetylcholinesterase enzyme, found in high concentrations in Alzheimer patient's brains, than the G4 form of the enzyme
- Butyrylcholinesterase action in the brain may not be relevant in individuals without Alzheimer disease or in early Alzheimer disease; in the later stages of the disease, enzyme actively increases as gliosis occurs
- Rivastigmine's effects on butyrylcholinesterase may be more relevant in later stages of Alzheimer disease, when gliosis is occurring
- ✳ May be more useful for later stages or for more rapidly progressive forms of Alzheimer disease, when gliosis increases butyrlylcholinesterase
- ✳ Butyrylcholinesterase actively could interfere with amyloid plaque formation, which contains this enzyme
- Some Alzheimer patients who fail to respond to another cholinesterase inhibitor may respond when switched to rivastigmine
- Some Alzheimer patients who fail to respond to rivastigmine may respond to another cholinesterase inhibitor
- To prevent potential clinical deterioration, generally switch from long-term treatment with one cholinesterase inhibitor to another without a washout period
- ✳ May slow the progression of mild cognitive impairment to Alzheimer disease
- ✳ May be useful for dementia with Lewy bodies (DLB, constituted by early loss of attentiveness and visual perception with possible hallucinations, Parkinson-like movement problems, fluctuating cognition such as daytime drowsiness and lethargy, staring into space for long periods, episodes of disorganized speech)
- May decrease delusion, apathy, agitation, and hallucinations in dementia with Lewy bodies
- ✳ May be useful for vascular dementia (e.g., acute onset with slow stepwise

progression that has plateaus, often with gait abnormalities, focal signs, imbalance, and urinary incontinence)
• May be helpful for dementia in Down's Syndrome
• Suggestions of utility in some cases of treatment-resistant bipolar disorder

• Theoretically, may be useful for ADHD, but not yet proven
• Theoretically, could be useful in any memory condition characterized by cholinergic deficiency (e.g., some cases of brain injury, cancer chemotherapy-induced cognitive changes, etc.)

 Suggested Reading

Bentue-Ferrer D, Tribut O, Polard E, Allain H. Clinically significant drug interactions with cholinesterase inhibitors: a guide for neurologists. CNS Drugs 2003;17:947–63.

Bonner LT, Peskind ER. Pharmacologic treatments of dementia. Med Clin North Am 2002;86:657–74.

Jones RW. Have cholinergic therapies reached their clinical boundary in Alzheimer's disease? Int J Geriatr Psychiatry 2003;18(Suppl 1): S7–S13.

Stahl SM. Cholinesterase inhibitors for Alzheimer's disease. Hosp Pract (Off Ed) 1998;33:131–6.

Stahl SM. The new cholinesterase inhibitors for Alzheimer's disease, part 1. J Clin Psychiatry 2000;61:710–11.

Stahl SM. The new cholinesterase inhibitors for Alzheimer's disease, part 2. J Clin Psychiatry 2000;61:813–14.

Williams BR, Nazarians A, Gill MA. A review of rivastigmine: a reversible cholinesterase inhibitor. Clin Ther 2003;25:1634–53.

SELEGILINE

THERAPEUTICS

Brands • Eldepryl
• Deprenyl
see index for additional brand names

Generic? Yes

Class
• Selective monoamine oxidase B (MAO-B) inhibitor

Commonly Prescribed For
(bold for FDA approved)
• **Parkinson's disease or symptomatic Parkinsonism (adjunctive)**
• Alzheimer disease and other dementias
• Treatment-resistant depression

How The Drug Works
• At recommended doses, selectively and irreversibly blocks monoamine oxidase type B (MAO-B) from breaking down dopamine
• This presumably boosts dopaminergic neurotransmission
• Above recommended doses, irreversibly blocks both monoamine oxidase A and monoamine oxidase B from breaking down norepinephrine, serotonin, and tyramine as well as dopamine and phenethylamine
• This presumably boosts noradrenergic, serotonergic, and dopaminergic neurotransmission as well as causes interaction with tyramine-containing foods

How Long Until It Works
• Can enhance the actions of levodopa in Parkinson's disease within a few weeks of initiating dosing
• Theoretical slowing of functional loss in both Parkinson's disease and Alzheimer disease is a provocative possibility under investigation and would take many months or more than a year to observe
• Onset of therapeutic actions in depression at high doses usually not immediate, but often delayed 2 to 4 weeks or longer in patients with treatment-resistant depression

If It Works
• Continue use in Parkinson's disease as long as there is evidence that selegiline is favorably enhancing the actions of levodopa
• Use of selegiline to slow functional loss in Parkinson's disease or Alzheimer disease would be long-term if proven effective for this use
• The goal of treatment in depression is complete remission of current symptoms as well as prevention of future relapses
• Treatment of depression most often reduces or even eliminates symptoms, but not a cure since symptoms can recur after medicine stopped
• Continue treatment of depression until all symptoms of depression are gone (remission)
• Once symptoms of depression are gone, continue treating for 1 year for the first episode of depression
• For second and subsequent episodes of depression, treatment may need to be indefinite

If It Doesn't Work
• Use alternate treatments for Parkinson's disease or Alzheimer disease
• Oral administration is not approved for treatment in depression, so lack of antidepressant response should lead to treatment with well-established antidepressants

Best Augmenting Combos for Partial Response or Treatment-Resistance
• Carbidopa-levodopa (for Parkinson's disease)
✳ Augmentation of selegiline has not been systematically studied in depression, and this is something for the expert, to be done with caution and with careful monitoring

Tests
• Patients should be monitored for changes in blood pressure
• Since nonselective MAO inhibitors are frequently associated with weight gain, before starting treatment for depression with high doses of selegiline, weigh all patients and determine if the patient is already overweight (BMI 25.0–29.9) or obese (BMI ≥30)

423

• Before giving a drug that can cause weight gain to an overweight or obese patient, consider determining whether the patient already has pre-diabetes (fasting plasma glucose 100–125 mg/dl), diabetes (fasting plasma glucose >126 mg/dl), or dyslipidemia (increased total cholesterol, LDL cholesterol and triglycerides; decreased HDL cholesterol), and treat or refer such patients for treatment, including nutrition and weight management, physical activity counseling, smoking cessation, and medical management

✻ Monitor weight and BMI during treatment

✻ While giving a drug to a patient who has gained >5% of initial weight, consider evaluating for the presence of pre-diabetes, diabetes, or dyslipidemia, or consider switching to a different antidepressant

SIDE EFFECTS

How Drug Causes Side Effects

• At recommended doses, dopamine increases in parts of the brain and body and at receptors other than those that cause therapeutic actions
• Serotonin and norepinephrine increase at high doses
• Side effects are generally immediate, but immediate side effects often disappear in time

Notable Side Effects

• Exacerbation of levodopa side effects, especially nausea, dizziness, abdominal pain, dry mouth, headache, dyskinesia, confusion, hallucinations, vivid dreams

 Life Threatening or Dangerous Side Effects

• Hypertensive crisis (especially when MAOIs are used with certain tyramine-containing foods or prohibited drugs) – reduced risk at low doses compared to nonselective MAOIs
• Theoretically, when used at high doses may induce seizures, mania, and suicidal ideation, as do nonselective MAOIs

Weight Gain

• Occurs in significant minority

Sedation

• Reported but not expected

What To Do About Side Effects

• Wait
• Wait
• Wait
• Lower the dose
• Switch to other anti-parkinsonian therapies (Parkinson's Disease)
• Switch after appropriate washout to an SSRI or newer antidepressant (depression)

Best Augmenting Agents for Side Effects

• Many side effects cannot be improved with an augmenting agent, especially at lower doses

DOSING AND USE

Usual Dosage Range

• Parkinson's disease/Alzheimer disease: 5–10 mg/day
• Depression: 30–60 mg/day

Dosage Forms

• Capsule 5 mg
• Tablet 5 mg scored

How to Dose

• Parkinson's disease: Initial 2.5 mg/day twice daily; increase to 5 mg twice daily; reduce dose of levodopa after 2–3 days

 Dosing Tips

✻ Dosage above 10 mg/day generally not recommended for Parkinson's disease
• Dosage of carbidopa-levodopa can at times be reduced by 10–30% after 2–3 days of administering selegiline 5–10 mg/day in Parkinson's disease
✻ At doses above 10 mg/day, selegiline may become nonselective and inhibit both MAO-A and MAO-B

✱ At doses above 30 mg/day, selegiline may have antidepressant properties
• Patients receiving high doses may need to be evaluated periodically for effects on the liver
✱ Doses above 10 mg/day may increase the risk of hypertensive crisis, tyramine interactions, and drug interactions similar to those of phenelzine and tranylcypromine
✱ A transdermal patch for delivery of 20–40 mg/day selegiline (e.g., 20mg/20cm²) is in late testing for depression and may prove to be a more viable treatment option for selegiline in depression than oral administration

Overdose
• Dizziness, anxiety, ataxia, insomnia, sedation, irritability, headache, cardiovascular effects, confusion, respiratory depression, coma

Long-Term Use
• MAOIs may lose efficacy long-term

Habit Forming
• Some patients have developed dependence to MAOIs
• Lack of evidence for abuse potential with selegiline

How to Stop
• Generally no need to taper, as the drug wears off slowly over 2–3 weeks

Pharmacokinetics
• Steady-state mean elimination half-life approximately 10 hours
• Clinical duration of action may be up to 21 days due to irreversible enzyme inhibition
• Major metabolite of orally administered selegiline is desmethylselegiline
• Other metabolites are L-methamphetamine and L-amphetamine
• Metabolite profile different for transdermal administration

 Drug Interactions
• Tramadol may increase the risk of seizures in patients taking an MAO inhibitor
• Selegiline may interact with opiate agonists to cause agitation, hallucination, or death
• Theoretically and especially at high doses, selegiline could cause a fatal "serotonin syndrome" when combined with drugs that block serotonin reuptake (e.g., SSRIs, SNRIs, sibutramine, tramadol, etc.), so do not use with a serotonin reuptake inhibitor or for up to 5 weeks after stopping the serotonin reuptake inhibitor
• Hypertensive crisis with headache, intracranial bleeding, and death may result from combining nonselective MAO inhibitors with sympathomimetic drugs (e.g., amphetamines, methylphenidate, cocaine, dopamine, epinephrine, norepinephrine, and related compounds methyldopa, levodopa, L-tryptophan, L-tyrosine, and phenylalanine
• Excitation, seizures, delirium, hyperpyrexia, circulatory collapse, coma, and death may result from combining nonselective MAO inhibitors with mepiridine or dextromethorphan
• Do not combine with another MAO inhibitor, alcohol, buspirone, bupropion, or guanethidine
• Adverse drug reactions can result from combining MAO inhibitors with tricyclic/tetracyclic antidepressants and related compounds, including carbamazepine, cyclobenzaprine, and mirtazapine, and should be avoided except by experts to treat difficult cases
• MAO inhibitors in combination with spinal anesthesia may cause combined hypotensive effects
• Combination of MAOIs and CNS depressants may enhance sedation and hypotension

 Other Warnings/ Precautions
• Although risk may be reduced with selective MAOIs, patient and prescriber must be vigilant to potential interactions with any drug, including antihypertensives and over-the-counter cough/cold preparations
• Over-the-counter medications to avoid include cough and cold preparations, including those containing dextromethorphan, nasal decongestants (tablets, drops, or spray), hay-fever medications, sinus medications, asthma inhalant medications, anti-appetite medications, weight reducing preparations, "pep" pills.

- Hypoglycemia may occur in diabetic patients receiving insulin or oral antidiabetic agents
- Use cautiously in patients receiving reserpine, anesthetics, disulfiram, metrizamide, anticholinergic agents
- Selegiline is not recommended for use in patients who cannot be monitored closely
- Monitor patients for activation of suicidal ideation, especially children and adolescents
- Although risk is reduced with selective MAOIs, foods that contain large amounts of tyramine or tryptophan, alcohol, and caffeine should be avoided
- Only use sympathomimetic agents or guanethidine with doses of selegiline below 10 mg/day

Do Not Use
- If patient is taking meperidine (pethidine)
- If patient is taking a sympathomimetic agent or taking guanethidine
- If patient is taking another MAOI
- If there is a proven allergy to selegiline

SPECIAL POPULATIONS

Renal Impairment
- Use with caution – drug may accumulate in plasma
- May require lower than usual adult dose

Hepatic Impairment
- May require lower than usual adult dose

Cardiac Impairment
- May require lower than usual adult dose

Elderly
- Initial dose should be lower than usual adult dose

Children and Adolescents
- Not recommended for use under age 16

Pregnancy
- Risk Category C [some animal studies show adverse effects, no controlled studies in humans]

- Not generally recommended for use during pregnancy, especially during first trimester
- Should evaluate patient for treatment with an antidepressant with a better risk/benefit ratio

Breast Feeding
- Some drug is found in mother's breast milk
- Immediate postpartum period is a high-risk time for depression, especially in women who have had prior depressive episodes, so drug may need to be reinstituted late in the third trimester or shortly after childbirth to prevent a recurrence during the postpartum period
- Should evaluate patient for treatment with an antidepressant with a better risk/benefit ratio

THE ART OF PSYCHOPHARMACOLOGY

Potential Advantages
- Parkinson's patients inadequately responsive to levodopa
- Treatment-resistant depression

Potential Disadvantages
- Patients with motor complications and fluctuations on levodopa treatment
- Patients with cardiac problems or hypertension
- Non-compliant patients

Primary Target Symptoms
- Motor symptoms (Parkinson's disease)
- Psychomotor disturbances (depression)
- Depressed mood (depression)
- Sleep and eating disturbances (depression)
- Somatic symptoms (depression)

Pearls
* Low doses may have minimal tyramine and drug interactions
- Generally used as an adjunctive treatment for Parkinson's disease after other drugs have lost efficacy
- At doses used for Parkinson's disease, virtually no risk of interactions with food
- Neuroprotective effects are possible but unproved
* Enhancement of levodopa action can occur for Parkinson's patients at low

doses, but antidepressant actions probably require high doses
* High doses may lose safety features
• High doses can be very expensive
• Because of its effects on dopamine, selegiline may be effective treatment for sexual dysfunction
* A transdermal patch for delivery of selegiline (Emsam) is in late testing for depression and may prove to be a more viable treatment option for selegiline in depression than oral administration
* Transdermal administration of high doses of selegiline may reduce the potential for tyramine-associated blood pressure reactions due to reduced inhibition of gastrointestinal MAO
* Transdermal administration of high doses of selegiline may improve the pharmacokinetic and active metabolite profile of this drug's use as an antidepressant
• MAOIs are generally reserved for second-line use after SSRIs, SNRIs, and combinations of newer antidepressants have failed
• Patient should be advised not to take any prescription or over-the-counter drugs without consulting their doctor because of possible drug interactions with the MAOI
• Headache is often the first symptom of hypertensive crisis
• Foods generally to avoid at high doses of selegiline, as they are usually high in tyramine content: dry sausage, pickled herring, liver, broad bean pods, sauerkraut, cheese, yogurt, alcoholic beverages, nonalcoholic beer and wine, chocolate, caffeine, meat and fish
• The rigid dietary restrictions may reduce compliance

* Myths about the danger of dietary tyramine can be exaggerated, but prohibitions against concomitant drugs often not followed closely enough
* MAOIs should be for the expert, especially if combining with agents of potential risk (e.g., stimulants, trazodone, TCAs)
* MAOIs should not be neglected as therapeutic agents for the treatment-resistant
• Although generally prohibited, a heroic but potentially dangerous treatment for severely treatment-resistant patients is for an expert to give a tricyclic/tetracyclic antidepressant other than clomipramine simultaneously with an MAO inhibitor for patients who fail to respond to numerous other antidepressants
• Use of MAOIs with clomipramine is always prohibited because of the risk of serotonin syndrome and death
• Amoxapine may be the preferred trycyclic/tetracyclic antidepressant to combine with an MAOI in heroic cases due to its theoretically protective 5HT2A antagonist properties
• If this option is elected, start the MAOI with the tricyclic/tetracyclic antidepressant simultaneously at low doses after appropriate drug washout, then alternately increase doses of these agents every few days to a week as tolerated
• Although very strict dietary and concomitant drug restrictions must be observed to prevent hypertensive crises and serotonin syndrome, the most common side effects of MAOI and tricyclic/tetracyclic combinations may be weight gain and orthostatic hypotension

Suggested Reading

Selegiline-transdermal—Somerset: Emsam. Drugs R D. 2003;4(1):59–60.

Kennedy SH. Continuation and maintenance treatments in major depression: the neglected role of monoamine oxidase inhibitors. J Psychiatry Neurosci. 1997;22:127–31.

Knoll J. (-)Deprenyl (Selegiline): past, present and future. Neurobiology (Bp) 2000;8:179–99.

Kuhn W, Muller T. The clinical potential of Deprenyl in neurologic and psychiatric disorders. J Neural Transm Suppl 1996;48:85–93.

SERTRALINE

THERAPEUTICS

Brands • Zoloft
see index for additional brand names

Generic? Not in U.S.

Class
- SSRI (selective serotonin reuptake inhibitor); often classified as an antidepressant, but it is not just an antidepressant

Commonly Prescribed For
(bold for FDA approved)
- **Major depressive disorder**
- **Premenstrual dysphoric disorder (PMDD)**
- **Panic disorder**
- **Posttraumatic stress disorder (PTSD)**
- **Social anxiety disorder (social phobia)**
- **Obsessive-compulsive disorder (OCD)**
- Generalized anxiety disorder (GAD)

How The Drug Works
- Boosts neurotransmitter serotonin
- Blocks serotonin reuptake pump (serotonin transporter)
- Desensitizes serotonin receptors, especially serotonin 1A receptors
- Presumably increases serotonergic neurotransmission
- ✱ Sertraline also has some ability to block dopamine reuptake pump (dopamine transporter), which could increase dopamine neurotransmission and contribute to its therapeutic actions
- Sertraline also has mild antagonist actions at sigma receptors

How Long Until It Works
- ✱ Some patients may experience increased energy or activation early after initiation of treatment
- Onset of therapeutic actions usually not immediate, but often delayed 2 to 4 weeks
- If it is not working within 6 to 8 weeks, it may require a dosage increase or it may not work at all
- May continue to work for many years to prevent relapse of symptoms

If It Works
- The goal of treatment is complete remission of current symptoms as well as prevention of future relapses
- Treatment most often reduces or even eliminates symptoms, but not a cure since symptoms can recur after medicine stopped
- Continue treatment until all symptoms are gone (remission) or significantly reduced (e.g., OCD, PTSD)
- Once symptoms gone, continue treating for 1 year for the first episode of depression
- For second and subsequent episodes of depression, treatment may need to be indefinite
- Use in anxiety disorders may also need to be indefinite

If It Doesn't Work
- Many patients only have a partial response where some symptoms are improved but others persist (especially insomnia, fatigue, and problems concentrating in depression)
- Other patients may be nonresponders, sometimes called treatment-resistant or treatment-refractory
- Some patients who have an initial response may relapse even though they continue treatment, sometimes called "poop-out"
- Consider increasing dose, switching to another agent or adding an appropriate augmenting agent
- Consider psychotherapy
- Consider evaluation for another diagnosis or for a comorbid condition (e.g., medical illness, substance abuse, etc.)
- Some patients may experience apparent lack of consistent efficacy due to activation of latent or underlying bipolar disorder, and require antidepressant discontinuation and a switch to a mood stabilizer

Best Augmenting Combos for Partial Response or Treatment-Resistance
- Trazodone, especially for insomnia
- In the U.S., sertraline (Zoloft) is commonly augmented with bupropion (Wellbutrin) with good results in a combination anecdotally called "Well-loft" (use combinations of antidepressants with caution as this may activate bipolar disorder and suicidal ideation)

- Mirtazapine, reboxetine, or atomoxetine (add with caution and at lower doses since sertraline could theoretically raise atomoxetine levels); use combinations of antidepressants with caution as this may activate bipolar disorder and suicidal ideation
- Modafinil, especially for fatigue, sleepiness, and lack of concentration
- Mood stabilizers or atypical antipsychotics for bipolar depression, psychotic depression, treatment-resistant depression, or treatment-resistant anxiety disorders
- Benzodiazepines
- If all else fails for anxiety disorders, consider gabapentin or tiagabine
- Hypnotics for insomnia
- Classically, lithium, buspirone, or thyroid hormone

Tests
- None for healthy individuals

SIDE EFFECTS

How Drug Causes Side Effects
- Theoretically due to increases in serotonin concentrations at serotonin receptors in parts of the brain and body other than those that cause therapeutic actions (e.g., unwanted actions of serotonin in sleep centers causing insomnia, unwanted actions of serotonin in the gut causing diarrhea, etc.)
* Increasing serotonin can cause diminished dopamine release and might contribute to emotional flattening, cognitive slowing, and apathy in some patients, although this could theoretically be diminished in some patients by sertraline's dopamine reuptake blocking properties
- Most side effects are immediate but often go away with time, in contrast to most therapeutic effects which are delayed and are enhanced over time
- Sertraline's possible dopamine reuptake blocking properties could contribute to agitation, anxiety, and undesirable activation, especially early in dosing

Notable Side Effects
- Sexual dysfunction (men: delayed ejaculation, erectile dysfunction; men and women: decreased sexual desire, anorgasmia)
- Gastrointestinal (decreased appetite, nausea, diarrhea, constipation, dry mouth)
- Mostly central nervous system (insomnia but also sedation, agitation, tremors, headache, dizziness)
- Note: patients with diagnosed or undiagnosed bipolar or psychotic disorders may be more vulnerable to CNS-activating actions of SSRIs
- Autonomic (sweating)
- Bruising and rare bleeding
- Rare hyponatremia (mostly in elderly patients and generally reversible on discontinuation of sertraline)
- Rare hypotension

 ### Life Threatening or Dangerous Side Effects
- Rare seizures
- Rare induction of mania and activation of suicidal ideation

Weight Gain

unusual · not unusual · common · problematic

- Reported but not expected
- Some patients may actually experience weight loss

Sedation

unusual · not unusual · common · problematic

- Reported but not expected
- Possibly activating in some patients

What To Do About Side Effects
- Wait
- Wait
- Wait
- If sertraline is activating, take in the morning to help reduce insomnia
- Reduce dose to 25 mg or even 12.5 mg until side effects abate, then increase dose as tolerated, usually to at least 50 mg/day
- In a few weeks, switch or add other drugs

Best Augmenting Agents for Side Effects
- Often best to try another SSRI or another antidepressant monotherapy prior to

resorting to augmentation strategies to treat side effects
- Trazodone or a hypnotic for insomnia
- Bupropion, sildenafil, vardenafil or tadalafil for sexual dysfunction
- Bupropion for emotional flattening, cognitive slowing, or apathy
- Mirtazapine for insomnia, agitation, and gastrointestinal side effects
- Benzodiazepines for jitteriness and anxiety, especially at initiation of treatment and especially for anxious patients
- Many side effects are dose-dependent (i.e., they increase as dose increases, or they reemerge until tolerance re-develops)
- Many side effects are time-dependent (i.e., they start immediately upon dosing and upon each dose increase, but go away with time)
- Activation and agitation may represent the induction of a bipolar state, especially a mixed dysphoric bipolar II condition sometimes associated with suicidal ideation, and require the addition of lithium, a mood stabilizer or an atypical antipsychotic, and/or discontinuation of sertraline

DOSING AND USE

Usual Dosage Range
- 50–200 mg/day

Dosage Forms
- Tablets 25 mg scored, 50 mg scored, 100 mg

How to Dose
- Depression and OCD: initial 50 mg/day; usually wait a few weeks to assess drug effects before increasing dose, but can increase once a week; maximum generally 200 mg/day; single dose
- Panic and PTSD: initial 25 mg/day; increase to 50 mg/day after 1 week thereafter, usually wait a few weeks to assess drug effects before increasing dose; maximum generally 200 mg/day; single dose

 Dosing Tips
- All tablets are scored, so to save costs, give 50 mg as half of 100 mg tablet, since

100 mg and 50 mg tablets cost about the same in many markets
- Give once daily, often in the mornings to reduce chances of insomnia
- Many patients ultimately require more than 50 mg dose per day
- Some patients are dosed above 200 mg
- Evidence that some treatment-resistant OCD patients may respond safely to doses up to 400 mg/day, but this is for experts and use with caution
- The more anxious and agitated the patient, the lower the starting dose, the slower the titration, and the more likely the need for a concomitant agent such as trazodone or a benzodiazepine
- If intolerable anxiety, insomnia, agitation, akathisia, or activation occur either upon dosing initiation or discontinuation, consider the possibility of activated bipolar disorder and switch to a mood stabilizer or atypical antipsychotic
- Utilize half a 25 mg tablet (12.5 mg) when initiating treatment in patients with a history of intolerance to previous antidepressants

Overdose
- Rarely lethal in monotherapy overdose; vomiting, sedation, heart rhythm disturbances, dilated pupils, agitation; fatalities have been reported in sertraline overdose combined with other drugs or alcohol

Long-Term Use
- Safe

Habit Forming
- No

How to Stop
- Taper to avoid withdrawal effects (dizziness, nausea, stomach cramps, sweating, tingling, dysesthesias)
- Many patients tolerate 50% dose reduction for 3 days, then another 50% reduction for 3 days, then discontinuation
- If withdrawal symptoms emerge during discontinuation, raise dose to stop symptoms and then restart withdrawal much more slowly

Pharmacokinetics
- Parent drug has 22–36 hour half-life

- Metabolite half-life 62–104 hours
- Inhibits CYP450 2D6 (weakly at low doses)
- Inhibits CYP450 3A4 (weakly at low doses)

 Drug Interactions

- Tramadol increases the risk of seizures in patients taking an antidepressant
- Can increase tricyclic antidepressant levels; use with caution with tricyclic antidepressants or when switching from a TCA to sertraline
- Can cause a fatal "serotonin syndrome" when combined with MAO inhibitors, so do not use with MAO inhibitors or for at least 14 days after MAOIs are stopped
- Do not start an MAO inhibitor for at least 2 weeks after discontinuing sertraline
- May displace highly protein bound drugs (e.g., warfarin)
- Can rarely cause weakness, hyperreflexia, and incoordination when combined with sumatriptan or possibly with other triptans, requiring careful monitoring of patient
- Via CYP450 2D6 inhibition, sertraline could theoretically interfere with the analgesic actions of codeine, and increase the plasma levels of some beta blockers and of atomoxetine
- Via CYP450 2D6 inhibition sertraline could theoretically increase concentrations of thioridazine and cause dangerous cardiac arrhythmias
- Via CYP450 3A4 inhibition, sertraline may increase the levels of alprazolam, buspirone, and triazolam
- Via CYP450 3A4 inhibition, sertraline could theoretically increase concentrations of certain cholesterol lowering HMG CoA reductase inhibitors, especially simvastatin, atorvastatin, and lovastatin, but not pravastatin or fluvastatin, which would increase the risk of rhabdomyolysis; thus, coadministration of sertraline with certain HMG CoA reductase inhibitors should proceed with caution
- Via CYP450 3A4 inhibition, sertraline could theoretically increase the concentrations of pimozide, and cause QTc prolongation and dangerous cardiac arrhythmias

 Other Warnings/ Precautions

- Add or initiate other antidepressants with caution for up to 2 weeks after discontinuing sertraline
- Use with caution in patients with history of seizures
- Use with caution in patients with bipolar disorder unless treated with concomitant mood stabilizing agent
- Monitor patients for activation of suicidal ideation, especially children and adolescents

Do Not Use

- If patient is taking an MAO inhibitor
- If patient is taking pimozide
- If patient is taking thioridazine
- Use of sertraline oral concentrate is contraindicated with disulfiram due to the alcohol content of the concentrate
- If there is a proven allergy to sertraline

SPECIAL POPULATIONS

Renal Impairment
- No dose adjustment
- Not removed by hemodialysis

Hepatic Impairment
- Lower dose or give less frequently, perhaps by half

Cardiac Impairment
- Preliminary research suggests that sertraline is safe in these patients
- Treating depression with SSRIs in patients with acute angina or following myocardial infarction may reduce cardiac events and improve survival as well as mood

Elderly
- Some patients may tolerate lower doses and/or slower titration better

 Children and Adolescents

- Use with caution, observing for activation of known or unknown bipolar disorder and/or suicidal ideation, and strongly consider informing parents or guardian of this risk so they can help observe child or adolescent patients

- Approved for use in OCD
- Ages 6–12: initial dose 25 mg/day
- Ages 13 and up: adult dosing
- Long-term effects, particularly on growth, have not been studied

Pregnancy

- Risk Category C [some animal studies show adverse effects, no controlled studies in humans]
- Not generally recommended for use during pregnancy, especially during first trimester
- Nonetheless, continuous treatment during pregnancy may be necessary and has not been proven to be harmful to the fetus
- At delivery there may be more bleeding in the mother and transient irritability or sedation in the newborn
- Must weigh the risk of treatment (first trimester fetal development, third trimester newborn delivery) to the child against the risk of no treatment (recurrence of depression, maternal health, infant bonding) to the mother and child
- For many patients this may mean continuing treatment during pregnancy
- Neonates exposed to SSRIs or SNRIs late in the third trimester have developed complications requiring prolonged hospitalization, respiratory support, and tube feeding; reported symptoms are consistent with either a direct toxic effect of SSRIs and SNRIs or, possibly, a drug discontinuation syndrome, and include respiratory distress, cyanosis, apnea, seizures, temperature instability, feeding difficulty, vomiting, hypoglycemia, hypotonia, hypertonia, hyperreflexia, tremor, jitteriness, irritability, and constant crying

Breast Feeding

- Some drug is found in mother's breast milk
- Trace amounts may be present in nursing children whose mothers are on sertraline
- Sertraline has shown efficacy in treating postpartum depression
- If child becomes irritable or sedated, breast feeding or drug may need to be discontinued
- Immediate postpartum period is a high-risk time for depression, especially in women who have had prior depressive episodes,

so drug may need to be reinstituted late in the third trimester or shortly after childbirth to prevent a recurrence during the postpartum period
- Must weigh benefits of breast feeding with risks and benefits of antidepressant treatment versus nontreatment to both the infant and the mother
- For many patients, this may mean continuing treatment during breast feeding

THE ART OF PSYCHOPHARMACOLOGY

Potential Advantages

- Patients with atypical depression (hypersomnia, increased appetite)
- Patients with fatigue and low energy
- Patients who wish to avoid hyperprolactinemia (e.g., pubescent children, girls and women with galactorrhea, girls and women with unexplained amenorrhea, postmenopausal women who are not taking estrogen replacement therapy)
- Patients who are sensitive to the prolactin-elevating properties of other SSRIs (sertraline is the one SSRI that generally does not elevate prolactin)

Potential Disadvantages

- Initiating treatment in anxious patients with some insomnia
- Patients with comorbid irritable bowel syndrome
- Can require dosage titration

Primary Target Symptoms

- Depressed mood
- Anxiety
- Sleep disturbance, both insomnia and hypersomnia (eventually, but may actually cause insomnia, especially short-term)
- Panic attacks, avoidant behavior, re-experiencing, hyperarousal

Pearls

✽ May be a first-line choice for atypical depression (e.g., hypersomnia, hyperphagia, low energy, mood reactivity)
✽ May block dopamine reuptake pump and enhance dopaminergic neurotransmission

- May block sigma 1 receptors, enhancing sertraline's anxiolytic actions
- Has more gastrointestinal effects, particularly diarrhea, than some other antidepressants
- Can cause cognitive and affective "flattening", although this could theoretically be diminished in some patients by sertraline's dopamine reuptake blocking properties
- May be more effective treatment for women with PTSD or depression than for men with PTSD or depression, but the clinical significance of this is unknown
- SSRIs may be less effective in women over 50, especially if they are not taking estrogen
- SSRIs may be useful for hot flushes in perimenopausal women
- For sexual dysfunction, can augment with bupropion, sildenafil, vardenafil, tadalafil, or switch to a non-SSRI such as bupropion or mirtazapine
- Some postmenopausal women's depression will respond better to sertraline plus estrogen augmentation than to sertraline alone
- Nonresponse to sertraline in elderly may require consideration of mild cognitive impairment or Alzheimer disease
- Not as well tolerated as some SSRIs for panic, especially when dosing is initiated, unless given with co-therapies such as benzodiazepines or trazodone
- Relative lack of effect on prolactin may make it a preferred agent for some children, adolescents, and women
- Some evidence suggests that sertraline treatment during only the luteal phase may be more effective than continuous treatment for patients with PMDD

Suggested Reading

DeVane CL, Liston HL, Markowitz JS. Clinical pharmacokinetics of sertraline. Clin Pharmacokinet. 2002;41:1247–66.

Flament MF, Lane RM, Zhu R, Ying Z. Predictors of an acute antidepressant response to fluoxetine and sertraline. International Clinical Psychopharmacology. 1999;14:259–275.

Khouzam HR, Emes R, Gill T, Raroque R. The antidepressant sertraline: a review of its uses in a range of psychiatric and medical conditions. Compr Ther. 2003;29:47–53.

McRae AL, Brady KT. Review of sertraline and its clinical applications in psychiatric disorders. Expert Opin Pharmacother. 2001;2:883–92.

SULPIRIDE

THERAPEUTICS

Brands • Dolmatil
see index for additional brand names

Generic? Yes

 Class

• Conventional antipsychotic (neuroleptic, benzamide, dopamine 2 antagonist)

Commonly Prescribed For
(bold for FDA approved)
• Schizophrenia
• Depression

 How The Drug Works

• Blocks dopamine 2 receptors, reducing positive symptoms of psychosis
• Blocks dopamine 3 and 4 receptors, which may contribute to sulpiride's actions
✳ Possibly blocks presynaptic dopamine 2 autoreceptors more potently at low doses, which could theoretically contribute to improving negative symptoms of schizophrenia as well as depression

How Long Until It Works

• Psychotic symptoms can improve within 1 week, but it may take several weeks for full effect on behavior

If It Works

• Most often reduces positive symptoms in schizophrenia but does not eliminate them
• Most schizophrenic patients do not have a total remission of symptoms but rather a reduction of symptoms by about a third
• Continue treatment in schizophrenia until reaching a plateau of improvement
• After reaching a satisfactory plateau, continue treatment for at least a year after first episode of psychosis in schizophrenia
• For second and subsequent episodes of psychosis in schizophrenia, treatment may need to be indefinite

If It Doesn't Work

• Consider trying one of the first-line atypical antipsychotics (risperidone, olanzapine, quetiapine, ziprasidone, aripiprazole, amisulpride)

• Consider trying another conventional antipsychotic
• If 2 or more antipsychotic monotherapies do not work, consider clozapine

 Best Augmenting Combos for Partial Response or Treatment-Resistance

• Augmentation of conventional antipsychotics has not been systematically studied
• Addition of a mood stabilizing anticonvulsant such as valproate, carbamazepine, or lamotrigine may be helpful in both schizophrenia and bipolar mania
• Augmentation with lithium in bipolar mania may be helpful
• Addition of a benzodiazepine, especially short-term for agitation

Tests

✳ Since conventional antipsychotics are frequently associated with weight gain, before starting treatment, weigh all patients and determine if the patient is already overweight (BMI 25.0–29.9) or obese (BMI ≥30)
• Before giving a drug that can cause weight gain to an overweight or obese patient, consider determining whether the patient already has pre-diabetes (fasting plasma glucose 100–125 mg/dl), diabetes (fasting plasma glucose >126 mg/dl), or dyslipidemia (increased total cholesterol, LDL cholesterol and triglycerides; decreased HDL cholesterol), and treat or refer such patients for treatment, including nutrition and weight management, physical activity counseling, smoking cessation, and medical management
✳ Monitor weight and BMI during treatment
✳ While giving a drug to a patient who has gained >5% of initial weight, consider evaluating for the presence of pre-diabetes, diabetes, or dyslipidemia, or consider switching to a different antipsychotic
• Monitoring elevated prolactin levels of dubious clinical benefit

SIDE EFFECTS

How Drug Causes Side Effects

- By blocking dopamine 2 receptors in the striatum, it can cause motor side effects
- By blocking dopamine 2 receptors in the pituitary, it can cause elevations in prolactin
- By blocking dopamine 2 receptors excessively in the mesocortical and mesolimbic dopamine pathways, especially at high doses, it can cause worsening of negative and cognitive symptoms (neuroleptic-induced deficit syndrome)
- Anticholinergic actions may cause sedation, blurred vision, constipation, dry mouth
- Antihistaminic actions may cause sedation, weight gain
- By blocking alpha 1 adrenergic receptors, it can cause dizziness, sedation, and hypotension
- Mechanism of weight gain and any possible increased incidence of diabetes or dyslipidemia with conventional antipsychotics is unknown

Notable Side Effects

- ✳ Extrapyramidal symptoms, akathisia
- ✳ Prolactin elevation, galactorrhea, amenorrhea
- Sedation, dizziness, sleep disturbance, headache, impaired concentration
- Dry mouth, nausea, vomiting, constipation, anorexia
- Impotence
- Rare tardive dyskinesia
- Rare hypomania
- Palpitations, hypertension
- Weight gain

Life Threatening or Dangerous Side Effects

- Rare neuroleptic malignant syndrome
- Rare seizures

Weight Gain

unusual not unusual common problematic

- Many experience and/or can be significant in amount

Sedation

unusual not unusual common problematic

- Many experience and/or can be significant in amount, especially at high doses

What To Do About Side Effects

- Wait
- Wait
- Wait
- For motor symptoms, add an anticholinergic agent
- Reduce the dose
- For sedation, give at night
- Switch to an atypical antipsychotic
- Weight loss, exercise programs, and medical management for high BMIs, diabetes, dyslipidemia

Best Augmenting Agents for Side Effects

- Benztropine or trihexyphenidyl for motor side effects
- Sometimes amantadine can be helpful for motor side effects
- Benzodiazepines may be helpful for akathisia
- Many side effects cannot be improved with an augmenting agent

DOSING AND USE

Usual Dosage Range

- Schizophrenia: 400–800 mg/day in 2 doses (oral)
- Predominantly negative symptoms: 50–300 mg/day (oral)
- Intramuscular injection: 600–800 mg/day
- Depression: 150–300 mg/day (oral)

Dosage Forms

- Different formulations may be available in different markets
- Tablet 200 mg, 400 mg, 500 mg
- Intramuscular injection 50 mg/mL, 100 mg/mL

How to Dose

- Initial 400–800 mg/day in 1–2 doses; may need to increase dose to control positive symptoms; maximum generally 2,400 mg/day

Dosing Tips

❋ Low doses of sulpiride may be more effective at reducing negative symptoms than positive symptoms in schizophrenia; high doses may be equally effective at reducing both symptom dimensions
❋ Lower doses are more likely to be activating; higher doses are more likely to be sedating
• Some patients receive more than 2,400 mg/day

Overdose
• Can be fatal; vomiting, agitation, hypotension, hallucinations, CNS depression, sinus tachycardia, arrhythmia, dystonia, dysarthria, hyperreflexia

Long-Term Use
• Apparently safe, but not well-studied

Habit Forming
• No

How to Stop
• Recommended to reduce dose over a week
• Slow down-titration (over 6 to 8 weeks), especially when simultaneously beginning a new antipsychotic while switching (i.e., cross-titration)
• Rapid discontinuation may lead to rebound psychosis and worsening of symptoms
• If antiparkinson agents are being used, they should be continued for a few weeks after sulpiride is discontinued

Pharmacokinetics
• Elimination half-life approximately 6–8 hours
• Excreted largely unchanged

 Drug Interactions
• Sulpiride may increase the effects of antihypertensive drugs
• CNS effects may be increased if sulpiride is used with other CNS depressants
• May decrease the effects of levodopa, dopamine agonists
• Antacids or sucralfate may reduce the absorption of sulpiride

 Other Warnings/ Precautions
• If signs of neuroleptic malignant syndrome develop, treatment should be immediately discontinued
• Use cautiously in patients with alcohol withdrawal or convulsive disorders because of possible lowering of seizure threshold
• Antiemetic effect of sulpiride may mask signs of other disorders or overdose; suppression of cough reflex may cause asphyxia
• Use with caution in patients with hypertension, cardiovascular disease, pulmonary disease, hyperthyroidism, urinary retention, glaucoma
• May exacerbate symptoms of mania or hypomania
• Use only with caution if at all in Parkinson's disease or Lewy Body dementia

Do Not Use
• If patient has pheochromocytoma
• If patient has prolactin-dependent tumor
• If patient is pregnant or nursing
• In children under age 15
• If there is a proven allergy to sulpiride

SPECIAL POPULATIONS

Renal Impairment
• Use with caution; drug may accumulate
• Sulpiride is eliminated by the renal route; in cases of severe renal insufficiency, the dose should be decreased and intermittent treatment or switching to another antipsychotic should be considered

Heptic Impairment
• Use with caution

Cardiac Impairment
• Use with caution

Elderly
• Some patients may tolerate lower doses better

 Children and Adolescents
• Not recommended for use under age 15
• 14 and older: recommended 3–5 mg/kg/day

SULPIRIDE (continued)

Pregnancy

- Potential risks should be weighed against the potential benefits, and sulpiride should be used only if deemed necessary
- Psychotic symptoms may worsen during pregnancy and some form of treatment may be necessary
- Atypical antipsychotics may be preferable to conventional antipsychotics or anticonvulsant mood stabilizers if treatment is required during pregnancy

Breast Feeding

- Some drug is found in mother's breast milk
- ✳ Recommended either to discontinue drug or bottle feed
- Immediate postpartum period is a high-risk time for relapse of psychosis

THE ART OF PSYCHOPHARMACOLOGY

Potential Advantages

- For negative symptoms in some patients

Potential Disadvantages

- Patients who cannot tolerate sedation at high doses
- Patients with severe renal impairment

Primary Target Symptoms

- Positive symptoms of psychosis
- Negative symptoms of psychosis
- Cognitive functioning
- Depressive symptoms
- Aggressive symptoms

Pearls

- ✳ There is some controversy over whether sulpiride is more effective than older conventionals at treating negative symptoms
- Sulpiride has been used to treat migraine associated with hormonal changes
- ✳ Some patients with inadequate response to clozapine may benefit from augmentation with sulpiride
- Sulpiride is poorly absorbed from the gastrointestinal tract and penetrates the blood brain barrier poorly, which can lead to highly variable clinical responses, especially at lower doses
- Small studies and clinical anecdotes suggest efficacy in depression and anxiety disorders ("neuroses") at low doses
- Patients have very similar antipsychotic responses to any conventional antipsychotic, which is different from atypical antipsychotics where antipsychotic responses of individual patients can occasionally vary greatly from one atypical antipsychotic to another
- Patients with inadequate responses to atypical antipsychotics may benefit from a trial of augmentation with a conventional antipsychotic such as sulpiride or from switching to a conventional antipsychotic such as sulpiride
- However, long-term polypharmacy with a combination of a conventional antipsychotic with an atypical antipsychotic may combine their side effects without clearly augmenting the efficacy of either
- Although a frequent practice by some prescribers, adding 2 conventional antipsychotics together has little rationale and may reduce tolerability without clearly enhancing efficacy

Suggested Reading

Caley CF, Weber SS. Sulpiride: an antipsychotic with selective dopaminergic antagonist properties. Ann Pharmacother 1995; 29 (2): 152–60.

Mauri MC, Bravin S, Bitetto A, Rudelli R, Invernizzi G. A risk-benefit assessment of sulpiride in the treatment of schizophrenia. Drug Saf 1996; 14 (5): 288–98.

O'Connor SE, Brown RA. The pharmacology of sulpiride—a dopamine receptor antagonist. Gen Pharmacol 1982; 13 (3): 185–93.

Soares BG, Fenton M, Chue P. Sulpiride for schizophrenia. Cochrane Database Syst Rev 2000; (2): CD001162.

TACRINE

THERAPEUTICS

Brands • Cognex
see index for additional brand names

Generic? Yes

Class
• Cholinesterase inhibitor (inhibits both acetylcholinesterase and butyrylcholinesterase); cognitive enhancer

Commonly Prescribed For
(bold for FDA approved)
• **Alzheimer disease**
• Memory disorders in other conditions
• Dementia

How The Drug Works
✱ Reversibly inhibits centrally-active acetylcholinesterase (AChE), making more acetylcholine available
• Increased availability of acetylcholine compensates in part for degenerating cholinergic neurons in neocortex that regulate memory
✱ Inhibits butyrylcholinesterase (BuChE)
• May release growth factors or interfere with amyloid deposition

How Long Until It Works
• May take up to 6 weeks before any improvement in baseline memory or behavior is evident
• May take months before any stabilization in degenerative course is evident

If It Works
• May improve symptoms and slow progression of disease, but does not reverse the degenerative process

If It Doesn't Work
• Consider adjusting dose, switching to a different cholinesterase inhibitor or adding an appropriate augmenting agent
• Reconsider diagnosis and rule out other conditions such as depression or a dementia other than Alzheimer disease

Best Augmenting Combos for Partial Response or Treatment-Resistance
• Atypical antipsychotics to reduce behavioral disturbances
• Antidepressants if concomitant depression, apathy, or lack of interest
• Memantine for moderate to severe Alzheimer disease
• Divalproex, carbamazepine, or oxcarbazepine for behavioral disturbances

Tests
✱ Serum hepatic transaminase levels should be monitored

SIDE EFFECTS

How Drug Causes Side Effects
• Peripheral inhibition of acetylcholinesterase can cause gastrointestinal side effects
• Peripheral inhibition of butyrylcholinesterase can cause gastrointestinal side effects
• Central inhibition of acetylcholinesterase may contribute to nausea, vomiting, weight loss, and sleep disturbances

Notable Side Effects
✱ Nausea, diarrhea, vomiting, appetite loss, increased gastric acid secretion, dyspepsia, weight loss
• Myalgia, rhinitis, rash

Life Threatening or Dangerous Side Effects
✱ Elevated hepatic transaminase
• Liver toxicity
• Rare seizures

Weight Gain

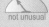
unusual   not unusual   common   problematic

• Reported but not expected
• Some patients may experience weight loss

Sedation

unusual   not unusual   common   problematic

• Reported but not expected

What To Do About Side Effects
- Wait
- Wait
- Wait
- Use slower dose titration
- Consider lowering dose, switching to a different agent or adding an appropriate augmenting agent

Best Augmenting Agents for Side Effects
- Many side effects cannot be improved with an augmenting agent

DOSING AND USE

Usual Dosage Range
- 40–160 mg/day

Dosage Forms
- Capsule 10 mg, 20 mg, 30 mg, 40 mg

How to Dose
- Initial 40 mg/day in 4 divided doses; dose should be maintained for 4 weeks; if tolerable after 4 weeks, dose should be increased to 80 mg/day in 4 divided doses; additional titration should occur at 4 week intervals if tolerable; maximum dose 160 mg/day
- If ALT is between 3 and 5 times the upper limit of normal, dose should be decreased by 40 mg/day and increased after ALT returns to normal
- If ALT is greater than 5 times the upper limit of normal, tacrine should be discontinued; rechallenge may occur after ALT returns to normal

 Dosing Tips
- Dose titration may need to be slowed to reduce adverse effects
- Dose titration should not be accelerated beyond the recommended regimen
- Taking tacrine with meals may reduce gastrointestinal effects; however, food decreases plasma concentrations of tacrine

Overdose
- Can be lethal; nausea, vomiting, excess salivation, sweating, hypotension, bradycardia, collapse, convulsions, muscle weakness (weakness of respiratory muscles can lead to death)

Long-Term Use
- Drug may lose effectiveness in slowing degenerative course of Alzheimer disease after 6 months
- Can be effective in some patients for several years

Habit Forming
- No

How to Stop
- May need to taper large doses
- Discontinuation may lead to notable deterioration in memory and behavior which may not be restored when drug is restarted or another cholinesterase inhibitor is initiated

Pharmacokinetics
- Metabolized principally by CYP450 1A2
- CYP450 1A2 inhibitor
- Short half-life, only a few hours

 Drug Interactions
- Tacrine may increase the effects of anesthetics and should be discontinued prior to surgery
- Tacrine may increase plasma levels of drugs metabolized by CYP450 1A2 (e.g., theophylline) and require dose adjustment
- Fluvoxamine and other CYP450 1A2 inhibitors may increase plasma levels of tacrine
- Tacrine may interact with anticholinergic agents and the combination may decrease the efficacy of both agents
- May have synergistic effect if administered with cholinomimetics (e.g., bethanechol)
- Cimetidine may increase tacrine plasma levels
- Tacrine plasma concentrations may be lower in smokers than in nonsmokers due to induction of CYP450 1A2
- Bradycardia may occur when tacrine is combined with beta blockers
- Tacrine may reduce the efficacy of levodopa in Parkinson's disease
- Not rational to combine with another cholinesterase inhibitor

Other Warnings/Precautions

- May exacerbate asthma or other pulmonary disease
- Increased gastric acid secretion may increase the risk of ulcers
- Bradycardia or heart block may occur in patients with or without cardiac impairment
- ✷ Tacrine may cause liver toxicity

Do Not Use

- If previous treatment with tacrine was discontinued because of treatment-associated jaundice, serum bilirubin >3 mg/dL, or hypersensitivity associated with ALT/SGPT elevation
- If there is a proven allergy to tacrine

SPECIAL POPULATIONS

Renal Impairment
- No dose adjustment

Hepatic Impairment
- Use with caution
- Potential for liver toxicity

Cardiac Impairment
- Should be used with caution

Elderly
- Some patients may tolerate lower doses better

Children and Adolescents
- Safety and efficacy have not been established

Pregnancy
- Risk Category C [no controlled studies in animals, no controlled studies in humans]
- ✷ Not recommended for use in pregnant women or in women of childbearing potential

Breast Feeding
- Unknown if tacrine is secreted in human breast milk, but all psychotropics assumed to be secreted in breast milk
- ✷ Recommended either to discontinue drug or bottle feed
- Tacrine is not recommended for use in nursing women

THE ART OF PSYCHOPHARMACOLOGY

Potential Advantages
- For some patients who fail to respond to several other cholinesterase inhibitors

Potential Disadvantages
- Hepatotoxicity
- Patients with gastrointestinal problems
- Patients who have difficulty taking medication several times a day

Primary Target Symptoms
- Memory loss in Alzheimer disease
- Behavioral symptoms in Alzheimer disease
- Memory loss in other dementias

Pearls
- ✷ Hepatotoxicity in up to a third of patients and 4 times daily dosing make tacrine a second-line treatment for Alzheimer disease
- ✷ Patients who discontinue treatment with tacrine because of ALT/SGPT elevation may be rechallenged with an initial dose of 40 mg 4 times per day maintained for 6 weeks before titration
- Treats behavioral and psychological symptoms of dementia as well as cognitive symptoms (i.e., especially apathy, disinhibition, delusions, anxiety, cooperation, pacing)
- Plasma concentrations of tacrine are higher in women than in men
- Women may experience cognitive symptoms in perimenopause as a result of hormonal changes that are not a sign of dementia or Alzheimer disease
- Some data that hormone replacement therapy in women with Alzheimer disease can enhance the effects of tacrine
- The first symptoms of Alzheimer disease are generally mood changes; thus, Alzheimer disease may initially be diagnosed as depression
- If treatment with antidepressants fails to improve apathy and depressed mood in the

elderly, it is possible that this represents early Alzheimer disease and a cholinesterase inhibitor may be helpful
• Cholinesterase inhibitors like tacrine depend upon the presence of intact targets

for acetylcholine for maximum effectiveness and thus may be most effective in the early stages of Alzheimer disease

Suggested Reading

Bentue-Ferrer D, Tribut O, Polard E, Allain H. Clinically significant drug interactions with cholinesterase inhibitors: a guide for neurologists. CNS Drugs 2003;17:947–63.

Bonner LT, Peskind ER. Pharmacologic treatments of dementia. Med Clin North Am 2002;86:657–74.

Jones RW. Have cholinergic therapies reached their clinical boundary in Alzheimer's disease? Int J Geriatr Psychiatry 2003;18(Suppl 1): S7–S13.

Oizilbash N, Birks J, Lopez-Arrieta J, Lewington S, Szeto S. Tacrine for Alzheimer's disease. Cochrane Database Syst Rev 2000;(3):CD000202.

Stahl SM. The new cholinesterase inhibitors for Alzheimer's disease, part 1. J Clin Psychiatry 2000;61:710–11.

Stahl SM. The new cholinesterase inhibitors for Alzheimer's disease, part 2. J Clin Psychiatry 2000;61:813–14.

TEMAZEPAM

Brands • Restoril
see index for additional brand names

Generic? Yes

 Class
• Benzodiazepine (hypnotic)

Commonly Prescribed For
(bold for FDA approved)
• **Short-term treatment of insomnia**

 How The Drug Works
• Binds to benzodiazepine receptors at the GABA-A ligand-gated chloride channel complex
• Enhances the inhibitory effects of GABA
• Boosts chloride conductance through GABA-regulated channels
• Inhibitory actions in sleep centers may provide sedative hypnotic effects

How Long Until It Works
• Generally takes effect in less than an hour, but can take longer in some patients

If It Works
• Improves quality of sleep
• Effects on total wake-time and number of nighttime awakenings may be decreased over time

If It Doesn't Work
• If insomnia does not improve after 7–10 days, it may be a manifestation of a primary psychiatric or physical illness such as obstructive sleep apnea or restless leg syndrome, which requires independent evaluation
• Increase the dose
• Improve sleep hygiene
• Switch to another agent

 Best Augmenting Combos for Partial Response or Treatment-Resistance
• Generally, best to switch to another agent
• Trazodone
• Agents with antihistamine actions (e.g., diphenhydramine, tricyclic antidepressants)

Tests
• In patients with seizure disorders, concomitant medical illness, and/or those with multiple concomitant long-term medications, periodic liver tests and blood counts may be prudent

How Drug Causes Side Effects
• Same mechanism for side effects as for therapeutic effects – namely due to excessive actions at benzodiazepine receptors
• Actions at benzodiazepine receptors that carry over to the next day can cause daytime sedation, amnesia, and ataxia
• Long-term adaptations in benzodiazepine receptors may explain the development of dependence, tolerance, and withdrawal

Notable Side Effects
✳ Sedation, fatigue, depression
✳ Dizziness, ataxia, slurred speech, weakness
✳ Forgetfulness, confusion
✳ Hyper-excitability, nervousness
• Rare hallucinations, mania
• Rare hypotension
• Hypersalivation, dry mouth
• Rebound insomnia when withdrawing from long-term treatment

 Life Threatening or Dangerous Side Effects
• Respiratory depression, especially when taken with CNS depressants in overdose
• Rare hepatic dysfunction, renal dysfunction, blood dyscrasias

Weight Gain

unusual   not unusual   common   problematic
• Reported but not expected

Sedation

unusual   not unusual   common   problematic
• Many experience and/or can be significant in amount

What To Do About Side Effects

- Wait
- To avoid problems with memory, only take temazepam if planning to have a full night's sleep
- Lower the dose
- Switch to a shorter-acting sedative hypnotic
- Switch to a non-benzodiazepine hypnotic
- Administer flumazenil if side effects are severe or life-threatening

Best Augmenting Agents for Side Effects

- Many side effects cannot be improved with an augmenting agent

DOSING AND USE

Usual Dosage Range

- 15 mg/day at bedtime

Dosage Forms

- Capsule 7.5 mg, 15 mg, 30 mg

How to Dose

- 15 mg/day at bedtime; may increase to 30 mg/day at bedtime if ineffective

 Dosing Tips

- Use lowest possible effective dose and assess need for continued treatment regularly
- Temazepam should generally not be prescribed in quantities greater than a 1-month supply
- Patients with lower body weights may require lower doses
- ✳ Because temazepam is slowly absorbed, administering the dose 1–2 hours before bedtime may improve onset of action and shorter sleep latency
- Risk of dependence may increase with dose and duration of treatment

Overdose

- Can be fatal in monotherapy; slurred speech, poor coordination, respiratory depression, sedation, confusion, coma

Long-Term Use

- Not generally intended for long-term use

Habit Forming

- Temazepam is a Schedule IV drug
- Some patients may develop dependence and/or tolerance; risk may be greater with higher doses
- History of drug addiction may increase risk of dependence

How to Stop

- If taken for more than a few weeks, taper to reduce chances of withdrawal effects
- Patients with history of seizure may seize upon sudden withdrawal
- Rebound insomnia may occur the first 1–2 nights after stopping
- For patients with severe problems discontinuing a benzodiazepine, dosing may need to be tapered over many months (i.e., reduce dose by 1% every 3 days by crushing tablet and suspending or dissolving in 100 ml of fruit juice and then disposing of 1 ml while drinking the rest; 3–7 days later, dispose of 2 ml, and so on). This is both a form of very slow biological tapering and a form of behavioral desensitization

Pharmacokinetics

- No active metabolites
- Half-life approximately 8–15 hours

 Drug Interactions

- Increased depressive effects when taken with other CNS depressants
- If temazepam is used with kava, clearance of either drug may be affected

 Other Warnings/ Precautions

- Insomnia may be a symptom of a primary disorder, rather than a primary disorder itself
- Some patients may exhibit abnormal thinking or behavioral changes similar to those caused by other CNS depressants (i.e., either depressant actions or disinhibiting actions)
- Some depressed patients may experience a worsening of suicidal ideation
- Use only with extreme caution in patients with impaired respiratory function or obstructive sleep apnea

- Temazepam should only be administered at bedtime

Do Not Use
- If patient is pregnant
- If patient has narrow angle-closure glaucoma
- If there is a proven allergy to temazepam or any benzodiazepine

Renal Impairment
- Recommended dose: 7.5 mg/day

Hepatic Impairment
- Recommended dose: 7.5 mg/day

Cardiac Impairment
- Dosage adjustment may not be necessary
- Benzodiazepines have been used to treat insomnia associated with acute myocardial infarction

Elderly
- Recommended dose: 7.5 mg/day

Children and Adolescents
- Safety and efficacy have not been established
- Long-term effects of temazepam in children/adolescents are unknown
- Should generally receive lower doses and be more closely monitored

Pregnancy
- Risk Category X [positive evidence of risk to human fetus; contraindicated for use in pregnancy]
- Infants whose mothers received a benzodiazepine late in pregnancy may experience withdrawal effects
- Neonatal flaccidity has been reported in infants whose mothers took a benzodiazepine during pregnancy

Breast Feeding
- Unknown if temazepam is secreted in human breast milk, but all psychotropics assumed to be secreted in breast milk

* Recommended either to discontinue drug or bottle feed
- Effects on infant have been observed and include feeding difficulties, sedation, and weight loss

Potential Advantages
- Patients with middle insomnia (nocturnal awakening)

Potential Disadvantages
- Patients with early insomnia (problems falling asleep)

Primary Target Symptoms
- Time to sleep onset
- Total sleep time
- Nighttime awakenings

 Pearls
- If tolerance develops, it may result in increased anxiety during the day and/or increased wakefulness during the latter part of the night
* Slow gastrointestinal absorption compared to other sedative benzodiazepines, so may be more effective for nocturnal awakening than for initial insomnia unless dosed 1–2 hours prior to bedtime
* Notable for delayed onset of action compared to some other sedative hypnotics

Suggested Reading

Ashton H. Guidelines for the rational use of benzodiazepines. When and what to use. Drugs 1994;48:25–40.

Fraschini F, Stankov B. Temazepam: pharmacological profile of a benzodiazepine and new trends in its clinical application. Pharmacol Res 1993;27:97–113.

Heel RC, Brogden RN, Speight TM, Avery GS. Temazepam: a review of its pharmacological properties and therapeutic efficacy as an hypnotic. Drugs 1981;21:321–40.

McElnay JC, Jones ME, Alexander B. Temazepam (Restoril, Sandoz Pharmaceuticals). Drug Intell Clin Pharm 1982;16:650–6.

THERAPEUTICS

Brands • Mellaril
see index for additional brand names

Generic? Yes

Class

• Conventional antipsychotic (neuroleptic, phenothiazine, dopamine 2 antagonist)

Commonly Prescribed For
(bold for FDA approved)
• **Schizophrenic patients who fail to respond to treatment with other antipsychotic drugs**

How The Drug Works

• Blocks dopamine 2 receptors, reducing positive symptoms of psychosis

How Long Until It Works
• Psychotic symptoms can improve within 1 week, but it may take several weeks for full effect on behavior

If It Works
• Is a second-line treatment option
✳ Should evaluate for switching to an antipsychotic with a better risk/benefit ratio

If It Doesn't Work
• Consider trying one of the first-line atypical antipsychotics (risperidone, olanzapine, quetiapine, ziprasidone, aripiprazole, amisulpride)
• Consider trying another conventional antipsychotic
• If 2 or more antipsychotic monotherapies do not work, consider clozapine

Best Augmenting Combos for Partial Response or Treatment-Resistance
✳ Augmentation of thioridazine has not been systematically studied and can be dangerous, especially with drugs that can either prolong QTc interval or raise thioridazine plasma levels

Tests
✳ Baseline ECG and serum potassium levels should be determined
✳ Periodic evaluation of ECG and serum potassium levels
• Serum magnesium levels may also need to be monitored
✳ Since conventional antipsychotics are frequently associated with weight gain, before starting treatment, weigh all patients and determine if the patient is already overweight (BMI 25.0–29.9) or obese (BMI ≥30)
• Before giving a drug that can cause weight gain to an overweight or obese patient, consider determining whether the patient already has pre-diabetes (fasting plasma glucose 100–125 mg/dl), diabetes (fasting plasma glucose >126 mg/dl), or dyslipidemia (increased total cholesterol, LDL cholesterol and triglycerides; decreased HDL cholesterol), and treat or refer such patients for treatment, including nutrition and weight management, physical activity counseling, smoking cessation, and medical management
✳ Monitor weight and BMI during treatment
✳ While giving a drug to a patient who has gained >5% of initial weight, consider evaluating for the presence of pre-diabetes, diabetes, or dyslipidemia, or consider switching to a different antipsychotic
• Should check blood pressure in the elderly before starting and for the first few weeks of treatment
• Monitoring elevated prolactin levels of dubious clinical benefit
• Phenothiazines may cause false-positive phenylketonuria results

SIDE EFFECTS

How Drug Causes Side Effects
• By blocking dopamine 2 receptors in the striatum, it can cause motor side effects
• By blocking dopamine 2 receptors in the pituitary, it can cause elevations in prolactin
• By blocking dopamine 2 receptors excessively in the mesocortical and mesolimbic dopamine pathways, especially at high doses, it can cause worsening of

negative and cognitive symptoms (neuroleptic-induced deficit syndrome)
- Anticholinergic actions may cause sedation, blurred vision, constipation, dry mouth
- Antihistaminic actions may cause sedation, weight gain
- By blocking alpha 1 adrenergic receptors, it can cause dizziness, sedation, and hypotension
- Mechanism of weight gain and any possible increased incidence of diabetes or dyslipidemia with conventional antipsychotics is unknown
- ✳ Mechanism of potentially dangerous QTc prolongation may be related to actions at ion channels

Notable Side Effects
- ✳ Neuroleptic-induced deficit syndrome
- ✳ Akathisia
- ✳ Priapism
- ✳ Extrapyramidal symptoms, Parkinsonism, tardive dyskinesia
- ✳ Galactorrhea, amenorrhea
- ✳ Pigmentary retinopathy at high doses
- Dizziness, sedation
- Dry mouth, constipation, blurred vision
- Decreased sweating
- Sexual dysfunction
- Hypotension
- Weight gain

 Life Threatening or Dangerous Side Effects
- Rare neuroleptic malignant syndrome
- Rare jaundice, agranulocytosis
- Rare seizures
- ✳ Dose-dependent QTc prolongation
- Ventricular arrhythmias and sudden death

Weight Gain

unusual   not unusual   common   problematic

- Many experience and/or can be significant in amount

Sedation

unusual   not unusual   common   problematic

- Many experience and/or can be significant in amount
- Sedation is usually transient

What To Do About Side Effects
- Wait
- Wait
- Wait
- For motor symptoms, add an anticholinergic agent
- Reduce the dose
- For sedation, give at night
- Switch to an atypical antipsychotic
- Weight loss, exercise programs, and medical management for high BMIs, diabetes, dyslipidemia

Best Augmenting Agents for Side Effects
- ✳ Augmentation of thioridazine has not been systematically studied and can be dangerous

DOSING AND USE

Usual Dosage Range
- 200–800 mg/day in divided doses

Dosage Forms
- Tablet 10 mg, 15 mg, 25 mg, 50 mg, 100 mg, 150 mg, 200 mg
- Liquid 30 mg/mL, 100 mg/mL
- Suspension 5 mg/mL, 20 mg/mL

How to Dose
- 50–100 mg 3 times a day; increase gradually; maximum 800 mg/day in divided doses

 Dosing Tips
- ✳ Prolongation of the QTc interval is dose-dependent, so start low and go slow while carefully monitoring QTc interval
- Pigmentary retinopathy has been reported in patients taking doses exceeding the recommended range

Overdose
- Sedation, confusion, respiratory depression, cardiac disturbance, hypotension, seizure, coma

Long-Term Use
- Some side effects may be irreversible (e.g., tardive dyskinesia)

Habit Forming
• No

How to Stop
• Slow down-titration (over 6 to 8 weeks), especially when simultaneously beginning a new antipsychotic while switching (i.e., cross-titration)
• Rapid discontinuation may lead to rebound psychosis and worsening of symptoms
• If antiparkinson agents are being used, they should be continued for a few weeks after thioridazine is discontinued

Pharmacokinetics
• Metabolized by CYP450 2D6

 Drug Interactions
• May decrease the effects of levodopa, dopamine agonists
• May increase the effects of antihypertensive drugs
• May enhance QTc prolongation of other drugs capable of prolonging QTc interval
✳ CYP450 2D6 inhibitors including paroxetine, fluoxetine, duloxetine, bupropion, sertraline, citalopram, and others can raise thioridazine to dangerous levels
✳ Fluvoxamine, propranolol, and pindolol also inhibit thioridazine metabolism and can raise thioridazine to dangerous levels
• Respiratory depression / arrest may occur if used with a barbiturate
• Additive effects may occur if used with CNS depressants
• Alcohol and diuretics may increase the risk of hypotension; epinephrine may lower blood pressure
• Some patients taking a neuroleptic and lithium have developed an encephalopathic syndrome similar to neuroleptic malignant syndrome

 Other Warnings/ Precautions
• If signs of neuroleptic malignant syndrome develop, treatment should be immediately discontinued
✳ Thioridazine can increase the QTc interval and potentially cause torsades de pointes-type arrhythmia or sudden death, especially in combination with drugs that raise its levels

• Use cautiously in patients with respiratory disorders, glaucoma, or urinary retention
• Avoid extreme heat exposure
• Antiemetic effect can mask signs of other disorders or overdose
• Use cautiously in patients with alcohol withdrawal or convulsive disorders because of possible lowering of seizure threshold
• Do not use epinephrine in event of overdose, as interaction with some pressor agents may lower blood pressure
• Use only with caution if at all in Parkinson's disease or Lewy Body dementia
• Observe for signs of pigmentary retinopathy, especially at higher doses
• Because thioridazine may dose-dependently prolong QTc interval, use with caution in patients who have bradycardia or who are taking drugs that can induce bradycardia (e.g., beta blockers, calcium channel blockers, clonidine, digitalis)
• Because thioridazine may dose-dependently prolong QTc interval, use with caution in patients who have hypokalemia and/or hypomagnesemia or who are taking drugs that can induce hypokalemia and/or magnesemia (e.g., diuretics, stimulant laxatives, intravenous amphotericin B, glucocorticoids, tetracosactide)

Do Not Use
• If patient is in a comatose state or has CNS depression
• If patient suffers from extreme hypertension/hypotension
✳ If QTc interval greater than 450 msec or if taking an agent capable of significantly prolonging QTc interval (e.g., pimozide, selected antiarrhythmics, moxifoxacin, and sparfloxacin)
✳ If there is a history of QTc prolongation or cardiac arrhythmia, recent acute myocardial infarction, uncompensated heart failure
✳ If patient is taking drugs that inhibit thioridazine metabolism, including CYP450 inhibitors
✳ If there is reduced CYP450 2D6 function, such as in patients who are 2D6 poor metabolizers
• If there is a proven allergy to thioridazine
• If there is a known sensitivity to any phenothiazine

THIORIDAZINE (continued)

Renal Impairment
• Use with caution

Hepatic Impairment
• Use with caution

Cardiac Impairment
• Thioridazine produces a dose-dependent prolongation of QTc interval, which may be enhanced by the existence of bradycardia, hypokalemia, congenital or acquired long QTc interval, which should be evaluated prior to administering thioridazine
• Use with caution if treating concomitantly with a medication likely to produce prolonged bradycardia, hypokalemia slowing of intracardiac conduction, or prolongation of the QTc interval
• Avoid thioridazine in patients with a known history of QTc prolongation, recent acute myocardial infarction, and uncompensated heart failure
✳ Risk/benefit ratio may not justify use in cardiac impairment

Elderly
• Some patients may tolerate lower doses better
• Elderly patients may be more sensitive to adverse effects, including agranulocytosis and leukopenia

Children and Adolescents
• Safety and efficacy not established under age 2
• Dose: initial 0.5 mg/kg/day in divided doses; increase gradually; maximum 3 mg/kg/day
• Risk/benefit ratio may not justify use in children or adolescents

Pregnancy
• Risk Category C [some animal studies show adverse effects, no controlled studies in humans]
• Reports of extrapyramidal symptoms, jaundice, hyperreflexia, hyporeflexia in infants whose mothers took a phenothiazine during pregnancy
• Psychotic symptoms may worsen during pregnancy and some form of treatment may be necessary

• Atypical antipsychotic may be preferable to conventional antipsychotics or anticonvulsant mood stabilizers if treatment is required during pregnancy
• Should evaluate for an antipsychotic with a better risk/benefit ratio if treatment is required during pregnancy

Breast Feeding
• Unknown if thioridazine is secreted in human breast milk, but all psychotropics assumed to be secreted in breast milk
✳ Recommended either to discontinue drug or bottle feed

Potential Advantages
• Only for patients who respond to this agent and not other antipsychotics

Potential Disadvantages
• Children
• Elderly
• Patients on other drugs
• Those with low CYP450 2D6 metabolism

Primary Target Symptoms
• Positive symptoms of psychosis in patients who fail to respond to treatment with other antipsychotics
• Motor and autonomic hyperactivity in patients who fail to respond to treatment with other antipsychotics
• Violent or aggressive behavior in patients who fail to respond to treatment with other antipsychotics

Pearls
✳ Generally, the benefits of thioridazine do not outweigh its risks for most patients
✳ Because of its effects on the QTc interval, thioridazine is not intended for use unless other options (at least 2 antipsychotics) have failed
• Thioridazine has not been systematically studied in treatment-refractory schizophrenia
✳ Phenotypic testing may be necessary in order to detect the 7% of the normal population for whom thioridazine is

contraindicated due to a genetic variant leading to reduced activity of CYP450 2D6
- Conventional antipsychotics are much less expensive than atypical antipsychotics
- Thioridazine causes less extrapyramidal symptoms than some other conventional antipsychotics
* Was once a preferred antipsychotic for children and the elderly, and for those whose symptoms benefited from a sedating low potency phenothiazine with a lower incidence of extrapyramidal symptoms
* However, now it is recognized that the dangers of cardiac arrhythmias and drug interactions outweigh the benefits of thioridazine, and it is now considered a second-line treatment if it is considered at all

 Suggested Reading

Frankenburg FR. Choices in antipsychotic therapy in schizophrenia. Harv Rev Psychiatry 1999;6:241–9.

Gardos G, Tecce JJ, Hartmann E, Bowers P, Cole JO. Treatment with mesoridazine and thioridazine in chronic schizophrenia: II. Potential predictors of drug response. Compr Psychiatry 1978;19:527–32.

Sultana A, Reilly J, Fenton M. Thioridazine for schizophrenia. Cochrane Database Syst Rev 2000;(3):CD001944.

Leucht S, Wahlbeck K, Hamann J, Kissling W. New generation antipsychotics versus low-potency conventional antipsychotics: a systematic review and meta-analysis. The Lancet 2003;361:1581–9.

THIOTHIXENE

THERAPEUTICS

Brands • Navane
see index for additional brand names

Generic? Yes

 Class
• Conventional antipsychotic (neuroleptic, thioxanthene, dopamine 2 antagonist)

Commonly Prescribed For
(bold for FDA approved)
• **Schizophrenia**
• Other psychotic disorders
• Bipolar disorder

 How The Drug Works
• Blocks dopamine 2 receptors, reducing positive symptoms of psychosis

How Long Until It Works
• Psychotic symptoms can improve within 1 week, but it may take several weeks for full effect on behavior

If It Works
• Most often reduces positive symptoms in schizophrenia but does not eliminate them
• Most schizophrenic patients do not have a total remission of symptoms but rather a reduction of symptoms by about a third
• Continue treatment in schizophrenia until reaching a plateau of improvement
• After reaching a satisfactory plateau, continue treatment for at least a year after first episode of psychosis in schizophrenia
• For second and subsequent episodes of psychosis in schizophrenia, treatment may need to be indefinite
• Reduces symptoms of acute psychotic mania but not proven as a mood stabilizer or as an effective maintenance treatment in bipolar disorder
• After reducing acute psychotic symptoms in mania, switch to a mood stabilizer and/or an atypical antipsychotic for mood stabilization and maintenance

If It Doesn't Work
• Consider trying one of the first-line atypical antipsychotics (risperidone, olanzapine, quetiapine, ziprasidone, aripiprazole, amisulpride)
• Consider trying another conventional antipsychotic
• If 2 or more antipsychotic monotherapies do not work, consider clozapine

 Best Augmenting Combos for Partial Response or Treatment-Resistance
• Augmentation of conventional antipsychotics has not been systematically studied
• Addition of a mood stabilizing anticonvulsant such as valproate, carbamazepine, or lamotrigine may be helpful in both schizophrenia and bipolar mania
• Augmentation with lithium in bipolar mania may be helpful
• Addition of a benzodiazepine, especially short-term for agitation

Tests
✳ Since conventional antipsychotics are frequently associated with weight gain, before starting treatment, weigh all patients and determine if the patient is already overweight (BMI 25.0–29.9) or obese (BMI ≥30)
• Before giving a drug that can cause weight gain to an overweight or obese patient, consider determining whether the patient already has pre-diabetes (fasting plasma glucose 100–125 mg/dl), diabetes (fasting plasma glucose >126 mg/dl), or dyslipidemia (increased total cholesterol, LDL cholesterol and triglycerides; decreased HDL cholesterol), and treat or refer such patients for treatment, including nutrition and weight management, physical activity counseling, smoking cessation, and medical management
✳ Monitor weight and BMI during treatment
✳ While giving a drug to a patient who has gained >5% of initial weight, consider evaluating for the presence of pre-diabetes, diabetes, or dyslipidemia, or consider switching to a different antipsychotic
• Monitoring elevated prolactin levels of dubious clinical benefit

SIDE EFFECTS

How Drug Causes Side Effects
- By blocking dopamine 2 receptors in the striatum, it can cause motor side effects
- By blocking dopamine 2 receptors in the pituitary, it can cause elevations in prolactin
- By blocking dopamine 2 receptors excessively in the mesocortical and mesolimbic dopamine pathways, especially at high doses, it can cause worsening of negative and cognitive symptoms (neuroleptic-induced deficit syndrome)
- Anticholinergic actions may cause sedation, blurred vision, constipation, dry mouth
- Antihistaminic actions may cause sedation, weight gain
- By blocking alpha 1 adrenergic receptors, it can cause dizziness, sedation, and hypotension
- Mechanism of weight gain and any possible increased incidence of diabetes or dyslipidemia with conventional antipsychotics is unknown

Notable Side Effects
- ❊ Neuroleptic-induced deficit syndrome
- ❊ Akathisia
- ❊ Extrapyramidal symptoms, Parkinsonism, tardive dyskinesia
- ❊ Galactorrhea, amenorrhea
- Sedation
- Dry mouth, constipation, vision disturbance, urrinary retention
- Hypotension, tachycardia
- Rare fine lenticular pigmentation

 Life Threatening or Dangerous Side Effects
- Rare neuroleptic malignant syndrome
- Rare seizures
- Rare blood dyscrasias
- Rare hepatic toxicity

Weight Gain

unusual · not unusual · common · problematic

- ❊ Reported but not expected

Sedation

unusual · not unusual · common · problematic

- Occurs in significant minority

What To Do About Side Effects
- Wait
- Wait
- Wait
- For motor symptoms, add an anticholinergic agent
- For sedation, take at night
- Reduce the dose
- Switch to an atypical antipsychotic
- Weight loss, exercise programs, and medical management for high BMIs, diabetes, dyslipidemia

Best Augmenting Agents for Side Effects
- Benztropine or trihexyphenidyl for motor side effects
- Sometimes amantadine can be helpful for motor side effects
- Benzodiazepines may be helpful for akathisia
- Many side effects cannot be improved with an augmenting agent

DOSING AND USE

Usual Dosage Range
- 15–30 mg/day

Dosage Forms
- Capsule 2 mg, 5 mg, 10 mg

How to Dose
- Initial 5–10 mg/day; maximum dose generally 60 mg/day; higher doses may be given in divided doses

 Dosing Tips
- When thiothixene is dosed too high, it can induce or worsen negative symptoms of schizophrenia
- Lower doses may provide the best benefit with fewest side effects in patients who respond to low doses

Overdose
- Muscle twitching, sedation, dizziness, CNS depression, rigidity, weakness, torticollis, dysphagia, hypotension, coma

Long-Term Use
- Some side effects may be irreversible (e.g., tardive dyskinesia)

Habit Forming
- No

How to Stop
- Slow down-titration (over 6 to 8 weeks), especially when simultaneously beginning a new antipsychotic while switching (i.e., cross-titration)
- Rapid discontinuation may lead to rebound psychosis and worsening of symptoms
- If antiparkinson agents are being used, they should be continued for a few weeks after thiothixene is discontinued

Pharmacokinetics
- Initial elimination half-life approximately 3.4 hours
- Terminal elimination half-life approximately 34 hours

 Drug Interactions
- Respiratory depression may occur when thiothixene is combined with lorazepam
- Additive effects may occur if used with CNS depressants
- May decrease the effects of levodopa, dopamine agonists
- Some patients taking a neuroleptic and lithium have developed an encephalopathic syndrome similar to neuroleptic malignant syndrome
- Combined use with epinephrine may lower blood pressure
- May increase the effects of antihypertensive drugs except for guanethidine, whose antihypertensive actions thiothixene may antagonize

 Other Warnings/ Precautions
- If signs of neuroleptic malignant syndrome develop, treatment should be immediately discontinued

- Use cautiously in patients with alcohol withdrawal or convulsive disorders because of possible lowering of seizure threshold
- Antiemetic effect can mask signs of other disorders or overdose
- Do not use epinephrine in event of overdose, as interaction with some pressor agents may lower blood pressure
- Use cautiously in patients with glaucoma, urinary retention
- Observe for signs of ocular toxicity (pigmentary retinopathy, lenticular pigmentation)
- Avoid extreme heat exposure
- Use only with caution if at all in Parkinson's disease or Lewy Body dementia

Do Not Use
- If patient has CNS depression, is in a comatose state, has circulatory collapse, or there is presence of blood dyscrasias
- If there is a proven allergy to thiothixene

SPECIAL POPULATIONS

Renal Impairment
- Use with caution

Hepatic Impairment
- Use with caution

Cardiac Impairment
- Thiothixene may cause or aggravate ECG changes

Elderly
- Some patients may tolerate lower doses better

 Children and Adolescents
- Safety and efficacy have not been established in children under age 12
- Generally consider second-line after atypical antipsychotics

 Pregnancy
- Use of thiothixene has not been studied in pregnant women

- Reports of extrapyramidal symptoms, jaundice, hyperreflexia, hyporeflexia in infants whose mothers took a phenothiazine during pregnancy
- Psychotic symptoms may worsen during pregnancy and some form of treatment may be necessary
- Atypical antipsychotics may be preferable to conventional antipsychotics or anticonvulsant mood stabilizers if treatment is required during pregnancy
- Thiothixene should generally not be used during the first trimester
- Thiothixene should only be used during pregnancy if clearly needed

Breast Feeding

- Unknown if thiothixene is secreted in human breast milk, but all psychotropics assumed to be secreted in breast milk
- ✱ Recommended either to discontinue drug or bottle feed

THE ART OF PSYCHOPHARMACOLOGY

Potential Advantages

- For patients who do not respond to other antipsychotics

Potential Disadvantages

- Patients with tardive dyskinesia
- Children
- Elderly

Primary Target Symptoms

- Positive symptoms of psychosis
- Negative symptoms of psychosis

 Pearls

- ✱ Although not systematically studied, may cause less weight gain than other antipsychotics
- Conventional antipsychotics are less expensive than atypical antipsychotics
- Patients have very similar antipsychotic responses to any conventional antipsychotic, which is different from atypical antipsychotics where antipsychotic responses of individual patients can occasionally vary greatly from one atypical antipsychotic to another
- Patients with inadequate responses to atypical antipsychotics may benefit from a trial of augmentation with a conventional antipsychotic such as thiothixene or from switching to a conventional antipsychotic such as thiothixene
- However, long-term polypharmacy with a combination of a conventional antipsychotic such as thiothixene with an atypical antipsychotic may combine their side effects without clearly augmenting the efficacy of either
- Although a frequent practice by some prescribers, adding 2 conventional antipsychotics together has little rationale and may reduce tolerability without clearly enhancing efficacy

 Suggested Reading

Huang CC, Gerhardstein RP, Kim DY, Hollister L. Treatment-resistant schizophrenia: controlled study of moderate- and high-dose thiothixene. Int Clin Psychopharmacol 1987;2:69–75.

Sterlin C, Ban TA, Jarrold L. The place of thiothixene among the thioxanthenes. Curr Ther Res Clin Exp 1972;14:205–14.

TIAGABINE

THERAPEUTICS

Brands • Gabitril
see index for additional brand names

Generic? No

 Class
• Anticonvulsant; selective GABA reuptake inhibitor (SGRI)

Commonly Prescribed For
(bold for FDA approved)
• **Partial seizures (adjunctive; adults and children 12 years and older)**
• Anxiety disorders
• Neuropathic pain/chronic pain

 How The Drug Works
• Selectively blocks reuptake of gamma-aminobutyric acid (GABA) by presynaptic and glial GABA transporters

How Long Until It Works
• Should reduce seizures by 2 weeks
• Not clear that it works in anxiety disorders or chronic pain but some patients may respond, and if they do, therapeutic actions can be seen by 2 weeks

If It Works
• The goal of treatment is complete remission of symptoms (e.g., seizures, anxiety)
• The goal of treatment of chronic neuropathic pain is to reduce symptoms as much as possible, especially in combination with other treatments
• Treatment of chronic neuropathic pain most often reduces but does not eliminate symptoms and is not a cure since symptoms usually recur after medicine stopped
• Continue treatment until all symptoms are gone or until improvement is stable and then continue treating indefinitely as long as improvement persists

If It Doesn't Work (for neuropathic pain or anxiety disorders)
• Many patients only have a partial response where some symptoms are improved but others persist

• Other patients may be nonresponders, sometimes called treatment-resistant or treatment-refractory
• May only be effective in a subset of patients with neuropathic pain or anxiety disorders, in some patients who fail to respond to other treatments, or it may not work at all
• Consider increasing dose, switching to another agent or adding an appropriate augmenting agent
• Consider biofeedback or hypnosis for pain
• Consider evaluation for another diagnosis or for a comorbid condition (e.g., medical illness, substance abuse, etc.)
• Switch to another agent with fewer side effects
• Consider evaluation for another diagnosis or for a comorbid condition (e.g., medical illness, substance abuse, etc.)

 Best Augmenting Combos for Partial Response or Treatment-Resistance
• Tiagabine is itself an augmenting agent for numerous other anticonvulsants in treating epilepsy
✱ For neuropathic pain, tiagabine can augment tricyclic antidepressants and SNRIs as well as gabapentin, other anticonvulsants, and even opiates if done by experts while carefully monitoring in difficult cases
• For anxiety, tiagabine is a second-line treatment to augment SSRIs, SNRIs, or benzodiazepines

Tests
• None for healthy individuals
• Tiagabine may bind to tissue that contains melanin, so for long-term treatment opthalmological checks may be considered

SIDE EFFECTS

How Drug Causes Side Effects
• CNS side effects may be due to excessive actions of GABA

Notable Side Effects
✱ Sedation, dizziness, asthenia, nervousness, difficulty concentrating,

speech/language problems, confusion, tremor
- Diarrhea, vomiting, nausea
- Ecchymosis, depression

 Life Threatening or Dangerous Side Effects
- Exacerbation of EEG abnormalities in epilepsy
- Status epilepticus in epilepsy (unknown if associated with tiagabine use)
- Sudden unexplained deaths have occurred in epilepsy (unknown if related to tiagabine use)

Weight Gain

unusual   not unusual   common   problematic

- Reported but not expected
- Some patients experience increased appetite

Sedation

unusual   not unusual   common   problematic

- Many experience and/or can be significant in amount

What To Do About Side Effects
- Wait
- Wait
- Wait
- Take more of the dose at night or all of the dose at night to reduce daytime sedation
- Lower the dose
- Switch to another agent

Best Augmenting Agents for Side Effects
- Many side effects cannot be improved with an augmenting agent

DOSING AND USE

Usual Dosage Range
- 32–56 mg/day in 2–4 divided doses for adjunctive treatment of epilepsy
- 2–12 mg/day for adjunctive treatment of chronic pain and anxiety disorders

Dosage Forms
- Tablet 2 mg, 4 mg, 12 mg, 16 mg, 20 mg

How to Dose
- Adjunct to enzyme-inducing antiepileptic drugs: initial 4 mg once daily; after 1 week can increase dose by 4–8 mg/day each week; maximum dose generally 56 mg/day in 2–4 divided doses
- Dosing for chronic pain or anxiety disorders not well established, but start as low as 2 mg at night, increasing by 2 mg increments every few days as tolerated to 8–12 mg/day

 Dosing Tips
- Usually administered as adjunctive medication to other anticonvulsants in the treatment of epilepsy
- ✳ Usually administered as adjunctive medication to benzodiazepines, SSRIs, and/or SNRIs in the treatment of anxiety disorders; and to SNRIs, gabapentin, other anticonvulsants, and even opiates in the treatment of chronic pain
- ✳ Dosing varies considerably among individual patients but is definitely at the lower end of the dosing spectrum for patients with chronic neuropathic pain or anxiety disorders (i.e., 2–12 mg either as a split dose or all at night)
- ✳ Patients with chronic neuropathic pain and anxiety disorders are far less tolerant of CNS side effects, so they require a much slower dosage titration as well as a lower maintenance dose
- Gastrointestinal absorption is markedly slowed by the concomitant intake of food, which also lessens the peak plasma concentrations
- ✳ Thus, for improved tolerability and consistent clinical actions, instruct patients to always take with food
- Side effects may increase with dose

Overdose
- No fatalities have been reported; sedation, agitation, confusion, speech difficulty, hostility, depression, weakness, myoclonus

Long-Term Use
- Safe

Habit Forming
- No

How to Stop
- Taper
- Epilepsy patients may seize upon withdrawal, especially if withdrawal is abrupt
- Discontinuation symptoms uncommon

Pharmacokinetics
- Primarily metabolized by CYP450 3A4
- Steady state concentrations tend to be lower in the evening than in the morning
- Half-life approximately 7–9 hours
- Renally excreted

 Drug Interactions
- Clearance of tiagabine may be reduced and thus plasma levels increased if taken with a non-enzyme inducing antiepileptic drug (e.g., valproate, gabapentin, lamotrigine), so tiagabine dose may need to be reduced
- CYP450 3A4 inducers such as carbamazepine can lower the plasma levels of tiagabine
- CYP450 3A4 inhibitors such as nefazodone, fluvoxamine, and fluoxetine could theoretically increase the plasma levels of tiagabine
- Clearance of tiagabine is increased if taken with an enzyme-inducing antiepileptic drug (e.g., carbamazepine, phenobarbital, phenytoin, primidone) and thus plasma levels are reduced; however, no dose adjustments are necessary for treatment of epilepsy as the dosing recommendations for epilepsy are based on adjunctive treatment with an enzyme-inducing antiepileptic drug
- Despite common actions upon GABA, no pharmacodynamic or pharmacokinetic interations have been shown when tiagabine is combined with the benzodiazepine triazolam or with alcohol
- However, sedating actions of any two sedative drugs given in combination can be additive

 Other Warnings/ Precautions
- Depressive effects may be increased by other CNS depressants (alcohol, MAOIs, other anticonvulsants, etc.)

- Tiagabine may bind to melanin, raising the possibility of long-term opthalmologic effects

Do Not Use
- If there is a proven allergy to tiagabine

Renal Impairment
- Although tiagabine is renally excreted, the pharmacokinetics of tiagabine in healthy patients and in those with impaired renal function are similar and no dose adjustment is recommended

Hepatic Impairment
- Clearance is decreased
- May require lower dose

Cardiac Impairment
- No dose adjustment recommended

Elderly
- Some patients may tolerate lower doses better

 Children and Adolescents
- Safety and efficacy not established under age 12
- Maximum recommended dose generally 32 mg/day in 2–4 divided doses

 Pregnancy
- Risk category C [some animal studies show adverse effects, no controlled studies in humans]
- Use in women of childbearing potential requires weighing potential benefits to the mother against the risks to the fetus
- Taper drug if discontinuing
- Seizures, even mild seizures, may cause harm to the embryo/fetus
- ✳ Lack of definitive evidence of efficacy for chronic neuropathic pain or anxiety disorders suggests risk/benefit ratio is in favor of discontinuing tiagabine during pregnancy for those indications

Breast Feeding
- Some drug is found in mother's breast milk

* Recommended either to discontinue drug or bottle feed
• If drug is continued while breast feeding, infant should be monitored for possible adverse effects
• If infant shows signs of irritability or sedation, drug may need to be discontinued

THE ART OF PSYCHOPHARMACOLOGY

Potential Advantages
• Treatment-resistant chronic neuropathic pain
• Treatment-resistant anxiety disorders

Potential Disadvantages
• May require 2–4 times a day dosing
• Needs to be taken with food

Primary Target Symptoms
• Incidence of seizures
• Pain
• Anxiety

 Pearls
• Well studied in epilepsy
• Much use is off-label
* Off-label use second-line and as an augmenting agent may be justified for treatment resistant anxiety disorders and neuropathic pain and also for fibromyalgia
* Off-label use for bipolar disorder may not be justified
* One of the few agents that enhances slow-wave delta sleep, which may be helpful in chronic neuropathic pain syndromes

 Suggested Reading

Backonja NM. Use of anticonvulsants for treatment of neuropathic pain. Neurology 2002 10;59(Suppl 2):S14–7.

Carta MG, Hardoy MC, Grunze H, Carpiniello B. The use of tiagabine in affective disorders. Pharmacopsychiatry 2002;35:33–4.

Evans EA. Efficacy of newer anticonvulsant medications in bipolar spectrum mood disorders. J Clin Psychiatry 2003;64(Suppl 8):9–14.

Lydiard RB. The role of GABA in anxiety disorders. J Clin Psychiatry 2003;64(Suppl 3):21–7.

Schmidt D, Gram L, Brodie M, Kramer G, Perucca E, Kalviainen R, Elger CE. Tiagabine in the treatment of epilepsy—a clinical review with a guide for the prescribing physician. Epilepsy Res. 2000; 41: 245–51.

Stahl SM. Psychopharmacology of anticonvulsants: do all anticonvulsants have the same mechanism of action? J Clin Psychiatry. 2004;65:149–50.

Stahl SM. Anticonvulsants as anxiolytics, part 1: tiagabine and other anticonvulsants with actions on GABA. J Clin Psychiatry. 2004;65:291–2.

TIANEPTINE

Brands • Coaxil
• Stablon
see index for additional brand names

Generic? No

Class
• Tricyclic antidepressant
• Serotonin reuptake enhancer

Commonly Prescribed For
(bold for FDA approved)
• Major depressive disorder
• Dysthymia
• Anxiety associated with depression, alcohol dependence

How The Drug Works
✳ Possibly increases serotonin uptake, but could also act similarly to agents that block serotonin reuptake

How Long Until It Works
• Onset of therapeutic actions usually not immediate, but often delayed 2 to 4 weeks
• If it is not working within 6 to 8 weeks for depression, it may require a dosage increase or it may not work at all
• May continue to work for many years to prevent relapse of symptoms

If It Works
• The goal of treatment is complete remission of current symptoms as well as prevention of future relapses
• Treatment most often reduces or even eliminates symptoms, but not a cure since symptoms can recur after medicine stopped
• Continue treatment until all symptoms are gone (remission)
• Once symptoms gone, continue treating for 1 year for the first episode of depression
• For second and subsequent episodes of depression, treatment may need to be indefinite

If It Doesn't Work
• Many patients only have a partial response where some symptoms are improved but others persist (especially insomnia, fatigue, and problems concentrating)
• Other patients may be nonresponders, sometimes called treatment-resistant or treatment-refractory
• Consider increasing dose, switching to another agent or adding an appropriate augmenting agent
• Consider psychotherapy
• Consider evaluation for another diagnosis or for a comorbid condition (e.g., medical illness, substance abuse, etc.)

Best Augmenting Combos for Partial Response or Treatment-Resistance
• Augmentation has not been systematically studied with tianeptine

Tests
• None for healthy individuals
✳ Since other tricyclic and tetracyclic antidepressants are frequently associated with weight gain, it is possible that this may also be the case for tianeptine; thus, before starting treatment, weigh all patients and determine if the patient is already overweight (BMI 25.0–29.9) or obese (BMI ≥30)
• Before giving a drug that can cause weight gain to an overweight or obese patient, consider determining whether the patient already has pre-diabetes (fasting plasma glucose 100–125 mg/dl), diabetes (fasting plasma glucose >126 mg/dl), or dyslipidemia (increased total cholesterol, LDL cholesterol and triglycerides; decreased HDL cholesterol), and treat or refer such patients for treatment, including nutrition and weight management, physical activity counseling, smoking cessation, and medical management
✳ Monitor weight and BMI during treatment
✳ While giving a drug to a patient who has gained >5% of initial weight, consider evaluating for the presence of pre-diabetes, diabetes, or dyslipidemia, or consider switching to a different antidepressant
• Theoretically, by analogy with other TCAs, EKGs may be useful for selected patients (e.g., those with personal or family history of QTc prolongation; cardiac arrhythmia; recent myocardial infarction; uncompensated heart failure; or taking agents that prolong QTc interval such as

pimozide, thioridazine, selected antiarrhythmics, moxifloxacin, sparfloxacin, etc.)
• On a theoretical basis and by analogy with other TCAs, patients at risk for electrolyte disturbances (e.g., patients on diuretic therapy) should have baseline and periodic serum potassium and magnesium measurements

SIDE EFFECTS

How Drug Causes Side Effects
✳ Mild anticholinergic activity (less than some other tricyclic antidepressants) could possibly lead to sedative effects, dry mouth, constipation, and blurred vision
• Most side effects are immediate but often go away with time
✳ Pharmacologic studies indicate tianeptine may not be a potent alpha 1antagonist or H1 antihistamine
• Theoretically, cardiac arrhythmias and seizures, especially in overdose, may be caused by blockade of ion channels

Notable Side Effects
• Headache, dizziness, insomnia, sedation
• Nausea, constipation, abdominal pain, dry mouth
• Abnormal dreams
• Rare hepatotoxicity
• Tachycardia

 Life Threatening or Dangerous Side Effects
• Theoretically, lowered seizure threshold and rare seizures
• Theoretically, rare induction of mania and activation of suicidal ideation
• Theoretically, could prolong QTc interval, but not well-studied

Weight Gain

unusual   not unusual   common   problematic
• Not well studied

Sedation

unusual   not unusual   common   problematic
• Occurs in significant minority

What To Do About Side Effects
• Wait
• Wait
• Wait
• Lower the dose
• In a few weeks, switch or add other drugs

Best Augmenting Agents for Side Effects
• Augmentation for side effects of tianeptine has not been systematically studied

DOSING AND USE

Usual Dosage Range
• 25–50 mg/day

Dosage Forms
• Tablet 12.5 mg

How to Dose
• 12.5 mg 3 times/day

 Dosing Tips
• Tianeptine's rapid elimination necessitates strict adherence to the dosing schedule
✳ Short half-life means multiple daily doses
✳ Although tianeptine has a tricyclic structure, it is dosed lower than usual TCA dosing

Overdose
• Effects are generally mild and nonfatal; unlikely to cause cardiovascular effects

Long-Term Use
• Safe

Habit Forming
• No

How to Stop
• Taper to avoid withdrawal symptoms
• Many patients tolerate 50% dose reduction for 3 days, then another 50% reduction for 3 days, then discontinuation
• If withdrawal symptoms emerge during discontinuation, raise dose to stop symptoms and then restart withdrawal much more slowly

Pharmacokinetics
- Not primarily metabolized by CYP 450 enzyme system
- Tianeptine is rapidly eliminated
- Half-life approximately 3 hours

 Drug Interactions
- Tramadol increases the risk of seizures in patients taking TCAs
- Activation and agitation, especially following switching or adding antidepressants, may represent the induction of a bipolar state, especially a mixed dysphoric bipolar II condition sometimes associated with suicidal ideation, and require the addition of lithium, a mood stabilizer or an atypical antipsychotic, and/or discontinuation of tianeptine
- Other drug interactions not well-studied

 Other Warnings/ Precautions
- Add or initiate other antidepressants with caution for up to 2 weeks after discontinuing tianeptine
- For elective surgery, tianeptine should be stopped 24–48 hours before general anesthesia is administered
- Generally, do not use with MAO inhibitors, including 14 days after MAOIs are stopped; do not start an MAOI until 2 weeks after discontinuing tianeptine
- Although not well studied for tianeptine, other TCAs can prolong QTc interval, especially at toxic doses, potentially causing torsade de pointes-type arrhythmia or sudden death; this has not been reported specifically for tianeptine
- Because other TCAs can prolong QTc interval, use with caution in patients who have bradycardia or who are taking drugs that can induce bradycardia (e.g., beta blockers, calcium channel blockers, clonidine, digitalis)
- Because other TCAs can prolong QTc interval, use with caution in patients who have hypokalemia and/or hypomagnesemia or who are taking drugs that can induce hypokalemia and/or magnesemia (e.g., diuretics, stimulant laxatives, intravenous amphotericin B, glucocorticoids, tetracosactide)

Do Not Use
- If patient is taking an MAO inhibitor
- If patient is pregnant or nursing
- On a theoretical basis, if patient is taking agents capable of significantly prolonging QTc interval (e.g., pimozide, thioridazine, selected antiarrhythmics, moxifloxacin, sparfloxacin)
- On a theoretical basis, if there is a history of QTc prolongation or cardiac arrhythmia, recent acute myocardial infarction, uncompensated heart failure
- If there is a proven allergy to tianeptine

SPECIAL POPULATIONS

Renal Impairment
- Dose should be reduced for severe impairment to 25 mg/day
- Dose reduction not necessary for patients on hemodialysis

Hepatic Impairment
- No dose adjustment necessary

Cardiac Impairment
- No dose adjustment necessary
- Safety of tianeptine in patients with cardiac impairment has not been specifically demonstrated
- TCAs have been reported to cause arrhythmias, prolongation of conduction time, orthostatic hypotension, sinus tachycardia, and heart failure, especially in the diseased heart
- Myocardial infarction and stroke have been reported with TCAs
- TCAs produce QTc prolongation, which may be enhanced by the existence of bradycardia, hypokalemia, congenital or acquired long QTc interval, which should be evaluated prior to administering tianeptine
- Avoid TCAs in patients with a known history of QTc prolongation, recent acute myocardial infarction, and uncompensated heart failure
- TCAs may cause a sustained increase in heart rate in patients with ischemic heart disease and may worsen (decrease) heart rate variability, an independent risk of mortality in cardiac populations
- ✱ Risk/benefit ratio may not justify use of TCAs in cardiac impairment

Elderly
• Dose should be reduced to 25 mg/day

Children and Adolescents
• Use with caution, observing for activation of known or unknown bipolar disorder and/or suicidal ideation, and strongly consider informing parents or guardian of this risk so they can help observe child or adolescent patients
• Has been used successfully to treat asthmatic symptoms in children
• Not recommended for use under age 15

Pregnancy
• Risk Category not formally assessed by the US FDA
• Not recommended for use during pregnancy

Breast Feeding
• Some drug is found in mother's breast milk
✳ Not recommended for use during pregnancy
• Immediate postpartum period is a high-risk time for depression, especially in women who have had prior depressive episodes, so drug may need to be reinstituted late in the third trimester or shortly after childbirth to prevent a recurrence during the postpartum period

• Must weigh benefits of breast feeding with risks and benefits of antidepressant treatment versus non-treatment to both the infant and the mother
• For many patients, this may mean continuing treatment during breast feeding

THE ART OF PSYCHOPHARMACOLOGY

Potential Advantages
• Elderly patients
• Alcohol withdrawal

Potential Disadvantages
• Patients who have difficulty being compliant with multiple daily dosing

Primary Target Symptoms
• Depressed mood
• Symptoms of anxiety

Pearls
✳ Possibly a unique mechanism of action
• However, mechanism of action not well understood
• Not marketed widely throughout the world, but mostly in France
✳ Effects on QTc prolongation not systematically studied

Suggested Reading

Ginestet D. Efficacy of tianeptine in major depressive disorders with or without melancholia. Eur Neuropsychopharmacol 1997;7 Suppl 3:S341–5.

Wagstaff AJ, Ormrod D, Spencer CM. Tianeptine: a review of its use in depressive disorders. CNS Drugs 2001;15(3):231–59.

Wilde MI, Benfield P. Tianeptine. A review of its pharmacodynamic and pharmacokinetic properties, and therapeutic efficacy in depression and coexisting anxiety and depression. Drugs 1995;49(3):411–39.

TOPIRAMATE

THERAPEUTICS

Brands
- Topamax
- Epitomax
- Topamac
- Topimax

see index for additional brand names

Generic? No

Class
- Anticonvulsant, voltage-sensitive sodium channel modulator

Commonly Prescribed For
(bold for FDA approved)
- **Partial onset seizures (adjunctive; adults and pediatric patients 2–16 years of age)**
- **Primary generalized tonic-clonic seizures (adjunctive; adults and pediatric patients 2–16 years of age)**
- **Seizures associated with Lennox-Gastaut Syndrome (2 years of age or older)**
- **Migraine prophylaxis**
- Bipolar disorder (adjunctive; no longer in development)
- Psychotropic drug-induced weight gain
- Binge-eating disorder

How The Drug Works
* Blocks voltage-sensitive sodium channels by an unknown mechanism
- Inhibits release of glutamate
- Potentiates activity of gamma-aminobutyric acid (GABA)
- Carbonic anhydrase inhibitor

How Long Until It Works
- Should reduce seizures by 2 weeks
- Not clear that it has mood stabilizing properties, but some bipolar patients may respond and if so, it may take several weeks to months to optimize an effect on mood stabilization

If It Works
- The goal of treatment is complete remission of symptoms (e.g., mania, seizures, migraine)
- Continue treatment until all symptoms are gone or until improvement is stable and then continue treating indefinitely as long as improvement persists
- Continue treatment indefinitely to avoid recurrence of mania, seizures, and headaches

If It Doesn't Work (for bipolar disorder)
* May only be effective in a subset of bipolar patients, in some patients who fail to respond to other mood stabilizers, or it may not work at all
* Consider increasing dose or switching to another agent with better demonstrated efficacy in bipolar disorder

 Best Augmenting Combos for Partial Response or Treatment-Resistance
- Topiramate is itself a second-line augmenting agent for numerous other anticonvulsants, lithium, and antipsychotics in treating bipolar disorder

Tests
* Baseline and periodic serum bicarbonate levels to monitor for hyperchloremic, non-anion gap metabolic acidosis (i.e., decreased serum bicarbonate below the normal reference range in the absence of chronic respiratory alkalosis)

SIDE EFFECTS

How Drug Causes Side Effects
- CNS side effects theoretically due to excessive actions at voltage-sensitive sodium channels
- Weak inhibition of carbonic anhydrase may lead to kidney stones and paresthesias
- Inhibition of carbonic anhydrase may also lead to metabolic acidosis

Notable Side Effects
* Sedation, asthenia, dizziness, ataxia, parasthesia, nervousness, nystagmus, tremor
* Nausea, appetite loss, weight loss
- Blurred or double vision, mood problems, problems concentrating, confusion, memory problems, psychomotor retardation, language problems, speech problems, fatigue, taste perversion

Life Threatening or Dangerous Side Effects

* Metabolic acidosis
* Kidney stones
- Secondary narrow angle-closure glaucoma
- Oligohidrosis and hyperthermia (more common in children)
- Sudden unexplained deaths have occurred in epilepsy (unknown if related to topiramate use)

Weight Gain

unusual   not unusual   common   problematic

- Reported but not expected
* Patients may experience weight loss

Sedation

unusual   not unusual   common   problematic

- Many experience and/or can be significant in amount

What To Do About Side Effects

- Wait
- Wait
- Wait
- Take at night to reduce daytime sedation
- Increase fluid intake to reduce the risk of kidney stones
- Switch to another agent

Best Augmenting Agents for Side Effects

- Many side effects cannot be improved with an augmenting agent

DOSING AND USE

Usual Dosage Range

- Adults: 200–400 mg/day in 2 divided doses for epilepsy; 50–300 mg/day for adjunctive treatment of bipolar disorder

Dosage Forms

- Tablet 25 mg, 100 mg, 200 mg
- Sprinkle capsule 15 mg, 25 mg

How to Dose

- Adults: initial 25–50 mg/day; increase each week by 50 mg/day; administer in 2 divided doses; maximum dose generally 1600 mg/day
- Seizures (ages 2–16): see Children and Adolescents

 Dosing Tips

- Adverse effects may increase as dose increases
- Topiramate is available in a sprinkle capsule formulation, which can be swallowed whole or sprinkled over approximately a teaspoon of soft food (e.g., applesauce); the mixture should be consumed immediately
- Bipolar patients are generally administered doses at the lower end of the dosing range
- Slow upward titration from doses as low as 25 mg/day can reduce the incidence of unacceptable sedation
- Many bipolar patients do not tolerate more than 200 mg/day
* Weight loss is dose-related but most patients treated for weight gain receive doses at the lower end of the dosing range

Overdose

- No fatalities have been reported in monotherapy; convulsions, sedation, speech disturbance, blurred or double vision, metabolic acidosis, impaired coordination, hypotension, abdominal pain, agitation, dizziness

Long-Term Use

- Probably safe
- Periodic monitoring of serum bicarbonate levels may be required

Habit Forming

- No

How to Stop

- Taper
- Epilepsy patients may seize upon withdrawal, especially if withdrawal is abrupt
* Rapid discontinuation may increase the risk of relapse in bipolar patients
* Discontinuation symptoms uncommon

Pharmacokinetics

- Elimination half-life approximately 21 hours
- Renally excreted

Drug Interactions

- Carbamazepine, phenytoin, and valproate may increase the clearance of topiramate, and thus decrease topiramate levels, possibly requiring a higher dose of topiramate
- Topiramate may increase the clearance of phenytoin and thus decrease phenytoin levels, possibly requiring a higher dose of phenytoin
- Topiramate may increase the clearance of valproate and thus decrease valproate levels, possibly requiring a higher dose of valproate
- Topiramate may increase plasma levels of metformin; also, metformin may reduce clearance of topiramate and increase topiramate levels
- Topiramate may interact with carbonic anhydrase inhibitors to increase the risk of kidney stones
- Topiramate may reduce the effectiveness of oral contraceptives

 Other Warnings/ Precautions

* If symptoms of metabolic acidosis develop (hyperventilation, fatigue, anorexia, cardiac arrhythmias, stupor), then dose may need to be reduced or treatment may need to be discontinued
- Depressive effects may be increased by other CNS depressants (alcohol, MAOIs, other anticonvulsants, etc.)
- Use with caution when combining with other drugs that predispose patients to heat-related disorders, including carbonic anhydrase inhibitors and anticholinergics

Do Not Use

- If there is a proven allergy to topiramate

SPECIAL POPULATIONS

Renal Impairment

- Topiramate is renally excreted, so the dose should be lowered by half
- Can be removed by hemodialysis; patients receiving hemodialysis may require supplemental doses of topiramate

Hepatic Impairment

- Drug should be used with caution

Cardiac Impairment

- Drug should be used with caution

Elderly

- Elderly patients may be more susceptible to adverse effects

 Children and Adolescents

- Approved for use in children age 2 and older for treatment of seizures
- Clearance is increased in pediatric patients
- Seizures (ages 2–16): initial 1–3 mg/kg/day at night; after 1 week increase by 1–3 mg/kg/day every 1–2 weeks with total daily dose administered in 2 divided doses; recommended dose generally 5–9 mg/kg/day in 2 divided doses

 Pregnancy

- Risk category C [some animal studies show adverse effects, no controlled studies in humans]
- Use in women of childbearing potential requires weighing potential benefits to the mother against the risks to the fetus
- Hypospadia has occurred in some male infants whose mothers took topiramate during pregnancy
* Lack of convincing efficacy for treatment of bipolar disorder suggests risk/benefit ratio is in favor of discontinuing topiramate in bipolar patients during pregnancy
* For bipolar patients, topiramate should generally be discontinued before anticipated pregnancies
- Taper drug if discontinuing
* For bipolar patients, given the risk of relapse in the postpartum period, mood stabilizer treatment, especially with agents with better evidence of efficacy than topiramate, should generally be restarted immediately after delivery if patient is unmedicated during pregnancy
* Atypical antipsychotics may be preferable to topiramate if treatment of bipolar disorder is required during pregnancy
- Bipolar symptoms may recur or worsen during pregnancy and some form of treatment may be necessary

• Seizures, even mild seizures, may cause harm to the embryo/fetus

Breast Feeding

• Some drug is found in mother's breast milk
✻ Recommended either to discontinue drug or bottle feed
• If drug is continued while breast feeding, infant should be monitored for possible adverse effects
• If infant shows signs of irritability or sedation, drug may need to be discontinued
✻ Bipolar disorder may recur during the postpartum period, particularly if there is a history of prior postpartum episodes of either depression or psychosis
✻ Relapse rates may be lower in women who receive prophylactic treatment for postpartum episodes of bipolar disorder
• Atypical antipsychotics and anticonvulsants such as valproate may be safer and more effective than topiramate during the postpartum period when treating nursing mother with bipolar disorder

THE ART OF PSYCHOPHARMACOLOGY

Potential Advantages

• Treatment-resistant bipolar disorder
• Patients who wish to avoid weight gain

Potential Disadvantages

• Efficacy in bipolar disorder uncertain
• Patients with a history of kidney stones or risks for metabolic acidosis

Primary Target Symptoms

• Incidence of seizures
• Unstable mood

 Pearls

• Side effects may actually occur less often in pediatric patients
• Has been studied in a wide range of psychiatric disorders, including bipolar disorder, posttraumatic stress disorder, binge-eating disorder, obesity and others

• Some anecdotes, case series, and open-label studies have been published and are widely known suggesting efficacy in bipolar disorder
✻ However, randomized clinical trials do not suggest efficacy in bipolar disorder; unfortunately these important studies have not been published by the manufacturer, who has dropped topiramate from further development as a mood stabilizer, though this is not widely known
✻ Misperceptions about topiramate's efficacy in bipolar disorder have led to its use in more patients than other agents with proven efficacy, such as lamotrigine
✻ Due to reported weight loss in some patients in trials with epilepsy, topiramate is commonly used to treat weight gain, especially in patients with psychotropic drug-induced weight gain
✻ Weight loss in epilepsy patients is dose related with more weight loss at high doses (mean 6.5 kg or 7.3% decline) and less weight loss at lower doses (mean 1.6 kg or 2.2% decline)
✻ Changes in weight were greatest in epilepsy patients who weighed the most at baseline (>100 kg), with mean loss of 9.6 kg or 8.4% decline, while those weighing <60 kg had only a mean loss of 1.3 kg or 2.5% decline
✻ Long-term studies demonstrate that weight losses in epilepsy patients were seen within the first 3 months of treatment and peaked at a mean of 6 kg after 12 to 18 months of treatment; however, weight tended to return to pretreatment levels after 18 months
✻ Some patients with psychotropic drug-induced weight gain may experience significant weight loss (>7% of body weight) with topiramate up to 200 mg/day for 3 months, but this is not typical, is not often sustained, and has not been systemically studied
• Early studies suggest potential efficacy in binge-eating disorder

Suggested Reading

Chengappa KR, Gershon S, Levine J. The evolving role of topiramate among other mood stabilizers in the management of bipolar disorder. Bipolar Disord. 2001; 3: 215–232.

Ormrod D, McClellan K. Topiramate: a review of its use in childhood epilepsy. Paediatr Drugs. 2001; 3: 293–319.

MacDonald KJ, Young LT. Newer antiepileptic drugs in bipolar disorder. CNS Drugs 2002;16:549–62.

Shank RP, Gardocki JF, Streeter AJ, Maryanoff BE. An overview of the preclinical aspects of topiramate: pharmacology, pharmacokinetics, and mechanism of action. Epilepsia. 2000; 41 (Suppl 1): S3–9.

Suppes T. Review of the use of topiramate for treatment of bipolar disorders. J Clin Psychopharmacol 2002;22:599–609.

TRANYLCYPROMINE

THERAPEUTICS

Brands • Parnate
see index for additional brand names

Generic? Not in U.S.

Class
• Monoamine oxidase inhibitor (MAOI)

Commonly Prescribed For
(bold for FDA approved)
• **Major depressive episode without melancholia**
• Treatment-resistant depression
• Treatment-resistant panic disorder
• Treatment-resistant social anxiety disorder

How The Drug Works
• Irreversibly blocks monoamine oxidase (MAO) from breaking down norepinephrine, serotonin, and dopamine
• This presumably boosts noradrenergic, serotonergic, and dopaminergic neurotransmission
✶ As the drug is structurally related to amphetamine, it may have some stimulant-like actions due to monoamine release and reuptake inhibition

How Long Until It Works
• Some patients may experience stimulant-like actions early in dosing
• Onset of therapeutic actions usually not immediate, but often delayed 2 to 4 weeks
• If it is not working within 6 to 8 weeks, it may require a dosage increase or it may not work at all
• May continue to work for many years to prevent relapse of symptoms

If It Works
• The goal of treatment is complete remission of current symptoms as well as prevention of future relapses
• Treatment most often reduces or even eliminates symptoms, but not a cure since symptoms can recur after medicine stopped
• Continue treatment until all symptoms are gone (remission)
• Once symptoms gone, continue treating for 1 year for the first episode of depression

• For second and subsequent episodes of depression, treatment may need to be indefinite
• Use in anxiety disorders may also need to be indefinite

If It Doesn't Work
• Many patients only have a partial response where some symptoms are improved but others persist (especially insomnia, fatigue, and problems concentrating)
• Other patients may be nonresponders, sometimes called treatment-resistant or treatment-refractory
• Some patients who have an initial response may relapse even though they continue treatment, sometimes called "poop-out"
• Consider increasing dose, switching to another agent or adding an appropriate augmenting agent
• Consider psychotherapy
• Consider evaluation for another diagnosis or for a comorbid condition (e.g., medical illness, substance abuse, etc.)
• Some patients may experience apparent lack of consistent efficacy due to activation of latent or underlying bipolar disorder, and require antidepressant discontinuation and a switch to a mood stabilizer

Best Augmenting Combos for Partial Response or Treatment-Resistance
✶ Augmentation of MAOIs has not been systematically studied, and this is something for the expert, to be done with caution and with careful monitoring
✶ A stimulant such as d-amphetamine or methylphenidate (with caution; may activate bipolar disorder and suicidal ideation; may elevate blood pressure)
• Lithium
• Mood stabilizing anticonvulsants
• Atypical antipsychotics (with special caution for those agents with monoamine reuptake blocking properties, such as ziprasidone and zotepine)

Tests
• Patients should be monitored for changes in blood pressure
• Patients receiving high doses or long-term treatment should have hepatic function evaluated periodically

SIDE EFFECTS

How Drug Causes Side Effects
- Theoretically due to increases in monoamines in parts of the brain and body and at receptors other than those that cause therapeutic actions (e.g., unwanted actions of serotonin in sleep centers causing insomnia, unwanted actions of norepinephrine on vascular smooth muscle causing hypertension, etc.)
- Side effects are generally immediate, but immediate side effects often disappear in time

Notable Side Effects
- Agitation, anxiety, insomnia, weakness, sedation, dizziness
- Constipation, dry mouth, nausea, diarrhea, change in appetite, weight gain
- Sexual dysfunction
- Orthostatic hypotension (dose-related); syncope may develop at high doses

 Life Threatening or Dangerous Side Effects
- Hypertensive crisis (especially when MAOIs are used with certain tyramine-containing foods or prohibited drugs)
- Induction of mania and activation of suicidal ideation
- Seizures
- Hepatotoxicity

Weight Gain

- Occurs in significant minority

Sedation

- Many experience and/or can be significant in amount
- Can also cause activation

What To Do About Side Effects
- Wait
- Wait
- Wait
- Lower the dose
- Take at night if daytime sedation; take in daytime if overstimulated at night

- Switch after appropriate washout to an SSRI or newer antidepressant

Best Augmenting Agents for Side Effects
- Trazodone (with caution) for insomnia
- Benzodiazepines for insomnia
- ❋ Single oral or sublingual dose of a calcium channel blocker (e.g., nifedipine) for urgent treatment of hypertension due to drug interaction or dietary tyramine
- Many side effects cannot be improved with an augmenting agent

DOSING AND USE

Usual Dosage Range
- 30 mg/day in divided doses

Dosage Forms
- Tablet 10 mg

How to Dose
- Initial 30 mg/day in divided doses; after 2 weeks increase by 10 mg/day each 1–3 weeks; maximum 60 mg/day

 Dosing Tips
- Orthostatic hypotension, especially at high doses, may require splitting into 3–4 daily doses
- Patients receiving high doses may need to be evaluated periodically for effects on the liver

Overdose
- Dizziness, sedation, ataxia, headache, insomnia, restlessness, anxiety, irritability; cardiovascular effects, confusion, respiratory depression, or coma may also occur

Long-Term Use
- May require periodic evaluation of hepatic function
- MAOIs may lose efficacy long-term

Habit Forming
- Some patients have developed dependence to MAOIs

How to Stop
• Generally no need to taper, as the drug wears off slowly over 2–3 weeks

Pharmacokinetics
• Clinical duration of action may be up to 21 days due to irreversible enzyme inhibition

 Drug Interactions
• Tramadol may increase the risk of seizures in patients taking an MAO inhibitor
• Can cause a fatal "serotonin syndrome" when combined with drugs that block serotonin reuptake (e.g., SSRIs, SNRIs, sibutramine, tramadol, etc.), so do not use with a serotonin reuptake inhibitor or for up to 5 weeks after stopping the serotonin reuptake inhibitor
• Hypertensive crisis with headache, intracranial bleeding, and death may result from combining MAO inhibitors with sympathomimetic drugs (e.g., amphetamines, methylphenidate, cocaine, dopamine, epinephrine, norepinephrine, and related compounds methyldopa, levodopa, L-tryptophan, L-tyrosine, and phenylalanine
• Excitation, seizures, delirium, hyperpyrexia, circulatory collapse, coma, and death may result from combining MAO inhibitors with mepiridine or dextromethorphan
• Do not combine with another MAO inhibitor, alcohol, buspirone, bupropion, or guanethidine
• Adverse drug reactions can result from combining MAO inhibitors with tricyclic/tetracyclic antidepressants and related compounds, including carbamazepine, cyclobenzaprine, and mirtazapine, and should be avoided except by experts to treat difficult cases
• MAO inhibitors in combination with spinal anesthesia may cause combined hypotensive effects
• Combination of MAOIs and CNS depressants may enhance sedation and hypotension

 Other Warnings/ Precautions
• Use requires low tyramine diet
• Patients taking MAO inhibitors should avoid high protein food that has undergone protein breakdown by aging, fermentation, pickling, smoking, or bacterial contamination
• Patients taking MAO inhibitors should avoid cheeses (especially aged varieties), pickled herring, beer, wine, liver, yeast extract, dry sausage, hard salami, pepperoni, Lebanon bologna, pods of broad beans (fava beans), yogurt, and excessive use of caffeine and chocolate
• Patient and prescriber must be vigilant to potential interactions with any drug, including antihypertensives and over-the-counter cough/cold preparations
• Over-the-counter medications to avoid include cough and cold preparations, including those containing dextromethorphan, nasal decongestants (tablets, drops, or spray), hay-fever medications, sinus medications, asthma inhalant medications, anti-appetite medications, weight reducing preparations, "pep" pills
• Hypoglycemia may occur in diabetic patients receiving insulin or oral antidiabetic agents
• Use cautiously in patients receiving reserpine, anesthetics, disulfiram, metrizamide, anticholinergic agents
• Tranylcypromine is not recommended for use in patients who cannot be monitored closely
• Monitor patients for activation of suicidal ideation, especially children and adolescents

Do Not Use
• If patient is taking meperidine (pethidine)
• If patient is taking a sympathomimetic agent or taking guanethidine
• If patient is taking another MAOI
• If patient is taking any agent that can inhibit serotonin reuptake (e.g., SSRIs, sibutramine, tramadol, milnacipran, duloxetine, venlafaxine, clomipramine, etc.)
• If patient is taking diuretics, dextromethorphan, buspirone, bupropion
• If patient has pheochromocytoma
• If patient has cardiovascular or cerebrovascular disease
• If patient has frequent or severe headaches
• If patient is undergoing elective surgery and requires general anesthesia
• If patient has a history of liver disease or abnormal liver function tests

- If patient is taking a prohibited drug
- If patient is not compliant with a low-tyramine diet
- If there is a proven allergy to tranylcypromine

SPECIAL POPULATIONS

Renal Impairment
- Use with caution – drug may accumulate in plasma
- May require lower than usual adult dose

Hepatic Impairment
- Tranylcypromine should not be used in patients with history of hepatic impairment or in patients with abnormal liver function tests

Cardiac Impairment
- Contraindicated in patients with any cardiac impairment

Elderly
- Initial dose lower than usual adult dose
- Elderly patients may have greater sensitivity to adverse effects

 Children and Adolescents
- Not generally recommended for use under age 18
- Use with caution, observing for activation of known or unknown bipolar disorder and/or suicidal ideation, and strongly consider informing parents or guardian of this risk so they can help observe child or adolescent patients

 Pregnancy
- Risk Category C [some animal studies show adverse effects, no controlled studies in humans]
- Not generally recommended for use during pregnancy, especially during first trimester
- Should evaluate patient for treatment with an antidepressant with a better risk/benefit ratio

Breast Feeding
- Some drug is found in mother's breast milk
- Effects on infant unknown

- Immediate postpartum period is a high-risk time for depression, especially in women who have had prior depressive episodes, so drug may need to be reinstituted late in the third trimester or shortly after childbirth to prevent a recurrence during the postpartum period
- Should evaluate patient for treatment with an antidepressant with a better risk/benefit ratio

THE ART OF PSYCHOPHARMACOLOGY

Potential Advantages
- Atypical depression
- Severe depression
- Treatment-resistant depression or anxiety disorders

Potential Disadvantages
- Requires compliance to dietary restrictions, concomitant drug restrictions
- Patients with cardiac problems or hypertension
- Multiple daily doses

Primary Target Symptoms
- Depressed mood
- Somatic symptoms
- Sleep and eating disturbances
- Psychomotor retardation
- Morbid preoccupation

 Pearls
- MAOIs are generally reserved for second-line use after SSRIs, SNRIs, and combinations of newer antidepressants have failed
- Patient should be advised not to take any prescription or over-the-counter drugs without consulting their doctor because of possible drug interactions with the MAOI
- Headache is often the first symptom of hypertensive crisis
- Foods generally to avoid as they are usually high in tyramine content: dry sausage, pickled herring, liver, broad bean pods, sauerkraut, cheese, yogurt, alcoholic beverages, nonalcoholic beer and wine, chocolate, caffeine, meat and fish
- The rigid dietary restrictions may reduce compliance

- Mood disorders can be associated with eating disorders (especially in adolescent females), and tranylcypromine can be used to treat both depression and bulimia
- MAOIs are a viable second-line treatment option in depression, but are not frequently used
* Myths about the danger of dietary tyramine can be exaggerated, but prohibitions against concomitant drugs often not followed closely enough
- Orthostatic hypotension, insomnia, and sexual dysfunction are often the most troublesome common side effects
* MAOIs should be for the expert, especially if combining with agents of potential risk (e.g., stimulants, trazodone, TCAs)
* MAOIs should not be neglected as therapeutic agents for the treatment-resistant
- Although generally prohibited, a heroic but potentially dangerous treatment for severely treatment-resistant patients is for an expert to give a tricyclic/tetracyclic

antidepressant other than clomipramine simultaneously with an MAO inhibitor for patients who fail to respond to numerous other antidepressants
- Use of MAOIs with clomipramine is always prohibited because of the risk of serotonin syndrome and death
- Amoxapine may be the preferred trycyclic/tetracyclic antidepressant to combine with an MAOI in heroic cases due to its theoretically protective 5HT2A antagonist properties
- If this option is elected, start the MAOI with the tricyclic/tetracyclic antidepressant simultaneously at low doses after appropriate drug washout, then alternately increase doses of these agents every few days to a week as tolerated
- Although very strict dietary and concomitant drug restrictions must be observed to prevent hypertensive crises and serotonin syndrome, the most common side effects of MAOI and tricyclic/tetracyclic combinations may be weight gain and orthostatic hypotension

 Suggested Reading

Baker GB, Coutts RT, McKenna KF, Sherry-McKenna RL. Insights into the mechanisms of action of the MAO inhibitors phenelzine and tranylcypromine: a review. J Psychiatry Neurosci 1992;17:206–14.

Kennedy SH. Continuation and maintenance treatments in major depression: the neglected role of monoamine oxidase inhibitors. J Psychiatry Neurosci 1997;22:127–31.

Lippman SB, Nash K. Monoamine oxidase inhibitor update. Potential adverse food and drug interactions. Drug Saf 1990;5:195–204.

Thase ME, Triyedi MH, Rush AJ. MAOIs in the contemporary treatment of depression. Neuropsychopharmacology 1995;12:185–219.

TRAZODONE

THERAPEUTICS

Brands • Desyrel
see index for additional brand names

Generic? Yes

Class
• SARI (serotonin 2 antagonist/reuptake inhibitor); antidepressant; hypnotic

Commonly Prescribed For
(bold for FDA approved)
• **Depression**
• Insomnia (primary and secondary)
• Anxiety

How The Drug Works
• Blocks serotonin 2A receptors potently
• Blocks serotonin reuptake pump (serotonin transporter) less potently

How Long Until It Works
✳ Onset of therapeutic actions in insomnia are immediate if dosing is correct
• Onset of therapeutic actions in depression usually not immediate, but often delayed 2 to 4 weeks whether given as an adjunct to another antidepressant or as a monotherapy
• If it is not working within 6 to 8 weeks for depression, it may require a dosage increase or it may not work at all
• May continue to work for many years to prevent relapse of symptoms in depression and to reduce symptoms of chronic insomnia

If It Works
✳ For insomnia, use possibly can be indefinite as there is no reliable evidence of tolerance, dependence, or withdrawal, but few long-term studies
• For secondary insomnia, if underlying condition (e.g., depression, anxiety disorder) is in remission, trazodone treatment may be discontinued if insomnia does not reemerge
• The goal of treatment for depression is complete remission of current symptoms of depression as well as prevention of future relapses

• Treatment most often reduces or even eliminates symptoms of depression, but is not a cure since symptoms can recur after medicine stopped
• Continue treatment until all symptoms of depression are gone (remission)
• Once symptoms of depression are gone, continue treating for 1 year for the first episode of depression
• For second and subsequent episodes of depression, treatment may need to be indefinite

If It Doesn't Work
• For insomnia, try escalating doses or switch to another agent
• Many patients only have a partial antidepressant response where some symptoms are improved but others persist (especially insomnia, fatigue, and problems concentrating)
• Other patients may be nonresponders, sometimes called treatment-resistant or treatment-refractory
• Consider increasing dose, switching to another agent or adding an appropriate augmenting agent for treatment of depression
• Consider psychotherapy
• Consider evaluation for another diagnosis or for a comorbid condition (e.g., medical illness, substance abuse, etc.)
• Some patients may experience apparent lack of consistent efficacy due to activation of latent or underlying bipolar disorder, and require antidepressant discontinuation and a switch to a mood stabilizer

Best Augmenting Combos for Partial Response or Treatment-Resistance
• Trazodone is not frequently used as a monotherapy for insomnia, but can be combined with sedative hypnotic benzodiazepines in difficult cases
• Trazodone is most frequently used in depression as an augmenting agent to numerous psychotropic drugs
• Trazodone can not only improve insomnia in depressed patients treated with antidepressants, but can also be an effective booster of antidepressant actions of other antidepressants (use combinations of antidepressants with caution as this may

activate bipolar disorder and suicidal ideation)
- Trazodone can also improve insomnia in numerous other psychiatric conditions (e.g., bipolar disorder, schizophrenia, alcohol withdrawal) and be added to numerous other psychotropic drugs (e.g., lithium, mood stabilizers, antipsychotics)

Tests
- None for healthy individuals

SIDE EFFECTS

How Drug Causes Side Effects
- Sedative effects may be due to antihistamine properties
- Blockade of alpha adrenergic 1 receptors may explain dizziness, sedation, and hypotension
- Most side effects are immediate but often go away with time

Notable Side Effects
- Nausea, vomiting, edema, blurred vision, constipation, dry mouth
- Dizziness, sedation, fatigue, headache, incoordination, tremor
- Hypotension, syncope
- Occasional sinus bradycardia (long-term)
- Rare rash

 Life Threatening or Dangerous Side Effects
- Rare priapism
- Rare seizures
- Rare induction of mania and acivation of suicidal ideation

Weight Gain

unusual   not unusual   common   problematic

- Reported but not expected

Sedation

unusual   not unusual   common   problematic

- Many experience and/or can be significant in amount

What To Do About Side Effects
- Wait

- Wait
- Wait
- Take larger dose at night to prevent daytime sedation
- Switch to another agent

Best Augmenting Agents for Side Effects
- Most side effects cannot be improved with an augmenting agent
- Activation and agitation may represent the induction of a bipolar state, especially a mixed dysphoric bipolar II condition sometimes associated with suicidal ideation, and require the addition of lithium, a mood stabilizer or an atypical antipsychotic, and/or discontinuation of trazodone

DOSING AND USE

Usual Dosage Range
- 150–600 mg/day

Dosage Forms
- Tablet 50 mg scored, 100 mg scored, 150 mg, 150 mg with pividone scored, 300 mg with pividone scored

How to Dose
- For depression as a monotherapy, initial 150 mg/day in divided doses; can increase every 3–4 days by 50 mg/day as needed; maximum 400 mg/day (outpatient) or 600 mg/day (inpatient), split into 2 daily doses
- For insomnia, initial 25–50 mg at bedtime; increase as tolerated, usually to 50–100 mg/day, but some patients may require up to full antidepressant dose range
- For augmentation of other antidepressants in the treatment of depression, dose as recommended for insomnia

 Dosing Tips
- Start low and go slow
- ✳ Patients can have carryover sedation, ataxia, and intoxicated-like feeling if dosed too aggressively, particularly when initiating dosing

✳ Do not discontinue trials if ineffective at low doses (<50 mg) as many patients with difficult cases may respond to higher doses (150–300 mg, even up to 600 mg in some cases)
- For relief of daytime anxiety, can give part of the dose in the daytime if not too sedating
- Although use as a monotherapy for depression is usually in divided doses due to its short half-life, use as an adjunct is often effective and best tolerated once daily at bedtime

Overdose
- Rarely lethal; sedation, vomiting, priapism, respiratory arrest, seizure, EKG changes

Long-Term Use
- Safe

Habit Forming
- No

How to Stop
- Taper is prudent to avoid withdrawal effects, but tolerance, dependence, and withdrawal effects have not been reliably demonstrated

Pharmacokinetics
- Metabolized by CYP450 3A4
- Half-life is biphasic; first phase is approximately 3–6 hours; second phase is approximately 5–9 hours

 Drug Interactions
- Tramadol increases the risk of seizures in patients taking an antidepressant
- Fluoxetine and other SSRIs may raise trazodone plasma levels
- Trazodone may block the hypotensive effects of some anti-hypertensive drugs
- Trazodone may increase digoxin or phenytoin concentrations
- Trazodone may interfere with the antihypertensive effects of clonidine
- Generally, do not use with MAO inhibitors, including 14 days after MAOIs are stopped
- Reports of increased and decreased prothrombin time in patients taking warfarin and trazodone

 Other Warnings/ Precautions
- Possibility of additive effects if trazodone is used with other CNS depressants
- Treatment should be discontinued if prolonged penile erection occurs because of the risk of permanent erectile dysfunction
- Advise patients to seek medical attention immediately if painful erections occur lasting more than one hour
- Generally, priapism reverses spontaneously, while penile blood flow and other signs being monitored, but in urgent cases, local phenylephrine injections or even surgery may be indicated
- Use with caution in patients with history of seizures
- Use with caution in patients with bipolar disorder unless treated with concomitant mood stabilizing agent
- Monitor patients for activation of suicidal ideation, especially children and adolescents

Do Not Use
- If patient is taking an MAO inhibitor, but see Pearls
- If there is a proven allergy to trazodone

SPECIAL POPULATIONS

Renal Impairment
- No dose adjustment necessary

Hepatic Impairment
- Drug should be used with caution

Cardiac Impairment
- Trazodone may be arrhythmogenic
- Monitor patients closely
- Not recommended for use during recovery from myocardial infarction

Elderly
- Elderly patients may be more sensitive to adverse effects and may require lower doses

 Children and Adolescents
- Use with caution, observing for activation of known or unknown bipolar disorder

and/or suicidal ideation, and strongly consider informing parents or guardian of this risk so they can help observe child or adolescent patients
- Safety and efficacy have not been established, but trazodone has been used for behavioral disturbances, depression, and night terrors
- Children require lower initial dose and slow titration
- Boys may be even more sensitive to having prolonged erections than adult men

 Pregnancy
- Risk Category C [some animal studies show adverse effects; no controlled studies in humans]
- Avoid use during first trimester
- Must weigh the risk of treatment (first trimester fetal development, third trimester newborn delivery) to the child against the risk of no treatment (recurrence of depression, maternal health, infant bonding) to the mother and child
- For many patients this may mean continuing treatment during pregnancy

Breast Feeding
- Some drug is found in mother's breast milk
- If child becomes irritable or sedated, breast feeding or drug may need to be discontinued
- Immediate postpartum period is a high-risk time for depression, especially in women who have had prior depressive episodes, so drug may need to be reinstituted late in the third trimester or shortly after childbirth to prevent a recurrence during the postpartum period
- Must weigh benefits of breast feeding with risks and benefits of antidepressant treatment versus non-treatment to both the infant and the mother
- For many patients, this may mean continuing treatment during breast feeding

THE ART OF PSYCHOPHARMACOLOGY

Potential Advantages
- For insomnia when it is preferred to avoid the use of dependence-forming agents

- As an adjunct to the treatment of residual anxiety and insomnia with other antidepressants
- Depressed patients with anxiety
- Patients concerned about sexual side effects or weight gain

Potential Disadvantages
- For patients with fatigue, hypersomnia
- For patients intolerant to sedating effects

Primary Target Symptoms
- Depression
- Anxiety
- Sleep disturbances

 Pearls
- May be less likely than some antidepressants to precipitate hypomania or mania
- Preliminary data suggest that trazodone may be effective treatment for drug-induced dyskinesias, perhaps in part because it reduces accompanying anxiety
- Trazodone may have some efficacy in treating agitation and aggression associated with dementia
- ✴ May cause sexual dysfunction only infrequently
- Can cause carryover sedation, sometimes severe, if dosed too high
- Often not tolerated as a monotherapy for moderate to severe cases of depression, as many patients cannot tolerate high doses (>150 mg)
- Do not forget to try at high doses, up to 600 mg/day, if lower doses well tolerated but ineffective
- ✴ For the expert psychopharmacologist, trazodone can be used cautiously for insomnia associated with MAO inhibitors, despite the warning – must be attempted only if patients closely monitored and by experts experienced in the use of MAOIs
- Priapism may occur in one in 8,000 men
- Early indications of impending priapism may be slow penile detumescence when awakening from REM sleep
- When using to treat insomnia, remember that insomnia may be a symptom of some other primary disorder, and not a primary disorder itself, and thus warrant evaluation

for comorbid psychiatric and/or medical conditions
• Rarely, patients may complain of visual "trails" or after-images on trazodone

 Suggested Reading

DeVane CL. Differential pharmacology of newer antidepressants. J Clin Psychiatry 1998;59 Suppl 20:85–93.

Haria M, Fitton A, McTavish D. Trazodone. A review of its pharmacology, therapeutic use in depression and therapeutic potential in other disorders. Drugs Aging 1994;4:331–55.

Rotzinger S, Bourin M, Akimoto Y, Coutts RT, Baker GB. Metabolism of some "second"- and "fourth"-generation antidepressants: iprindole, viloxazine, bupropion, mianserin, maprotiline, trazodone, nefazodone, and venlafaxine. Cell Mol Neurobiol 1999;19:427–42.

TRIAZOLAM

THERAPEUTICS

Brands • Halcion
see index for additional brand names

Generic? Yes

 Class
• Benzodiazepine (hypnotic)

Commonly Prescribed For
(bold for FDA approved)
• **Short-term treatment of insomnia**

 How The Drug Works
• Binds to benzodiazepine receptors at the GABA-A ligand-gated chloride channel complex
• Enhances the inhibitory effects of GABA
• Boosts chloride conductance through GABA-regulated channels
• Inhibitory actions in sleep centers may provide sedative hypnotic effects

How Long Until It Works
• Generally takes effect in less than an hour

If It Works
• Improves quality of sleep
• Effects on total wake-time and number of nighttime awakenings may be decreased over time

If It Doesn't Work
• If insomnia does not improve after 7–10 days, it may be a manifestation of a primary psychiatric or physical illness such as obstructive sleep apnea or restless leg syndrome, which requires independent evaluation
• Increase the dose
• Improve sleep hygiene
• Switch to another agent

 Best Augmenting Combos for Partial Response or Treatment-Resistance
• Generally, best to switch to another agent
• Trazodone
• Agents with antihistamine actions (e.g., diphenhydramine, tricyclic antidepressants)

Tests
• In patients with seizure disorders, concomitant medical illness, and/or those with multiple concomitant long-term medications, periodic liver tests and blood counts may be prudent

SIDE EFFECTS

How Drug Causes Side Effects
• Same mechanism for side effects as for therapeutic effects – namely due to excessive actions at benzodiazepine receptors
• Actions at benzodiazepine receptors that carry over to the next day can cause daytime sedation, amnesia, and ataxia
• Long-term adaptations in benzodiazepine receptors may explain the development of dependence, tolerance, and withdrawal

Notable Side Effects
✱ Sedation, fatigue, depression
✱ Dizziness, ataxia, slurred speech, weakness
✱ Forgetfulness, confusion
✱ Hyper-excitability, nervousness
✱ Anterograde amnesia
• Rare hallucinations, mania
• Rare hypotension
• Hypersalivation, dry mouth
• Rebound insomnia when withdrawing from long-term treatment

 Life Threatening or Dangerous Side Effects
• Respiratory depression, especially when taken with CNS depressants in overdose
• Rare hepatic dysfunction, renal dysfunction, blood dyscrasias

Weight Gain

unusual | not unusual | common | problematic
• Reported but not expected

Sedation

unusual | not unusual | **common** | problematic
• Many experience and/or can be significant in amount

What To Do About Side Effects

- Wait
- To avoid problems with memory, only take triazolam if planning to have a full night's sleep
- Lower the dose
- Switch to a shorter-acting sedative hypnotic
- Switch to a non-benzodiazepine hypnotic
- Administer flumazenil if side effects are severe or life-threatening

Best Augmenting Agents for Side Effects

- Many side effects cannot be improved with an augmenting agent

DOSING AND USE

Usual Dosage Range

- 0.125–0.25 mg/day at bedtime for 7–10 days

Dosage Forms

- Tablet 0.125 mg, 0.25 mg

How to Dose

- Initial 0.125 or 0.25 mg/day at bedtime; may increase cautiously to 0.5 mg/day if ineffective; maximum dose generally 0.5 mg/day

 Dosing Tips

- Use lowest possible effective dose and assess need for continued treatment regularly
- ✳ Many patients cannot tolerate 0.5 mg dose (e.g., developing anterograde amnesia)
- Triazolam should generally not be prescribed in quantities greater than a 1-month supply
- Some side effects (sedation, dizziness, lightheadedness, amnesia) seem to increase with dose
- Patients with lower weights may require only a 0.125 mg dose
- Risk of dependence may increase with dose and duration of treatment
- ✳ Higher doses associated with more behavioral problems and anterograde amnesia

Overdose

- Can be fatal in monotherapy; poor coordination, confusion, seizure, slurred speech, sedation, coma, respiratory depression

Long-Term Use

- Not generally intended for long-term use
- Increased wakefulness during the latter part of night (wearing off) or an increase in daytime anxiety (rebound) may occur because of short half-life

Habit Forming

- Triazolam is a Schedule IV drug
- Some patients may develop dependence and/or tolerance; risk may be greater with higher doses
- History of drug addiction may increase risk of dependence

How to Stop

- If taken for more than a few weeks, taper to reduce chances of withdrawal effects
- Patients with seizure history may seize upon sudden withdrawal
- Rebound insomnia may occur the first 1–2 nights after stopping
- For patients with severe problems discontinuing a benzodiazepine, dosing may need to be tapered over many months (i.e., reduce dose by 1% every 3 days by crushing tablet and suspending or dissolving in 100 ml of fruit juice and then disposing of 1 ml while drinking the rest; 3–7 days later, dispose of 2 ml, and so on). This is both a form of very slow biological tapering and a form of behavioral desensitization

Pharmacokinetics

- Half-life 1.5–5.5 hours
- Inactive metabolites

 Drug Interactions

- CYP450 3A inhibitors such as nefazodone, fluoxetine, and fluvoxamine may decrease clearance of triazolam and raise triazolam levels significantly
- Ranitidine may increase plasma concentrations of triazolam
- Increased depressive effects when taken with other CNS depressants

Other Warnings/ Precautions

- Insomnia may be a symptom of a primary disorder, rather than a primary disorder itself
- Some patients may exhibit abnormal thinking or behavioral changes similar to those caused by other CNS depressants (i.e., either depressant actions or disinhibiting actions)
- Some depressed patients may experience a worsening of suicidal ideation
- Use only with extreme caution in patients with impaired respiratory function or obstructive sleep apnea
- Triazolam should only be administered at bedtime
- Grapefruit juice could increase triazolam levels

Do Not Use

- If patient is pregnant
- If patient has narrow angle-closure glaucoma
- If patient is taking ketoconazole, itraconazole, nefazodone, or other potent CYP450 3A4 inhibitors
- If there is a proven allergy to triazolam or any benzodiazepine

SPECIAL POPULATIONS

Renal Impairment

- Drug should be used with caution

Hepatic Impairment

- Drug should be used with caution

Cardiac Impairment

- Benzodiazepines have been used to treat insomnia associated with acute myocardial infarction

Elderly

- Recommended initial dose: 0.125 mg
- May be more sensitive to adverse effects

Children and Adolescents

- Safety and efficacy have not been established
- Long-term effects of triazolam in children/adolescents are unknown

- Should generally receive lower doses and be more closely monitored

Pregnancy

- Risk Category X [positive evidence of risk to human fetus; contraindicated for use in pregnancy]
- Infants whose mothers received a benzodiazepine late in pregnancy may experience withdrawal effects
- Neonatal flaccidity has been reported in infants whose mothers took a benzodiazepine during pregnancy

Breast Feeding

- Unknown if triazolam is secreted in human breast milk, but all psychotropics assumed to be secreted in breast milk
- ✳ Recommended either to discontinue drug or bottle feed
- Effects on infant have been observed and include feeding difficulties, sedation, and weight loss

THE ART OF PSYCHOPHARMACOLOGY

Potential Advantages

- Short-acting

Potential Disadvantages

- Patients on concomitant CYP450 3A4 inhibitors
- Patients with terminal insomnia (early morning awakenings)

Primary Target Symptoms

- Time to sleep onset
- Total sleep time
- Nighttime awakenings

Pearls

- ✳ The shorter half-life should prevent impairments in cognitive and motor performance during the day as well as daytime sedation
- ✳ If tolerance develops, the short half-life of elimination may result in increased anxiety during the day and/or increased wakefulness during the latter part of the night

- The short half-life may minimize the risk of drug interactions with agents taken during the day (e.g., alcohol)
✳ However, the risk of drug interactions with alcohol taken at night may be greater than for some other sedative hypnotics, especially for anterograde amnesia
✳ Anterograde amnesia may be more likely with triazolam than with other sedative benzodiazepines
- Because of its short half-life and inactive metabolites, triazolam may be preferred

over some benzodiazepines for patients with liver disease
✳ The risk of unusual behaviors or hallucinations may be greater with triazolam than with other sedative benzodiazepines
- Clearance of triazolam may be slightly faster in women than in men
- Women taking oral progesterone may be more sensitive to the effects of triazolam

Suggested Reading

Jonas JM, Coleman BS, Sheridan AQ, Kalinske RW. Comparative clinical profiles of triazolam versus other shorter-acting hypnotics. J Clin Psychiatry 1992;53(Suppl):19–31.

Lobo BL, Greene WL. Zolpidem: distinct from triazolam? Ann Pharmacother 1997; 31:625–32.

Rothschild AJ. Disinhibition, amnestic reactions, and other adverse reactions secondary to triazolam: a review of the literature. J Clin Psychiatry 1992; 53(Suppl):69–79.

Yuan R, Flockhart DA, Balian JD. Pharmacokinetic and pharmacodynamic consequences of metabolism-based drug interactions with alprazolam, midazolam, and triazolam. J Clin Pharmacol 1999;39:1109–25.

TRIFLUOPERAZINE

THERAPEUTICS

Brands • Stelazine
see index for additional brand names

Generic? Yes

 Class

- Conventional antipsychotic (neuroleptic, phenothiazine, dopamine 2 antagonist)

Commonly Prescribed For
(bold for FDA approved)

- **Schizophrenia (oral, intramuscular)**
- **Non-psychotic anxiety (short-term, second-line)**
- Other psychotic disorders
- Bipolar disorder

 How The Drug Works

- Blocks dopamine 2 receptors, reducing positive symptoms of psychosis

How Long Until It Works

- Psychotic symptoms can improve within 1 week, but it may take several weeks for full effect on behavior

If It Works

- Most often reduces positive symptoms in schizophrenia but does not eliminate them
- Most schizophrenic patients do not have a total remission of symptoms but rather a reduction of symptoms by about a third
- Continue treatment in schizophrenia until reaching a plateau of improvement
- After reaching a satisfactory plateau, continue treatment for at least a year after first episode of psychosis in schizophrenia
- For second and subsequent episodes of psychosis in schizophrenia, treatment may need to be indefinite
- Reduces symptoms of acute psychotic mania but not proven as a mood stabilizer or as an effective maintenance treatment in bipolar disorder
- After reducing acute psychotic symptoms in mania, switch to a mood stabilizer and/or an atypical antipsychotic for mood stabilization and maintenance

If It Doesn't Work

- Consider trying one of the first-line atypical antipsychotics (risperidone, olanzapine, quetiapine, ziprasidone, aripiprazole, amisulpride)
- Consider trying another conventional antipsychotic
- If 2 or more antipsychotic monotherapies do not work, consider clozapine

 Best Augmenting Combos for Partial Response or Treatment-Resistance

- Augmentation of conventional antipsychotics has not been systematically studied
- Addition of a mood stabilizing anticonvulsant such as valproate, carbamazepine, or lamotrigine may be helpful in both schizophrenia and bipolar mania
- Augmentation with lithium in bipolar mania may be helpful
- Addition of a benzodiazepine, especially short-term for agitation

Tests

* Since conventional antipsychotics are frequently associated with weight gain, before starting treatment, weigh all patients and determine if the patient is already overweight (BMI 25.0–29.9) or obese (BMI ≥30)
- Before giving a drug that can cause weight gain to an overweight or obese patient, consider determining whether the patient already has pre-diabetes (fasting plasma glucose 100–125 mg/dl), diabetes (fasting plasma glucose >126 mg/dl), or dyslipidemia (increased total cholesterol, LDL cholesterol and triglycerides; decreased HDL cholesterol), and treat or refer such patients for treatment, including nutrition and weight management, physical activity counseling, smoking cessation, and medical management
* Monitor weight and BMI during treatment
* While giving a drug to a patient who has gained >5% of initial weight, consider evaluating for the presence of pre-diabetes, diabetes, or dyslipidemia, or consider switching to a different antipsychotic

- Should check blood pressure in the elderly before starting and for the first few weeks of treatment
- Monitoring elevated prolactin levels of dubious clinical benefit
- Phenothiazines may cause false-positive phenylketonuria results

SIDE EFFECTS

How Drug Causes Side Effects
- By blocking dopamine 2 receptors in the striatum, it can cause motor side effects
- By blocking dopamine 2 receptors in the pituitary, it can cause elevations in prolactin
- By blocking dopamine 2 receptors excessively in the mesocortical and mesolimbic dopamine pathways, especially at high doses, it can cause worsening of negative and cognitive symptoms (neuroleptic-induced deficit syndrome)
- Anticholinergic actions may cause sedation, blurred vision, constipation, dry mouth
- Antihistaminic actions may cause sedation, weight gain
- By blocking alpha 1 adrenergic receptors, it can cause dizziness, sedation, and hypotension
- Mechanism of weight gain and any possible increased incidence of diabetes or dyslipidemia with conventional antipsychotics is unknown

Notable Side Effects
✳ Neuroleptic-induced deficit syndrome
✳ Akathisia
✳ Rash
✳ Priapism
✳ Extrapyramidal symptoms, Parkinsonism, tardive dyskinesia, tardive dystonia
✳ Galactorrhea, amenorrhea
- Dizziness, sedation
- Dry mouth, constipation, blurred vision, urinary retention
- Decreased sweating
- Sexual dysfunction
- Hypotension

 Life Threatening or Dangerous Side Effects
- Rare neuroleptic malignant syndrome

- Rare jaundice, agranulocytosis
- Rare seizures

Weight Gain

unusual   not unusual   common   problematic

✳ Reported but not expected

Sedation

unusual   not unusual   common   problematic

- Many experience and/or can be significant in amount
- Sedation is usually transient

What To Do About Side Effects
- Wait
- Wait
- Wait
- For motor symptoms, add an anticholinergic agent
- Reduce the dose
- For sedation, give at night
- Switch to an atypical antipsychotic
- Weight loss, exercise programs, and medical management for high BMIs, diabetes, dyslipidemia

Best Augmenting Agents for Side Effects
- Benztropine or trihexyphenidyl for motor side effects
- Sometimes amantadine can be helpful for motor side effects
- Benzodiazepines may be helpful for akathisia
- Many side effects cannot be improved with an augmenting agent

DOSING AND USE

Usual Dosage Range
- Oral: Psychosis: 15–20 mg/day

Dosage Forms
- Tablet 1 mg, 2 mg, 5 mg, 10 mg
- Vial 2 mg/mL
- Concentrate 10 mg/mL

How to Dose
- Psychosis: oral: initial 2–5 mg twice a day; increase gradually over 2–3 weeks

- Psychosis: intramuscular: 1–2 mg every 4–6 hours; generally do not exceed 6 mg/day
- Anxiety: initial 1–2 mg/day; maximum 6 mg/day

 Dosing Tips

✳ Use only low doses and short-term for anxiety because trifluoperazine is now a second-line treatment and has the risk of tardive dyskinesia
- Concentrate contains sulfites that may cause allergic reactions, particularly in patients with asthma
- Many patients can be dosed once a day

Overdose
- Extrapyramidal symptoms, sedation, seizures, coma, hypotension, respiratory depression

Long-Term Use
- Some side effects may be irreversible (e.g., tardive dyskinesia)
- Not intended to treat anxiety long-term (i.e., longer than 12 weeks)

Habit Forming
- No

How to Stop
- Slow down-titration of oral formulation (over 6 to 8 weeks), especially when simultaneously beginning a new antipsychotic while switching (i.e., cross-titration)
- Rapid oral discontinuation may lead to rebound psychosis and worsening of symptoms
- If antiparkinson agents are being used, they should be continued for a few weeks after trifluoperazine is discontinued

Pharmacokinetics
- Mean elimination half-life approximately 12.5 hours

 Drug Interactions
- May decrease the effects of levodopa, dopamine agonists
- May increase the effects of antihypertensive drugs except for guanethidine, whose antihypertensive actions trifluoperazine may antagonize
- Additive effects may occur if used with CNS depressants
- Alcohol and diuretics may increase the risk of hypotension; epinephrine may lower blood pressure
- Phenothiazines may reduce effects of anticoagulants
- Some patients taking a neuroleptic and lithium have developed an encephalopathic syndrome similar to neuroleptic malignant syndrome
- If used with propranolol, plasma levels of both drugs may rise

 Other Warnings/ Precautions
- If signs of neuroleptic malignant syndrome develop, treatment should be immediately discontinued
- Use cautiously in patients with alcohol withdrawal or convulsive disorders because of possible lowering of seizure threshold
- Use with caution in patients with respiratory disorders, glaucoma, or urinary retention
- Avoid undue exposure to sunlight
- Avoid extreme heat exposure
- Antiemetic effect may mask signs of other disorders or overdose; suppression of cough reflex may cause asphyxia
- Do not use epinephrine in event of overdose as interaction with some pressor agents may lower blood pressure
- Use only with caution if at all in Parkinson's disease or Lewy Body dementia

Do Not Use
- If patient is in a comatose state or has CNS depression
- If there is the presence of blood dyscrasias, bone marrow depression, or liver disease
- If there is a proven allergy to trifluoperazine
- If there is a known sensitivity to any phenothiazine

SPECIAL POPULATIONS

Renal Impairment
• Use with caution

Hepatic Impairment
• Not recommended for use

Cardiac Impairment
• Dose should be lowered
• Do not use parenteral administration unless necessary

Elderly
• Lower doses should be used and patient should be monitored closely

 ### Children and Adolescents
• Not recommended for use under age 6
• Children should be closely monitored when taking trifluoperazine
• Oral: initial 1 mg; increase gradually; maximum 15 mg/day except in older children with severe symptoms
• Intramuscular: 1 mg once or twice a day
• Generally consider second-line after atypical antipsychotics

 ### Pregnancy
• Risk Category C [some animal studies show adverse effects, no controlled studies in humans]
• Reports of extrapyramidal symptoms, jaundice, hyperreflexia, hyporeflexia in infants whose mothers took a phenothiazine during pregnancy
• Trifluoperazine should only be used during pregnancy if clearly needed
• Psychotic symptoms may worsen during pregnancy and some form of treatment may be necessary
• Atypical antipsychotics may be preferable to conventional antipsychotics or anticonvulsant mood stabilizers if treatment is required during pregnancy

Breast Feeding
• Some drug is found in mother's breast milk.
✳ Recommended either to discontinue drug or bottle feed

THE ART OF PSYCHOPHARMACOLOGY

Potential Advantages
• Intramuscular formulation for emergency use

Potential Disadvantages
• Patients with tardive dyskinesia
• Children
• Elderly

Primary Target Symptoms
• Positive symptoms of psychosis
• Motor and autonomic hyperactivity
• Violent or aggressive behavior

 ### Pearls
• Trifluoperazine is a higher potency phenothiazine
✳ Although not systematically studied, may cause less weight gain than other antipsychotics
• Less risk of sedation and orthostatic hypotension but greater extrapyramidal symptoms than with low potency phenothiazines
• Conventional antipsychotics are much less expensive than atypical antipsychotics
• Patients have very similar antipsychotic responses to any conventional antipsychotic, which is different from atypical antipsychotics where antipsychotic responses of individual patients can occasionally vary greatly from one atypical antipsychotic to another
• Patients with inadequate responses to atypical antipsychotics may benefit from a trial of augmentation with a conventional antipsychotic such as trifluoperazine or from switching to a conventional antipsychotic such as trifluoperazine
• However, long-term polypharmacy with a combination of a conventional antipsychotic such as trifluoperazine with an atypical antipsychotic may combine their side effects without clearly augmenting the efficacy of either
• Although a frequent practice by some prescribers, adding 2 conventional antipsychotics together has little rationale and may reduce tolerability without clearly enhancing efficacy

Suggested Reading

Doongaji DR, Satoskar RS, Sheth AS, Apte JS, Desai AB, Shah BR. Centbutindole vs trifluoperazine: a double-blind controlled clinical study in acute schizophrenia. J Postgrad Med 1989; 35: 3–8.

Frankenburg FR. Choices in antipsychotic therapy in schizophrenia. Harv Rev Psychiatry 1999; 6: 241–9.

Kiloh LG, Williams SE, Grant DA, Whetton PS. A double-blind comparative trial of loxapine and trifluoperazine in acute and chronic schizophrenic patients. J Int Med Res 1976; 4: 441–8.

TRIMIPRAMINE

THERAPEUTICS

Brands • Surmontil
see index for additional brand names

Generic? Yes

Class

- Tricyclic antidepressant (TCA)
- Serotonin and norepinephrine/noradrenaline reuptake inhibitor

Commonly Prescribed For
(bold for FDA approved)

- **Depression**
- **Endogenous depression**
- Anxiety
- Insomnia
- Neuropathic pain/chronic pain
- Treatment-resistant depression

How The Drug Works

- Boosts neurotransmitters serotonin and norepinephrine/noradrenaline
- Blocks serotonin reuptake pump (serotonin transporter), presumably increasing serotonergic neurotransmission
- Blocks norepinephrine reuptake pump (norepinephrine transporter), presumably increasing noradrenergic neurotransmission
- Presumably desensitizes both serotonin 1A receptors and beta adrenergic receptors
- Since dopamine is inactivated by norepinephrine reuptake in frontal cortex, which largely lacks dopamine transporters, trimipramine can increase dopamine neurotransmission in this part of the brain

How Long Until It Works

- May have immediate effects in treating insomnia, agitation, or anxiety
- Onset of therapeutic actions usually not immediate, but often delayed 2 to 4 weeks
- If it is not working within 6 to 8 weeks for depression, it may require a dosage increase or it may not work at all
- May continue to work for many years to prevent relapse of symptoms

If It Works

- The goal of treatment of depression is complete remission of current symptoms as well as prevention of future relapses
- The goal of treatment of chronic neuropathic pain is to reduce symptoms as much as possible, especially in combination with other treatments
- Treatment of depression most often reduces or even eliminates symptoms, but not a cure since symptoms can recur after medicine stopped
- Treatment of chronic neuropathic pain may reduce symptoms, but rarely eliminates them completely, and is not a cure since symptoms can recur after medicine is stopped
- Continue treatment of depression until all symptoms are gone (remission)
- Once symptoms of depression are gone, continue treating for 1 year for the first episode of depression
- For second and subsequent episodes of depression, treatment may need to be indefinite
- Use in anxiety disorders and chronic pain may also need to be indefinite, but long-term treatment is not well studied in these conditions

If It Doesn't Work

- Many depressed patients only have a partial response where some symptoms are improved but others persist (especially insomnia, fatigue, and problems concentrating)
- Other depressed patients may be nonresponders, sometimes called treatment-resistant or treatment-refractory
- Consider increasing dose, switching to another agent or adding an appropriate augmenting agent
- Consider psychotherapy
- Consider evaluation for another diagnosis or for a comorbid condition (e.g., medical illness, substance abuse, etc.)
- Some patients may experience apparent lack of consistent efficacy due to activation of latent or underlying bipolar disorder, and require antidepressant discontinuation and a switch to a mood stabilizer

Best Augmenting Combos for Partial Response or Treatment-Resistance

- Lithium, buspirone, thyroid hormone (for depression)
- Gabapentin, tiagabine, other anticonvulsants, even opiates if done by experts while monitoring carefully in difficult cases (for chronic pain)

Tests

- None for healthy individuals
- ✱ Since tricyclic and tetracyclic antidepressants are frequently associated with weight gain, before starting treatment, weigh all patients and determine if the patient is already overweight (BMI 25.0–29.9) or obese (BMI ≥30)
- Before giving a drug that can cause weight gain to an overweight or obese patient, consider determining whether the patient already has pre-diabetes (fasting plasma glucose 100–125 mg/dl), diabetes (fasting plasma glucose >126 mg/dl), or dyslipidemia (increased total cholesterol, LDL cholesterol and triglycerides; decreased HDL cholesterol), and treat or refer such patients for treatment, including nutrition and weight management, physical activity counseling, smoking cessation, and medical management
- ✱ Monitor weight and BMI during treatment
- ✱ While giving a drug to a patient who has gained >5% of initial weight, consider evaluating for the presence of pre-diabetes, diabetes, or dyslipidemia, or consider switching to a different antipsychotic
- EKGs may be useful for selected patients (e.g., those with personal or family history of QTc prolongation; cardiac arrhythmia; recent myocardial infarction; uncompensated heart failure; or taking agents that prolong QTc interval such as pimozide, thioridazine, selected antiarrhythmics, moxifloxacin, sparfloxacin, etc.)
- Patients at risk for electrolyte disturbances (e.g., patients on diuretic therapy) should have baseline and periodic serum potassium and magnesium measurements

SIDE EFFECTS

How Drug Causes Side Effects

- Anticholinergic activity may explain sedative effects, dry mouth, constipation, and blurred vision
- Sedative effects and weight gain may be due to antihistamine properties
- Blockade of alpha adrenergic 1 receptors may explain dizziness, sedation, and hypotension
- Cardiac arrhythmias and seizures, especially in overdose, may be caused by blockade of ion channels

Notable Side Effects

- Blurred vision, constipation, urinary retention, increased appetite, dry mouth, nausea, diarrhea, heartburn, unusual taste in mouth, weight gain
- Fatigue, weakness, dizziness, sedation, headache, anxiety, nervousness, restlessness
- Sexual dysfunction (impotence, change in libido)
- Sweating, rash, itching

Life Threatening or Dangerous Side Effects

- Paralytic ileus, hyperthermia (TCAs + anticholinergic agents)
- Lowered seizure threshold and rare seizures
- Orthostatic hypotension, sudden death, arrhythmias, tachycardia
- QTc prolongation
- Hepatic failure, extrapyramidal symptoms
- Increased intraocular pressure
- Rare induction of mania and activation of suicidal ideation

Weight Gain

unusual — not unusual — common — problematic

- Many experience and/or can be significant in amount
- Can increase appetite and carbohydrate craving

Sedation

unusual — not unusual — common — problematic

- Many experience and/or can be significant in amount

- Tolerance to sedative effects may develop with long-term use

What To Do About Side Effects
- Wait
- Wait
- Wait
- Lower the dose
- Switch to an SSRI or newer antidepressant

Best Augmenting Agents for Side Effects
- Many side effects cannot be improved with an augmenting agent

DOSING AND USE

Usual Dosage Range
- 50–150 mg/day

Dosage Forms
- Capsule 25 mg, 50 mg, 100 mg

How to Dose
- Initial 25 mg/day at bedtime; increase by 75 mg every 3–7 days
- 75 mg/day in divided doses; increase to 150 mg/day; maximum 200 mg/day; hospitalized patients may receive doses up to 300 mg/day

 Dosing Tips
- If given in a single dose, should generally be administered at bedtime because of its sedative properties
- If given in split doses, largest dose should generally be given at bedtime because of its sedative properties
- If patients experience nightmares, split dose and do not give large dose at bedtime
- Patients treated for chronic pain may only require lower doses
- If intolerable anxiety, insomnia, agitation, akathisia, or activation occur either upon dosing initiation or discontinuation, consider the possibility of activated bipolar disorder, and switch to a mood stabilizer or an atypical antipsychotic

Overdose
- Death may occur; CNS depression, convulsions, cardiac dysrhythmias, severe hypotension, ECG changes, coma

Long-Term Use
- Safe

Habit Forming
- No

How to Stop
- Taper to avoid withdrawal effects
- Even with gradual dose reduction some withdrawal symptoms may appear within the first 2 weeks
- Many patients tolerate 50% dose reduction for 3 days, then another 50% reduction for 3 days, then discontinuation
- If withdrawal symptoms emerge during discontinuation, raise dose to stop symptoms and then restart withdrawal much more slowly

Pharmacokinetics
- Substrate for CYP450 2D6, 2C19, and 2C9
- Half-life approximately 7–23 hours

 Drug Interactions
- Tramadol increases the risk of seizures in patients taking TCAs
- Use of TCAs with anticholinergic drugs may result in paralytic ileus or hyperthermia
- Fluoxetine, paroxetine, bupropion, duloxetine, and other CYP450 2D6 inhibitors may increase TCA concentrations
- Cimetidine may increase plasma concentrations of TCAs and cause anticholinergic symptoms
- Phenothiazines or haloperidol may raise TCA blood concentrations
- May alter effects of antihypertensive drugs; may inhibit hypotensive effects of clonidine
- Use with sympathomimetic agents may increase sympathetic activity
- Methylphenidate may inhibit metabolism of TCAs
- Activation and agitation, especially following switching or adding antidepressants, may represent the induction of a bipolar state, especially a mixed dysphoric bipolar II condition sometimes associated with suicidal

ideation, and require the addition of lithium, a mood stabilizer or an atypical antipsychotic, and/or discontinuation of trimipramine

Other Warnings/ Precautions

- Add or initiate other antidepressants with caution for up to 2 weeks after discontinuing trimipramine
- Generally, do not use with MAO inhibitors, including 14 days after MAOIs are stopped; do not start an MAOI until 2 weeks after discontinuing trimipramine, but see Pearls
- Use with caution in patients with history of seizures, urinary retention, narrow angle-closure glaucoma, hyperthyroidism
- TCAs can increase QTc interval, especially at toxic doses which can be attained not only by overdose but also by combining with drugs that inhibit TCA metabolism via CYP450 2D6, potentially causing torsade de pointes-type arrhythmia or sudden death
- Because TCAs can prolong QTc interval, use with caution in patients who have bradycardia or who are taking drugs that can induce bradycardia (e.g., beta blockers, calcium channel blockers, clonidine, digitalis)
- Because TCAs can prolong QTc interval, use with caution in patients who have hypokalemia and/or hypomagnesemia or who are taking drugs that can induce hypokalemia and/or magnesemia (e.g., diuretics, stimulant laxatives, intravenous amphotericin B, glucocorticoids, tetracosactide)

Do Not Use

- If patient is recovering from myocardial infarction
- If patient is taking agents capable of significantly prolonging QTc interval (e.g., pimozide, thioridazine, selected antiarrhythmics, moxifloxacin, sparfloxacin)
- If there is a history of QTc prolongation or cardiac arrhythmia, recent acute myocardial infarction, uncompensated heart failure
- If patient is taking drugs that inhibit TCA metabolism, including CYP450 2D6 inhibitors, except by an expert

- If there is reduced CYP450 2D6 function, such as patients who are poor 2D6 metabolizers, except by an expert and at low doses
- If there is a proven allergy to trimipramine

Renal Impairment

- Use with caution; may need to lower dose

Hepatic Impairment

- Use with caution; may need to lower dose

Cardiac Impairment

- TCAs have been reported to cause arrhythmias, prolongation of conduction time, orthostatic hypotension, sinus tachycardia, and heart failure, especially in the diseased heart
- Myocardial infarction and stroke have been reported with TCAs
- TCAs produce QTc prolongation, which may be enhanced by the existence of bradycardia, hypokalemia, congenital or acquired long QTc interval, which should be evaluated prior to administering trimipramine
- Use with caution if treating concomitantly with a medication likely to produce prolonged bradycardia, hypokalemia, slowing of intracardiac conduction, or prolongation of the QTc interval
- Avoid TCAs in patients with a known history of QTc prolongation, recent acute myocardial infarction, and uncompensated heart failure
- TCAs may cause a sustained increase in heart rate in patients with ischemic heart disease and may worsen (decrease) heart rate variability, an independent risk of mortality in cardiac populations
- Since SSRIs may improve (increase) heart rate variability in patients following a myocardial infarct and may improve survival as well as mood in patients with acute angina or following a myocardial infarction, these are more appropriate agents for cardiac population than tricyclic/tetracyclic antidepressants
- ✱ Risk/benefit ratio may not justify use of TCAs in cardiac impairment

Elderly

- May be more sensitive to anticholinergic, cardiovascular, hypotensive, and sedative effects
- Initial dose 50 mg/day; increase gradually up to 100 mg/day

Children and Adolescents

- Use with caution, observing for activation of known or unknown bipolar disorder and/or suicidal ideation, and strongly consider informing parents or guardian of this risk so they can help observe child or adolescent patients
- Not recommended for use under age 12
- Several studies show lack of efficacy of TCAs for depression
- May be used to treat enuresis or hyperactive/impulsive behaviors
- Some cases of sudden death have occurred in children taking TCAs
- Adolescents: initial dose 50 mg/day; increase gradually up to 100 mg/day

Pregnancy

- Risk Category C [some animal studies show adverse effects, no controlled studies in humans]
- Crosses the placenta
- Adverse effects have been reported in infants whose mothers took a TCA (lethargy, withdrawal symptoms, fetal malformations)
- Must weigh the risk of treatment (first trimester fetal development, third trimester newborn delivery) to the child against the risk of no treatment (recurrence of depression, maternal health, infant bonding) to the mother and child
- For many patients this may mean continuing treatment during pregnancy

Breast Feeding

- Some drug is found in mother's breast milk
- ✱ Recommended either to discontinue drug or bottle feed
- Immediate postpartum period is a high-risk time for depression, especially in women who have had prior depressive episodes, so drug may need to be reinstituted late in the third trimester or shortly after

childbirth to prevent a recurrence during the postpartum period
- Must weigh the risk of treatment (first trimester fetal development, third trimester newborn delivery) to the child against the risk of no treatment (recurrence of depression, maternal health, infant bonding) to the mother and child
- For many patients this may mean continuing treatment during breast feeding

THE ART OF PSYCHOPHARMACOLOGY

Potential Advantages

- Patients with insomnia, anxiety
- Severe or treatment-resistant depression

Potential Disadvantages

- Pediatric and geriatric patients
- Patients concerned with weight gain and sedation

Primary Target Symptoms

- Depressed mood
- Symptoms of anxiety
- Somatic symptoms

Pearls

- ✱ May be more useful than some other TCAs for patients with anxiety, sleep disturbance, and depression with physical illness
- ✱ May be more sedating than some other TCAs
- Tricyclic antidepressants are often a first-line treatment option for chronic pain
- Tricyclic antidepressants are no longer generally considered a first-line option for depression because of their side effect profile
- Tricyclic antidepressants continue to be useful for severe or treatment-resistant depression
- TCAs may aggravate psychotic symptoms
- Alcohol should be avoided because of additive CNS effects
- Underweight patients may be more susceptible to adverse cardiovascular effects
- Children, patients with inadequate hydration, and patients with cardiac

disease may be more susceptible to TCA-induced cardiotoxicity than healthy adults

- For the expert only: although generally prohibited, a heroic but potentially dangerous treatment for severely treatment-resistant patients is for an expert to give a tricyclic/tetracyclic antidepressant other than clomipramine simultaneously with an MAO inhibitor for patients who fail to respond to numerous other antidepressants
- If this option is elected, start the MAOI with the tricyclic/tetracyclic antidepressant simultaneously at low doses after appropriate drug washout, then alternately increase doses of these agents every few days to a week as tolerated
- Although very strict dietary and concomitant drug restrictions must be observed to prevent hypertensive crises and serotonin syndrome, the most common side effects of MAOI and tricyclic/tetracyclic antidepressant combinations may be weight gain and orthostatic hypotension
- Patients on tricyclics should be aware that they may experience symptoms such as photosensitivity or blue-green urine

- SSRIs may be more effective than TCAs in women, and TCAs may be more effective than SSRIs in men
- Since tricyclic/tetracyclic antidepressants are substrates for CYP450 2D6, and 7% of the population (especially Caucasians) may have a genetic variant leading to reduced activity of 2D6, such patients may not safely tolerate normal doses of tricyclic/tetracyclic antidepressants and may require dose reduction
- Phenotypic testing may be necessary to detect this genetic variant prior to dosing with a tricyclic/tetracyclic antidepressant, especially in vulnerable populations such as children, elderly, cardiac populations, and those on concomitant medications
- Patients who seem to have extraordinarily severe side effects at normal or low doses may have this phenotypic CYP450 2D6 variant and require low doses or switching to another antidepressant not metabolized by 2D6

Suggested Reading

Anderson IM. Meta-analytical studies on new antidepressants. Br Med Bull. 2001; 57:161–178.

Anderson IM. Selective serotonin reuptake inhibitors versus tricyclic antidepressants: a meta-analysis of efficacy and tolerability. J Aff Disorders. 2000;58:19–36.

Berger M, Gastpar M. Trimipramine: a challenge to current concepts on antidepressives. Eur Arch Psychiatry Clin Neurosci. 1996;246:235–9.

Lapierre YD. A review of trimipramine. 30 years of clinical use. Drugs. 1989;38 (Suppl 1):17–24;discussion 49–50.

THERAPEUTICS

Brands
- Depakene
- Depacon
- Depakote, Depakote ER

see index for additional brand names

Generic? Yes (not for Depakote ER)

 Class
- Anticonvulsant, mood stabilizer, migraine prophylaxis, voltage-sensitive sodium channel modulator

Commonly Prescribed For
(bold for FDA approved)
- **Mania (divalproex only)**
- **Complex partial seizures that occur either in isolation or in association with other types of seizures (monotherapy and adjunctive)**
- **Simple and complex absence seizures (monotherapy and adjunctive)**
- **Multiple seizure types which include absence seizures (adjunctive)**
- **Migraine prophylaxis (divalproex, divalproex ER)**
- Maintenance treatment of bipolar disorder
- Bipolar depression
- Psychosis, schizophrenia (adjunctive)

 How The Drug Works
- ✳ Blocks voltage-sensitive sodium channels by an unknown mechanism
- Increases brain concentrations of gamma-aminobutyric acid (GABA) by an unknown mechanism

How Long Until It Works
- For acute mania, effects should occur within a few days
- May take several weeks to months to optimize an effect on mood stabilization
- Should also reduce seizures and improve migraine within a few weeks

If It Works
- The goal of treatment is complete remission of symptoms (e.g., mania, seizures, migraine)
- Continue treatment until all symptoms are gone or until improvement is stable and then continue treating indefinitely as long as improvement persists
- Continue treatment indefinitely to avoid recurrence of mania, depression, seizures, and headaches

If It Doesn't Work (for bipolar disorder)
- ✳ Many patients only have a partial response where some symptoms are improved but others persist or continue to wax and wane without stabilization of mood
- Other patients may be nonresponders, sometimes called treatment-resistant or treatment-refractory
- Consider checking plasma drug level, increasing dose, switching to another agent or adding an appropriate augmenting agent
- Consider adding psychotherapy
- Consider the presence of noncompliance and counsel patient
- Switch to another mood stabilizer with fewer side effects
- Consider evaluation for another diagnosis or for a comorbid condition (e.g., medical illness, substance abuse, etc.)

 Best Augmenting Combos for Partial Response or Treatment-Resistance (for bipolar disorder)
- Lithium
- Atypical antipsychotics (especially risperidone, olanzapine, quetiapine, ziprasidone, and aripiprazole)
- ✳ Lamotrigine (with caution and at half the dose in the presence of valproate because valproate can double lamotrigine levels)
- ✳ Antidepressants (with caution because antidepressants can destabilize mood in some patients, including induction of rapid cycling or suicidal ideation; in particular consider bupropion; also SSRIs, SNRIs, others; generally avoid TCAs, MAOIs)

Tests
- ✳ Before starting treatment, platelet counts and liver function tests
- Consider coagulation tests prior to planned surgery or if there is a history of bleeding
- During the first few months of treatment, regular liver function tests and platelet

counts; this can be shifted to once or twice a year for the remainder of treatment
- Plasma drug levels can assist monitoring of efficacy, side effects, and compliance
* Since valproate is frequently associated with weight gain, before starting treatment, weigh all patients and determine if the patient is already overweight (BMI 25.0–29.9) or obese (BMI ≥30)
- Before giving a drug that can cause weight gain to an overweight or obese patient, consider determining whether the patient already has pre-diabetes (fasting plasma glucose 100–125 mg/dl), diabetes (fasting plasma glucose >126 mg/dl), or dyslipidemia (increased total cholesterol, LDL cholesterol and triglycerides; decreased HDL cholesterol), and treat or refer such patients for treatment, including nutrition and weight management, physical activity counseling, smoking cessation, and medical management
* Monitor weight and BMI during treatment
* While giving a drug to a patient who has gained >5% of initial weight, consider evaluating for the presence of pre-diabetes, diabetes, or dyslipidemia, or consider switching to a different agent

SIDE EFFECTS

How Drug Causes Side Effects
- CNS side effects theoretically due to excessive actions at voltage-sensitive sodium channels

Notable Side Effects
* Sedation, tremor, dizziness, ataxia, asthenia, headache
* Abdominal pain, nausea, vomiting, diarrhea, reduced appetite, constipation, dyspepsia, weight gain
* Alopecia (unusual)
- Polycystic ovaries (controversial)
- Hyperandrogenism, hyperinsulinemia, lipid dysregulation (controversial)
- Decreased bone mineral density (controversial)

Life Threatening or Dangerous Side Effects
- Rare hepatotoxicity with liver failure sometimes severe and fatal, particularly in children under 2
- Rare pancreatitis, sometimes fatal

Weight Gain

- Many experience and/or can be significant in amount
- Can become a health problem in some

Sedation

- Frequent and can be significant in amount
- Some patients may not tolerate it
- Can wear off over time
- Can reemerge as dose increases and then wear off again over time

What To Do About Side Effects
- Wait
- Wait
- Wait
- Take at night to reduce daytime sedation, especially with divalproex ER
- Lower the dose
- Switch to another agent

Best Augmenting Agents for Side Effects
* Propranolol 20–30 mg 2–3 times/day may reduce tremor
* Multivitamins fortified with zinc and selenium may help reduce alopecia
- Many side effects cannot be improved with an augmenting agent

DOSING AND USE

Usual Dosage Range
- Mania: 1200–1500 mg/day
- Migraine: 500–1000 mg/day
- Epilepsy: 10–60 mg/kg/day

Dosage Forms
- Tablet [delayed release, as divalproex sodium (Depakote)] 125 mg, 250 mg, 500 mg

- Tablet [extended release, as divalproex sodium (Depakote ER)] 250 mg, 500 mg
- Capsule [sprinkle, as divalproex sodium (Depakote Sprinkle)] 125 mg
- Capsule [as valproic acid (Depakene)] 250 mg
- Injection [as sodium valproate (Depacon)] 100 mg/mL (5 mL)
- Syrup [as sodium valproate (Depakene)] 250 mg/5mL (5 mL, 50 mL, 480 mL)

How to Dose

- Usual starting dose for mania or epilepsy is 15 mg/kg in 2 divided doses (once daily for extended release valproate)
- Acute mania (adults): initial 1000 mg/day; increase dose rapidly; maximum dose generally 60 mg/kg/day
- For less acute mania, may begin at 250–500 mg the first day, and then titrate upward as tolerated
- Migraine (adults): initial 500 mg/day, maximum recommended dose 1000 mg/day
- Epilepsy (adults): initial 10–15 mg/kg/day; increase by 5–10 mg/kg/week; maximum dose generally 60 mg/kg/day

 Dosing Tips

- ✳ Oral loading with 20–30 mg/kg/day may reduce onset of action to 5 days or less and may be especially useful for treatment of acute mania in inpatient settings
- Given the half-life of immediate release valproate (e.g., Depakene, Depakote), twice daily dosing is probably ideal
- Extended release valproate (e.g., Depakote ER) can be given once daily
- However, extended release valproate is only about 80% as bioavailable as immediate release valproate, producing plasma drug levels 10–20% lower than with immediate release valproate
- ✳ Thus, the dose of extended release valproate may need to be higher (by about one-third) when converting patients to the ER formulation
- Depakote (divalproex sodium) is an enteric-coated stable compound containing both valproic acid and sodium valproate
- ✳ Divalproex immediate release formulation reduces gastrointestinal side effects compared to generic valproate

- ✳ Divalproex ER improves gastrointestinal side effects and alopecia compared to immediate release divalproex or generic valproate
- The amide of valproic acid is available in Europe [valpromide (Depamide)]
- Trough plasma drug levels >45 µg/ml may be required for either antimanic effects or anticonvulsant actions
- Trough plasma drug levels up to 100 µg/ml are generally well tolerated
- Trough plasma drug levels up to 125 µg/ml may be required in some acutely manic patients
- Dosages to achieve therapeutic plasma levels vary widely, often between 750–3000 mg/day

Overdose

- Fatalities have been reported; coma, restlessness, hallucinations, sedation, heart block

Long-Term Use

- Requires regular liver function tests and platelet counts

Habit Forming

- No

How to Stop

- Taper; may need to adjust dosage of concurrent medications as valproate is being discontinued
- Patients may seize upon withdrawal, especially if withdrawal is abrupt
- ✳ Rapid discontinuation increases the risk of relapse in bipolar disorder
- Discontinuation symptoms uncommon

Pharmacokinetics

- Mean terminal half-life 9–16 hours
- Metabolized primarily by the liver, approximately 25% dependent upon CYP450 system

 Drug Interactions

- ✳ Lamotrigine dose should be reduced by perhaps 50% if used with valproate, as valproate inhibits metabolism of lamotrigine and raises lamotrigine plasma levels, theoretically increasing the risk of rash

- Plasma levels of valproate may be <u>lowered</u> by carbamazepine, phenytoin, ethosuximide, phenobarbital, rifampin
- Aspirin may inhibit metabolism of valproate and <u>increase</u> valproate plasma levels
- Plasma levels of valproate may also be <u>increased</u> by felbamate, chlorpromazine, fluoxetine, fluvoxamine, topiramate, cimetidine, erythromycin, and ibuprofen
- Valproate inhibits metabolism of ethosuximide, phenobarbital, and phenytoin, and can thus <u>increase</u> their plasma levels
- No likely pharmacokinetic interactions of valproate with lithium or atypical antipsychotics
- Use of valproate with clonazepam may cause absence status

 Other Warnings/ Precautions

✱ Be alert to the following symptoms of hepatotoxicity that require immediate attention: malaise, weakness, lethargy, facial edema, anorexia, vomiting, yellowing of the skin and eyes

✱ Be alert to the following symptoms of pancreatitis that require immediate attention: abdominal pain, nausea, vomiting, anorexia

✱ Teratogenic effects in developing fetuses such as neural tube defects may occur with valproate use

✱ Somnolence may be more common in the elderly and may be associated with dehydration, reduced nutritional intake, and weight loss, requiring slower dosage increases, lower doses, and monitoring of fluid and nutritional intake

- Use in patients with thrombocytopenia is not recommended; patients should report easy bruising or bleeding
- Evaluate for urea cycle disorders, as hyperammonemic encephalopathy, sometimes fatal, has been associated with valproate administration in these uncommon disorders; urea cycle disorders, such as ormithine transcarbamylase deficiency, are associated with unexplained encephalopathy, mental retardation, elevated plasma ammonia, cyclical vomiting, and lethargy

Do Not Use
- If patient has pancreatitis
- If patient has serious liver disease
- If patient has urea cycle disorder
- If there is a proven allergy to valproic acid, valproate, or divalproex

SPECIAL POPULATIONS

Renal Impairment
- No dose adjustment necessary

Hepatic Impairment
- Contraindicated

Cardiac Impairment
- No dose adjustment necessary

Elderly
- Reduce starting dose and titrate slowly; dosing is generally lower than in healthy adults

✱ Sedation in the elderly may be more common and associated with dehydration, reduced nutritional intake, and weight loss
- Monitor fluid and nutritional intake

 Children and Adolescents

✱ Not generally recommended for use under age 10 for bipolar disorder except by experts and when other options have been considered
- Children under age 2 have significantly increased risk of hepatotoxicity, as they have a markedly decreased ability to eliminate valproate compared to older children and adults
- Use requires close medical supervision

 Pregnancy

- Risk category D [positive evidence of risk to human fetus; potential benefits may still justify its use during pregnancy]

✱ Use during first trimester may raise risk of neural tube defects (e.g., spina bifida) or other congenital anomalies
- Use in women of childbearing potential requires weighing potential benefits to the mother against the risks to the fetus

* If drug is continued, monitor clotting parameters and perform tests to detect birth defects
* If drug is continued, start on folate 1 mg/day early in pregnancy to reduce risk of neural tube defects
* If drug is continued, consider vitamin K during the last 6 weeks of pregnancy to reduce risks of bleeding
• Taper drug if discontinuing
• Seizures, even mild seizures, may cause harm to the embryo/fetus
* For bipolar patients, valproate should generally be discontinued before anticipated pregnancies
• Recurrent bipolar illness during pregnancy can be quite disruptive
* For bipolar patients, given the risk of relapse in the postpartum period, mood stabilizer treatment such as valproate should generally be restarted immediately after delivery if patient is unmedicated during pregnancy
* Atypical antipsychotics may be preferable to lithium or anticonvulsants such as valproate if treatment of bipolar disorder is required during pregnancy
• Bipolar symptoms may recur or worsen during pregnancy and some form of treatment may be necessary

Breast Feeding
• Some drug is found in mother's breast milk
* Generally considered safe to breast feed while taking valproate
• If drug is continued while breast feeding, infant should be monitored for possible adverse effects
• If infant shows signs of irritability or sedation, drug may need to be discontinued
* Bipolar disorder may recur during the postpartum period, particularly if there is a history of prior postpartum episodes of either depression or psychosis
* Relapse rates may be lower in women who receive prophylactic treatment for postpartum episodes of bipolar disorder
• Atypical antipsychotics and anticonvulsants such as valproate may be safer than lithium during the postpartum period when breast feeding

THE ART OF PSYCHOPHARMACOLOGY

Potential Advantages
• Manic phase of bipolar disorder
• Works well in combination with lithium and/or atypical antipsychotics
• Patients for whom therapeutic drug monitoring is desirable

Potential Disadvantages
• Depressed phase of bipolar disorder
• Patients unable to tolerate sedation or weight gain
• Multiple drug interactions
• Multiple side effect risks
• Pregnant patients

Primary Target Symptoms
• Unstable mood
• Incidence of migraine
• Incidence of partial complex seizures

 Pearls (for bipolar disorder)

* Valproate is a first-line treatment option that may be best for patients with mixed states of bipolar disorder or for patients with rapid-cycling bipolar disorder
* Seems to be more effective in treating manic episodes than depressive episodes in bipolar disorder (treats from above better than it treats from below)
* May also be more effective in preventing manic relapses than in preventing depressive episodes (stabilizes from above better than it stabilizes from below)
• Only a third of bipolar patients experience adequate relief with a monotherapy, so most patients need multiple medications for best control
• Useful in combination with atypical antipsychotics and/or lithium for acute mania
* May also be useful for bipolar disorder in combination with lamotrigine, but must reduce lamotrigine dose by half when combined with valproate
• Usefulness for bipolar disorder in combination with anticonvulsants other than lamotrigine is not well demonstrated; such combinations can be expensive and are possibly ineffective or even irrational
* May be useful as an adjunct to atypical antipsychotics for rapid onset of action in schizophrenia

✳ Used to treat aggression, agitation, and impulsivity not only in bipolar disorder and schizophrenia but also in many other disorders, including dementia, personality disorders, and brain injury
- Patients with acute mania tend to tolerate side effects better than patients with hypomania or depression
- Multivitamins fortified with zinc and selenium may help reduce alopecia
- Association of valproate with polycystic ovaries is controversial and may be related to weight gain, obesity, or epilepsy
- Nevertheless, may wish to be cautious in administering valproate to women of child bearing potential, especially adolescent female bipolar patients, and carefully monitor weight, endocrine status, and ovarian size and function

✳ In women of child bearing potential who are or are likely to become sexually active, should inform about risk of harm to the fetus and monitor contraceptive status
- Association of valproate with decreased bone mass is controversial and may be related to activity levels, exposure to sunlight, and epilepsy, and might be prevented by supplemental vitamin D 2000 Iu/day and calcium 600–1000 mg/day

Suggested Reading

Bowden CL. Valproate. Bipolar Disorders 2003;5:189–202.

Emilien G, Maloteaux JM, Seghers A, Charles G. Lithium compared to valproic acid and carbamazepine in the treatment of mania: a statistical meta-analysis. Eur Neuropsychopharmacol. 1996;6:245–52.

Landy SH, McGinnis J. Divalproex sodium—review of prophylactic migraine efficacy, safety and dosage, with recommendations. Tenn Med. 1999;92:135–6.

Macritchie KA, Geddes JR, Scott J, Haslam DR, Goodwin GM. Valproic acid, valproate and divalproex in the maintenance treatment of bipolar disorder. Cochrane Database Syst Rev. 2001;(3):CD003196.

Strakowski SM, DelBello MP, Adler CM. Comparative efficacy and tolerability of drug treatments for bipolar disorder. CNS Drugs. 2001;15:701–18.

VENLAFAXINE

THERAPEUTICS

Brands • Effexor
• Effexor XR
see index for additional brand names

Generic? No

Class
• SNRI (dual serotonin and norepinephrine reuptake inhibitor); often classified as an antidepressant, but it is not just an antidepressant

Commonly Prescribed For
(bold for FDA approved)
• **Depression**
• **Generalized anxiety disorder (GAD)**
• **Social anxiety disorder (social phobia)**
• Panic disorder
• Posttraumatic stress disorder (PTSD)
• Premenstrual dysphoric disorder (PMDD)

How The Drug Works
• Boosts neurotransmitters serotonin, norepinephrine/noradrenaline, and dopamine
• Blocks serotonin reuptake pump (serotonin transporter), presumably increasing serotonergic neurotransmission
• Blocks norepinephrine reuptake pump (norepinephrine transporter), presumably increasing noradrenergic neurotransmission
• Presumably desensitizes both serotonin 1A receptors and beta adrenergic receptors
• Since dopamine is inactivated by norepinephrine reuptake in frontal cortex, which largely lacks dopamine transporters, venlafaxine can increase dopamine neurotransmission in this part of the brain
• Weakly blocks dopamine reuptake pump (dopamine transporter), and may increase dopamine neurotransmission

How Long Until It Works
• Onset of therapeutic actions usually not immediate, but often delayed 2 to 4 weeks
• If it is not working within 6 to 8 weeks for depression, it may require a dosage increase or it may not work at all
• By contrast, for generalized anxiety, onset of response and increases in remission

rates may still occur after 8 weeks, and for up to 6 months after initiating dosing
• May continue to work for many years to prevent relapse of symptoms

If It Works
• The goal of treatment is complete remission of current symptoms as well as prevention of future relapses
• Treatment most often reduces or even eliminates symptoms, but not a cure since symptoms can recur after medicine stopped
• Continue treatment until all symptoms are gone (remission), especially in depression and whenever possible in anxiety disorders
• Once symptoms gone, continue treating for 1 year for the first episode of depression
• For second and subsequent episodes of depression, treatment may need to be indefinite
• Use in anxiety disorders may also need to be indefinite

If It Doesn't Work
• Many patients only have a partial response where some symptoms are improved but others persist (especially insomnia, fatigue, and problems concentrating)
• Other patients may be nonresponders, sometimes called treatment-resistant or treatment-refractory
• Some patients who have an initial response may relapse even though they continue treatment, sometimes called "poop-out"
• Consider increasing dose, switching to another agent or adding an appropriate augmenting agent
• Consider psychotherapy
• Consider evaluation for another diagnosis or for a comorbid condition (e.g., medical illness, substance abuse, etc.)
• Some patients may experience apparent lack of consistent efficacy due to activation of latent or underlying bipolar disorder, and require antidepressant discontinuation and a switch to a mood stabilizer

 ### Best Augmenting Combos for Partial Response or Treatment-Resistance
✱ Mirtazapine ("California rocket fuel"; a potentially powerful dual serotonin and norepinephrine combination, but observe

for activation of bipolar disorder and suicidal ideation)
- Bupropion, reboxetine, nortriptyline, desipramine, maprotiline, atomoxetine (all potentially powerful enhancers of noradrenergic action, but observe for activation of bipolar disorder and suicidal ideation)
- Modafinil, especially for fatigue, sleepiness, and lack of concentration
- Mood stabilizers or atypical antipsychotics for bipolar depression, psychotic depression or treatment-resistant depression
- Benzodiazepines
- If all else fails for anxiety disorders, consider gabapentin or tiagabine
- Hypnotics or trazodone for insomnia
- Classically, lithium, buspirone, or thyroid hormone

Tests
- Check blood pressure before initiating treatment and regularly during treatment

SIDE EFFECTS

How Drug Causes Side Effects
- Theoretically due to increases in serotonin and norepinephrine concentrations at receptors in parts of the brain and body other than those that cause therapeutic actions (e.g., unwanted actions of serotonin in sleep centers causing insomnia, unwanted actions of norepinephrine on acetylcholine release causing constipation and dry mouth, etc.)
- Most side effects are immediate but often go away with time

Notable Side Effects
- Most side effects increase with higher doses, at least transiently
- Headache, nervousness, insomnia, sedation
- Nausea, diarrhea, decreased appetite
- Sexual dysfunction (abnormal ejaculation/orgasm, impotence)
- Asthenia, sweating
- SIADH (syndrome of inappropriate antidiuretic hormone secretion)
- Hyponatremia
- Dose-dependent increase in blood pressure

 Life Threatening or Dangerous Side Effects
- Rare seizures
- Rare induction of hypomania and activation of suicidal ideation

Weight Gain

unusual | not unusual | common | problematic
- Reported but not expected
- Possible weight loss, especially short-term

Sedation

unusual | not unusual | common | problematic
- Occurs in significant minority
- May also be activating in some patients

What To Do About Side Effects
- Wait
- Wait
- Wait
- Lower the dose
- In a few weeks, switch or add other drugs

Best Augmenting Agents for Side Effects
- Often best to try another antidepressant monotherapy prior to resorting to augmentation strategies to treat side effects
- Trazodone or a hypnotic for insomnia
- Bupropion, sildenafil, vardenafil, or tadalafil for sexual dysfunction
- Benzodiazepines for jitteriness and anxiety, especially at initiation of treatment and especially for anxious patients
- Mirtazapine for insomnia, agitation, and gastrointestinal side effects
- Many side effects are dose-dependent (i.e., they increase as dose increases, or they reemerge until tolerance re-develops)
- Many side effects are time-dependent (i.e., they start immediately upon dosing and upon each dose increase, but go away with time)
- Activation and agitation may represent the induction of a bipolar state, especially a mixed dysphoric bipolar II condition sometimes associated with suicidal ideation, and require the addition of lithium, a mood stabilizer or an atypical antipsychotic, and/or discontinuation of venlafaxine

DOSING AND USE

Usual Dosage Range
- Depression: 75–225 mg/day, once daily (extended release) or divided into 2–3 doses (immediate release)
- GAD: 150–225 mg/day

Dosage Forms
- Capsule (extended release) 37.5 mg, 75 mg, 150 mg
- Tablet 25 mg scored, 37.5 mg scored, 50 mg scored, 75 mg scored, 100 mg scored

How to Dose
- Initial dose 37.5 mg once daily (extended release) or 25–50 mg divided into 2–3 doses (immediate release) for a week, if tolerated; increase daily dose generally no faster than 75 mg every 4 days until desired efficacy is reached; maximum dose generally 375 mg/day
- Usually try doses at 75 mg increments for a few weeks prior to incrementing by an additional 75 mg

 Dosing Tips
- At all doses, potent serotonin reuptake blockade
- 75–225 mg/day may be predominantly serotonergic in some patients, and dual serotonin and norepinephrine acting in other patients
- 225–375 mg/day is dual serotonin and norepinephrine acting in most patients
- ✳ Thus, nonresponders at lower doses should try higher doses to be assured of the benefits of dual SNRI action
- At very high doses (e.g., >375 mg/day), dopamine reuptake blocked as well in some patients
- Up to 600 mg/day has been given for heroic cases
- Venlafaxine has an active metabolite O-desmethylvenlafaxine (ODV), which is formed as the result of CYP450 2D6
- Thus, CYP450 2D6 inhibition reduces the formation of ODV, but this is of uncertain clinical significance
- ✳ Consider checking plasma levels of ODV and venlafaxine in nonresponders who tolerate high doses, and if plasma levels are low, experts can prudently prescribe doses above 375 mg/day while monitoring closely
- Do not break or chew venlafaxine XR capsules, as this will alter controlled release properties
- ✳ For patients with severe problems discontinuing venlafaxine, dosing may need to be tapered over many months (i.e., reduce dose by 1% every 3 days by crushing tablet and suspending or dissolving in 100 mL of fruit juice, and then disposing of 1 mL while drinking the rest; 3–7 days later, dispose of 2 mL, and so on). This is both a form of very slow biological tapering and a form of behavioral desensitization
- For some patients with severe problems discontinuing venlafaxine, it may be useful to add an SSRI with a long half-life, especially fluoxetine, prior to taper of venlafaxine; while maintaining fluoxetine dosing, first slowly taper venlafaxine and then taper fluoxetine
- Be sure to differentiate between re-emergence of symptoms requiring re-institution of treatment and withdrawal symptoms

Overdose
- Rarely lethal; may cause no symptoms; possible symptoms include sedation, convulsions, rapid heartbeat

Long-Term Use
- See doctor regularly to monitor blood pressure, especially at doses >225 mg/day

Habit Forming
- No

How to Stop
- Taper to avoid withdrawal effects (dizziness, nausea, stomach cramps, sweating, tingling, dysesthesias)
- Many patients tolerate 50% dose reduction for 3 days, then another 50% reduction for 3 days, then discontinuation
- If withdrawal symptoms emerge during discontinuation, raise dose to stop symptoms and then restart withdrawal much more slowly
- ✳ Withdrawal effects can be more common or more severe with venlafaxine than with some other antidepressants

Pharmacokinetics
- Parent drug has 3–7 hour half-life
- Active metabolite has 9–13 hour half-life

 Drug Interactions
- Tramadol increases the risk of seizures in patients taking an antidepressant
- Can cause a fatal "serotonin syndrome" when combined with MAO inhibitors, so do not use with MAO inhibitors or for at least 14 days after MAOIs are stopped
- Do not start an MAO inhibitor for at least 2 weeks after discontinuing venlafaxine
- Concomitant use with cimetidine may reduce clearance of venlafaxine and raise venlafaxine levels
- Could theoretically interfere with the analgesic actions of codeine or possibly with other triptans
- Few known adverse drug interactions

⚠ Other Warnings/ Precautions
- Use with caution in patients with history of seizures
- Use with caution in patients with bipolar disorder unless treated with concomitant mood stabilizing agent
- Monitor patients for activation of suicidal ideation, especially children and adolescents

Do Not Use
- If patient has uncontrolled narrow angle-closure glaucoma
- If patient is taking an MAO inhibitor
- If there is a proven allergy to venlafaxine

SPECIAL POPULATIONS

Renal Impairment
- Lower dose by 25–50%
- Patients on dialysis should not receive subsequent dose until dialysis is completed

Hepatic Impairment
- Lower dose by 50%

Cardiac Impairment
- Drug should be used with caution
- Venlafaxine has a dose-dependent effect on blood pressure

Elderly
- Some patients may tolerate lower doses better

 Children and Adolescents
- Use with caution, observing for activation of known or unknown bipolar disorder and/or suicidal ideation, and strongly consider informing parents or guardian of this risk so they can help observe child or adolescent patients
- Not specifically approved, but preliminary data suggest that venlafaxine is effective in children and adolescents with depression, anxiety disorders, and ADHD

 Pregnancy
- Risk Category C [some animal studies show adverse effects, no controlled studies in humans]
- Not generally recommended for use during pregnancy, especially during first trimester
- Nonetheless, continuous treatment during pregnancy may be necessary and has not been proven to be harmful to the fetus
- Must weigh the risk of treatment (first trimester fetal development, third trimester newborn delivery) to the child against the risk of no treatment (recurrence of depression, maternal health, infant bonding) to the mother and child
- For many patients this may mean continuing treatment during pregnancy
- Neonates exposed to SSRIs or SNRIs late in the third trimester have developed complications requiring prolonged hospitalization, respiratory support, and tube feeding; reported symptoms are consistent with either a direct toxic effect of SSRIs and SNRIs or, possibly, a drug discontinuation syndrome, and include respiratory distress, cyanosis, apnea, seizures, temperature instability, feeding difficulty, vomiting, hypoglycemia, hypotonia, hypertonia, hyperreflexia, tremor, jitteriness, irritability, and constant crying

Breast Feeding
- Some drug is found in mother's breast milk
- Trace amounts may be present in nursing children whose mothers are on venlafaxine

- If child becomes irritable or sedated, breast feeding or drug may need to be discontinued
- Immediate postpartum period is a high-risk time for depression, especially in women who have had prior depressive episodes, so drug may need to be reinstituted late in the third trimester or shortly after childbirth to prevent a recurrence during the postpartum period
- Must weigh benefits of breast feeding with risks and benefits of antidepressant treatment versus non-treatment to both the infant and the mother
- For many patients, this may mean continuing treatment during breast feeding

THE ART OF PSYCHOPHARMACOLOGY

Potential Advantages
- Patients with retarded depression
- Patients with atypical depression
- Patients with comorbid anxiety
- Patients with depression may have higher remission rates on SNRIs than on SSRIs
- Depressed patients with somatic symptoms, fatigue, and pain
- Patients who do not respond or remit on treatment with SSRIs

Potential Disadvantages
- Patients sensitive to nausea
- Patients with borderline or uncontrolled hypertension

Primary Target Symptoms
- Depressed mood
- Energy, motivation, and interest
- Sleep disturbance
- Anxiety

 Pearls

✳ May be effective in patients who fail to respond to SSRIs, and may be one of the preferred treatments for treatment-resistant depression

✳ May be used in combination with other antidepressants for treatment-refractory cases
- XR formulation improves tolerability, reduces nausea, and requires only once-daily dosing
- May be effective in a broad array of anxiety disorders
- May be effective in adult ADHD
- Not studied in stress urinary incontinence

✳ Has greater potency for serotonin reuptake blockade than for norepinephrine reuptake blockade, but this is of unclear clinical significance as a differentiating feature from other SNRIs

✳ In vitro binding studies tend to underestimate in vivo potency for reuptake blockade, as they do not factor in the presence of high concentrations of an active metabolite, higher oral mg dosing, or the lower protein binding which can increase functional drug levels at receptor sites
- Effective dose range is broad (i.e., 75 mg to 375 mg in many difficult cases, and up to 600 mg or more in heroic cases)

✳ Preliminary studies in neuropathic pain and fibromyalgia suggest potential efficacy
- Efficacy as well as side effects (especially nausea and increased blood pressure) are dose-dependent
- Blood pressure increases rare for XR formulation in doses up to 225 mg
- More withdrawal reactions reported upon discontinuation than for some other antidepressants
- May be helpful for hot flushes in perimenopausal women
- May be associated with higher depression remission rates than SSRIs

Suggested Reading

Hackett D. Venlafaxine XR in the treatment of anxiety. Acta Psychiatrica Scandinavica 2000; 406[suppl]:30–35.

Sheehan DV. Attaining remission in generalized anxiety disorder: venlafaxine extended release comparative data. J Clin Psychiatry 2001;62 Suppl 19:26–31.

Smith D, Dempster C, Glanville J, Freemantle N, Anderson I. Efficacy and tolerability of venlafaxine compared with selective serotonin reuptake inhibitors and other antidepressants: a meta-analysis. Br J Psychiatry 2002; 180:396–404.

Wellington K, Perry CM. Venlafaxine extended-release: a review of its use in the management of major depression. CNS Drugs 2001; 15:643–69.

ZALEPLON

THERAPEUTICS

Brands • Sonata
see index for additional brand names

Generic? No

 Class
• Non-benzodiazepine hypnotic; alpha 1 isoform antagonist of GABA-A/benzodiazepine receptors

Commonly Prescribed For
(bold for FDA approved)
• **Short-term treatment of insomnia**

 How The Drug Works
• Binds selectively to a subtype of the benzodiazepine receptor, the alpha 1 isoform
• May enhance GABA inhibitory actions that provide sedative hypnotic effects more selectively than other actions of GABA
• Boosts chloride conductance through GABA-regulated channels
• Inhibitory actions in sleep centers may provide sedative hypnotic effects

How Long Until It Works
• Generally takes effect in less than an hour

If It Works
• Improves quality of sleep
• Effects on total wake-time and number of nighttime awakenings may be decreased over time

If It Doesn't Work
• If insomnia does not improve after 7–10 days, it may be a manifestation of a primary psychiatric or physical illness such as obstructive sleep apnea or restless leg syndrome, which requires independent evaluation
• Increase the dose
• Improve sleep hygiene
• Switch to another agent

 Best Augmenting Combos for Partial Response or Treatment-Resistance
• Generally, best to switch to another agent
• Trazodone

• Agents with antihistamine actions (e.g., diphenhydramine, tricyclic antidepressants)

Tests
• None for healthy individuals

SIDE EFFECTS

How Drug Causes Side Effects
• Actions at benzodiazepine receptors that carry over to the next day can cause daytime sedation, amnesia, and ataxia
• Long-term adaptations of zaleplon not well studied, but chronic studies of other alpha 1 selective non-benzodiazepine hypnotics suggest lack of notable tolerance or dependence developing over time

Notable Side Effects
* Sedation
* Dizziness, ataxia
* Dose-dependent amnesia
* Hyper-excitability, nervousness
• Rare hallucinations
• Headache
• Decreased appetite

 Life Threatening or Dangerous Side Effects
• Respiratory depression, especially when taken with other CNS depressants in overdose

Weight Gain

unusual   not unusual   common   problematic

• Reported but not expected

Sedation

unusual   not unusual   common   problematic

• Many experience and/or can be significant in amount

What To Do About Side Effects
• Wait
• To avoid problems with memory, do not take zaleplon if planning to sleep for less than 4 hours
• Lower the dose
• Administer flumazenil if side effects are severe or life-threatening

Best Augmenting Agents for Side Effects
- Many side effects cannot be improved with an augmenting agent

DOSING AND USE

Usual Dosage Range
- 10 mg/day at bedtime for 7–10 days

Dosage Forms
- Capsule 5 mg, 10 mg

How to Dose
- Initial 10 mg/day at bedtime; may increase to 20 mg/day at bedtime if ineffective; maximum dose generally 20 mg/day

 Dosing Tips
- Patients with lower body weights may require only a 5 mg dose
- Zaleplon should generally not be prescribed in quantities greater than a 1-month supply
- Risk of dependence may increase with dose and duration of treatment
- ✱ However, treatment with alpha 1 selective non-benzodiazepine hypnotics may cause less tolerance or dependence than benzodiazepine hypnotics

Overdose
- No fatalities reported with zaleplon; fatalities have occurred with other sedative hypnotics; sedation, confusion, ataxia, hypotension, respiratory depression, coma

Long-Term Use
- Not generally intended for long-term use
- Increased wakefulness during the latter part of night (wearing off) or an increase in daytime anxiety (rebound) may occur because of short half-life

Habit Forming
- Zaleplon is a Schedule IV drug
- Some patients may develop dependence and/or tolerance; risk may be greater with higher doses
- History of drug addiction may increase risk of dependence

How to Stop
- Rebound insomnia may occur the first night after stopping
- If taken for more than a few weeks, taper to reduce chances of withdrawal effects

Pharmacokinetics
- Terminal phase elimination half-life approximately 1 hour (ultra-short half-life)

 Drug Interactions
- Increased depressive effects when taken with other CNS depressants
- Cimetidine may increase plasma concentrations of zaleplon, requiring a lower initial dose of zaleplon (5 mg/day)
- CYP450 3A4 inducers such as carbamazepine may reduce the effectiveness of zaleplon

 Other Warnings/ Precautions
- Insomnia may be a symptom of a primary disorder, rather than a primary disorder itself
- Some patients may exhibit abnormal thinking or behavioral changes similar to those caused by other CNS depressants (i.e., either depressant actions or disinhibiting actions)
- Some depressed patients may experience a worsening of suicidal ideation
- Use only with extreme caution in patients with impaired respiratory function or obstructive sleep apnea
- Zaleplon should only be administered at bedtime

Do Not Use
- If there is a proven allergy to zaleplon

SPECIAL POPULATIONS

Renal Impairment
- No dose adjustment necessary
- Use with caution in patients with severe impairment

Hepatic Impairment
- Mild to moderate impairment: recommended dose 5 mg

- Not recommended for use in patients with severe impairment

Cardiac Impairment
- Zaleplon has not been studied in patients with cardiac impairment, but dose adjustment may not be necessary

Elderly
- Recommended dose: 5 mg

 Children and Adolescents
- Safety and efficacy have not been established
- Long-term effects of zaleplon in children/adolescents are unknown
- Should generally receive lower doses and be more closely monitored

 Pregnancy
- Risk category C [some animal studies show adverse effects, no controlled studies in humans]
- Infants whose mothers took sedative hypnotics during pregnancy may experience some withdrawal symptoms
- Neonatal flaccidity has been reported in infants whose mothers took sedative hypnotics during pregnancy

Breast Feeding
- Some drug is found in mother's breast milk
- ✳ Recommended either to discontinue drug or bottle feed

THE ART OF PSYCHOPHARMACOLOGY

Potential Advantages
- Those needing short duration of action

Potential Disadvantages
- Those needing longer duration of action
- More expensive than some other sedative hypnotics

Primary Target Symptoms
- Time to sleep onset
- Total sleep time
- Nighttime awakenings

 Pearls
- Zaleplon has not been shown to increase the total time asleep or to decrease the number of awakenings
- ✳ May be preferred over benzodiazepines because of its rapid onset of action, short duration of effect, and safety profile
- ✳ Popular for uses requiring short half-life (e.g., dosing in the middle of the night, sleeping on airplanes, jet lag)
- ✳ May not be ideal for patients who desire immediate hypnotic onset and eat just prior to bedtime
- Not a benzodiazepine itself, but binds to benzodiazepine receptors
- May have fewer carryover side effects than some other sedative hypnotics
- May not have sufficient efficacy in patients with severe chronic insomnia resistant to some other sedative hypnotics
- May cause less dependence than some other sedative hypnotics, especially in those without a history of substance abuse
- ✳ Zaleplon is not absorbed as quickly if taken with high fat foods, which may reduce onset of action

 Suggested Reading

Dooley M, Plosker GL. Zaleplon: a review of its use in the treatment of insomnia. Drugs 2000; 60:413–45.

Heydorn WE. Zaleplon – a review of a novel sedative hypnotic used in the treatment of insomnia. Expert Opin Invest Drugs 2000; 9:841–58.

Mangano RM. Efficacy and safety of zaleplon at peak plasma levels. Int J Clin Pract Suppl 2001;116:9–13.

Weitzel KW, Wickman JM, Augustin SG, Strom JG. Zaleplon: a pyrazolopyrimidine sedative-hypnotic agent for the treatment of insomnia. Clin Ther 2000;22:1254–67.

ZIPRASIDONE

THERAPEUTICS

Brands • Geodon
see index for additional brand names

Generic? Not in U.S. or Europe

 Class

- Atypical antipsychotic (serotonin-dopamine antagonist; second generation antipsychotic; also a mood stabilizer)

Commonly Prescribed For
(bold for FDA approved)
- **Schizophrenia**
- **Delaying relapse in schizophrenia**
- **Acute agitation in schizophrenia (intramuscular)**
- **Acute mania**
- Other psychotic disorders
- Bipolar maintenance
- Bipolar depression
- Behavioral disturbances in dementias
- Behavioral disturbances in children and adolescents
- Disorders associated with problems with impulse control

 How The Drug Works

- Blocks dopamine 2 receptors, reducing positive symptoms of psychosis and stabilizing affective symptoms
- Blocks serotonin 2A receptors, causing enhancement of dopamine release in certain brain regions and thus reducing motor side effects and possibly improving cognitive and affective symptoms
- Interactions at a myriad of other neurotransmitter receptors may contribute to ziprasidone's efficacy
- ✳ Specifically, interactions at 5HT2C and 5HT1A receptors may contribute to efficacy for cognitive and affective symptoms in some patients
- ✳ Specifically, interactions at 5HT1D receptors and at serotonin, norepinephrine, and dopamine transporters (especially at high doses) may contribute to efficacy for affective symptoms in some patients

How Long Until It Works
- Psychotic symptoms can improve within 1 week, but it may take several weeks for full effect on behavior as well as on cognition and affective stabilization
- Classically recommended to wait at least 4–6 weeks to determine efficacy of drug, but in practice some patients require up to 16–20 weeks to show a good response, especially on cognitive symptoms

If It Works
- Most often reduces positive symptoms in schizophrenia but does not eliminate them
- Can improve negative symptoms, as well as aggressive, cognitive, and affective symptoms in schizophrenia
- Most schizophrenic patients do not have a total remission of symptoms but rather a reduction of symptoms by about a third
- Perhaps 5–15% of schizophrenic patients can experience an overall improvement of greater than 50–60%, especially when receiving stable treatment for more than a year
- Such patients are considered super-responders or "awakeners" since they may be well enough to be employed, live independently, and sustain long-term relationships
- Many bipolar patients may experience a reduction of symptoms by half or more
- Continue treatment until reaching a plateau of improvement
- After reaching a satisfactory plateau, continue treatment for at least a year after first episode of psychosis
- For second and subsequent episodes of psychosis, treatment may need to be indefinite
- Even for first episodes of psychosis, it may be preferable to continue treatment indefinitely to avoid subsequent episodes
- Treatment may not only reduce mania but also prevent recurrences of mania in bipolar disorder

If It Doesn't Work
- Try one of the other atypical antipsychotics (risperidone, olanzapine, quetiapine, aripiprazole, amisulpride)
- If 2 or more antipsychotic monotherapies do not work, consider clozapine
- If no first-line atypical antipsychotic is effective, consider higher doses or augmentation with valproate or lamotrigine
- Some patients may require treatment with a conventional antipsychotic

- Consider noncompliance and switch to another antipsychotic with fewer side effects or to an antipsychotic that can be given by depot injection
- Consider initiating rehabilitation and psychotherapy
- Consider presence of concomitant drug abuse

Best Augmenting Combos for Partial Response or Treatment-Resistance

- Valproic acid (valproate, divalproex, divalproex ER)
- Other mood stabilizing anticonvulsants (carbamazepine, oxcarbazepine, lamotrigine)
- Lithium
- Benzodiazepines

Tests

Before starting an atypical antipsychotic

✳ Weigh all patients and track BMI during treatment
- Get baseline personal and family history of obesity, dyslipidemia, hypertension, and cardiovascular disease
✳ Get waist circumference (at umbilicus), blood pressure, fasting plasma glucose, and fasting lipid profile
- Determine if the patient is
  - overweight (BMI 25.0–29.9)
  - obese (BMI ≥30)
  - has pre-diabetes (fasting plasma glucose 100–125 mg/dl)
  - has diabetes (fasting plasma glucose >126 mg/dl)
  - has hypertension (BP >140/90 mm Hg)
  - has dyslipidemia (increased total cholesterol, LDL cholesterol, and triglycerides; decreased HDL cholesterol)
- Treat or refer such patients for treatment, including nutrition and weight management, physical activity counseling, smoking cessation, and medical management

Monitoring after starting an atypical antipsychotic

✳ BMI monthly for 3 months, then quarterly
✳ Blood pressure, fasting plasma glucose, fasting lipids within 3 months and then annually, but earlier and more frequently for patients with diabetes or who have gained >5% of initial weight

- Treat or refer for treatment and consider switching to another atypical antipsychotic for patients who become overweight, obese, pre-diabetic, diabetic, hypertensive, or dyslipidemic while receiving an atypical antipsychotic
✳ Even in patients without known diabetes, be vigilant for the rare but life threatening onset of diabetic ketoacidosis, which always requires immediate treatment, by monitoring for the rapid onset of polyuria, polydipsia, weight loss, nausea, vomiting, dehydration, rapid respiration, weakness and clouding of sensorium, even coma
- Routine EKGs for screening or monitoring of dubious clinical value
- EKGs may be useful for selected patients (e.g., those with personal or family history of QTc prolongation; cardiac arrhythmia; recent myocardial infarction; uncompensated heart failure; or those taking agents that prolong QTc interval such as pimozide, thioridazine, selected antiarrhythmics, moxifloxacin, sparfloxacin, etc.)
- Patients at risk for electrolyte disturbances (e.g., patients on diuretic therapy) should have baseline and periodic serum potassium and magnesium measurements

SIDE EFFECTS

How Drug Causes Side Effects

- By blocking alpha 1 adrenergic receptors, it can cause dizziness, sedation, and hypotension, especially at high doses
- By blocking dopamine 2 receptors in the striatum, it can cause motor side effects (unusual)
✳ Mechanism of any possible weight gain is unknown; weight gain is not common with ziprasidone and may thus have a different mechanism from atypical antipsychotics for which weight gain is common or problematic
✳ Mechanism of any possible increased incidence of diabetes or dyslipidemia is unknown; early experience suggests these complications are not clearly associated with ziprasidone and if present may therefore have a different mechanism from that of atypical antipsychotics associated

with an increased incidence of diabetes and dyslipidemia

Notable Side Effects

✳ Some patients may experience activating side effects at very low to low doses
• Dizziness, extrapyramidal symptoms, sedation, dystonia
• Nausea, dry mouth
• Asthenia, skin rash
• Rare tardive dyskinesia (much reduced risk compared to conventional antipsychotics)
• Orthostatic hypotension

 ### Life Threatening or Dangerous Side Effects

• Rare neuroleptic malignant syndrome (much reduced risk compared to conventional antipsychotics)
• Rare seizures

Weight Gain

unusual   not unusual   common   problematic

• Reported in a few patients, especially those with low BMIs, but not expected
• Less frequent and less severe than for most other antipsychotics

Sedation

unusual   not unusual   common   problematic

• Some patients experience
• May be less than for some antipsychotics, more than for others
• Usually transient and at higher doses
• Can be activating at low doses

What To Do About Side Effects

• Wait
• Wait
• Wait
• Usually dosed twice daily, so take more of the total daily dose at bedtime to help reduce daytime sedation
• Anticholinergics may reduce motor side effects when present
• Weight loss, exercise programs, and medical management for high BMIs, diabetes, dyslipidemia
✳ For activating side effects at low doses, raise the dose

✳ For sedating side effects at high doses, lower the dose
• Switch to another atypical antipsychotic

Best Augmenting Agents for Side Effects

• Benztropine or trihexyphenidyl for motor side effects
• Many side effects cannot be improved with an augmenting agent

DOSING AND USE

Usual Dosage Range

• Schizophrenia: 40–200 mg/day (in divided doses) orally
• Bipolar disorder: 80–160 mg/day (in divided doses) orally
• 10–20 mg intramuscularly

Dosage Forms

• Capsules 20 mg, 40 mg, 60 mg, 80 mg
• Injection 20 mg/mL

How to Dose

• Schizophrenia (according to manufacturer): initial oral dose 20 mg twice a day; however, 40 mg twice a day or 60 mg twice a day may be better tolerated in many patients (less activation); maximum approved dose 100 mg twice a day
• Biplar disorder (according to manufacturer): initial oral dose 40 mg twice a day; on day 2 increase to 60 or 80 mg twice a day
• For intramuscular formulation, recommended dose is 10–20 mg given as required; doses of 10 mg may be administered every 2 hours; doses of 20 mg may be administered every 4 hours; maximum daily dose 40 mg intramuscularly; should not be administered for more than 3 consecutive days

 ### Dosing Tips

✳ **More may be much more:** clinical practice suggests ziprasidone often under-dosed, then switched prior to adequate trials, perhaps due to unjustified fears of QTc prolongation

* Dosing many patients at 20–40 mg twice a day is too low and in fact activating, perhaps due to potent 5HT2C antagonist properties
* Paradoxically, such activation is often reduced by increasing the dose to 60–80 mg twice a day, perhaps due to increasing amounts of dopamine 2 receptor antagonism
* Best efficacy in schizophrenia and bipolar disorder is at doses >120 mg/day, but only a minority of patients are adequately dosed in clinical practice
* Doses up to 80 mg twice a day may have a lower cost than some other atypical antipsychotics
* Recommended to be taken with food because food can double bioavailability by increasing absorption and thus increasing plasma drug levels
* Some patients respond better to doses >160 mg/day and up to 320 mg/day in 2 divided doses (i.e., 80–160 mg twice a day)
* Although studies suggest patients switching to ziprasidone from another antipsychotic can do well with rapid cross-titration, clinical experience suggests many patients do best by building up a full dose of ziprasidone (>120 mg/day) added to the maintenance dose of the first antipsychotic for up to 3 weeks prior to slow down-titration of the first antipsychotic
* QTc prolongation at 320 mg/day not significantly greater than at 160 mg/day
* Rather than raise the dose above these levels in acutely agitated patients requiring acute antipsychotic actions, consider augmentation with a benzodiazepine or conventional antipsychotic, either orally or intramuscularly
* Rather than raise the dose above these levels in partial responders, consider augmentation with a mood stabilizing anticonvulsant, such as valproate or lamotrigine
* Children and elderly should generally be dosed at the lower end of the dosage spectrum
* Ziprasidone intramuscular can be given short-term, both to initiate dosing with oral ziprasidone or another oral antipsychotic and to treat breakthrough agitation in patients maintained on oral antipsychotics

* QTc prolongation of intramuscular ziprasidone is the same or less than with intramuscular haloperidol

Overdose

* Rarely lethal in monotherapy overdose; sedation, slurred speech, transitory hypertension

Long-Term Use

* Approved to delay relapse in long-term treatment of schizophrenia
* Often used for long-term maintenance in bipolar disorder and various behavioral disorders

Habit Forming

* No

How to Stop

* Slow down-titration of oral formulation (over 6 to 8 weeks), especially when simultaneously beginning a new antipsychotic while switching (i.e. cross-titration)
* Rapid oral discontinuation may lead to rebound psychosis and worsening of symptoms

Pharmacokinetics

* Mean half-life 6.6 hours
* Protein binding >99%
* Metabolized by CYP450 3A4

 Drug Interactions

* Neither CYP450 3A4 nor CYP450 2D6 inhibitors significantly affect ziprasidone plasma levels
* Little potential to affect metabolism of drugs cleared by CYP450 enzymes
* May enhance the effects of antihypertensive drugs
* May antagonize levodopa, dopamine agonists
* May enhance QTc prolongation of other drugs capable of prolonging QTc interval

 Other Warnings/ Precautions

* Ziprasidone prolongs QTc interval more than some other antipsychotics

- Use with caution in patients with conditions that predispose to hypotension (dehydration, overheating)
- Priapism has been reported
- Dysphagia has been associated with antipsychotic use, and ziprasidone should be used cautiously in patients at risk for aspiration pneumonia

Do Not Use

- If patient is taking agents capable of significantly prolonging QTc interval (e.g., pimozide, thioridazine, selected antiarrhythmics, moxifloxacin, sparfloxacin)
- If there is a history of QTc prolongation or cardiac arrhythmia, recent acute myocardial infarction, uncompensated heart failure
- If there is a proven allergy to ziprasidone

SPECIAL POPULATIONS

Renal Impairment

- No dose adjustment necessary
- Not removed by hemodialysis
- Intramuscular formulation should be used with caution

Hepatic Impairment

- No dose adjustment necessary

Cardiac Impairment

- Ziprasidone is contraindicated in patients with a known history of QTc prolongation, recent acute myocardial infarction, and uncompensated heart failure
- Should be used with caution in other cases of cardiac impairment because of risk of orthostatic hypotension

Elderly

- Some patients may tolerate lower doses better

Children and Adolescents

- Not officially recommended for patients under age 18
- Clinical experience and early data suggest ziprasidone may be safe and effective for behavioral disturbances in children and adolescents

- Children and adolescents using ziprasidone may need to be monitored more often than adults and may tolerate lower doses better

Pregnancy

- Risk Category C [some animal studies show adverse effects, no controlled studies in humans]
- Psychotic symptoms may worsen during pregnancy and some form of treatment may be necessary
- Ziprasidone may be preferable to anticonvulsant mood stabilizers if treatment is required during pregnancy

Breast Feeding

- Unknown if ziprasidone is secreted in human breast milk, but all psychotropics assumed to be secreted in breast milk
- ✳ Recommended either to discontinue drug or bottle feed
- Infants of women who choose to breast feed while on ziprasidone should be monitored for possible adverse effects

THE ART OF PSYCHOPHARMACOLOGY

Potential Advantages

- Some cases of psychosis and bipolar disorder refractory to treatment with other antipsychotics
- ✳ Patients concerned about gaining weight
- ✳ Patients with diabetes
- Patients requiring rapid relief of symptoms (intramuscular injection)
- Patients switching from intramuscular ziprasidone to an oral preparation

Potential Disadvantages

- Patients noncompliant with twice daily dosing
- ✳ Patients noncompliant with dosing with food

Primary Target Symptoms

- Positive symptoms of psychosis
- Negative symptoms of psychosis
- Cognitive symptoms
- Unstable mood (both depression and mania)
- Aggressive symptoms

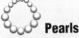

Pearls

✳ QTc prolongation fears are often exaggerated and not justified since QTc prolongation with ziprasidone is not dose-related and few drugs have any potential to increase ziprasidone's plasma levels

✳ Efficacy may be underestimated since ziprasidone is mostly under-dosed (<120 mg/day) in clinical practice

✳ Well-accepted in clinical practice when wanting to avoid weight gain because less weight gain than most other atypical antipsychotics

✳ May not have diabetes or dyslipidemia risk, but monitoring is still indicated

• Less sedation than some antipsychotics, more than others (at moderate to high doses)

✳ More activating than some other antipsychotics at low doses

• One of the least expensive atypical antipsychotics within recommended therapeutic dosing range

• Anecdotal reports of utility in treatment-resistant cases, especially when adequately dosed

✳ One of only 2 atypical antipsychotics with a short-acting intramuscular dosage formulation

Suggested Reading

Bantick RA, Deakin JF, Grasby PM. The 5-HT1A receptor in schizophrenia: a promising target for novel atypical neuroleptics? J Psychopharmacol 2001;15:37–46.

Gunasekara NS, Spencer CM, Keating GM. Spotlight on ziprasidone in schizophrenia and schizoaffective disorder. CNS Drugs 2002;16:645–52.

Keck PE Jr, McElroy SL, Arnold LM. Ziprasidone: a new atypical antipsychotic. Expert Opin Pharmacother 2001;2:1033–42.

Taylor D. Ziprasidone in the management of schizophrenia : the QT interval issue in context. CNS Drugs 2003;17:423–30.

Yatham LN. Efficacy of atypical antipsychotics in mood disorders. J Clin Psychopharmacol 2003;23(3 Suppl 1):S9–14.

ZOLPIDEM

THERAPEUTICS

Brands • Ambien
see index for additional brand names

Generic? No

 Class
• Non-benzodiazepine hypnotic; alpha 1 isoform selective antagonist of GABA-A/benzodiazepine receptors

Commonly Prescribed For
(bold for FDA approved)
• **Short-term treatment of insomnia**

 How The Drug Works
• Binds selectively to a subtype of the benzodiazepine receptor, the alpha 1 isoform
• May enhance GABA inhibitory actions that provide sedative hypnotic effects more selectively than other actions of GABA
• Boosts chloride conductance through GABA-regulated channels
• Inhibitory actions in sleep centers may provide sedative hypnotic effects

How Long Until It Works
• Generally takes effect in less than an hour

If It Works
• Improves quality of sleep
• Effects on total wake-time and number of nighttime awakenings may be decreased over time

If It Doesn't Work
• If insomnia does not improve after 7–10 days, it may be a manifestation of a primary psychiatric or physical illness such as obstructive sleep apnea or restless leg syndrome, which requires independent evaluation
• Increase the dose
• Improve sleep hygiene
• Switch to another agent

 Best Augmenting Combos for Partial Response or Treatment-Resistance
• Generally, best to switch to another agent
• Trazodone

• Agents with antihistamine actions (e.g., diphenhydramine, tricyclic antidepressants)

Tests
• None for healthy individuals

SIDE EFFECTS

How Drug Causes Side Effects
• Actions at benzodiazepine receptors that carry over to the next day can cause daytime sedation, amnesia, and ataxia
• Long-term adaptations of zolpidem not well studied, but chronic studies of other alpha 1 selective non-benzodiazepine hypnotics suggest lack of notable tolerance or dependence developing over time

Notable Side Effects
✳ Sedation
✳ Dizziness, ataxia
✳ Dose-dependent amnesia
✳ Hyper-excitability, nervousness
• Rare hallucinations
• Diarrhea, nausea
• Headache

 Life Threatening or Dangerous Side Effects
• Respiratory depression, especially when taken with other CNS depressants in overdose

Weight Gain

unusual   not unusual   common   problematic
• Reported but not expected

Sedation

unusual   not unusual   **common**   problematic
• Many experience and/or can be significant in amount

What To Do About Side Effects
• Wait
• To avoid problems with memory, only take zolpidem if planning to have a full night's sleep
• Lower the dose
• Switch to a shorter-acting sedative hypnotic

- Administer flumazenil if side effects are severe or life-threatening

Best Augmenting Agents for Side Effects
- Many side effects cannot be improved with an augmenting agent

DOSING AND USE

Usual Dosage Range
- 10 mg/day at bedtime for 7–10 days

Dosage Forms
- Tablet 5 mg

How to Dose
- 10 mg/day at bedtime

Dosing Tips
* Zolpidem is not absorbed as quickly if taken with food, which could reduce onset of action
- Patients with lower body weights may require only a 5 mg dose
- Zolpidem should generally not be prescribed in quantities greater than a 1-month supply
- Risk of dependence may increase with dose and duration of treatment
* However, treatment with alpha 1 selective non-benzodiazepine hypnotics may cause less tolerance or dependence than benzodiazepine hypnotics

Overdose
- No fatalities reported with zolpidem monotherapy; sedation, ataxia, confusion, hypotension, respiratory depression, coma

Long-Term Use
- Not generally intended for long-term use
- Increased wakefulness during the latter part of night (wearing off) or an increase in daytime anxiety (rebound) may occur

Habit Forming
- Zolpidem is a Schedule IV drug
- Some patients may develop dependence and/or tolerance; risk may be greater with higher doses
- History of drug addiction may increase risk of dependence

How to Stop
- Although rebound insomnia could occur, this effect has not generally been seen with therapeutic doses of zolpidem
- If taken for more than a few weeks, taper to reduce chances of withdrawal effects

Pharmacokinetics
- Short elimination half-life (approximately 2.5 hours)

Drug Interactions
- Increased depressive effects when taken with other CNS depressants
- Sertraline may increase plasma levels of zolpidem
- Rifampin may decrease plasma levels of zolpidem

Other Warnings/ Precautions
- Insomnia may be a symptom of a primary disorder, rather than a primary disorder itself
- Some patients may exhibit abnormal thinking or behavioral changes similar to those caused by other CNS depressants (i.e., either depressant actions or disinhibiting actions)
- Some depressed patients may experience a worsening of suicidal ideation
- Use only with extreme caution in patients with impaired respiratory function or obstructive sleep apnea
- Zolpidem should only be administered at bedtime
- Temporary memory loss may occur at doses above 10 mg/night

Do Not Use
- If there is a proven allergy to zolpidem

SPECIAL POPULATIONS

Renal Impairment
- No dose adjustment necessary
- Patients should be monitored

Hepatic Impairment
- Recommended dose 5 mg
- Patients should be monitored

Cardiac Impairment
• No available data

Elderly
• Recommended initial dose: 5 mg
• Elderly may have increased risk for falls, confusion

 Children and Adolescents
• Safety and efficacy have not been established
• Long-term effects of zolpidem in children/adolescents are unknown
• Should generally receive lower doses and be more closely monitored

 Pregnancy
• Risk category B [animal studies do not show adverse effects, no controlled studies in humans]
• Infants whose mothers took sedative hypnotics during pregnancy may experience some withdrawal symptoms
• Neonatal flaccidity has been reported in infants whose mothers took sedative hypnotics during pregnancy

Breast Feeding
• Some drug is found in mother's breast milk
✳ Recommended either to discontinue drug or bottle feed

THE ART OF PSYCHOPHARMACOLOGY

Potential Advantages
• Patients who require long-term treatment

Potential Disadvantages
• More expensive than some other sedative hypnotics

Primary Target Symptoms
• Time to sleep onset
• Total sleep time
• Nighttime awakenings

 Pearls
✳ One of the most popular sedative hypnotic agents in psychopharmacology
• Zolpidem has been shown to increase the total time asleep and to reduce the amount of nighttime awakenings
✳ May be preferred over benzodiazepines because of its rapid onset of action, short duration of effect, and safety profile
• Clearance of zolpidem may be slightly slower in women than in men
• May not be ideal for patients who desire immediate hypnotic onset and eat just prior to bedtime
• Not a benzodiazepine itself, but binds to benzodiazepine receptors
• May have fewer carryover side effects than some other sedative hypnotics
• May cause less dependence than some other sedative hypnotics, especially in those without a history of substance abuse

 Suggested Reading

Holm KJ, Goa KL. Zolpidem: an update of its pharmacology, therapeutic efficacy and tolerability in the treatment of insomnia. Drugs 2000;59:865–89.

Rush CR. Behavioral pharmacology of zolpidem relative to benzodiazepines: a review. Pharmacol Biochem Behav 1998;61:253–69.

Soyka M, Bottlender R, Moller HJ. Epidemiological evidence for a low abuse potential of zolpidem. Pharmacopsychiatry 2000;33:138–41.

Toner LC, Tsambiras BM, Catalano G, Catalano MC, Cooper DS. Central nervous system side effects associated with zolpidem treatment. Clin Neuropharmacol 2000;23:54–8.

ZONISAMIDE

Brands • Zonegran
• Excegran
see index for additional brand names

Generic? Not in U.S.

 Class

• Anticonvulsant, voltage-sensitive sodium channel modulator; T-type calcium channel modulator; structurally a sulfonamide

Commonly Prescribed For
(bold for FDA approved)
• **Adjunct therapy for partial seizures in adults with epilepsy**
• Bipolar disorder
• Chronic neuropathic pain
• Migraine
• Parkinson's disease
• Psychotropic drug-induced weight gain
• Binge-eating disorder

 How The Drug Works

• Unknown
• Modulates voltage-sensitive sodium channels by an unknown mechanism
• Also modulates T-type calcium channels
• Blocks glutamate release
• Facilitates dopamine and serotonin release
• Inhibits MAO-B
• Inhibits carbonic anhydrase

How Long Until It Works
• Should reduce seizures by 2 weeks
• Onset of action as well as convincing therapeutic efficacy have not been demonstrated for uses other than adjunctive treatment of partial seizures

If It Works
• The goal of treatment is complete remission of symptoms (e.g., seizures, pain, mania, migraine)
• Would currently only be expected to work in a subset of patients for conditions other than epilepsy as an adjunctive treatment to agents with better demonstration of efficacy

If It Doesn't Work (for conditions other than epilepsy)
• May only be effective in patients who fail to respond to agents with proven efficacy, or it may not work at all
• Consider increasing dose or switching to another agent with better demonstrated efficacy

 Best Augmenting Combos for Partial Response or Treatment-Resistance

• Zonisamide is itself a second-line augmenting agent to numerous other agents in treating conditions other than epilepsy, such as bipolar disorder, chronic neuropathic pain, and migraine

Tests
• Consider baseline and periodic monitoring of renal function

How Drug Causes Side Effects
• CNS side effects theoretically due to excessive actions at voltage-sensitive ion channels
• Weak inhibition of carbonic anhydrase may lead to kidney stones
• Serious rash theoretically an allergic reaction

Notable Side Effects
✳ Sedation, depression, difficulty concentrating, agitation, irritability, psychomotor slowing, dizziness, ataxia
• Headache
• Nausea, anorexia, abdominal pain, vomiting
• Kidney stones
• Elevated serum creatinine and blood urea nitrogen

 Life Threatening or Dangerous Side Effects

• Rare serious rash (Stevens Johnson syndrome, toxic epidermal necrolysis) (sulfonamide)
• Rare oligohidrosis and hyperthermia (pediatric patients)
• Rare blood dyscrasias (aplastic anemia; agranulocytosis)
• Sudden hepatic necrosis

- Sudden unexplained deaths have occurred (unknown if related to zonisamide use)

Weight Gain

unusual | not unusual | common | problematic

- Reported but not expected
- ✱ Patients may experience weight loss

Sedation

unusual | not unusual | common | problematic

- Many experience and/or can be significant in amount
- Dose-related
- Can wear off with time but may not wear off at high doses

What To Do About Side Effects

- Wait
- Wait
- Wait
- Take more of the dose at night to reduce daytime sedation
- Lower the dose
- Switch to another agent

Best Augmenting Agents for Side Effects

- Many side effects cannot be improved with an augmenting agent

DOSING AND USE

Usual Dosage Range

- 100–600 mg/day in 1–2 doses

Dosage Forms

- Capsule 25 mg, 50 mg, 100 mg

How to Dose

- Initial 100 mg/day; after 2 weeks can increase to 200 mg/day; dose can be increased by 100 mg/day every 2 weeks if necessary and tolerated; maximum dose generally 600 mg/day; maintain stable dose for at least 2 weeks before increasing dose

 Dosing Tips

- ✱ Most clinical experience is at doses up to 400 mg/day

- No evidence from controlled trials of increasing response over 400 mg/day
- However, some patients may tolerate and respond to doses up to 600 mg/day
- Little experience with doses greater than 600 mg/day
- Side effects may increase notably at doses greater than 300 mg/day
- For intolerable sedation, can give most of the dose at night and less during the day

Overdose

- No fatalities; bradycardia, hypotension, respiratory depression

Long-Term Use

- Safe
- Consider periodic monitoring of blood urea nitrogen and creatinine

Habit Forming

- No

How to Stop

- Taper
- Epilepsy patients may seize upon withdrawal, especially if withdrawal is abrupt
- Rapid discontinuation may increase the risk of relapse in bipolar patients
- Discontinuation symptoms uncommon

Pharmacokinetics

- Plasma elimination half-life approximately 63 hours
- Metabolized in part by CYP450 3A4
- Partially eliminated renally

 Drug Interactions

- Agents that inhibit CYP450 3A4 (such as nefazodone, fluvoxamine, and fluoxetine) may decrease the clearance of zonisamide, and increase plasma zonisamide levels, possibly requiring lower doses of zonisamide
- Agents that induce CYP450 3A4 (such as carbamazepine) may increase the clearance of zonisamide and decrease plasma zonisamide levels, possibly requiring higher doses of zonisamide
- Enzyme-inducing antiepileptic drugs (carbamazepine, phenytoin, phenobarbital, and primidone) may decrease plasma levels of zonisamide

- Theoretically, zonisamide may interact with carbonic anhydrase inhibitors to increase the risk of kidney stones

 Other Warnings/ Precautions

- Depressive effects may be increased by other CNS depressants (alcohol, MAOIs, other anticonvulsants, etc.)
- Use with caution when combining with other drugs that predispose patients to heat-related disorders, including carbonic anhydrase inhibitors and anticholinergics
- ✳ Life-threatening rashes have developed in association with zonisamide use; zonisamide should generally be discontinued at the first sign of serious rash
- Patient should be instructed to report any symptoms of hypersensitivity immediately (fever; flu-like symptoms; rash; blisters on skin or in eyes, mouth, ears, nose, or genital areas; swelling of eyelids, conjunctivitis, lymphadenopathy)
- Patients should be monitored for signs of unusual bleeding or bruising, mouth sores, infections, fever, and sore throat, as there may be an increased risk of aplastic anemia and agranulocytosis with zonisamide

Do Not Use

- If there is a proven allergy to zonisamide or sulfonamides

SPECIAL POPULATIONS

Renal Impairment

- Zonisamide is primarily renally excreted
- Use with caution
- May require slower titration

Hepatic Impairment

- Use with caution
- May require slower titration

Cardiac Impairment

- No specific recommendations

Elderly

- Some patients may tolerate lower doses better
- Elderly patients may be more susceptible to adverse effects

 Children and Adolescents

- Cases of oligohidrosis and hyperthermia have been reported
- Not approved for use in children
- Use in children for the expert only, with close monitoring, after other options have failed

 Pregnancy

- Risk category C [some animal studies show adverse effects, no controlled studies in humans]
- Use in women of childbearing potential requires weighing potential benefits to the mother against the risks to the fetus
- Taper drug if discontinuing
- Seizures, even mild seizures, may cause harm to the embryo/fetus
- Lack of convincing efficacy for treatment of conditions other than epilepsy suggests risk/benefit ratio is in favor of discontinuing zonisamide during pregnancy for these indications

Breast Feeding

- Unknown if zonisamide is secreted in human breast milk, but all psychotropics assumed to be secreted in breast milk
- ✳ Recommended either to discontinue drug or bottle feed
- If drug is continued while breast feeding, infant should be monitored for possible adverse effects
- If child becomes irritable or sedated, breast feeding or drug may need to be discontinued

THE ART OF PSYCHOPHARMACOLOGY

Potential Advantages

- Treatment-resistant conditions
- Patients who wish to avoid weight gain

Potential Disadvantages

- Poor documentation of efficacy for off-label uses
- Patients noncompliant with twice daily dosing

Primary Target Symptoms

- Seizures

- Numerous other symptoms for off-label uses
- Patients with a history of kidney stones

 Pearls

- Well studied in epilepsy
- ✳ Much off-label use is based upon theoretical considerations rather than clinical experience or compelling efficacy studies
- Early studies suggest efficacy in binge-eating disorder
- Early studies suggest possible efficacy in migraine
- Early studies suggest possible utility in Parkinson's disease
- Preclinical studies suggest possible utility in neuropathic pain
- Early studies suggest some therapeutic potential for mood stabilizing
- Chronic intake of caffeine may lower brain zonisamide concentrations and attenuate its anticonvulsant effects
- ✳ Due to reported weight loss in some patients in trials with epilepsy, some patients with psychotropic-induced weight gain are treated with zonisamide
- Utility for this indication is not clear nor has it been systematically studied

 Suggested Reading

Chadwick DW, Marson AG. Zonisamide add-on for drug-resistant partial epilepsy. Cochrane Database Syst Rev. 2002;(2):CD001416.

Glauser TA, Pellock JM. Zonisamide in pediatric epilepsy: review of the Japanese experience. J Child Neurol. 2002;17:87–96.

Jain KK. An assessment of zonisamide as an anti-epileptic drug. Expert Opin Pharmacother. 2000;1:1245–60.

Leppik IE. Three new drugs for epilepsy: levetiracetam, oxcarbazepine, and zonisamide. J Child Neurol. 2002;17 Suppl 1:S53–7.

ZOPICLONE

THERAPEUTICS

Brands • Imovane
see index for additional brand names

Generic? No

 Class
• Non-benzodiazepine hypnotic; alpha 1 isoform selective antagonist of GABA-A/ benzodiazepine receptors

Commonly Prescribed For
(bold for FDA approved)
• Short-term treatment of insomnia

 How The Drug Works
• May bind selectively to a subtype of the benzodiazepine receptor, the alpha 1 isoform
• May enhance GABA inhibitory actions that provide sedative hypnotic effects more selectively than other actions of GABA
• Boosts chloride conductance through GABA-regulated channels
• Inhibitory actions in sleep centers may provide sedative hypnotic effects

How Long Until It Works
• Generally takes effect in less than an hour

If It Works
• Improves quality of sleep
• Effects on total wake-time and number of nighttime awakenings may be decreased over time

If It Doesn't Work
• If insomnia does not improve after 7–10 days, it may be a manifestation of a primary psychiatric or physical illness such as obstructive sleep apnea or restless leg syndrome, which requires independent evaluation
• Increase the dose
• Improve sleep hygiene
• Switch to another agent

 Best Augmenting Combos for Partial Response or Treatment-Resistance
• Generally, best to switch to another agent
• Trazodone

• Agents with antihistamine actions (e.g., diphenhydramine, tricyclic antidepressants)

Tests
• None for healthy individuals

SIDE EFFECTS

How Drug Causes Side Effects
• Actions at benzodiazepine receptors that carry over to the next day can cause daytime sedation, amnesia, and ataxia
✳ Long-term adaptations of zopiclone, a mixture of an active S enantiomer and an inactive R enantiomer, have not been well studied, but chronic studies of the active isomer eszopiclone suggest lack of notable tolerance or dependence developing over time

Notable Side Effects
✳ Sedation
✳ Dizziness, ataxia
✳ Dose-dependent amnesia
✳ Hyper-excitability, nervousness
• Dry mouth, loss of appetite, constipation, bitter taste
• Impaired vision

 Life Threatening or Dangerous Side Effects
• Respiratory depression, especially when taken with other CNS depressants in overdose

Weight Gain

unusual   not unusual   common   problematic
• Reported but not expected

Sedation

unusual   not unusual   common   problematic
• Many experience and/or can be significant in amount

What To Do About Side Effects
• Wait
• To avoid problems with memory, only take zopiclone if planning to have a full night's sleep
• Lower the dose

• Switch to a shorter-acting sedative hypnotic
• Administer flumazenil if side effects are severe or life-threatening

Best Augmenting Agents for Side Effects
• Many side effects cannot be improved with an augmenting agent

DOSING AND USE

Usual Dosage Range
• 7.5 mg at bedtime

Dosage Forms
• Tablet 7.5 mg scored

How to Dose
• No titration, take dose at bedtime

Dosing Tips
• Zopiclone should generally not be prescribed in quantities greater than a 1-month supply
• Risk of dependence may increase with dose and duration of treatment
• However, chronic treatment with alpha 1 selective non-benzodiazepine hypnotics may cause less tolerance or dependence than benzodiazepine hypnotics

Overdose
• Can be fatal; clumsiness, mood changes, sedation, weakness, breathing trouble, unconsciousness

Long-Term Use
• Not generally intended for use past 4 weeks

Habit Forming
• Some patients may develop dependence and/or tolerance; risk may be greater with higher doses
• History of drug addiction may increase risk of dependence

How to Stop
• Rebound insomnia may occur the first night after stopping
• If taken for more than a few weeks, taper to reduce chances of withdrawal effects

Pharmacokinetics
• Metabolized by CYP450 3A4
• Terminal elimination half-life approximately 3.5–6.5 hours

Drug Interactions
• Increased depressive effects when taken with other CNS depressants
• Theoretically, inhibitors of CYP450 3A4, such as nefazodone and fluvoxamine, could increase plasma levels of zopiclone

Other Warnings/ Precautions
• Insomnia may be a symptom of a primary disorder, rather than a primary disorder itself
• Some patients may exhibit abnormal thinking or behavioral changes similar to those caused by other CNS depressants (i.e., either depressant actions or disinhibiting actions)
• Some depressed patients may experience a worsening of suicidal ideation
• Use only with extreme caution in patients with impaired respiratory function or obstructive sleep apnea
• Zopiclone should only be administered at bedtime

Do Not Use
• If patient has myasthenia gravis
• If patient has severe respiratory impairment
• If patient has had a stroke
• If there is a proven allergy to zopiclone

SPECIAL POPULATIONS

Renal Impairment
• Increased plasma levels
• May need to lower dose

Hepatic Impairment
• Increased plasma levels
• Recommended dose 3.75 mg

Cardiac Impairment
• Dosage adjustment may not be necessary

Elderly
• May be more susceptible to adverse effects

- Initial dose 3.75 mg at bedtime; can increase to usual adult dose if necessary and tolerated

Children and Adolescents
- Safety and efficacy have not been established
- Long-term effects of zopiclone in children/adolescents are unknown
- Should generally receive lower doses and be more closely monitored

Pregnancy
- Risk category C [some animal studies show adverse effects, no controlled studies in humans]
- Infants whose mothers took sedative hypnotics during pregnancy may experience some withdrawal symptoms
- Neonatal flaccidity has been reported in infants whose mothers took sedative hypnotics during pregnancy

Breast Feeding
- Some drug is found in mother's breast milk
- ✱ Recommended either to discontinue drug or bottle feed

THE ART OF PSYCHOPHARMACOLOGY

Potential Advantages
- Those who require long-term treatment

Potential Disadvantages
- More expensive than some other sedative hypnotics

Primary Target Symptoms
- Time to sleep onset
- Nighttime awakenings
- Total sleep time

Pearls
- ✱ May be preferred over benzodiazepines because of its rapid onset of action, short duration of effect, and safety profile
- Zopiclone does not appear to be a highly dependence-causing drug, at least not in patients with no history of drug abuse
- Rebound insomnia does not appear to be common
- Not a benzodiazepine itself, but binds to benzodiazepine receptors
- May have fewer carryover side effects than some other sedative hypnotics
- The active enantiomer of zopiclone, eszopiclone, has received an approvable letter from the United States Food and Drug Administration

Suggested Reading

Fernandez C, Martin C, Gimenez F, Farinotti R. Clinical pharmacokinetics of zopiclone. Clin Pharmacokinet 1995;29:431–41.

Hajak G. A comparative assessment of the risks and benefits of zopiclone: a review of 15 years' clinical experience. Drug Saf 1999; 21:457–69.

Noble S, Langtry HD, Lamb HM. Zopiclone. An update of its pharmacology, clinical efficacy and tolerability in the treatment of insomnia. Drugs 1998;55:277–302.

ZOTEPINE

THERAPEUTICS

Brands • Lodopin
• Zoleptil
see index for additional brand names

Generic? No

Class

• Atypical antipsychotic (serotonin-dopamine antagonist)

Commonly Prescribed For

(bold for FDA approved)
• Schizophrenia
• Other psychotic disorders
• Mania

How The Drug Works

• Blocks dopamine 2 receptors, reducing positive symptoms of psychosis
• Blocks serotonin 2A receptors, causing enhancement of dopamine release in certain brain regions and thus reducing motor side effects and possibly improving cognitive and affective symptoms
• Interactions at a myriad of other neurotransmitter receptors may contribute to zotepine's efficacy
✶ Specifically inhibits norepinephrine uptake

How Long Until It Works

• Psychotic symptoms can improve within 1 week, but it may take several weeks for full effect on behavior as well as on cognition and affective stabilization
• Classically recommended to wait at least 4–6 weeks to determine efficacy of drug, but in practice some patients require up to 16–20 weeks to show a good response, especially on cognitive symptoms

If It Works

• Most often reduces positive symptoms in schizophrenia but does not eliminate them
• Can improve negative symptoms, as well as aggressive, cognitive, and affective symptoms in schizophrenia
• Most schizophrenic patients do not have a total remission of symptoms but rather a reduction of symptoms by about a third

• Perhaps 5–15% of schizophrenic patients can experience an overall improvement of greater than 50–60%, especially when receiving stable treatment for more than a year
• Such patients are considered super-responders or "awakeners" since they may be well enough to be employed, live independently, and sustain long-term relationships
• Many bipolar patients may experience a reduction of symptoms by half or more
• Continue treatment until reaching a plateau of improvement
• After reaching a satisfactory plateau, continue treatment for at least a year after first episode of psychosis
• For second and subsequent episodes of psychosis, treatment may need to be indefinite
• Even for first episodes of psychosis, it may be preferable to continue treatment indefinitely to avoid subsequent episodes
• Treatment may not only reduce mania but also prevent recurrences of mania in bipolar disorder

If It Doesn't Work

• Consider trying one of the first-line atypical antipsychotics (risperidone, olanzapine, quetiapine, ziprasidone, aripiprazole, amisulpride)
• If 2 or more antipsychotic monotherapies do not work, consider clozapine
• If no first-line atypical antipsychotic is effective, consider higher doses or augmentation with valproate or lamotrigine
• Some patients may require treatment with a conventional antipsychotic
• Consider noncompliance and switch to another antipsychotic with fewer side effects or to an antipsychotic that can be given by depot injection
• Consider initiating rehabilitation and psychotherapy
• Consider presence of concomitant drug abuse

 Best Augmenting Combos for Partial Response or Treatment-Resistance

• Augmentation of zotepine has not been systematically studied
• Valproic acid (valproate, divalproex, divalproex ER)

- Other mood stabilizing anticonvulsants (carbamazepine, oxcarbazepine, lamotrigine)
- Lithium
- Benzodiazepines

Tests

✳ Although risk of diabetes and dyslipidemia with zotepine has not been systematically studied, monitoring as for all other atypical antipsychotics is suggested

Before starting an atypical antipsychotic

✳ Weigh all patients and track BMI during treatment
- Get baseline personal and family history of obesity, dyslipidemia, hypertension, and cardiovascular disease
✳ Get waist circumference (at umbilicus), blood pressure, fasting plasma glucose, and fasting lipid profile
- Determine if the patient is
  - overweight (BMI 25.0–29.9)
  - obese (BMI ≥30)
  - has pre-diabetes (fasting plasma glucose 100–125 mg/dl)
  - has diabetes (fasting plasma glucose >126 mg/dl)
  - has hypertension (BP >140/90 mm Hg)
  - has dyslipidemia (increased total cholesterol, LDL cholesterol, and triglycerides; decreased HDL cholesterol)
- Treat or refer such patients for treatment, including nutrition and weight management, physical activity counseling, smoking cessation, and medical management

Monitoring after starting an atypical antipsychotic

✳ BMI monthly for 3 months, then quarterly
✳ Blood pressure, fasting plasma glucose, fasting lipids within 3 months and then annually, but earlier and more frequently for patients with diabetes or who have gained >5% of initial weight
- Treat or refer for treatment and consider switching to another atypical antipsychotic for patients who become overweight, obese, pre-diabetic, diabetic, hypertensive, or dyslipidemic while receiving an atypical antipsychotic
✳ Even in patients without known diabetes, be vigilant for the rare but life threatening onset of diabetic ketoacidosis, which always requires immediate treatment, by

monitoring for the rapid onset of polyuria, polydipsia, weight loss, nausea, vomiting, dehydration, rapid respiration, weakness and clouding of sensorium, even coma
- EKGs may be useful for selected patients (e.g., those with personal or family history of QTc prolongation; cardiac arrhythmia; recent myocardial infarction; uncompensated heart failure; or those taking agents that prolong QTc interval such as pimozide, thioridazine, selected antiarrhythmics, moxifloxacin, sparfloxacin, etc.)
- Patients at risk for electrolyte disturbances (e.g., patients on diuretic therapy) should have baseline and periodic serum potassium and magnesium measurements
- Patients with suspected hematologic abnormalities may require a white blood cell count before initiating treatment
- Monitor liver function tests in patients with established liver disease
- Should check blood pressure in the elderly before starting and for the first few weeks of treatment

SIDE EFFECTS

How Drug Causes Side Effects

- By blocking alpha 1 adrenergic receptors, it can cause dizziness, sedation, and hypotension
- By blocking histamine 1 receptors in the brain, it can cause sedation and weight gain
- By blocking dopamine 2 receptors in the striatum, it can cause motor side effects
- By blocking dopamine 2 receptors in the pituitary, it can cause elevations in prolactin
- Mechanism of weight gain and possible increased incidence of dyslipidemia and diabetes of atypical antipsychotics is unknown

Notable Side Effects

- Atypical antipsychotics may increase the risk for diabetes and dyslipidemia, although the specific risks associated with zotepine are unknown
- Agitation, anxiety, depression, asthenia, headache, insomnia, sedation, hypo/hyperthermia

- Constipation, dry mouth, dyspepsia, weight gain
- Tachycardia, hypotension, sweating, blurred vision
- Rare tardive dyskinesia
- Dose-related hyperprolactinemia

 Life Threatening or Dangerous Side Effects
- Rare neuroleptic malignant syndrome
- Rare seizures (risk increases with dose, especially over 300 mg/day)
- Blood dyscrasias
- Dose-dependent QTc prolongation

Weight Gain

unusual   not unusual   **common**   problematic

- Many experience and/or can be significant in amount

Sedation

unusual   not unusual   **common**   problematic

- Many experience and/or can be significant in amount

What To Do About Side Effects
- Wait
- Wait
- Wait
- For motor symptoms, add an anticholinergic agent
- Take more of the dose at bedtime to help reduce daytime sedation
- Weight loss, exercise programs, and medical management for high BMIs, diabetes, dyslipidemia
- Reduce the dose
- Switch to a first-line atypical antipsychotic

Best Augmenting Agents for Side Effects
- Benztropine or trihexyphenidyl for motor side effects
- Sometimes amantadine can be helpful for motor side effects
- Benzodiazepines may be helpful for akathisia
- Many side effects cannot be improved with an augmenting agent

DOSING AND USE

Usual Dosage Range
- 75–300 mg/day in 3 divided doses

Dosage Forms
- Tablet 25 mg, 50 mg, 100 mg

How to Dose
- Initial 75 mg/day in 3 doses; can increase every 4 days; maximum 300 mg/day in 3 doses

 Dosing Tips
- Slow initial titration can minimize hypotension
- No formal studies, but some patients may do well on twice daily dosing rather than 3 times daily dosing
- * Dose-related QTc prolongation, so use with caution, especially at high doses

Overdose
- Can be fatal, especially in mixed overdoses; seizures, coma

Long-Term Use
- Can be used to delay relapse in long-term treatment of schizophrenia

Habit Forming
- No

How to Stop
- Slow down-titration (over 6 to 8 weeks), especially when simultaneously beginning a new antipsychotic while switching (i.e., cross-titration)
- Rapid discontinuation may lead to rebound psychosis and worsening of symptoms
- If antiparkinson agents are being used, they should be continued for a few weeks after zotepine is discontinued

Pharmacokinetics
- Metabolized by CYP450 3A4 and CYP450 1A2
- Active metabolite norzotepine

 Drug Interactions
- Combined use with phenothiazines may increase risk of seizures

- Can decrease the effects of levodopa, dopamine agonists
- Epinephrine may lower blood pressure
- May interact with hypotensive agents due to alpha 1 adrenergic blockade
- May enhance QTc prolongation of other drugs capable of prolonging QTc interval
- Plasma concentrations increased by diazepam, fluoxetine
- Zotepine may increase plasma levels of phenytoin
- May increase risk of bleeding if used with anticoagulants
- Theoretically, dose may need to be raised if given in conjunction with CYP450 1A2 inducers (e.g., cigarette smoke)
- Theoretically, dose may need to be lowered if given in conjunction with CYP450 1A2 inhibitors (e.g., fluvoxamine) in order to prevent dangers of dose-dependent QTc prolongation
- Theoretically, dose may need to be lowered if given in conjunction with CYP450 3A4 inhibitors (e.g., fluvoxamine, nefazodone, fluoxetine) in order to prevent dangers of dose-dependent QTc prolongation

Other Warnings/ Precautions

- Not recommended for use with sibutramine
- Use cautiously in patients with alcohol withdrawal or convulsive disorders because of possible lowering of seizure threshold
- If signs of neuroleptic malignant syndrome develop, treatment should be immediately discontinued
- Because zotepine may dose-dependently prolong QTc interval, use with caution in patients who have bradycardia or who are taking drugs that can induce bradycardia (e.g., beta blockers, calcium channel blockers, clonidine, digitalis)
- Because zotepine may dose-dependently prolong QTc interval, use with caution in patients who have hypokalemia and or hypomagnesemia or who are taking drugs than can induce hypokalemia and/or magnesemia (e.g., diuretics, stimulant laxatives, intravenous amphotericin B, glucocorticoids, tetracosactide)
- Because zotepine dose-dependently prolongs QTc interval, use with caution in patients taking any agent capable of

increasing zotepine plasma levels (e.g., diazepam, CYP450 1A2 inhibitors and CYP450 3A4 inhibitors)

Do Not Use
- If patient has epilepsy or family history of epilepsy
- If patient has gout or history of nephrolithiasis
- If patient is taking other CNS depressants
- If patient is taking high doses of other antipsychotics
- If patient is taking agents capable of significantly prolonging QTc interval (e.g., pimozide; thioridazine; selected antiarrhythmics such as quinidine, disopyramide, amiodarone, and sotalol; selected antibiotics such as moxifloxacin and sparfloxacin)
- If there is a history of QTc prolongation or cardiac arrhythmia, recent acute myocardial infarction, uncompensated heart failure
- If patient is pregnant or breast feeding
- If there is a proven allergy to zotepine

SPECIAL POPULATIONS

Renal Impairment
- Recommended starting dose 25 mg twice a day; recommended maximum dose generally 75 mg twice a day

Hepatic Impairment
- Recommended starting dose 25 mg twice a day; recommended maximum dose generally 75 mg twice a day
- May require weekly monitoring of liver function during the first few months of treatment

Cardiac Impairment
- Drug should be used with caution
- Zotepine produces a dose-dependent prolongation of QTc interval, which may be enhanced by the existence of bradycardia, hypokalemia, congenital or acquired long QTc interval, which should be evaluated prior to administering zotepine
- Use with caution if treating concomitantly with a medication likely to produce prolonged bradycardia, hypokalemia, slowing of intracardiac conduction, or prolongation of the QTc interval

• Avoid zotepine in patients with a known history of QTc prolongation, recent acute myocardial infraction, and uncompensated heart failure

Elderly
• Recommended starting dose 25 mg twice a day; recommended maximum dose generally 75 mg twice a day

 Children and Adolescents
• Not recommended under age 18

 Pregnancy
• Insufficient data in humans to determine risk
• Zotepine is not recommended during pregnancy

Breast Feeding
• Zotepine is not recommended during breast feeding
• Immediate postpartum period is a high-risk time for relapse of psychosis, so may consider treatment with another antipsychotic

Potential Advantages
• Norepinephrine reuptake blocking actions have theoretical benefits for cognition (attention) and for depression

Potential Disadvantages
• Patients not compliant with 3 times daily dosing
• Patients requiring rapid onset of antipsychotic action
• Patients with uncontrolled seizures

Primary Target Symptoms
• Positive symptoms of psychosis
• Negative symptoms of psychosis
• Cognitive functioning
• Depressive symptoms

 Pearls
✳ Zotepine inhibits norepinephrine reuptake, which may have implications for treatment of depression, as well as for cognitive symptoms of schizophrenia
• Risks of diabetes and dyslipidemia not well-studied for zotepine, but known significant weight gain suggests the need for careful monitoring during zotepine treatment
• Not as well investigated in bipolar disorder, but its mechanism of action suggests efficacy in acute bipolar mania

 Suggested Reading

Ackenheil M. [The biochemical effect profile of zotepine in comparison with other neuroleptics]. Fortschr Neurol Psychiatr 1991; 59 Suppl 1: 2–9.

Fenton M, Morris S, De-Silva P, Bagnall A, Cooper SJ, Gammelin G, Leitner M. Zotepine for schizophrenia. Cochrane Database Syst Rev 2000; (2): CD001948.

Stanniland C, Taylor D. Tolerability of atypical antipsychotics. Drug Saf 2000; 22 (3): 195–214.

ZUCLOPENTHIXOL

THERAPEUTICS

Brands • Clopixol
• Clopixol-Acuphase
see index for additional brand names

Generic? No

Class

• Conventional antipsychotic (neuroleptic, thioxanthene, dopamine 2 antagonist)

Commonly Prescribed For
(bold for FDA approved)

• **Acute schizophrenia (oral, acetate injection)**
• **Maintenance treatment of schizophrenia (oral, decanoate injection)**
• Bipolar disorder
• Aggression

How The Drug Works

• Blocks dopamine 2 receptors, reducing positive symptoms of psychosis

How Long Until It Works

• For injection, psychotic symptoms can improve within a few days, but it may take 1–2 weeks for notable improvement
• For oral formulation, psychotic symptoms can improve within 1 week, but may take several weeks for full effect on behavior

If It Works

• Most often reduces positive symptoms in schizophrenia but does not eliminate them
• Most schizophrenic patients do not have a total remission of symptoms but rather a reduction of symptoms by about a third
• Continue treatment in schizophrenia until reaching a plateau of improvement
• After reaching a satisfactory plateau, continue treatment for at least a year after first episode of psychosis in schizophrenia
• For second and subsequent episodes of psychosis in schizophrenia, treatment may need to be indefinite
• Reduces symptoms of acute psychotic mania but not proven as a mood stabilizer or as an effective maintenance treatment in bipolar disorder
• After reducing acute psychotic symptoms in mania, switch to a mood stabilizer

and/or an atypical antipsychotic for mood stabilization and maintenance

If It Doesn't Work

• Consider trying one of the first-line atypical antipsychotics (risperidone, olanzapine, quetiapine, ziprasidone, aripiprazole, amisulpride)
• Consider trying another conventional antipsychotic
• If 2 or more antipsychotic monotherapies do not work, consider clozapine

Best Augmenting Combos for Partial Response or Treatment-Resistance

• Augmentation of conventional antipsychotics has not been systematically studied
• Addition of a mood stabilizing anticonvulsant such as valproate, carbamazepine, or lamotrigine may be helpful in both schizophrenia and bipolar mania
• Augmentation with lithium in bipolar mania may be helpful
• Addition of a benzodiazepine, especially short-term for agitation

Tests

✳ Since conventional antipsychotics are frequently associated with weight gain, before starting treatment, weigh all patients and determine if the patient is already overweight (BMI 25.0–29.9) or obese (BMI ≥30)
• Before giving a drug that can cause weight gain to an overweight or obese patient, consider determining whether the patient already has pre-diabetes (fasting plasma glucose 100–125 mg/dl), diabetes (fasting plasma glucose >126 mg/dl), or dyslipidemia (increased total cholesterol, LDL cholesterol and triglycerides; decreased HDL cholesterol), and treat or refer such patients for treatment, including nutrition and weight management, physical activity counseling, smoking cessation, and medical management
✳ Monitor weight and BMI during treatment
✳ While giving a drug to a patient who has gained >5% of initial weight, consider evaluating for the presence of pre-diabetes, diabetes, or dyslipidemia, or consider switching to a different antipsychotic

- Should check blood pressure in the elderly before starting and for the first few weeks of treatment
- Monitoring elevated prolactin levels of dubious clinical benefit

SIDE EFFECTS

How Drug Causes Side Effects
- By blocking dopamine 2 receptors in the striatum, it can cause motor side effects
- By blocking dopamine 2 receptors in the pituitary, it can cause elevations in prolactin
- By blocking dopamine 2 receptors excessively in the mesocortical and mesolimbic dopamine pathways, especially at high doses, it can cause worsening of negative and cognitive symptoms (neuroleptic-induced deficit syndrome)
- Anticholinergic actions may cause sedation, blurred vision, constipation, dry mouth
- Antihistaminic actions may cause sedation, weight gain
- By blocking alpha 1 adrenergic receptors, it can cause dizziness, sedation, and hypotension
- Mechanism of weight gain and any possible increased incidence of diabetes or dyslipidemia with conventional antipsychotics is unknown

Notable Side Effects
- ✳ Extrapyramidal symptoms
- ✳ Tardive dyskinesia (risk increases with duration of treatment and with dose)
- ✳ Priapism
- ✳ Galactorrhea, amenorrhea
- Rare lens opacity
- Sedation, dizziness
- Dry mouth, constipation, vision problems
- Hypotension
- Weight gain

Life Threatening or Dangerous Side Effects
- Rare neuroleptic malignant syndrome
- Rare neutropenia
- Rare respiratory depression
- Rare agranulocytosis
- Rare seizures

Weight Gain

unusual | not unusual | common | problematic

- Many experience and/or can be significant in amount
- Some people may lose weight

Sedation

unusual | not unusual | common | problematic

- Many experience and/or can be significant in amount
- Acetate formulation may be associated with an initial sedative response

What To Do About Side Effects
- Wait
- Wait
- Wait
- For motor symptoms, add an anticholinergic agent
- Reduce the dose
- For sedation, take at night
- Switch to an atypical antipsychotic
- Weight loss, exercise programs, and medical management for high BMIs, diabetes dyslipidemia

Best Augmenting Agents for Side Effects
- Benztropine or trihexyphenidyl for motor side effects
- Sometimes amantadine can be helpful for motor side effects
- Benzodiazepines may be helpful for akathisia
- Many side effects cannot be improved with an augmenting agent

DOSING AND USE

Usual Dosage Range
- Oral 20–60 mg/day
- Acetate 50–150 mg every 2–3 days
- Decanoate 150–300 mg every 2–4 weeks

Dosage Forms
- Tablet 10 mg, 25 mg, 40 mg
- Acetate 50 mg/mL (equivalent to zuclopenthixol 45.25 mg/mL), 100 mg/2 mL (equivalent to zuclopenthixol 45.25 mg/mL)

- Decanoate 200 mg/mL (equivalent to zuclopenthixol 144.4 mg/mL), 500 mg/mL (equivalent to zuclopenthixol 361.1 mg/mL)

How to Dose
- Oral: initial 10–15 mg/day in divided doses; can increase by 10–20 mg/day every 2–3 days; maintenance dose can be administered as a single nighttime dose; maximum dose generally 100 mg/day
- Injection should be administered intramuscularly in the gluteal region in the morning
- Acetate generally should be administered every 2–3 days; some patients may require a second dose 24–48 hours after the first injection; duration of treatment should not exceed 2 weeks; maximum cumulative dosage should not exceed 400 mg; maximum number of injections should not exceed 4
- Decanoate: initial dose 100 mg; after 1–4 weeks administer a second injection of 100–200 mg; maintenance treatment is generally 100–600 mg every 1–4 weeks

 Dosing Tips
- Onset of action of the intramuscular acetate formulation following a single injection is generally 2–4 hours; duration of action is generally 2–3 days
- Zuclopenthixol acetate is not intended for long-term use, and should not generally be used for longer than 2 weeks; patients requiring treatment longer than 2 weeks should be switched to a depot or oral formulation of zuclopenthixol or another antipsychotic
- When changing from zuclopenthixol acetate to maintenance treatment with zuclopenthixol decanoate, administer the last injection of acetate concomitantly with the initial injection of decanoate
- The peak of action for the decanoate is usually 4–9 days, and doses generally have to be administered every 2–3 weeks

Overdose
- Sedation, convulsions, extrapyramidal symptoms, coma, hypotension, shock, hypo/hyperthermia

Long-Term Use
- Zuclopenthixol decanoate is intended for maintenance treatment
- Some side effects may be irreversible (e.g., tardive dyskinesia)

Habit Forming
- No

How to Stop
- Slow down-titration of oral formulation (over 6 to 8 weeks), especially when simultaneously beginning a new antipsychotic while switching (i.e., cross-titration)
- Rapid oral discontinuation may lead to rebound psychosis and worsening of symptoms
- If antiparkinson agents are being used, they should be continued for a few weeks after zuclopenthixol is discontinued

Pharmacokinetics
- Metabolized by CYP450 2D6
- For oral formulation, elimination half-life approximately 20 hours
- For acetate, rate limiting half-life approximately 32 hours
- For decanoate, rate limiting half-life approximately 17–21 days with multiple doses

 Drug Interactions
- Theoretically, concomitant use with CYP450 2D6 inhibitors (such as paroxetine and fluoxetine) could raise zuclopenthixol plasma levels and require dosage reduction
- CNS effects may be increased if used with other CNS depressants
- If used with anticholinergic agents, may potentiate their effects
- Combined use with epinephrine may lower blood pressure
- Zuclopenthixol may block the antihypertensive effects of drugs such as guanethidine, but may enhance the actions of other antihypertensive drugs
- Using zuclopenthixol with metoclopramide or piperazine may increase the risk of extrapyramidal symptoms
- Zuclopenthixol may antagonize the effects of levodopa and dopamine agonists

- Some patients taking a neuroleptic and lithium have developed an encephalopathic syndrome similar to neuroleptic malignant syndrome

 Other Warnings/ Precautions

- If signs of neuroleptic malignant syndrome develop, treatment should be immediately discontinued
- Use with caution in patients with epilepsy, glaucoma, urinary retention
- Decanoate should not be used with clozapine because it cannot be withdrawn quickly in the event of serious adverse effects such as neutropenia
- Possible antiemetic effect of zuclopenthixol may mask signs of other disorders or overdose; suppression of cough reflex may cause asphyxia
- Use only with great caution if at all in Parkinson's disease or Lewy Body dementia
- Observe for signs of ocular toxicity (pigmentary retinopathy and lenticular and corneal deposits)
- Avoid undue exposure to sunlight
- Avoid extreme heat exposure
- Do not use epinephrine in event of overdose as interaction with some pressor agents may lower blood pressure

Do Not Use

- If patient is taking a large concomitant dose of a sedative hypnotic
- If patient is taking guanethidine or a similar acting compound
- If patient has CNS depression, is comatose, or has subcortical brain damage
- If patient has acute alcohol, barbiturate, or opiate intoxication
- If patient has narrow angle-closure glaucoma
- If patient has phaeochromocytoma, circulatory collapse, or blood dyscrasias
- In case of pregnancy
- If there is a proven allergy to zuclopenthixol

Renal Impairment

- Use with caution

Hepatic Impairment

- Use with caution

Cardiac Impairment

- Use with caution

Elderly

- Some patients may tolerate lower doses better
- Maximum acetate dose 100 mg

 Children and Adolescents

- Safety and efficacy have not been established in children under age 18
- Preliminary open-label data show that oral zuclopenthixol may be effective in reducing aggression in mentally impaired children

 Pregnancy

- Not recommended for use during pregnancy
- Psychotic symptoms may worsen during pregnancy and some form of treatment may be necessary
- Atypical antipsychotics may be preferable to conventional antipsychotics or anticonvulsant mood stabilizers if treatment is required during pregnancy

Breast Feeding

- Some drug is found in mother's breast milk
- ✳ Recommended either to discontinue drug or bottle feed
- Infants of women who choose to breast feed should be monitored for possible adverse effects

Potential Advantages

- Non-compliant patients (decanoate)
- Emergency use (acute injection)

Potential Disadvantages

- Children
- Elderly
- Patients with tardive dyskinesia

Primary Target Symptoms

- Positive symptoms of psychosis
- Negative symptoms of psychosis

• Aggressive symptoms

 Pearls

• Zuclopenthixol depot may reduce risk of relapse more than some other depot conventional antipsychotics, but it may also be associated with more adverse effects

• Can combine acute injection with depot injection in the same syringe for rapid onset and long duration effects when initiating treatment

• Zuclopenthixol may have serotonin 2A antagonist properties, but these have never been systematically investigated for atypical antipsychotic properties at low doses

• Patients have very similar antipsychotic responses to any conventional antipsychotic, which is different from atypical antipsychotics where antipsychotic responses of individual patients can occasionally vary greatly from one atypical antipsychotic to another

• Patients with inadequate responses to atypical antipsychotics may benefit from a trial of augmentation with a conventional antipsychotic such as zuclopenthixol or from switching to a conventional antipsychotic such as zuclopenthixol

• However, long-term polypharmacy with a combination of a conventional antipsychotic such as zuclopenthixol with an atypical antipsychotic may combine their side effects without clearly augmenting the efficacy of either

• Although a frequent practice by some prescribers, adding 2 conventional antipsychotics together has little rationale and may reduce tolerability without clearly enhancing efficacy

 Suggested Reading

Coutinho E, Fenton M, Adams C, Campbell C. Zuclopenthixol acetate in psychiatric emergencies: looking for evidence from clinical trials. Schizophr Res 2000;46:111–8.

Coutinho E, Fenton M, Quraishi S. Zuclopenthixol decanoate for schizophrenia and other serious mental illnesses. Cochrane Database Syst Rev 2000;(2):CD001164.

Fenton M, Coutinho ES, Campbell C. Zuclopenthixol acetate in the treatment of acute schizophrenia and similar serious mental illnesses. Cochrane Database Syst Rev 2000;(2):CD000525.

Index by Drug Name

Digton (sulpiride), *435*
Diligan (hydroxyzine), *219*
Dinalexin (fluoxetine), *175*
Dipromal (valproate), *499*
Discimer (trifluoperazine), *487*
Distedon (diazepam), *109*
divalproex (valproate), *499*
Divial (lorazepam), *265*
Dixarit (clonidine), *81*
Dixibon (sulpiride), *435*
Dizac (diazepam), *109*
Dobren (sulpiride), *435*
Dobupal (venlafaxine), *505*
Dogmatil (sulpiride), *435*
Dogmatyl (sulpiride), *435*
Dolmatil (sulpiride), *435*
Domical (amitriptyline), *13*
Dominans (nortriptyline), *329*
Domnamid (estazolam), *163*
DOM-trazodone (trazodone), *477*
donepezil, *133*
Doneurin (doxepin), *145*
Donix (lorazepam), *265*
Dopress (Dothiepin), *139*
Doral (quazepam), *397*
Dorken (clorazepate), *87*
Dorm (lorazepam), *265*
Dormalin (quazepam), *397*
Dormapam (temazepam), *443*
Dorme (quazepam), *397*
Dormicum (midazolam), *291*
Dormodor (flurazepam), *191*
Dothep (Dothiepin), *139*
dothiepin, *139*
Doxal (doxepin), *145*
Doxedyn (doxepin), *145*
doxepin, *145*
Dozic (haloperidol), *213*
Drenian (diazepam), *109*
Dresent (sulpiride), *435*
Ducene (diazepam), *109*
duloxetine, *151*
Dumirox (fluvoxamine), *195*
Dumozolam (triazolam), *483*
Dumyrox (fluvoxamine), *195*
Duraclon (clonidine), *81*
Duradiazepam (diazepam), *109*
Duralith (lithium), *247*
Duraperidol (haloperidol), *213*
Durazepam (oxazepam), *341*
Durazolam (lorazepam), *265*
Dutonin (nefazodone), *323*
Dynalert (pemoline), *357*
Dynamin (pemoline), *357*
Eclorion (sulpiride), *435*
Edronax (reboxetine), *407*
Efectin (venlafaxine), *505*

Efexir (venlafaxine), *505*
Efexor (venlafaxine), *505*
Efexor XL (venlafaxine), *505*
Effexor (venlafaxine), *505*
Effexor XR (venlafaxine), *505*
Effiplen (buspirone), *43*
Egibren (selegiline), *423*
Eglonyl (sulpiride), *435*
Elavil (amitriptyline), *13*
Elavil Plus (amitriptyline), *13*
Eldepryl (selegiline), *423*
Elenium (chlordiazepoxide), *53*
Eliwel (amitriptyline), *13*
Elopram (citalopram), *63*
Elroquil N (hydroxyzine), *219*
Elperil (thioridazine), *447*
Emdalen (lofepramine), *253*
Endep (amitriptyline), *13*
Enimon (sulpiride), *435*
Epial (carbamazepine), *47*
Epilim (valproate), *499*
Epitol (carbamazepine), *47*
Epitomax (topiramate), *465*
Equilid (sulpiride), *435*
Equitam (lorazepam), *265*
Ergenyl (valproate), *499*
Eridan (diazepam), *109*
Erocap (fluoxetine), *175*
Ergocalm (lorazepam), *265*
escitalopram, *157*
Esculid (diazepam), *109*
Esilgan (estazolam), *163*
Esipride (sulpiride), *435*
Eskalith (lithium), *247*
Eskalith CR (lithium), *247*
Eskazine (trifluoperazine), *487*
Esparon (alprazolam), *1*
estazolam, *163*
Ethipam (diazepam), *103*
Ethipramine (imipramine), *223*
Euhypnos (temazepam), *443*
Euipnos (temazepam), *443*
Eurosan (diazepam), *109*
Eutimil (paroxetine), *351*
Eutimox (fluphenazine), *185*
Evacalm (diazepam), *109*
Everiden (valproate), *499*
Exan (buspirone), *43*
Excegran (zonisamide), *525*
Exelon (rivastigmine), *417*
Exogran (zonisamide), *525*
Exostrept (fluoxetine), *175*
Fardalan (sulpiride), *435*
Fargenor (chlordiazepoxide), *53*
Faustan (diazepam), *109*
Faverin (fluvoxamine), *195*
Felicium (fluoxetine), *175*

Seroquel (quetiapine), *401*
Seroxal (paroxetine), *351*
Seroxat (paroxetine), *351*
Serpax (oxazepam), *341*
Sertofren (desipramine), *103*
sertraline, *429*
Serzone (nefazodone), *323*
Setous (zotepine), *523*
Sevinol (fluphenazine), *185*
Sevium (haloperidol), *213*
SK-Pramine (imipramine), *223*
Sibason (diazepam), *109*
Sicorelax (diazepam), *109*
Sigacalm (oxazepam), *341*
Sigaperidol (haloperidol), *213*
Signopam (temazepam), *443*
Sinequan (doxepin), *145*
Sinquan (doxepin), *145*
Sinquane (doxepin), *145*
Siqualone (fluphenazine), *185*
Siqualone decanoat (fluphenazine), *185*
Siqualone Enantat (fluphenazine), *185*
Sirtal (carbamazepine), *47*
Sobile (oxazepam), *341*
Sobril (oxazepam), *341*
Socian (amisulpride), *7*
Softramal (clorazepate), *87*
Solarix (moclobemide), *307*
Solian (amisulpride), *7*
Solidon (chlorpromazine), *57*
Solis (diazepam), *109*
Somagerol (lorazepam), *265*
Somapam (temazepam), *443*
Somatarax (hydroxyzine), *219*
Somniton (triazolam), *483*
Somnium (lorazepam), *265*
Somnol (flurazepam), *191*
Somnubene (flunitrazepam), *171*
Sonata (zaleplon), *511*
Songar (triazolam), *483*
Sovigen (zolpidem), *521*
Sporalon (trifluoperazine), *487*
Stablon (tianeptine), *461*
Stalleril (thioridazine), *447*
Spasmilan (buspirone), *43*
Spasmo Praxiten (oxazepam), *341*
Stamoneurol (sulpiride), *435*
Staurodorm (flurazepam), *191*
Staurodorm Neu (flurazepam), *191*
Stazepine (carbamazepine), *47*
Stedon (diazepam), *109*
Stelabid (trifluoperazine), *487*
Stelabid forte (trifluoperazine), *487*
Stelabid mite (trifluoperazine), *487*
Stelazine (trifluoperazine), *487*
Stelbid (trifluoperazine), *487*
Stelbid forte (trifluoperazine), *487*

Stelium (trifluoperazine), *487*
Stelminal (amitriptyline), *13*
Stephadilat (fluoxetine), *175*
Stesolid (diazepam), *109*
Stilnoct (zolpidem), *521*
Stilnox (zolpidem), *521*
Stimul (pemoline), *357*
Strattera (atomoxetine), *31*
Stressigal (buspirone), *43*
Sulamid (amisulpride), *7*
Sulp (sulpiride), *435*
Sulparex (sulpiride), *435*
Sulpiphar (sulpiride), *435*
Sulpirid (sulpiride), *435*
sulpiride, *435*
Sulpiryd (sulpiride), *435*
Sulpitil (sulpiride), *435*
Sulpivert (sulpiride), *435*
Sulpril (sulpiride), *435*
Suprium (sulpiride), *435*
Surmontil (trimipramine), *493*
Suxidina (oxazepam), *341*
Sylador (haloperidol), *213*
Symbyax (olanzapine-fluoxetine combination), *335*
Synedil (sulpiride), *435*
Synedil Fort (sulpiride), *435*
Syneudon 50 (amitriptyline), *13*
tacrine, *439*
Tafil (alprazolam), *1*
Tagonis (paroxetine), *351*
Tardotol (carbamazepine), *47*
Taro-Carbamazepine (carbamazepine), *47*
Tatanka (alprazolam), *1*
Tatig (sertraline), *429*
Tavor (lorazepam), *265*
Tazepam (oxazepam), *341*
Tegretal (carbamazepine), *47*
Tegretol (carbamazepine), *47*
Tegretol LP (carbamazepine), *47*
Teledomin (milnacipran), *295*
Temador (temazepam), *443*
Temaze (temazepam), *443*
temazepam, *443*
Temesta (lorazepam), *265*
Temodal (quazepam), *397*
Temporal Slow (carbamazepine), *47*
Temporol (carbamazepine), *47*
Temtabs (temazepam), *443*
Tenox (temazepam), *443*
Tenso-Timelets (clonidine), *81*
Tensispes (buspirone), *43*
Tensium (diazepam), *109*
Tensopam (diazepam), *109*
Tepavil (sulpiride), *435*
Tepazepam (diazepam), *109*
Tepazepam (sulpiride), *435*
Teperin (amitriptyline), *13*

Index by Use

Excessive sleepiness in narcolepsy,
obstructive sleep apnea/hypopnea syndrome,
shift work sleep disorder
 modafinil, *313*

Fibromyalgia
 amitriptyline, *13*
 duloxetine, *151*
 milnacipran, *295*
 pregabalin, *387*

Generalized anxiety disorder
 alprazolam, *1*
 citalopram, *63*
 duloxetine, *151*
 escitalopram, *157*
 fluoxetine, *175*
 fluvoxamine, *195*
 mirtazapine, *301*
 paroxetine, *351*
 pregabalin, *387*
 sertraline, *429*
 tiagabine (adjunct), *457*
 venlafaxine, *505*

Hypertension
 clonidine, *81*

Insomnia
 alprazolam, *1*
 amitriptyline, *13*
 amoxapine, *19*
 clomipramine, *69*
 clonazepam, *75*
 desipramine, *103*
 diazepam, *109*
 dothiepin, *139*
 doxepin, *145*
 estazolam, *163*
 flunitrazepam, *171*
 flurazepam, *191*
 hydroxyzine, *219*
 imipramine, *223*
 lofepramine, *253*
 lorazepam, *265*
 maprotiline, *277*
 nortriptyline, *329*
 quazepam, *397*
 temazepam, *443*
 trazodone, *477*
 triazolam, *483*
 trimipramine, *493*
 zaleplon, *511*
 zolpidem, *521*
 zopiclone, *529*

Intractable hiccups
 chlorpromazine, *57*

Mania
 alprazolam (adjunct), *1*
 aripiprazole, *25*
 chlorpromazine, *57*
 clonazepam (adjunct), *75*
 lamotrigine, *235*
 levetiracetam, *243*
 lithium, *247*
 lorazepam (adjunct), *265*
 olanzapine, *355*
 quetiapine, *401*
 risperidone, *411*
 valproate (divalproex), *499*
 ziprasidone, *515*
 zotepine, *533*

Migraine
 topiramate, *465*
 valproate (divalproex), *499*

Muscle spasm
 diazepam, *109*
 lorazepam, *265*

Narcolepsy
 d,l-amphetamine, *115*
 d,l-methylphenidate, *121*
 d-amphetamine, *97*
 d-methylphenidate, *127*
 modafinil, *313*

Nausea/vomiting
 chlorpromazine, *57*
 hydroxyzine, *219*
 perphenazine, *365*

Neuropathic pain/chronic pain
 amitriptyline, *13*
 amoxapine, *19*
 carbamazepine, *47*
 clomipramine, *69*
 clonidine (adjunct), *81*
 desipramine, *103*
 dothiepin, *139*
 doxepin, *145*
 duloxetine, *151*
 gabapentin, *201*
 imipramine, *223*
 lamotrigine, *235*
 levetiracetam, *243*
 lofepramine, *253*
 maprotiline, *277*
 memantine, *283*
 milnacipran, *295*

Index by Class

Abbreviations

5HT	serotonin
ACH	acetylcholine
ACHE	acetylcholinesterase
ADHD	attention deficit hyperactivity disorder
ALT	alanine aminotransferase
ALPT	total serum alkaline phosphatase
AST	aspartate aminotransferase
BID	twice a day
BMI	body mass index
BuChE	butyrylcholinesterase
CMI	clomipramine
CNS	central nervous system
CYP450	cytochrome P450
De-CMI	desmethyl-clomipramine
DA	dopamine
dl	deciliter
DLB	dementia with Lewy bodies
ECG	electrocardiogram
EEG	electroencephalogram
EKG	electrocardiogram
EPS	extrapyramidal side effects
ERT	estrogen replacement therapy
FDA	Food and Drug Administration
FSH	follicle-stimulating hormone
GAD	generalized anxiety disorder
GI	gastrointestinal
HDL	high-density lipoprotein
HMG CoA	beta-hydroxy-beta-methylglutaryl Coenzyme A
HRT	hormone replacement therapy
IM	intramuscular
IV	intravenous
LDL	low-density lipoprotein
LH	luteinizing hormone
Lb	pound
MAO	monoamine oxidase
MAOI	monoamine oxidase inhibitor
mCPP	meta-chloro-phenyl-piperazine
mg	milligram
mL	milliliter
mm Hg	millimeters of mercury
MDD	major depressive disorder

NE	norepinephrine
NMDA	N-methyl-d-aspartate
OCD	obsessive-compulsive disorder
ODV	O-desmethylvenlafaxine
PET	positron emission tomography
PK	pharmacokinetic
PMDD	premenstrual dysphoric disorder
PMS	premenstrual syndrome
PTSD	posttraumatic stress disorder
QD	once a day
QHS	once a day at bedtime
QID	four times a day
RIMA	reversible inhibitor of monoamine oxidase A
SNRI	dual serotonin and norepinephrine reuptake inhibitor
SSRI	selective serotonin reuptake inhibitor
TCA	tricyclic antidepressant
TID	three times a day
TSH	thyroid stimulating hormone

FDA Use-In-Pregnancy Ratings

Category A: Controlled studies show no risk: adequate, well-controlled studies in pregnant women have failed to demonstrate risk to the fetus

Category B: No evidence of risk in humans: either animal findings show risk, but human findings do not; or, if no adequate human studies have been performed, animal findings are negative

Category C: Risk cannot be ruled out: human studies are lacking, and animal studies are either positive for fetal risk or lacking as well. However, potential benefits may outweigh risks

Category D: Positive evidence of risk: investigational or postmarketing data show risk to the fetus. Nevertheless, potential benefits may outweigh risks

Category X: Contraindicated in pregnancy: studies in animals or humans, or investigational or postmarketing reports, have shown fetal risk that clearly outweighs any possible benefit to the patient